Fungal Disease

BASIC AND CLINICAL DERMATOLOGY

Series Editors

ALAN R. SHALITA, M.D.

Professor and Chairman
Department of Dermatology
State University of New York
Health Science Center at Brooklyn
Brooklyn, New York

DAVID A. NORRIS, M.D.

Director of Research
Professor of Dermatology
The University of Colorado
Health Sciences Center
Denver, Colorado

1. Cutaneous Investigation in Health and Disease: Noninvasive Methods and Instrumentation, *edited by Jean-Luc Lévêque*
2. Irritant Contact Dermatitis, *edited by Edward M. Jackson and Ronald Goldner*
3. Fundamentals of Dermatology: A Study Guide, *Franklin S. Glickman and Alan R. Shalita*
4. Aging Skin: Properties and Functional Changes, *edited by Jean-Luc Lévêque and Pierre G. Agache*
5. Retinoids: Progress in Research and Clinical Applications, *edited by Maria A. Livrea and Lester Packer*
6. Clinical Photomedicine, *edited by Henry W. Lim and Nicholas A. Soter*
7. Cutaneous Antifungal Agents: Selected Compounds in Clinical Practice and Development, *edited by John W. Rippon and Robert A. Fromtling*
8. Oxidative Stress in Dermatology, *edited by Jürgen Fuchs and Lester Packer*
9. Connective Tissue Diseases of the Skin, *edited by Charles M. Lapière and Thomas Krieg*
10. Epidermal Growth Factors and Cytokines, *edited by Thomas A. Luger and Thomas Schwarz*
11. Skin Changes and Diseases in Pregnancy, *edited by Marwali Harahap and Robert C. Wallach*
12. Fungal Disease: Biology, Immunology, and Diagnosis, *edited by Paul H. Jacobs and Lexie Nall*

ADDITIONAL VOLUMES IN PREPARATION

Fungal Disease

Biology, Immunology, and Diagnosis

edited by

Paul H. Jacobs
Lexie Nall
Stanford University School of Medicine
Stanford, California

Marcel Dekker, Inc. New York • Basel • Hong Kong

Library of Congress Cataloging-in-Publication Data

Fungal disease : biology, immunology, and diagnosis / edited by Paul
H. Jacobs, Lexie Nall.
p. cm. — Basic and clinical dermatology ; 12)
Includes bibliographical references and index.
ISBN 0-8247-9402-8 (alk. paper)
1. Mycoses. 2. Mycoses—Immunological aspects. 3. Mycoses-
-Diagnosis. I. Jacobs, Paul H. II. Nall, Lexie.
III. Series.
[DNLM: 1. Mycoses—immunology. 2. Mycoses—drug therapy.
3. Antifungal Agents—therapeutic use. 4. Fungi—pathogenicity.
W1 CL69L v.12 1997 / WC 450 F9788 1997]
QR245.F853 1997
616.9'69—dc20
DNLM/DLC
for Library of Congress

96-18673
CIP

The publisher offers discounts on this book when ordered in bulk quantities. For more information, write to Special Sales/Professional Marketing at the address below.

This book is printed on acid-free paper.

MARCEL DEKKER, INC.
270 Madison Avenue, New York, New York 10016

Current printing (last digit):
10 9 8 7 6 5 4 3 2 1

PRINTED IN THE UNITED STATES OF AMERICA

Preface

This text consists of chapters written by world renowned researchers and clinicians. Its purpose is to present to the reader the pertinent basic science studies in a common-sense, practical manner for the clinician, who today is faced with an exponential increase in fungal infections in the immunocompromised patient, the elderly, and the ever-increasing AIDS population. It presents the latest in state-of-the-art data in clinical mycology for the practitioner and indicates areas for future investigations and therapies.

We briefly describe many of the chapters in the book to indicate the broad range of material: Dr. Borgers covers in detail the ultrastructure of fungi with his unequaled electron microscopy work. Cell-mediated immunity is simplified by Dr. Cassone, while Dr. Hay covers immunology, and Dr. Hearn, the structure and function of the fungal cell wall. Dr. Nilius stresses the importance of iron acquisition in aspergillosis, Dr. Odds records the methodology of strain typing of *Candida,* and Dr. Domer spells out immunomodulation by *Candida*. Dr. Segal gives the basis for *Candida* adherence and penetration. Fungal enzymes and their relationship to pathogenesis are documented by Dr. Ogawa. Dr. Richardson's article is related to neutrophils in cryptococcal infections, and Dr. Ruiz-Herrera's, to the biology of mucoralis agents. Discussion of immune and clinical responses to paracoccidioid organisms is the contribution by Drs. San-Blas and San-Blas.

Dr. Seeliger presents insight into the pathogenesis of *Aspergillus,* and Dr. Steele, into the proteinase gene identification of the organism. Dr. Takahashi's treatise covers fungicidal activity in tissue, and Dr. Vanden Bossche's explains the determinants of polymorphism. Dr. Wagner delineates the mechanisms of cutaneous defense. And the significant breakthrough that at last has occurred in the treatment of onychomycosis is thoroughly documented by Dr. De Donker. Drs. Korting and Braun-Falco underscore the important treatment adjunct through the use of liposomes. And Dr. Wheat discusses susceptibility to histoplasmosis.

Are *Pityrosporum orbiculare* and *ovale* the same organism? Dr. Faergemann offers his views.

Taxonomy is included in Dr. McGinnis's study. Dr. Polonelli reviews vaccine development and use. Dr. Sigler acquaints us with some of the lesser known fungi that may cause problems in the future, and Dr. Van Cutsem covers animal models. Azole drug resistance in *Candida* is Dr. Warnock's study, while Dr. Iwata explains the mechanism of azole resistance. And although systemic allylamines are not yet approved in the United States, Dr. Elewski informs us of their application in other countries.

Dr. Cauwenbergh discusses exciting future research and therapies.

We feel that this text not only presents the current status of medical mycology, but will serve as a stimulus for future investigators and clinicians.

Paul H. Jacobs
Lexie Nall

Contents

II. HOST DEFENSE AND RESPONSE TO FUNGI

III. FUNGAL INVASION AND IMMUNITY

Contributors

Patrick Boiron, Ph.D. Senior Scientist, Unit of Mycology, Institut Pasteur, Paris, France

Marcel Borgers, Ph.D. Department of Life Sciences, Janssen Research Foundation, Beerse, Belgium

Otto Braun-Falco Professor of Dermatology, Departments of Dermatology and Venerology, Dermatologische Klinik, Universität Munchen, Munchen, Germany

Cristina Cantelli, Ph.D. Researcher, Institute of Microbiology, Faculty of Medicine and Surgery, University of Parma, Parma, Italy

Antonio Cassone, Ph.D., M.D. Head, Laboratory of Bacteriology and Medical Mycology, Istituto Superiore di Sanità, Rome, Italy

Geert Cauwenbergh Vice President, Research and Development, Consumer Products Worldwide, Johnson & Johnson, Skillman, New Jersey

Kenichiro Chikakane, M.D. Department of Dermatology, School of Medicine, Teikyo University, Tokyo, Japan

Stefania Conti, Ph.D. Institute of Microbiology, Faculty of Medicine and Surgery, University of Parma, Parma, Italy

Piet de Doncker, Ph.D. Clinical Research Manager, Janssen Research Foundation, Beerse, Belgium

Judith E. Domer, Ph.D. Professor of Microbiology and Immunology, and Associate Dean, Graduate School, Tulane University, New Orleans, Louisiana

Boni E. Elewski, M.D. Associate Professor, Department of Dermatology, Case Western Reserve University, Cleveland, Ohio

Jan Faergemann, M.D., Ph.D. Assistant Professor, Department of Dermatology, Sahlgrens University Hospital, Gothenburg, Sweden

Paola Fisicaro, Ph.D. Researcher, Institute of Microbiology, Faculty of Medicine and Surgery,University of Parma, Parma, Italy

Mara Gerloni, Ph.D. Researcher, Institute of Microbiology, Faculty of Medicine and Surgery, University of Parma, Parma, Italy

Roderick James Hay, D.M., F.R.C.P., M.R.C.Path Mary Dunhill Professor of Cutaneous Medicine, St. John's Institute of Dermatology, Guy's Hospital, London, England

Veronica M. Hearn, M.Sc., Ph.D. Research Fellow, Department of Microbiology, Leeds University, Leeds, West Yorkshire, England

Kazuo Iwata, M.D., Ph.D. University of Tokyo, Tokyo, Japan

Paul H. Jacobs, M.D., F.A.C.P. Professor Emeritus, Department of Dermatology, Stanford University School of Medicine, Stanford, California

Elizabeth M. Johnson, B.Sc., Ph.D. PHLS Mycology Reference Laboratory, Public Health Laboratory, Bristol, England

Masato Kashima, M.D., Ph.D. St. Marianna Medical College, Tokyo, Japan

Hans Christian Korting, M.D., Ph.D. Professor, Department of Dermatology, Ludwig-Maximilians-Universität, Munchen, Germany

Walter Magliani Institute of Microbiology, Faculty of Medicine and Surgery, University of Parma, Parma, Italy

Michael R. McGinnis, Ph.D. Professor and Associate Director, WHO Collaborating Center for Tropical Diseases, and Director, Medical Mycology Research Center, Department of Pathology, University of Texas Medical Branch, Galveston, Texas

Angela M. Nilius, Ph.D. Senior Research Microbiologist, Department of Anti-Infective Microbiology, Abbott Laboratories, Abbott Park, Illinois

Frank C. Odds, Ph.D., M.R.C.Path Director, Department of Bacteriology and Mycology, Janssen Research Foundation, Beerse, Belgium

Hideoki Ogawa, M.D., Ph.D. Professor and Chairman, Department of Dermatology, Juntendo University School of Medicine, Tokyo, Japan

Allan C. Pier, D.V.M., Ph.D. Professor of Veterinary Mycology (Emeritus), Department of Veterinary Sciences, University of Wyoming, Laramie, Wyoming

Luciano Polonelli, Ph.D. Full Professor in Microbiology, Institute of Microbiology, Faculty of Medicine and Surgery, University of Parma, Parma, Italy

Judith C. Rhodes, Ph.D. Associate Professor, Departments of Pathology and Laboratory Medicine, University of Cincinnati, Cincinnati, Ohio

Malcolm D. Richardson, B.Sc., Ph.D., M.R.C.Path Mycology Reference Laboratory, Department of Dermatology, University of Glasgow and Western Infirmary, Glasgow, Scotland

Jose Ruiz-Herrera, Q.B.P., Ph.D. Professor, Ingenieria Genetica, and Genetica y Biologia Molecular, Centro de Investigación y de Estudios Avanzados del IPN, Irapuato, Mexico

Felipe San-Blas, Ph.D. Investigador Emerito, Centro de Microbiología y Biología Celular, Instituto Venezolano de Investigaciones Científicas (IVIC), Caracas, Venezuela

Gioconda San-Blas, Ph.D. Investigador Titular, Centro de Microbiología y Biología Celular, Instituto Venezolano de Investigaciones Científicas (IVIC), Caracas, Venezuela

Hana Sandovsky-Losica, Ph.D. Department of Human Microbiology, Sackler School of Medicine, Tel-Aviv University, Tel-Aviv, Israel

Heinz Seeliger Emeritus Professor of Hygiene and Microbiology, Institute of Hygiene, University of Würzburg, Wüzburg, Germany

Esther Segal, Ph.D. Professor, Department of Human Microbiology, Sackler School of Medicine, Tel-Aviv University, Tel-Aviv, Israel

Lynne Sigler, M.Sc. Associate Professor, Departments of Medical Microbiology and Immunology, and Devonian Botanic Garden, University of Alberta, Edmonton, Alberta, Canada

Peter G. Sohnle, M.D. Chief, Division of Infectious Diseases, Department of Medicine, Medical College of Wisconsin, and Milwaukee Veterans Affairs Medical Center, Milwaukee, Wisconsin

Paul E. Steele, M.D. Assistant Professor, Departments of Pathology and Laboratory Medicine, University of Cincinnati, Cincinnati, Ohio

Saundra Lemaster Stringer, Ph.D. Departments of Molecular Genetics, Biochemistry, and Microbiology, University of Cincinnati, Cincinnati, Ohio

Hisashi Takahashi, M.D. Department of Dermatology, School of Medicine, Teikyo University, Tokyo, Japan

Ryoji Tsuboi, M.D., Ph.D. Assistant Professor, Department of Dermatology, Juntendo University School of Medicine, Tokyo, Japan

Jan Van Cutsem Honorary Director, Department of Bacteriology and Mycology, and Senior Consultant, Janssen Research Foundation, Beerse, Belgium

Hugo Vanden Bossche Director, Department of Comparative Biochemistry, Janssen Research Foundation, Beerse, Belgium

David K. Wagner, M.D. Associate Professor, Department of Medicine, Medical College of Wisconsin, Milwaukee, Wisconsin

David W. Warnock, B.Sc., Ph.D., F.R.C.Path PHLS Mycology Reference Laboratory, Public Health Laboratory, Bristol, England

Shinichi Watanabe, M.D., Ph.D. Professor, Department of Dermatology, School of Medicine, Teikyo University, Tokyo, Japan

L. Joseph Wheat, M.D. Professor of Medicine, Department of Internal Medicine, Indiana University, Indianapolis, Indiana

Fungal Disease

1

An Overview: Antifungal Treatment

PAUL H. JACOBS
Stanford University School of Medicine
Stanford, California

There are perhaps over 100,000 species of fungi, but less than 100 cause disease in humans. What are the factors in humans and fungi that promote or prevent these mycotic diseases?

1. Geographic Habitat

Climatic conditions play an obvious role in the presence or absence of certain organisms. In the United States, *Coccidioides immitis* is found in the arid lower Sonoran life zones, while *Histoplasma capsulatum* prefers the more moist areas of the middle United States and the East Coast. Sporotrichosis occurs only in the tropical or temperate regions of the world. *Blastomyces braziliensis* is fairly well limited to South and Central America. North and South America have a greater variety of systemic pathogens than any other continent, for unknown reasons. It is true that certain organisms are present in specific localities; however, with travel as common as it is today, clinicians worldwide must be alert to the possibility that their patients can have what in their home area would be considered rare mycotic diseases.

2. Animal Hosts

Although most fungi probably originated in the soil, many have lost the ability to survive in soil but have found, instead, various animals to be their ideal habitats. Humans who associate with these animals, then, can become infected with the zoophilic organisms. Once infected, the human may then further transmit the organism to other humans or even back to an animal. *Microsporum canis*, *Microsporum manum*, *Trichophyton mentagrophytes*, and *Trichophyton verrucosum* are examples. Other fungi seem to exist in humans and are mainly spread from human to human. *Trichophyton rubrum*, *Trichophyton tonsurans*, and *Microsporum audouinii* are examples of these anthropophilic fungi.

3. Heredity

Obviously heredity is a factor. Coccidioidomycosis is a frequent and severe disease in African Americans and especially in Filipinos, more so than in other racial groups. Tokelau (tinea imbricata) only occurs in natives, while visitors from other parts of the globe appear to be immune to *Trichophyton concentricum* infections. It is not unusual for clinicians to see *T. rubrum* infections in one parent and the offspring, but it is extremely rare to find the infection in both parents despite intimate contact.

4. Occupation

The environment of the work area is a definite factor in mycotic diseases. This was dramatically demonstrated by the outbreak of histoplasmosis in Ohio following a soil-moving project. Veterinarian workers have a higher incidence of sporotrichosis, and animal handlers are at risk from *M. canis*, *M. manum*, and *T. verrucosum* infections.

Immunocompromised patients are susceptible to *Aspergillus fumigatus*, which is found in abundance wherever decaying vegetative matter exists.

5. Sex

The female seems to be more resistant to *Coccidioides immitis* than the male but more susceptible to *Histoplasma*.

6. Age

Evidence exists to show that both the young and the aged are more susceptible to histoplasmosis and that, in the old-old age group, superficial fungal infections are the rule rather than the exception.

7. Trauma

Skin penetration can afford a route of infection in mycetomas, chromoblastomycosis, sporotrichosis, and other infections. The debilitating effects of surgical procedures and radiation are often followed by extensive involvement with *Pityrosporum*, dermatophytes, and *Candida*.

8. Nutrition and Hygiene

These are further obvious factors.

9. Diseases

Patients with diabetes, lymphoma, or leukemia and, more recently, acquired immunodeficiency syndrome (AIDS) all have an increased frequency and severity of fungal infections. Perhaps these immunocompromised patients should be given prophylactic therapy with the new, potent oral antifungal drugs now available so as to reduce the incidence and severity of fungal infections in these patients.

10. Drugs

Antineoplastics and the new, more potent antibiotics play a part, and the frequent use of systemic and topical corticosteroid therapy has produced a host of compromised patients vulnerable to mycotic diseases. When patients are given high doses of corticosteroids or potent immunosuppressive drugs, are they told to avoid exposure to decaying vegetative waste? *Aspergillus fumigatus* is invariably present in decaying vegetative matter. Should these patients also be considered for prophylactic therapy with the new oral antifungal medicines?

One must use care in prescribing topical corticosteroids, especially under occlusion, lest they convert a superficial tinea to a Majocchi's granuloma. The astute physician will test with a simple potassium hydroxide direct preparation to first rule out the presence of mycelia.

11. Organism

Changes can occur in the fungi themselves. Perhaps this explains the disappearance of *Microsporum audouinii* epidemics that occurred in the past. Certainly the recent increase of infections with *Coccidioides* in California raises the possibility of an increased pathogenicity of the organism or at least of changes in the local environment, favoring the proliferation of the organism and the spread of the disease.

One should also be alert to the possibility of a previously considered nonpathogen becoming pathogenic and producing disease, especially in the immunosuppressed individual.

12. Mechanics of Infection

For an infection to occur, there must first be adherence of the organism. It must then be capable of penetration and finally to overcome or at least resist the defense mechanisms of the host. In this text, the mechanisms of adherence and penetration and their relationship to the host defenses are covered in detail.

13. Natural disasters

These may also play an important role, exemplified by the outbreak of coccidioidomycosis in the Los Angeles area following the recent earthquake, which caused arthrospores to be disseminated along with the dust caused by the tremor.

14. Therapy

Worldwide, probably the oldest and most frequently used antifungal drug was salicylic acid, which is still used in poorer societies. In the middle of this century, several more potent agents became available to the practitioner; nystatin, griseofulvin, flucytosine, and amphotericin B. These are further being replaced by the azoles, allylamines, and morpholenes. The triazoles itraconazole and fluconazole, with their broad spectrum of action, low toxicity, and effectiveness both for therapy and prophylaxis, are the paragons among antifungal drugs today.

What will the future bring? The organism and the individual will continue to change. Will investigation of marine and plant antifungals lead to new and dramatic nostrums? Will the chemist, by altering the basic molecules of present-day drugs, produce new and more potent drugs? Certainly the development of liposomal amphotericin B has reduced the toxicity of this drug.

Finally, will investigation yield the means to change the resistance of the individual? Certainly veterinary researchers have shown that a vaccine can be used to reduce *T. verrucosum* infections in animals.

Can vaccines or other innovative ways and means be developed to change individuals and make them resistant to the mycoses?

Each and every chapter of this text presents innumerable stimulating ideas and possibilities for future study and investigation.

2

Taxonomy of Medically Important Fungi

MICHAEL R. McGINNIS
WHO Collaborating Center for Tropical Diseases and University of Texas Medical Branch Galveston, Texas

I. INTRODUCTION

Taxonomy is concerned with the orderly classification of organisms as a means to show their presumed natural relationships. Decisions regarding the classification of fungi are based upon the experiences and perspectives of the taxonomists who are proposing the classification schemes. There are no committees or other official bodies that determine which classification scheme will serve as the accepted one. Even though controversy may exist at times, the freedom of each taxonomist to voice his or her own perspective and opinion ensures that the search for new knowledge having taxonomic usefulness is not restricted.

Nomenclature deals with the naming of organisms, which is the task to be completed after all of the taxonomic decisions have been made. Unlike taxonomy, there are specific rules in the International Code of Botanical Nomenclature (ICBN) that must be followed in order to validly name a fungus. Such rules ensure that all fungi are named in a consistent manner utilizing internationally agreed upon standards. Taxonomists are obligated to follow the rules of nomenclature, which are reevaluated during each International Botanical Congress. Even though some of the rules may not be acceptable to everyone, they must be followed, or names being proposed could be rejected as being invalid. The requirement for a permanently preserved specimen to serve as the nomenclatural type, the requirement for either a diagnosis or description of a new fungus being in Latin rather than a modern language like English, and the use of the term *division* rather than *phylum* often results in emotional debates. A living culture under certain conditions may serve as a type.

Characters selected by various taxonomists to be used in proposing classification schemes are chosen based upon the experiences of the investigator. Characters judged to be important by one individual or group of individuals may have entirely different usefulness in classifying fungi than others. Because the fundamental goal of any classification scheme is to show phylogenetic relatedness, the use of a diagnosis instead of a description becomes more important. Much of the molecular data being gathered tend to strengthen the value of the diagnosis as a means to compare and contrast fungi and to more clearly understand their relatedness to each other. The importance of the nomenclatural type, that is, the permanently preserved specimen, assumes greater meaning when it is realized that the name given to a particular fungus is attached to that type. It is often forgotten that the nomenclatural type may not be typical of the taxon. This may be the case when the number of isolates being studied is too small. The true range of variation may not be evident because the isolate used to prepare the nomenclatural type may actually represent the outer boundaries for the taxon. In proposing new classifications, a major danger exists when only one or only a very limited number of isolates are characterized using molecular approaches such as 18S rDNA gene sequences or phylogenetic relatedness. If the isolate being studied by molecular tools is not central to the concept for the taxon, the concept for the taxon can be changed, because the molecular data will be used as the new central reference point. Many fungi that are morphologically similar may be polyphyletic in origin.

II. WHAT ARE FUNGI?

Mycologists study organisms that possess similar biologic properties using similar techniques and approaches. The majority of these organisms are phylogenetically related and definable in the kingdom Fungi. The fungi can be viewed from two basic perspectives: as a group of biologically similar organisms having different phylogenetic relationships or as a group of phylogenetically similar organisms that are taxonomically classified within a single kingdom (1,2). Mycologists study *Pythium insidiosum* using mycologic techniques, yet the microorganism is an oomycete classified in the kingdom Chromista. This seems reasonable because its biology resembles that of a fungus and it meets the needs of the users who have pragmatic interests. Barr (3) has suggested that assemblages of polyphyletic organisms that make up logical groups should be studied together for the benefit of scientists having particular needs in common. He has suggested that a "union of fungi" could be created that contains the organisms historically studied by mycologists that phylogenetically are classified in the kingdoms Fungi, Chromista, and Protoctista.

Classification systems may be either biologic or phylogenetic. Taxonomy attempts to classify fungi based upon phylogenetic relatedness. The traditional approach to studying fungi has been biologically based; hence mycologists have studied organisms currently classified in the kingdoms Fungi, Chromista, Protoctista, and Monera. The contemporary approach to studying fungi is phylogenetically orientated, which means that only organisms classified in the kingdom Fungi (Table 1) are considered to be fungi. Molecular analysis is often the driving force behind this approach to defining what is or is not a fungus.

Fungi are eukaryotic organisms whose vegetative growth may range from filamentous hyphae to solitary vegetative cells that are easily maintained (4) for long periods of time. Each of their nuclei contains a nucleolus and several chromosomes contained within a nuclear membrane, which usually persists during nuclear division. Fungal cells have mitochondria, 80S ribosomes, centrioles, and other subcellular structures. Only the chytrids have motile cells possessing single whiplash posterior flagella that are of the 9 + 2 fibril construction.

Fungal cell walls are approximately 80% polysaccharides, 3–20% proteins, lipids, pigments, and inorganic salts. The structural components consists primarily of chitin and β- and α-glucans, chitosan, glycoproteins, polyuronides, lipids, pigments, and inorganic salts (5). The cell wall is important because it provides shape and form for the fungus, protection against injury and osmotic lysis, as well as damage from some types of large macromolecules. When the fungi are supplied with carbon and nitrogen sources and essential minerals, they are able to synthesize their own proteins, and most amino acids and vitamins. All fungi synthesize lysine by the L-α-adipic acid pathway (6).

Owing to the fact that some microorganisms have not been cultivated in the laboratory, their inclusion with the fungi is still speculative. Based upon their morphology in tissue, *Rhinosporidium seeberi* and *Loboa loboi* are thought to be fungi. Even though these microorganisms have not been cultivated in vitro, they are studied by mycologists. Recently, employing molecular data, *Pneumocystis carinii* has been reclassified among the fungi and removed from the protozoans.

Table 1 The Six Kingdoms of Organisms[a]

Kingdoms	Principal features	Representative members
Monera	Prokaryotic; absorptive nutrition; mitotic apparatus absent; asexual reproduction by binary fission	Bacteria and blue-green algae
Protoctista[b]	Eukaryotic; ingestive, absorptive or photoautotrophic nutrition; mitotic reproduction; DNA and RNA; unicellular or multicellular; flagella or cilia with microtubules in 9 + 2 pattern	Protozoans, plasmodiophorids, protostelids, mycetozoans
Chromista	Eukaryotic; absorptive or photoautotrophic nutrition; thrust-reversing tubular ciliary mastigonemes present or absent, if absent, chloroplast, endoplasmic reticulum present; golgi cisternae stacked into dictyosomes, mitochondrial cristae tubular; plastids enclosed by membranes continuous with nuclear envelope; lysine synthesis by the diaminopimelic acid pathway	Brown algae, labyrinthulids, hyphochytrids, thraustochytrids, oomycetes
Fungi	Eukaryotic; absorptive nutrition; zygotic meiosis; unicellular or filamentous; posterior whiplash-type flagella present (chytrids), cilia absent; cell walls chitinous; mitochondrial cristae non-discordal platelike; lysine synthesis by the L-α-adipic acid biosynthetic pathway	Chytridiomycetes, zygomycetes, ascomycetes, basidiomycetes, fungi imperfecti, lichens
Plantae	Eukaryotic; photoautotrophic nutrition; tissue highly differentiated; diploid phase arising from embryophyte	Liverworts, mosses, vascular plants
Animalia	Eukaryotic; heterotrophic nutrition; gametic meiosis; multicellular; develop from diploid blastula, gastrulation occurs	Sponges, coelenterates, worms, arthropods, echinoderms, mammals, etc.

[a] Modified from Refs. 71 and 72.

[b] Protozoa sensu Cavalier Smith, Protista sensu Whittaker.

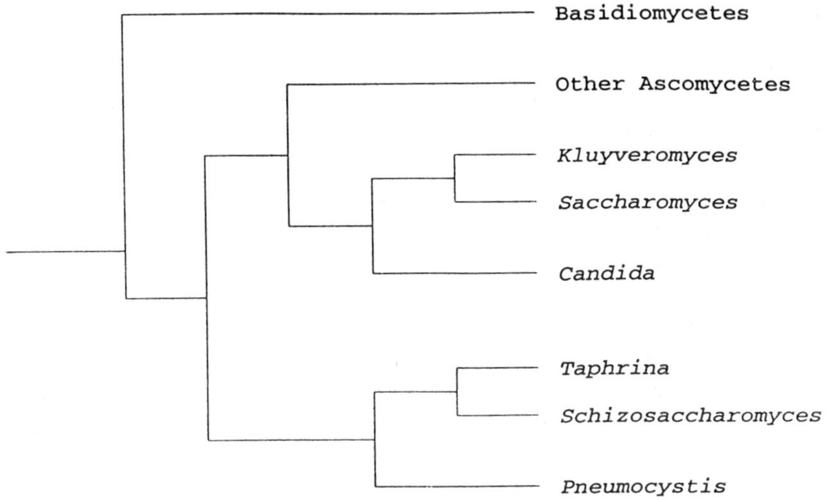

Figure 1 Relationship of *Pneumocystis carinii* to other fungi based upon 18S rDNA sequences. This tree depicts general relationships, but distances are not accurately portrayed. (From Ref. 10.)

Pneumocystis carinii has been historically treated as a protozoan because of its amoeboid appearance with filopodia as well as its therapeutic response to pentamidine, trimethoprim-sulfamethoxazole, and pyrimethamine-sulfadiazine but not to antifungal agents like amphotericin B and the azoles. Factors in favor of a fungal classification include 16S and 18S rRNA gene sequences, thymidylate synthase gene sequence and gene location that are similar to other fungi, and the dihydrofolate reductase gene, which is neither physically nor genetically linked to thymidylate synthase. Ludewig et al. (7) have recently shown that pentamidine in low concentrations inhibit *Saccaromyces cerevisiae* growth. This shows that both *P. carinii* and other fungi can be inhibited by this one antimicrobic agent.

Wakefield et al. (8) have suggested that *P. carinii* is closely related to the ustomycetous red yeasts, that is, the basidiomycetes. In response to their proposal, Taylor and Bowman (9) provided a scholarly discussion of the most ideal phylogenetic placement for *P. carinii* among the ascomycetes (Fig. 1). It appears that *P. carinii* diverged early along with the early ascomycetes. This conclusion is based upon 18S rRNA gene sequence data.

III. ORIGIN OF FUNGI

Using 18S rDNA gene sequence-based phylogenies, the chytrids have been shown to be the first fungi to evolve. The terrestrial fungi separated from the chytrids approximately 550 ± 150 million years ago (10). This age is estimated from a phylogeny inferred from 18S rRNA gene sequence data and pairwise percent substitution data from a DNA sequence distance matrix that was calibrated to a geologic time scale using fungal data obtained from the fossil record. It is unfortunate that the fossil record does not contain more preserved fungi.

The zygomycetes diverged from the ancestor that gave rise to the ascomycetes and basidiomycetes (11). The ascomycetes and basidiomycetes appear to have evolved from the same common ancestor approximately 400 ± 125 million years ago (10). Among the more recent fungi, the genera *Aspergillus* and *Penicillium* separated from each other approximately 60 million years ago, whereas *Sporothrix schenckii* became asexual from its probable teleomorph *Ophiostoma stenoceras* about 20 million years ago. *Pneumocystis carinii* has its fungal roots back nearly 300 million years.

During the evolution of the fungi (Fig. 2), a number of important steps occurred. The introduction of a chitinous cell wall is seen in the Chytridio-

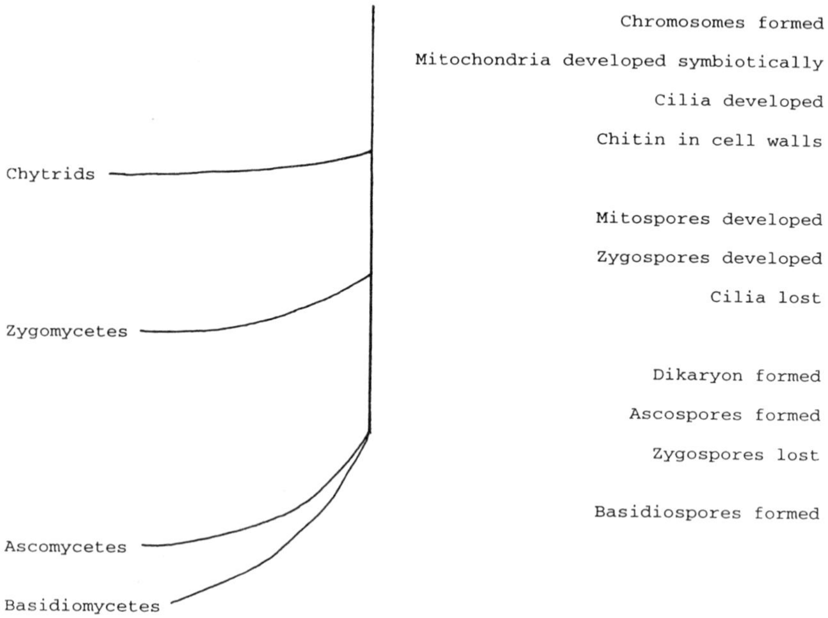

Figure 2 Some events in the evolution of fungi. (From Ref. 68.)

mycota. The Zygomycota developed mitospores that formed in sporangia and meiospores known as the zygospores. With the separation of the Ascomycota and Basidiomycota, the zygospore was lost, meiotic endospores (ascospores) and meiotic expospores (basidiospores) were developed, and fruiting bodies formed.

Among the fungi, the order Onygenales is one of the most important groups because several dimorphic fungi and the dermatophytes have their roots in this group (Fig. 3). Even though sexual reproduction is unknown in *Coccidioides immitis*, 18S (small-subunit) rDNA gene sequence data shows that it is a close relative to *Ajellomyces capsulatus* (anamorph *Histoplasma capsulatum*), *A. dermatitidis* (anamorph *Blastomyces dermatitidis*), and especially close to *Uncinocarpus reesii*. The family Onygenaceae contains these fungi, whereas the dermatophytes are classified in the family Arthrodermataceae. Both molecular and morphologic data support the single genus *Arthroderma* for the teleomorph of *Trichophyton*

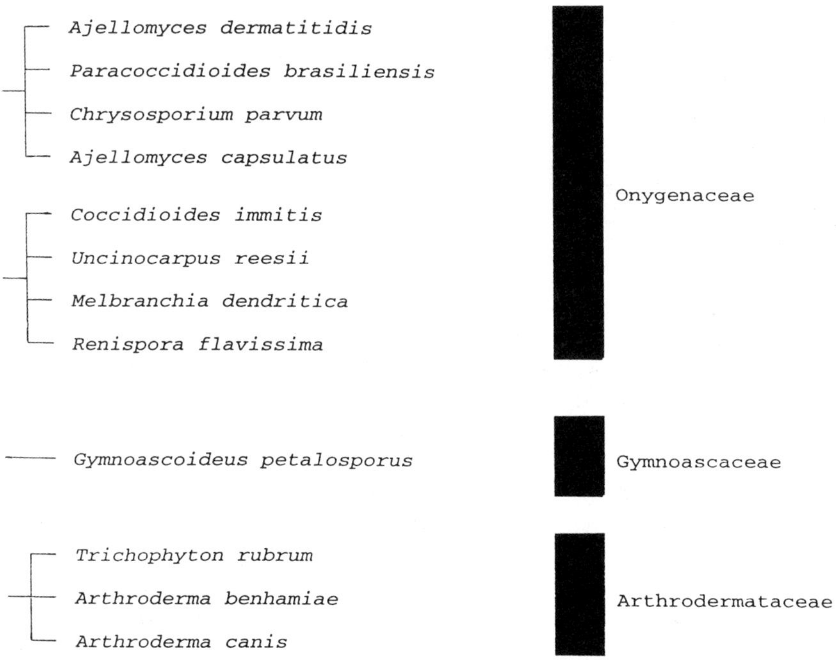

Figure 3 Relationship of some members of the Onygenales based upon 18S rDNA sequences. This tree depicts general relationships, but distances are not accurately portrayed. (From Refs. 10, 11, and 69.)

spp. and *Microsporum* spp. (12). Weitzman et al. (13) recently transferred all of the species classified in the genus *Nannizzia* to the genus *Arthroderma*.

It is often difficult to appreciate evolution exhibited by some fungi because the morphologic expression exhibited by these fungi is simple and often convergent. When the fossil record is searched for fungi, the preserved record of fungi and their changes is sparse. Fungi demonstrate a tremendous diversity, which is often related or controlled by their adaptation to specific ecologic niches. The study of several fungi with molecular tools used to evaluate their nucleic acids has resulted in fragmentary or equivocal data (14).

IV. HOLOMORPH CONCEPT

There are two independent classification systems for the fungi. The system based upon sexual (meiotic) structures or teleomorphs is the most central one because it not only allows for the classification of fungi but is used to develop phylogenetic relationships among individual species as well as between groups at various taxonomic levels. A teleomorph is any reproductive structure that is morphologically, karyologically, or both specialized for the production of sexual spores or their homologues, whether by normal sexual means or by some similar process.

Some fungi are known by only asexual (mitotic) or somatic reproduction. Asexual structures or anamorphs maybe either specialized or generalized, but they are neither karyologically nor morphologically involved in sexual reproduction. Some fungi may form more than a single anamorph. The term *synanamorph* is used to describe such a fungus. From a practical perspective, fungi having synanamorphs become difficult to classify, especially if a teleomorph is unknown. The term *holomorph* refers to the entire or whole fungus, including all of its morphologic forms.

To avoid confusion in using these two different concepts, form-division, form-classes, form-orders, form-families, form-genera, and form-species are commonly used for the various anamorphs or conidial states. The prefix *form-* usually denotes that these groups are intended neither to show nor to imply phylogenetic (natural) relationships but only to serve as groupings for morphologically similar imperfect fungi, so that one mycologist can effectively communicate with another. Even though the prefix *form-* was established for fossils, it is used by many mycologists for the Fungi Imperfecti. Imperfect fungi are "imperfect" only in the sense that their perfect stages (teleomorphs) are yet unknown. In essence, the concept of Fungi Imperfecti is like a file cabinet in which everything is in an organized format but the individual components are not necessarily meant to be related to each other. The term Fungi Imperfecti is preferred for these asexual fungi, rather than the term Deuteromycota. The term Deuteromycota implies that these fungi have equal taxonomic status to the other fungi classified upon their teleomorphs. There is a trend to replace terms such as Fungi Imperfecti and Deuteromycota by the expression *mitotic fungi* or *mitotic holomorph*, so that it becomes clear that phylogenetic relatedness is not implied. An interesting situation exists because the rules of nomenclature are being applied to an asexual portion of a fungus rather than one characterized by sexual reproduction.

The expression *pleomorphic* has different meanings to the taxonomist and the medical mycologist (15). *Pleomorphic* to the medical mycologist refers to dermatophytes that exhibit morphologic changes—including reduced conidiation, loss of pigmentation, and white tufts of aerial hyphae upon prolonged maintenance in culture—which results from molecular-level changes in the colony, like genetic mutations. *Pleomorphic*, *pleomorphism*, and *pleomorphy* refer to single organisms that possess different forms, such as teleomorphs, anamorphs, or synanamorphs in various combinations.

There are no universal characteristics applying to all fungi. Each group possesses its own particular characteristics, which may or may not have taxonomic value in another group of fungi. There are few characters that have applicability in all circumstances. The most useful characters are those that can be used most of the time. For this reason, no one character should be used in identifying or describing a fungus.

V. PLEOMORPHIC ANAMORPHIC DEMATIACEOUS FUNGI WITH LOCULOASCOMYCETOUS AFFINITIES

To illustrate some of the contemporary thought regarding fungal taxonomy, I would like to discuss an important monophylogenic group of dematiaceous (melanized) fungi having either known or suspected loculoascomycetous affinities.

Just recently, Pappagianis and Ajello (16) shown that the *demat* in *dematiaceous* is epistemologically incorrect. Even though this is the case, the term *dematiaceous* will be used in this discussion to describe fungi having olive-to-brown-to-black colonies due to the presence of melanin. Many dematiaceous, anamorphic fungi are postulated to have phylogenetic affinities with teleomorphic members of the class Loculoascomycetes within the Ascomycotina. These fungi present a number of interesting taxonomic challenges because their asexual nature dictates their inclusion in the Fungi Imperfecti. Recent chitin synthase gene sequences (17,18) and partial 18S rDNA sequence data (19) have revealed a particular clade of fungi known to consist of taxa classified in the loculoascomycetous families Diaporthaceae, Dimeriaceae, and Herpotrichiellaceae, order Diaporthales, and the imperfect genera *Exophiala*, *Fonsecaea*, *Phaeoannellomyces*, *Phaeococcomyces*, *Phialophora*, *Ramichloridium*, *Rhinocladiella*, and *Wangiella*. Members of this group of fungi are saprophytes of secondary incidence rather than primary degraders of cellulose, lignin, starch, pectin, and chitin (20) as well as etiologic agents of phaeohypomycosis, chromoblastomycosis, and mycetoma in humans (6). Phenotypically, members of this clade are primarily recognized for their dematiaceous and pleomorphic nature.

The anamorphic members of this clade morphologically reflect the effect of environmental pressures and ecologic niches, making relatedness among individual isolates and phylogenetic relatedness among taxa difficult to appreciate. Owing to the fact that their different morphologic forms (yeasts and molds) have been studied using different morphologic, physiologic, and molecular methods and criteria, the concept of a single fungus has been lost. Either similarity or dissimilarity in morphologic form appears to be simply a reflection of a response to specific environmental conditions.

Perhaps the best example of morphologic diversity in this group of fungi is the imperfect pleomorphic fungus *Wangiella dermatitidis* (Fig. 4). *Wangiella dermatitidis* has provided a great deal of insight regarding morphogenesis and the regulatory mechanisms involved (1,21–24). Depending on environmental conditions, this black yeast is capable of forming yeast cells that reproduce by either multilateral blastoconidia or percurrent proliferation, moniliform hyphae, pseudohyphae, hyphae, annellidic conidiogenous cells that are intercalary, terminal, or both, phialidic conidiogenous cells that are intercalary, terminal, or both and may or may not have collarettes, sympodially proliferating conidiogenous cells, conidia in balls or in acropetal chains, endoconidia, muriform cells, sporodochia, and teleomorph initials. By simple modifications of the in vitro culture conditions, this fungus can be induced to form each of the above structures (22,25–36).

Many of the synanamorphs produced by *W. dermatitidis* are also exhibited by other members of the clade, as well as some fungi that have not been adequately studied. The latter include species classified in the anamorphic genera *Botryomyces*, *Hyphozyma*, *Phaeoannellomyces*, *Phaeococcomyces*, *Phaeotheca*, and *Sarcinomyces*. *Exophiala jeanselmei* and *W. dermatitidis* are two pleomorphic anamorphic black yeast members of this clade that are known to form bodies resembling the ascomata of *Capronia* (Dothideales, Herpotrichiellaceae) (22,37) (Fig. 5). Similar bodies have been observed in *Fonsecaea pedrosoi* (38), *Phaeoannellomyces*

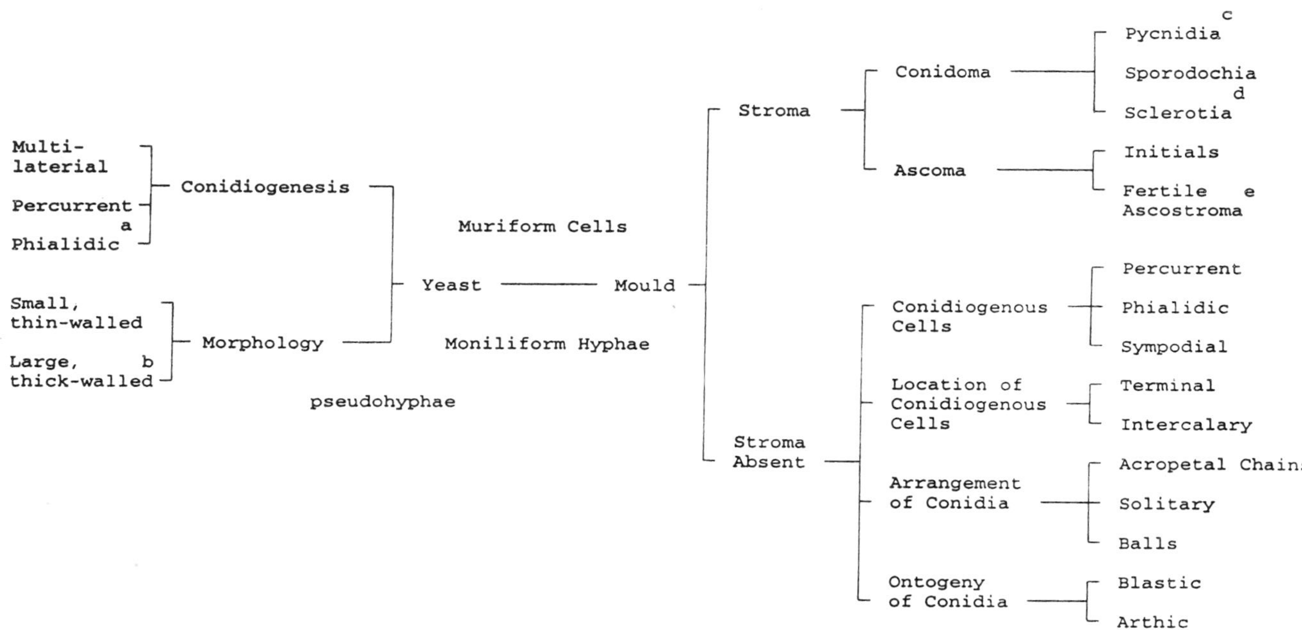

Figure 4 Pleomorphy of *Waginella dermatitidis*. (From Refs. 21, 22, 25–36, and 39.) [a] two-celled structures with distinct collarettes seen in *Phialophora verrucosa*; [b] frequently seen in *Exophiala spinifera*; [c] pycnidia seen in *Phaeoannellomyces werneckii*; [d] sclerotia seen in *Exophiala jeanselmei*; [e] fertile ascostroma of *Capronia* spp. reported for *Exophiala* spp.

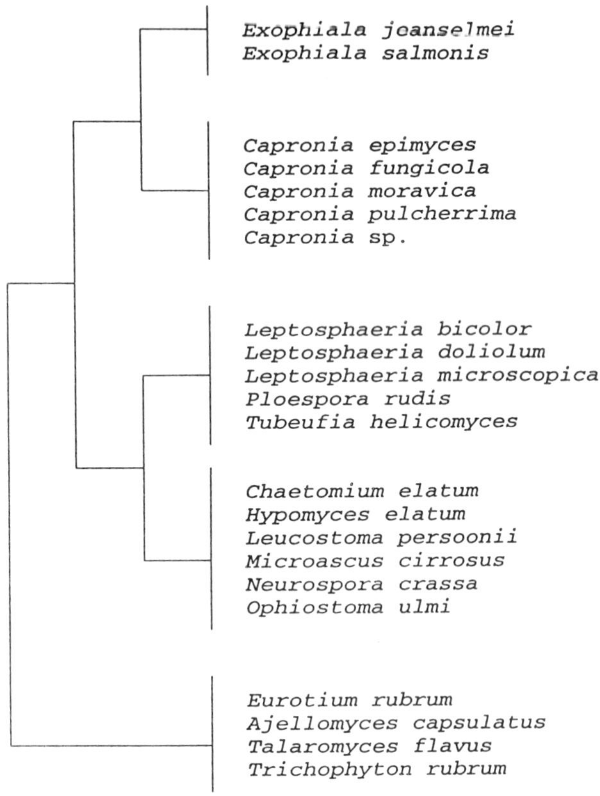

Figure 5 Phylogenetic tree based upon partial 18S rDNA sequences. This tree depicts general relationships, but distances are not accurately portrayed. (From Ref. 19.)

werneckii (39), and *Phialophora verrucosa* (40), which are also members of this clade. Unnamed *Exophiala* anamorphs are produced by *Capronia acutiseta*, *C. coronata*, *C. fungicola*, *C. mansonii*, *C. spinifera*, *C. villosa*, and *Valsaria insitiva* (Diaporthales, Diaporthaceae) (41,42). *Ramichloridium* spp. and *Rhinocladiella* spp. have been associated with taxa such as *C. parasitica*, *C. fungicola*, *Thecotheus pelletieri* (Pezizales, Ascobolaceae), and *Wentiomyces javanicus* (Dothideales, Dimeriaceae) (43,46). Even though *Rhinocladiella atrovirens* (44) is stated to be produced by *Acanthostigmella brevispina* (Dothideales, Herpotrichiellaceae), the illustration presented of its anamorphic form is clearly a taxon other than *R. atrovirens*.

Members of this clade are initially recognized by their dark color. The dark color is due to melanin, which is formed by the oxidative polymerization of 1,8-dihydroxynaphthalene (DHN) via pentaketide metabolism. The biosynthetic pathway was first demonstrated in *Verticillium dahliae* by using melanin-deficient mutants (45). Melanin biosynthesis may be either constitutive or nonconstitutive. For those members of this clade tested, they produce DHN melanin constitutively (46–48). Melanin is always present in the cell walls of their vegetative form. Hence, constitutive DHN melanin biosynthesis appears to provide another means to recognize members of this group.

Empiric evidence for the presence of a DHN melanin pathway is most easily provided by the use of the compound tricyclazole. The inhibition of DHN melanin synthesis using tricyclazole causes the accumulation of relatively large amounts of 2-hydroxyjuglone and flaviolin, which provides a simple method to recognize fungi that produce DHN melanin (49–57). Tricyclazole inhibits DHN synthesis by inhibiting either the reductase enzymes for 1,3,8-trihydroxynaphthalene or the pathway between 1,3,6,8-tetrahydroxy-naphthalene and scytalone. The specific inhibition is dependent upon the concentration of the inhibitor. The effect of tricyclazole mimics the *brm-2* and *brm-4* mutations in *V. dahliae*. At 42 mM, tricyclazole prevents the formation of melanin in the cell walls of *Cladophialophora bantiana* (syn. *Cladosporium trichoides*, *Xylohypha bantiana*), *Cladosporium carrionii* (syn. *Cladosporium carrionii*), *E. jeanselmei*, *Fonsecaea compacta*, *F. pedrosoi*, *P. werneckii*, *Phialophora richardsiae*, *Phialophora verrucosa*, *W. dermatitidis*, and other black fungi (46,47,54). These taxa are all members of the clade with the exception of *Ph. richardsiae*. DHN melanin has been found only in a few Ascomycotina and allied Fungi Imperfecti, but not in the Basidiomycotina nor Zygomycotina (46,54).

One published report regarding a phylogenetic study of dematiaceous fungi using rDNA sequences comes from a symposium review (23). Their data from partial 18S rDNA sequences of 23 taxa indicate that species of *Capronia* and those of *Exophiala* not having a known teleomorphic state form a loculoascomycetous, monophyletic group. The data clearly show that this loculoascomycetous clade is distinct from the Pleosporales and unitunicate pyrenomycetes (58). However, the data cannot adequately determine inter-familial relationships among *Capronia* and *Exophiala* species. Interestingly, the type strains of *E. salmonis* and *E. jeanselmei* form a monophyletic group within this clade, but their exact relationship to *Capronia* remains unknown (Fig. 5).

Chitin, the β-(1,4)-linked polymer of *N*-acetylglucosamine, is an important structural polysaccharide of the fungal cell wall. Three genes that encode distinct chitin synthases (Chs) have been cloned from both *Saccharomyces cerevisiae* and *Candida albicans* (59,60–66). These three Chs are responsible for the synthesis of chitin in different stages of the life cycle and cell cycle of these fungi.

Comparison of the derived amino acid sequences of the chitin synthase genes (CHS) from *S. cerevisiae* and *C. albicans* revealed a number of highly conserved regions. Degenerate PCR primers, based upon amino acid sequences, have been made to amplify one of these conserved coding regions using genomic DNA of a variety of fungi. These same primers were also used more recently to identify *CHS* homologues from the dematiaceous fungi, *W. dermatitidis*, *Ph. verrucosa*, *F. pedrosoi*, and *Sporothrix schenckii*. Three *CHS* homologs were identified in *W. dermatitidis* and *S. schenckii* and two in *Ph. verrucosa* and *F. pedrosoi* (17,18,24,67). Multiple sequence alignments showed that each homologue fell into one of three distinct Chs classes. The information obtained from *CHS* gene analysis was also useful in phylogenetic studies of these and other fungi (17,67). These data parallel the results obtained from 18S rDNA sequence analysis and strongly suggest that the dematiaceous fungi form a single monophyletic group.

"Holomorph" is an all-inclusive concept that reflects the entire reality of the fungus. It includes all of its forms and potentialities, regardless of whether they are latent, expressed, known, or unknown. Holomorph diversity in a single fungus can be expressed as three fundamental evolutionary units (Fig. 6) (68). The principal unit is the mitotic holomorph, which is characterized by asexual reproduction. The vegetative growth, which occurs in all fungi, is the platform from which the other two units may occur. The meiotic holomorph is the state formed by sexual reproduction. When both sexual and asexual states occur in the same fungus, the third unit, known as the pleomorphic holomorph, exists. Each of these holomorphs may morphologically evolve independently of each other. An overriding concern of many mycologists involves the idea that eventually a mitotic holomorph will express a meiotic holomorph, thereby becoming a pleomorphic holomorph. Subsequently, the name reflecting the mitotic holomorph could be eliminated. Such an expectation is unrealistic, because in many fungi sexual reproduction may have been lost, or even replaced, by processes like parasexuality, gene transfer, and heterokaryotic transfer.

Some mitotic fungi will be difficult to accommodate in a phylogenetically based classification system because they are polyphyletic. Methods must be found that will allow meiotic and mitotic holomorphs to be inte-

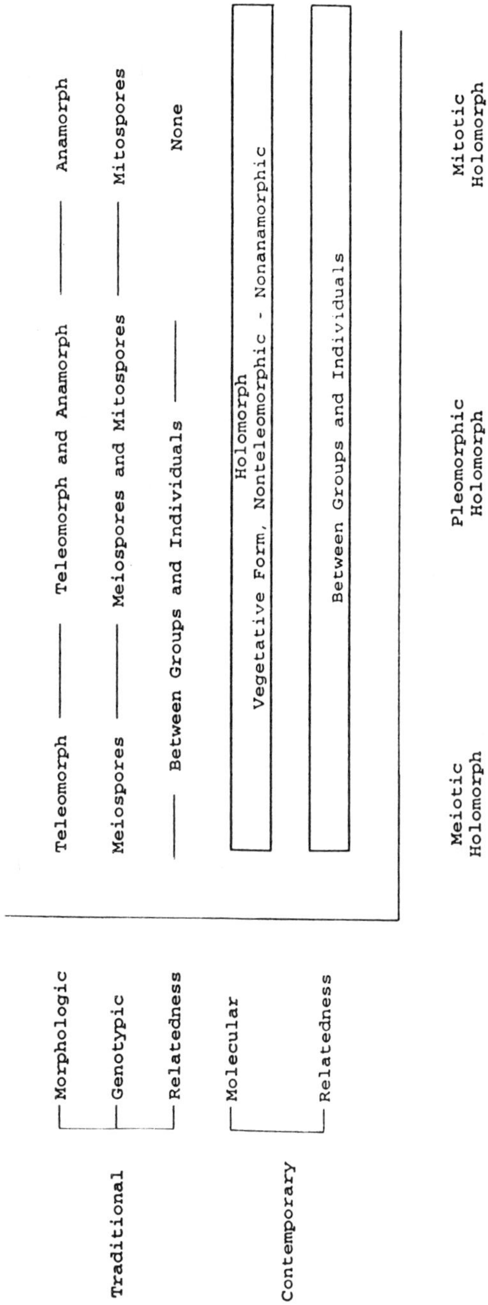

Figure 6 Holomorphic concept. (Based partly on Ref. 62.)

grated into a single classification system that reflects the holomorph. It is important to remember that, too often, the holomorph is based upon what we know and not necessarily upon its entire reality. Historically, when the terms *teleomorph* and *anamorph* were proposed as a means to help characterize the holomorph—that is, the whole fungus—they were used to refer to organs of reproduction without a karyologic connotation (69,70).

Yet another consideration occurs when anamorphic species are found as components of pleomorphic holomorphs. It is often assumed that other morphologically similar fungi that do not form sexual stages should have similar meiotic holomorphs because asexual morphologic similarity still implies relatedness to many taxonomists. For example, *Scedosporium prolificans* and *Scedosporium apiospermum* strongly resemble each other. *Scedosporium apiospermum* is the mitotic holomorph of *Pseudallescheria boydii*, whereas there is no meiotic holomorph known for *S. prolificans*. Recently, molecular characterization of 18S rDNA from each of these species has properly aligned the isolates of the mitotic holomorph *S. apiospermum* with *P. boydii* (71,72). This confirmed earlier results from previous DNA-DNA hybridization studies (73). In contrast, rDNA studies of a morphologically similar fungus to *S. prolificans* and *S. apiospermum* shows that its meiotic holomorph lies in the ascomycetous genus *Petriella* Curzi (71).

The superficial similarity or dissimilarity seen in these and many other fungi does not necessarily reflect phylogenetic relatedness. The anamorphs formed may have evolved at different stages in the evolutionary process of several different fungi to result in the forms that we see today. The recognition of a single fungus in this clade having mold-yeast phenotypes is typically lost owing to the fact that these forms are studied by different investigators who use different techniques with different purposes and priorities. Phenotypic classification of this group is difficult and controversial because of its complexity, owing to its artificial nature. Such a system does not allow the individual to be recognized, nor its relatedness to others.

During the next few years, molecular data will resolve many taxonomic and phylogenetic problems. Molecular data have been extremely valuable in confirming many phylogenetic proposals based upon the study of teleomorphs. They also provide a useful tool to speculate where a number of the anamorphic fungi should occur within various phylogenic trees.

REFERENCES

1. Christensen T. Plants, animals, algae and fungi: four non-taxonomic group designations. Taxon 1990;39:93–94.

2. Vilgalys R, Hibbett DS. Phylogenetic classification of fungi and our Linnaean heritage. In: Reynolds DR, Taylor JW, eds. The Fungal Holomorph: Mitotic, Meiotic, and Pleomorphic Speciation in Fungal Systematics, CAB International, Wallingford, UK, 1993:256–260.
3. Barr DJS. Evolution and kingdoms of organisms from the perspective of a mycologist. Mycologia 1992;84:1–11.
4. Pasarell L, McGinnis, MR. Viability of fungal cultures maintained at −70°C. J Clin Microbiol 1992;30:1000–1004.
5. Ruiz-Herrera J. Fungal Cell Wall: Structure, Synthesis, and Assembly. Boca Raton, FL: CRC Press, 1992.
6. McGinnis MR. Laboratory Handbook of Medical Mycology. New York: Academic Press, 1980.
7. Ludewig G, Williams JM, Li Y, Staben C. Effects of pentamidine isethionate on Saccharomyces cerevisiae. Antimicrob Agents Chemother 1994;38: 1123–1128.
8. Wakefield AE, Peters SE, Banerji S, et al. Pneumocystis carinii shows DNA homology with the ustomycetous red yeast fungi. Mol Microbiol 1992;6: 1903–1911.
9. Taylor JW, Bowman BH. Pneumocystis carinii and the ustomycetous red yeast fungi. Mol Microbiol 1993;8:425–427.
10. Berbee ML, Taylor JW. Dating the evolutionary radiations of the true fungi. Can J Bot 1993;71:1114–1127.
11. Bowman B, Taylor JW, Brownlee AG, et al. Molecular evolution of the fungi: Relationships of the basidiomycetes, ascomycetes, and chytridiomycetes. Mol Biol Evol 1992;9:285–296.
12. Bowman BH, Taylor JW, White TJ. Molecular evolution of the fungi. Mol Biol Evol 1992;9:893–904.
13. Weitzman I, McGinnis MR, Padhye AA, Ajello L. The genus Arthroderma and its later synonym Nannizzia. Mycotaxon 1986;25:505–518.
14. Bruns TD, White TJ, Taylor JW. Fungal molecular systematics. Annu Rev Ecol Syst 1991;22:525–564.
15. McGinnis MR, Salkin IF. A clinical user perspective of anamorphs and teleomorphs. In: Reynolds DR, Taylor JW, eds. The Fungal Holomorph: Mitotic, Meiotic, and Pleomorphic Speciation in Fungal Systematics. Wallingford, UK: CAB International, 1993:87–92.
16. Pappagianis D, Ajello L. Dematiaceous–A mycologic misnomer? J Med Vet Mycol 1994;32:319–321.
17. Chua SS, Momany M, Mendoza L, Szaniszlo PJ. Identification of three chitin synthase genes in the dimorphic fungal pathogen Sporothrix schenckii. Curr Microbiol 1994;29:151–156.
18. Peng M, Karuppayil SM, Mendoza L, et al. Use of PCR to identify coding sequences for zymogenic and nonzymogenic chitin isozymes in Phialophora verrucosa. Curr Genet 1995;27:517–523.
19. de Hoog GS, Sigler L, Untereiner WA, et al. Changing taxonomic concepts and their impact on nomenclatural stability. J Med Vet Mycol (suppl 1) 1994; 32:113–122.

20. Domsch KH, Gams W, Anderson T. Compendium of Soil Fungi, Vol 1. New York: Academic Press, 1989.
21. Cooper CR Jr, Szaniszlo PJ. Evidence for two cell division cycle (CDC) genes that govern yeast bud emergence in the pathogenic fungus Wangiella dermatitidis. Infect Immun 1993;61:2069–2081.
22. de Hoog GS, Takeo, K, Yoshida S, et al. Pleoanamorphic life cycle of Exophiala (Wangiella) dermatitidis. Antonie van Leeuwenhoek 1994;65:143–153.
23. Jacobs CW, Szaniszlo PJ. Microtubule function and its relation to cellular development and the yeast cell cycle in Wangiella dermatitidis. Arch Microbiol 1992;133:155–161.
24. Szaniszlo PJ, Momany M. Chitin, chitin synthase and chitin synthase conserved region homologues in Wangiella dermatitidis. In Maresca B, Kobayashi GS, Yamaguchi H, eds. Molecular Biology and Its Application to Medical Mycology. Berlin and Heidelberg: Springer-Verlag, 1993:229–242.
25. Geis PA, Jacobs CW. Polymorphism of Wangiella dermatitidis. In: Szaniszlo PJ, ed., Fungal Dimorphism: With Emphasis on Fungi Pathogenic for Humans. New York: Plenum Press, 1985:205–233.
26. Matsumoto T, Matsuda T, McGinnis, MR. A previously undescribed synanamorph of Wangiella dermatitidis. J Med Vet Mycol 1990;28:437–444.
27. Dixon DM, Szaniszlo PJ, Polak A. Dihydroxynaphthalene (DHN) melanin and its relationship with virulence in the early stages of phaeohyphomycosis. In: Cole GT, Hoch HC, eds. Fungal Spore and Disease Initiation in Plants and Animals. New York: Plenum Press, 1991:297–318.
28. McGinnis MR. Wangiella dermatitidis, a correction. Mycotaxon 1997;6: 367–369.
29. McGinnis MR, Schell WA, Carson J. Phaeoannellomyces and the Phaeococcomycetaceae, new dematiaceous blastomycete taxa. Sabouraudia 1985;23: 179–188.
30. McGinnis MR Wangiella, a new genus to accommodate Hormiscium dermatitidis. Mycotaxon 1977;5:353–363.
31. McGinnis MR, Sigler L, Bowman BH, et al. Impact of conidiogenesis, teleomorph connections, pleomorphism and molecular genetics on evolving hyphomycete systematics. J Med Vet Mycol 1992;30:261–269.
32. Nishimura K, Miyaji M. Studies on a saprophyte of Exophiala dermatitidis isolated from a humidifier. Mycopathologia 1982;77:173–181.
33. Nishimura K, Miyaji M. Studies on the phylogenesis of pathogenic "black yeasts." Mycopathologia 1983;81:135–144.
34. Oujezdsky KB, Grove SN, Szaniszlo, PJ. Morphological and structural changes during yeast-to-mold conversion of Phialophora dermatitidis. Mycologia 1973;66:537–542.
35. Szaniszlo PJ, Geis PA, Jacobs CW, et al. Cell-wall changes associated with yeast-to-multicellular-form conversion in Wangiella dermatitidis. In: Schlessinger D, ed. Microbiology—1983. Washington, DC: American Society for Microbiology, 1983:239–244.
36. Szaniszlo PJ, Hsieh PH, Marlowe JD. Induction and ultrastructure of the

multicellular (sclerotic) morphology in Phialophora dermatitidis. Mycologia 1976;68:117–130.

37. Szaniszlo PJ, Jacobs CW, Geis PA. Dimorphism: Morphological and biochemical aspects. In: Howard D, ed. Fungi Pathogenic for Humans and Animals, Part A (Biology). New York: Marcel Dekker, 1983:323–436.
38. Szaniszlo PJ, Mendoza L, Karuppayil SM. Clues about chromoblastomycotic and other dematiaceous fungal pathogens based on Wangiella as a model. In: Vanden Bossche H, Odds FC, Kerridge D, eds. Dimorphic Fungi in Biology and Medicine. New York: Plenum Press, 1993:241–255.
39. Untereiner WA. A simple method for the in vitro production of pseudothecia in species of Capronia. Mycologia 1994;86:290–295.
40. Karrer H, Conant, NF. A cleistothecium-like structure found in Hormodendrum pedrosoi. Mycologia 1953;45:693–697.
41. Borelli D. Aureobasidium werneckii: Acervuli, sporodochia, and pycnidia. PAHO Sci. Publ. 1977;356:79–90.
42. Ajello L, Runyon L. Abortive "perithecial" reproduction by Phialophora verrucosa. Mycologia 1953;45:947–950.
43. Bell AA, Puhalla JE, Tolmsoff WJ, Stipanovic RD. Use of mutants to establish (+)-scytalone as an intermediate in melanin biosynthesis by Verticillium dahliae. Can J Microbiol 1976;22:787–799.
44. Müller E, Petrini O, Fisher PJ, et al. Taxonomy and anamorphs of the Herpotrichiellaceae with notes on generic synonym. Trans Br Mycol Soc 1987;88: 63–74.
45. Conway KE. Ascocarp ontogeny and imperfect state of Thecotheus (Pezizales, Ascomycetes). Mycologia 1975;67:241–252.
46. Joly P. Sur quelques champignons foliicoles du Kentia forsteriansa. Rev Mycol 1965;30:42–51.
47. Barr ME, Rogerson CT. Two new species of loculoascomycetes. Mycotaxon 1983;17:247–252.
48. Bell AA, Wheeler MH. Biosynthesis and functions of fungal melanins. Annu Rev Phytopathol 1986;24:411–451.
49. Taylor BE, Wheeler MH, Szaniszlo PJ. Evidence for pentaketide melanin biosynthesis in dematiaceous human pathogenic fungi. Mycologia 1987;79: 320–322.
50. Wheeler MH, Bell AA. Melanins and their importance in pathogenic fungi. In: McGinnis MR, ed. Current Topics in Medical Mycology, vol. 2. New York: Springer-Verlag, 1988:338–387.
51. Geis PA, Wheeler MH, Szaniszlo PJ. Pentaketide metabolites of melanin synthesis in the dematiaceous fungus Wangiella dermatitidis. Arch Microbiol 1984;137:324–328.
52. Stipanovic RD, Wheeler MH. Accumulation of 3,3′-biflaviolin, a melanin shunt product, by tricyclazole-treated Thielaviopsis basicola. Pestic Biochem Physiol 1980;13:198–201.
53. Tokousbalides MC, Sisler, HD. Site of inhibition by tricyclazole in the melanin biosynthetic pathway of Verticillium dahliae. Pestic Biochem Physiol 1979;11:64–73.

54. Wheeler MH. Melanin biosynthesis in Verticillium dahliae: Dehydration and reduction reactions in cell-free homogenates. Exp Mycol 1979;6:171–179.
55. Wheeler MH, Stipanovic RD. Melanin biosynthesis and the metabolism of flaviolin and 2-hydroxyjuglone in Wangiella dermatitidis. Arch Microbiol 1985;142:234–241.
56. Wheeler MH, Stipanovic RD. Melanin biosynthesis in Thielaviopsis basicola. Exp Mycol 1979;3:340–350.
57. Woloshuk CP, Sisler HD, Tokousbalides MC, Dulky SR. Melanin biosynthesis in Pyricularia oryzae: Site of tricyclazole inhibition and pathogenesis of melanin-deficient mutants. Pestic Biochem Physiol 1980;14:256–264.
58. de Hoog GS, McGinnis, MR. Ascomycetous black yeasts. Stud Mycol 1987; 30:187–199.
59. Au-Young J, Robbins PW. Isolation of a chitin synthase (CHS1) from Candida albicans by expression in Saccharomyces cerevisiae. Mol Microbiol 1990;4:197–207.
60. Bulawa CE. CSD2, CSD3, and CSD4, genes required for chitin synthesis in Saccharomyces cerevisiae: The CSD2 gene product is related to chitin synthases and to developmentally regulated proteins in Rhizobium species and Xenopus laevis. Mol Cell Biol 1992;12:1764–1776.
61. Bulawa CE, Slater M, Cabib E, et al. The S cerevisiae structural gene for chitin synthase is not required for chitin synthesis in vivo. Cell 1986;46: 213–225.
62. Chen-Wu J, Zwicker J, Bowen AR, Robbins PW. Expression of chitin synthase genes during yeast and hyphal growth phases of Candida albicans. Mol Microbiol 1992;6:497–502.
63. Shaw JA, Mol PC, Bowers B, et al. The function of chitin synthases 2 and 3 in the Saccharomyces cerevisiae cell cycle. J Cell Biol 1991;114:111–123.
64. Silverman SJ. Similar and different domains of chitin synthase 1 and 2 of S cerevisiae: Two isozymes with distinct functions. Yeast 1989;5:495–467.
65. Silverman SJ, Sburlati A, Slater ML, Cabib E. Chitin synthase 2 is essential for septum formation and cell division in Saccharomyces cerevisiae. Proc Natl Acad Sci USA 1988;85:4735–4739.
66. Sudoh M, Nagahashi S, Doi M, et al. Cloning of the chitin synthase 3 gene from Candida albicans and its expression during yeast-hyphal transition. Mol Gen Genet 1993;241:351–358.
67. Bowen AR, Chen-Wu JL, Momany M, et al. Classification of fungal chitin synthases. Proc Natl Acad Sci USA 1992;89:519–523.
68. Reynolds DR. The fungal holomorph: An overview. In: Reynolds DR, Taylor JW, eds. The Fungal Holomorph: Mitotic, Meiotic, and Pleomorphic Speciation in Fungal Systematics, Wallingford, UK: CAB International, 1993: 15–25.
69. Hennebert GL. Towards a natural classification of the fungi. In: Reynolds DR, Taylor JW, eds. The Fungal Holomorph: Mitotic, Meiotic, and Pleomorphic Speciation in Fungal Systematics. Wallingford, UK: CAB International, 1993:283–294.

70. Weresub LK, Hennebert GL. Anamorph and teleomorph: Terms for organs of reproduction rather than karyological phases. Mycotaxon 1979;8:181–186.
71. Cooper CR Jr, Salkin IF, McGinnis, MR. Development of a species-specific probe for Scedosporium prolificans (abstr). Ann Mtg Am Soc Microbiol, Washington, DC, 1995.
72. Lennon PA, Cooper CR Jr, Salkin IF, Lee SB. Ribosomal DNA internal transcribed spacer analysis supports synonymy of Scedosporium inflatum and Lomentospora prolificans. J Clin Microbiol 1994;32:2413–2416.
73. Guého E, de Hoog GS. Taxonomy of the medical species of Pseudallescheria and Scedosporium. J Mycol Med 1991;118:3–9.
74. Hawksworth, DL. The fungal dimension of biodiversity: Magnitude, significance, and conservation. Mycol Res 1991;95:641–655.
75. Margulis L, Schwartz KV. Five Kingdoms. San Francisco: Freeman, 1982.
76. Cavalier-Smith T. The kingdom Chromista: Origin and systematics. Prog Phycol Res 1986;4:309–347.

3

Structure and Function of the Fungal Cell Wall

VERONICA M. HEARN
Leeds University
Leeds, West Yorkshire, England

I. INTRODUCTION

The fungal wall performs many functions, determining cell shape, serving a protective role, and containing specific adhesive molecules for attachment and subsequent invasion of the host. In addition, antibiotic potency is heavily dependent on the wall composition of the organism (1). The wall is a layered structure with an outer surface that consists of totally amorphous material, with the skeletal component located toward the inner side of the wall. The matrix polysaccharides are mostly water-soluble and include α-linked glucans and glycoproteins. Skeletal polysaccharides are water-insoluble and include chitin and β-linked glucans. The association of wall composition with cell shape has long been recognized (2,3). The formation and structural modifications of the chitin/β-glucan complex play an essential role in fungal morphogenesis (4).

Lipids and melanins are minor components in many fungi, but this does not minimize their significance (5). Melanins may render organisms resistant to lysis; observations suggest that its presence has an inhibitory effect on classic phagocytosis (6,7). *Fonsecaea pedrosoi* has been reported to have both melanin and sialylated constituents on the external layers of its cell wall, where they may play an important role in the pathogenicity of this fungus (8). α-Glucan has been strongly implicated in the virulence of *Paracoccidioides brasiliensis* and *Histoplasma capsulatum* (9,10). It may also perform a protective function.

It is important to realize that the cell surface is a dynamic structure (11). Its composition is influenced by a variety of environmental conditions, including temperature, and also by the developmental stage of the fungus (12). The variations in *Candida albicans* adhesion with changes in medium composition highlight the potential of this organism for cell-surface modification in vivo. It offers one explanation why *C. albicans* has a greater ability to attach to tissues than other *Candida* species (13). It has also been suggested that modulation of antigen expression may provide the fungus with a potent means of evading the host's immune response or minimize its consequences (14).

The fungal wall and the host response have been studied from many aspects. In this chapter, an attempt has been made to compare a number of fungal pathogens, emphasizing both their common structural features and their differences and relating these, where possible, to performance and function. All fungi discussed here contain chitin in their walls, while many of them share cross-reacting galactomannan structures. Others, in contrast, possess special components such as the glucuronoxylomannan of *Cryptococcus* and the rhamnomannans of *Sporothrix schenckii*. The complement system is thought to play a significant role in resistance to a variety of medically important fungi (15). The alternative complement pathway (ACP), which is stimulated by certain polysaccharides, seems to play a primary role in resistance to infection by promoting phagocytosis (16). Inhibition of ACP is mediated by surface components of the pathogens (17). In cellular defense mechanisms, phagocytosis may proceed via different routes; interaction occurs with fungi in ways that are in part determined by the surface composition of the organism. Primary and opportunistic fungal pathogens to be discussed in the text include dimorphic, filamentous, and yeastlike representatives. For information outside the scope of this chapter, a number of excellent reviews are available (15,18–20).

II. *Candida*

A. Structural Composition

The cell wall of *C. albicans* contains polysaccharides, protein, and lipid with phosphorus as a minor component. Mannans represent 35 to 40% and β-glucans account for 47 to 60% of the total dry weight (21,22). The organization of the components of the cell wall of *C. albicans* has been investigated (23,24). Inner wall layers, which contain much of the wall glucan and chitin, maintain the rigidity of the cell wall (25). Gale (26) has demonstrated a possible role for the glucan of *C. albicans* in the development of resistance to amphotericin B. Recently, the determination of plasma (1 → 3)-β-D-glucan has been proposed as an aid in the diagnosis of deep-seated mycoses (27).

The protein component of *C. albicans* cell wall is heterogeneous in composition, differs between morphological forms, and may be differently distributed within the wall (28,29). It has been reported that not all proteins are glycoproteins; in addition, the carbohydrate structure of glycoproteins is not always the same (28,30). It has further been shown that not all glycoproteins contain detectable phosphate and that at least one 19–20-kDa protein may be phosphorylated in the absence of carbohydrate (31). A structure peculiar to *C. albicans* has been identified as a 14–18-kDa phospholipomannan containing β-1,2-linked oligomannosides (32).

B. Mannan Immunochemistry

Reports from different centers on the chemical analysis of the mannans of *C. albicans* support a model consisting of a backbone of α-1,6-linked mannopyranosyl units heavily substituted with side chains of mannose attached via α-1,2 and α-1,3 bonds. Mannans are the major cell wall antigens of *Candida* and readily induce antibody formation (33). Antimannan antibodies help the host to resist disseminated candidiasis (34). Intact phosphopeptidomannan of *C. albicans* serotype A shows reactivity to factor sera 1, 4, 5, and 6 of "Candida Check" on enzyme-linked immunosorbent assay (ELISA). *Candida albicans* serotype B strain involves antigenic factor 13b instead of factor 6 (35). It has been shown that phosphate-bound β-1,2-linked oligomannosyl residues correspond to antigenic factor 5, found in strains of *C. albicans* serotypes A and B, *Candida stellatoidea*, *Candida tropicalis*, and *Candida glabrata* (36,37). The structure responsible for the serotype specificity of *C. albicans* A (i.e., antigen 6) is thought to reside in terminal oligomannosyl residues containing both β-1,2 and α-1,2 linkages. Antigenic factor 6 is shared by *C. glabrata* and, theoretically, by *C. tropicalis*, and *C. stellatoidea* type II (38). *Candida guilliermondii*, in addition to β-1,2 linked oligomannosides contains α-1,3 linkages (39). Surface antigen 4 (located in a glycoprotein-rich cell wall layer), is present in *C. albicans*, *C. tropicalis*, *C. guilliermondii*, *C. pseudotropicalis*, and *C. parapsilosis* (40).

An immunomodulatory role for *C. albicans* 0-linked oligomannosides against human lymphocytic proliferation induced in vitro, has been demonstrated (41). Recent results have shown the synthesis of human antibodies against these oligomannosides or related structures; this could have important implications for the effect of these molecules on lymphoid cells (42). The lymphokine interleukin-2 (IL-2), which is necessary for the generation of an optimal cell-mediated immune response, has an affinity for high mannose groups. It has been shown to bind to sites of the surface of *C. albicans* blastoconidia (43).

C. Mannoproteins

Cell-surface antigenic characters of *Candida* are dynamic and influenced by the environment and developmental stages of the fungus (44–49). Some studies have addressed the question of possible antigen gain or loss in vivo (50–51). The fact that antigenic variation may be transitory and unevenly distributed within the cellular population has been noted (52). The involvement of mannoproteins in *Candida* cell wall variability has also been noted by Poulain (53). Besides being an integral constituent of the fungal cell wall, mannoproteins are released into the external medium during growth of *C. albicans*. These secretory constituents must therefore be seen as an essential adjunct to, and interplaying with, the mannoproteins present on the cell surface in the host-parasite relationship (54). A mannoprotein constituent of *C. albicans* that elicits different levels of delayed-type hypersensitivity, cytokine production, and anticandidial protection in mice has been described (55).

Antigenic determinants expressed exclusively or predominantly on either yeast or hyphal *Candida* have been generally characterized as high-molecular-mass mannoproteins (56–58). However, the absence of a reactive epitope on the yeast cell surface of *C. albicans* does not exclude the possibility that this epitope is expressed intracellularly in this morphological phase (59–62). An acidic mannoprotein fraction of 65-kDa molecular mass, has been proposed as an immunodominant antigen that is ordinarily expressed as a target of anticandidal cell-mediated immunity in healthy humans (63).

D. Adhesion Properties

The interaction of *C. albicans* with host cells and host-cell ligands represents a crucial step in the initiation of the disease process (64). Strains of *C. albicans* possess long, filamentous cell surface appendages termed fimbriae that act as adhesins. A major glycoprotein structure has been isolated and partially characterized (65). A mucous cell-wall coating is secreted by both blastospores and hyphae of *C. albicans*. It may play an important role in virulence, since increased proliferation of this outer wall layer during cell adherence has been established (66). Colonization of mucosal surfaces by *Candida* requires adherence of these organisms to epithelial cells (67–69). It has been shown that germinating cells of *C. albicans* were significantly more adhesive than their nongerminating counterparts (70).

The rate of antigenic shedding during germ tube formation is significantly different to what is seen during yeast growth (54). Its has been suggested that changes in cell surface expression of certain antigens, perhaps proteins and mannoproteins of apparent molecular mass between 20 and 67 kDa, may be connected with hydrophobicity changes of the cell surface (60,71). Hydrophobic cells are more likely to bind to epithelial cells and display a more generalized binding pattern to host tissues than do hydrophilic cells (72). The authors reported that surface hydrophobicity appeared to contribute to the total number of bound yeasts by promoting yeast coadhesion (13,73). Hydrophobic and hydrophilic yeast cells are obtained by growth of the organism at 23°C and 37°C, respectively (74). Cells grown at 25°C were significantly more adhesive to buccal epithelial cells (BECs) than cells grown at 37°C. However, growth temperature alone is not responsible for the differences seen in adherence between hydrophobic and hydrophilic strains (75). At a molecular level, *Candida*–host cell interaction is mediated by cell surface mannans and mannoproteins (76,77). Mannoproteins of the organism recognize either fucosyl or glucosamine glycosides of epithelial cells (78). A chitin-soluble extract from *C. albicans* cell walls inhibited in vitro adhesion of *C. albicans* to human epithelial vaginal cells (79). Inhibition of adhesion of *C. albicans* clinical isolates to human BECs by fucosyl α-1,2-galacosyl β-bearing complex carbohydrates has been reported (80). Using isolated, perfused mouse liver, it was found that lectins with binding specificities for mannose, *N*-acetyl-galactosamine and galactose increased hepatic trapping and killing of *C. albicans* (81). Adherence of *C. albicans* to human BECs has also been linked to antigen 6, found only in *C. albicans* serotype A cells. *Candida albicans* serotype B has significantly lower adherence than serotype A, *C. tropicalis* and *C. glabrata*, all of which bear antigen 6 (82). Another category of cell-host interaction is the recognition of arginine-glycine-aspartic acid–containing peptides of endothelial cells or their extracellular matrix proteins (83). This amino acid sequence is found in many mammalian cell proteins such as iC3b (a complement C3 conversion product), fibrinogen, fibronectin and laminin. *Candida* binds avidly to extracellular matrix proteins such as laminin and fibronectin in vitro (84–87). A 58-kDa mannoprotein which binds to fibrinogen has been identified in both yeast and hyphal cells of *C. albicans* (57). Fukayama and Calderone (88) suggested an adhesive function for 55–60 and 165-kDa proteins in a wild-type strain of *C. albicans*. The lack of these antigens on the surface of the spontaneous avirulent mutant of this strain, suggested to the authors that the virulence of the native strain might be related to its greater adherence properties.

In two separate studies it has been suggested that a glycoprotein on the yeast cell surface of *C. albicans* may be involved in adhesion to salivary mucin (89,90).

E. Cell-Mediated Immunity

A glycomannoprotein from the cell wall of *C. albicans* yeast cell wall enhanced polymorphonuclear leukocytes (PMNL) inhibition of candidal growth in vitro as potently as lipopolysaccharide. It stimulated release of lactoferrin which inhibited candidal growth in absence of PMNL (91).

Both mannoprotein and glucan components of *Candida* cell wall activate natural killer cell activity in the peritoneal cavity of a murine model. A role has been suggested for NK cells in host protection against disseminated candidiasis (92). Mannoprotein constituents of the cell wall of *C. albicans* have been shown to stimulate tumor necrosis factor from murine macrophages in vitro (93). A similar role has been reported for the phospholipomannan 14–18-kDa antigen (94). The hyphal form of *C. albicans* acts as a macrophage-stimulating agent (95). After contact with a cloned macrophage line Y-Candida, but not H-Candida proteinaceous, cell wall components are profoundly modified (96).

F. Complement

The importance of complement in the phagocytosis and killing of *C. albicans* by both mononuclear phagocytic cells and PMNL is long established (97). The ACP is primarily responsible for this enhancement of phagocytosis (98).

There is evidence that the C3d-binding protein (CR2) is expressed in vivo on both yeast and filamentous forms of *C. albicans* (99). The purified receptor consists of a doublet of 60 and 66–68 kDa (100). *Candida albicans* and *C. stellatoidea*, in contrast to other *Candida* species, bind iC3b and C3d but not C3b components of complement (101). The CR2 protein also recognizes host cell matrix proteins, such as laminin (102). Avirulent clones of *C. albicans* had reduced ability to recognize the CR2 ligand C3d while recognition of iC3b was unaffected (103).

The expression of the C3bi-binding protein is restricted to the pseudohyphae of the dimorphic fungi. The expression of this receptor is temperature-dependent. *Candida albicans* grown at 30°C bound strongly to this component of complement, but not when grown at 38.5°C (104). The isolated iC3b receptor (CR3) is a protein of approximately 42 kDa. The authors suggest that this molecule also exists in glycosylated forms of 55 and 66 kDa (105). Despite the apparent differences in molecular mass, it is uncertain whether a single protein or different proteins recognize iC3b and C3d. Recent investigations indicate that *C. albicans* CR3 behaves as an adhesive in recognizing endothelial cells (106).

III. *Cryptococcus neoformans*

A. Structural Composition

The cell envelope of *Cryptococcus neoformans* consists of a rigid cell wall, mainly glucans, acapsular polysaccharide, glucuronoxylomannan (GXM), composed of an O-acetylated α (1,3) linked mannan backbone with xylose and glucuronic acid side chains and two minor constituents, namely, galactoxylomannan (GalXM) and mannoprotein (MP). Glucuronoxylomannan, a viscous polysaccharide, represents approximately 88% of the capsular mass, while GalXM and MP make up approximately 12% (107,108). The GalXM consists of xylose:mannose:galactose in a molar ratio of 1.0:1.5:1.8. Mannoprotein consists of xylose:mannose:galactose in a molar ratio of 1.0:7.6:0.8 and contains approximately 20% peptide (109). *Cryptococcus neoformans* exists in two varieties defining four serotypes *C. neoformans* var. *neoformans* (serotypes A and D) and *C. neoformans* var. *gattii* (serotypes B and C). Glucuronoxylomannan is responsible for the serotype specificity of *C. neoformans* (110,111). Immunological and chemical results indicate that there is heterogeneity within all four serotypes (112–114). Mannoprotein modulates delayed-type hypersensitivity, whereas GalXM elicits little immune response (115). The cell wall of nonencapsulated *Cryptococcus* contains 86% glucose, 7.3% *N*-acetylglucosamine, and no mannose (115).

B. Pathogenicity

Melanization has been linked to virulence in *C. neoformans* (116,117). Synthesis of melanin is partly accomplished by phenol oxidase enzymes. The activity of phenol oxidase produced in cultures at 37°C (a growth temperature used to differentiate *C. neoformans* from other nonpathogenic *Cryptococcus* species) was lower than that of its counterpart produced at 25°C. The enzymes produced at these two temperatures differed in both their electrophoretic mobilities and in their carbohydrate composition. Thus a given strain of *C. neoformans* produced different species of phenol oxidase under different culture conditions (118). While the activity of phenol oxidase was depressed at 37°C, it was compensated by a reciprocal increase in superoxide dismutase (119).

Virulence, a factor that varied widely among strains of *C. neoformans*, has also been linked to the size of the polysaccharide capsule (120). Capsular size is influenced by the strains, the medium used, and the age of the culture. It has been shown that cryptococcal polysaccharide synthesis is increased by limitation of ferric iron availability and by dissolved CO_2 (121,122).

C. Adhesion Properties

Lung is the primary site of infection by *Cryptococcus*; therefore factors that influence adherence and internalization of *Cryptococcus* by lung epithelial cells are important. The process was optimal at a growth temperature of 37°C, using stationary-phase cells and a medium supplemented with 1% glucose (123). Treating the yeast cells with trypsin reduced adherence, while sugars—principally *N*-acetylglucosamine, sucrose, and lactose—had a similar effect (124). *N*-Acetylglucosamine has a similar ability to disrupt adherence of *Candida albicans* to endothelial cells (125).

D. Immunochemistry and Immunology

Glucuronoxylomannan has been shown to be the capsular component responsible for inhibiting phagocytosis of *C. neoformans* (126). There is general agreement that GXM is the *Cryptococcus* antigen responsible for the induction of immunological unresponsiveness in cryptococcocis (127,128). Acapsular strains of *C. neoformans* are far more sensitive to the cell-mediated immune system of the host (129,130). Lymphocytes that responded to an acapsular strain had the response suppressed by the addition of pure polysaccharide (131). Both the GalXM and MP are produced by acapsular mutants of *C. neoformans*. The cell wall MP of many nonpathogenic yeasts is surface-exposed. In contrast, current evidence indicates that *Cryptococcus* MP is a nonstructural element of the cell wall and is located on its inner side (132).

In humans the development of anticapsular antibodies is correlated with improved prognosis (133). Specific anticapsular antibodies enhance natural killer cell inhibition of *C. neoformans* growth (134). Binding of antibody to the capsule of *C. neoformans* may prevent adhesion of the fungus to glycosphingolipid receptors on endothelial cells, thereby decreasing infectivity (135).

Three murine IgM monoclonal antibodies (mAbs), each recognizing different epitopes within the capsular polysaccharide, varied in their ability to prolong survival. This raises the possibility that epitope specificity is an important determinant of protective efficacy. There is some indication that acetyl groups are either part of the epitope recognized or necessary for the structural integrity of the epitope (136).

E. Complement

Occlusion of antigenic sites at the cryptococcal cell wall is a newly recognized biological property of its capsule (137). It has been reported that normal human serum contains antibodies that react with the cell wall of nonencapsulated yeast cells, while encapsulated *Cryptococcus* does so to a lesser extent (138). Normal human serum opsonization of non-encapsulated *Cryptococcus* for phagocytosis by macrophages is due solely to the activity of the complement system (139). It has been claimed that activation of complement by encapsulated *Cryptococcus* proceeds via the ACP only (140).

IV. *Blastomyces dermatitidis*

A. Structural Composition

The conidia of the thermally dimorphic fungus *Blastomyces dermatitidis* are converted to the invasive yeast forms at body temperature. An α-1,3 glucan is the major glycan of the yeast form wall with β-1,3 glucan a minor component. Chitin comprises about 37% of the yeast wall. In the mycelial form of *B. dermatitidis*, the α-1,3 glucan and chitin contents are reduced with a corresponding increase in β-1,3 glucan. Galactomannan (GM) is also increased in mycelial cell walls (15).

There is extensive sharing of cell wall determinants in *B. dermatitidis* and other dimorphic fungi. This is exemplified by the crude alkali and water-soluble antigen (B-ASWS) of *B. dermatitidis* yeast cells, the antigen initially developed by Cox and Larsh (141) for cellular studies of this organism. Acquired resistance to *B. dermatitidis* involves a T-cell response. Recently, a surface protein (WI-1) has been purified from the yeast phase, possessing epitopes that showed minimal cross-reactivity with antibodies from patients with histoplasmosis, coccidioidomycosis, and sporotrichosis. The molecule has an apparent molecular mass of 120 kDa and is nonglycosylated (142,143). Peripheral blood lymphocytes from blastomycosis patients proliferated in response to this protein at levels comparable with B-ASWS. It appears to share important T-cell epitopes with B-ASWS.

B. Cell-Mediated Immunity

Mutants of reduced virulence of *B. dermatitidis* that expressed more WI-1 antigen on their surfaces than the wild-type strain greatly facilitated their recognition and binding by human macrophages and may contribute to more rapid ingestion and killing by the host (144). Reduced virulence has also been associated with low levels of surface α-1,3-glucan (145).

Thermally dimorphic fungal pathogens are resistant to significant killing by human PMNs and may confer primary pathogenicity on these organisms (146). A suggestion that high levels of catalase may enhance the resistance of some strains of *B. dermatitidis* to in vitro killing by PMNs has been proposed (147).

The size of *B. dermatitidis* relative to that of PMN makes internalization almost impossible and makes conditions suboptimal for deposition of myloperoxidase (MPO), leading to the inefficient generation of MPO system products. In contrast, *C. albicans* is readily phagocytosed and is very efficient in generating MPO products. This may be partly accounted for by the affinity of MPO for mannan-rich outer cell wall components, which are rare in the α-1,3-glucan rich outer wall of *B. dermatitidis* (148). It has been reported that PMNs were not fungistatic for nonphagocytosable *B. dermatitidis* but had the opposite effect of enhancing its replication in vitro (149). This contrasts markedly with *H. capsulatum* where fungistatic activity of human neutrophils against this organism correlates with phagocytosis (150).

V. *Coccidioides immitis*

A. Morphogenesis and Cell Wall–Associated Proteinases

Infection by *C. immitis* occurs as a result of inhalation of arthroconidia, which are converted to the parasitic phase in the lungs of the infected host. These spherules undergo segementation into endospores, which are released and disseminate within the host. The changes in cellular form which occur during *C. immitis* morphogenesis are largely dictated by changes in the structure and composition of the cell wall (151).

Much research has been concerned with the proteolytic activity associated with the wall of *C. immitis*. A chymotrypsinlike serine proteinase of apparent molecular mass 34 kDa has been described. It has been found in spherule envelope, segmentation wall, and endospore wall. The apparent high affinity of this 34-kDa glycoprotein for walls of actively growing cells of *C. immitis* led the authors to suggest that the enzyme may participate in cell-wall plasticization and/or in cell-wall turnover (152). An inhibitor of this enzyme that coexists in the spherule wall may have regulatory properties (151).

A trypsinlike serine proteinase has been found in the saprophytic phase. The nonreduced form of this glycoprotein enzyme (38 kDa) demonstrated tube precipitin (TP) antibody reactivity in the immunodiffusion test (ID-

TP). Primary infection by *C. immitis* is accompanied by the production of TP antibody (153). The TP antigen can be released from intact spherules with chitinase (154). It has been found to be localized predominantly in the inner cell wall layer of saprobic- and parasitic-phase cells. Tube precipitin antigen is a high-molecular-mass, heat-stable polysaccharide or polysaccharide-protein complex (155). It gives a reaction of partial identity when tested against sera of patients with histoplasmosis (156).

B. Cell-Mediated Immunity

An alkali-soluble, water soluble fraction of mycelial and spherule cell wall was found to be reactive in eliciting cell-mediated immune responses. Much of this activity appeared to be associated with a polymeric mannoprotein antigen (Ag2). Subcutaneous vaccination of mice with this alkali-soluble, water-soluble fraction induced protective immunity, much of it again thought to be due to Ag2. Spherule was found to be significantly more protective than mycelium (157). In contrast, high doses of antigen can suppress the immune response; results implicate Ag2 and/or TP antigen as immunosuppressive agent(s) (158).

Recently a murine mAb has been developed which recognizes a peptide epitope that is specific to Ag2 and is also present on an Ag2-derived, 33-kDa peptide from spherule wall (159,160). Soluble conidial-wall fraction from arthroconidia of *C. immitis* has been shown to elicit a vigorous, antigen-specific proliferative response from immune mouse lymph node T cells. This reaction was associated with components of molecular mass of 43–66 kDa (161).

Thus it appears that wall fractions of *C. immitis* are reservoirs of biologically active components that have important functions in fungal morphogenesis as well as playing significant roles in fungal-host interactions.

VI. *Histoplasma capsulatum*

A. Structural Composition

The major components of the *H. capsulatum* cell wall are α-1,3 glucan, β-1,3 glucan, and chitin. In comparison with other dimorphic fungal pathogens, *H. capsulatum* yeast types have a high chitin content in their walls. The β-1,3 glucan may be enmeshed in chitin fibrils (162). Galactomannan, though a minor wall component, is the only known antigenic polysaccharide in *H. capsulatum* (163). It is considered, from immunoelectronmicroscopy studies, to form an amorphous outer wall layer. The mannan backbone consists of α-1,6–linked mannopyranosyl units with α-1,2-linked oligomannosyl side chains and galactofuranosyl residues as nonreducing termini (164). It may thus be considered a GM-I-type heteropolysaccharide that cross-reacts with the GMs of *B. dermatitidis* and *P. brasiliensis*. The preparation and partial characterization of a 62-kDa glycoprotein antigen (heat shock protein 60) from *H. capsulatum* wall and membrane, which protects mice against pulmonary histoplasmosis, has been described (165,166).

B. Cell-Mediated Immunity

The occurrence of four surface factors and five yeast form serotypes has been recognized in *H. capsulatum* (167). Chemotype 2 isolates of *H. capsulatum* contain high amounts of α-1,3-glucan, which is completely absent in other isolates. This lack of α-1,3 glucan from the cell wall occurs in avirulent variants of *H. capsulatum* (168). However, it may not be entirely absent (144). Recently it was found that when hamster trachea epithelial cells were incubated with α-1,3 glucan-positive strains, they appeared to switch, within 24 hr, to cells lacking glucan in their cell walls and incapable of killing macrophages. The authors suggested that these cells in natural histoplasmosis could constitute a reservoir of organisms capable of causing chronic or latent infections found in this disease (169). It is the yeast form of *H. capsulatum* that is responsible for the various disease states. T lymphocytes play a critical role in limiting the replication of *H. capsulatum* yeast cells in macrophages (170). A detergent-soluble extract of cell wall and membranes of *H. capsulatum* yeast cells yielded fractions of apparent molecular mass of 53–64 and 69–82 kDa capable of causing proliferation by a murine T-cell line (171).

VII. *Paracoccidioides brasiliensis*

A. Morphogenesis and Structural Composition

The main constituents of the cell wall of both the yeast and mycelial phases of *P. brasiliensis* are polysaccharides, comprising hexoses and amino sugars, proteins and lipids. The cell wall α- and β-1,3-glucans of *P. brasiliensis* play a role in morphology and dimorphism, since the former is found only in the yeast (Y) form while the latter is found mainly in the mycelial (M) phase (172). It has been suggested that when the Y phase is growing at 37°C, β-glucan synthetase activity must be depressed to a minimum. Under these conditions α-glucan begins to be synthesized, securing the round shape of the yeast cell. The strategic arrangement of α-glucan, which is located more externally on the cell wall, protects β-glucan from metabolism by the host (175). More chitin is found in the Y than in the M form, while the GM is relatively evenly distributed between the two phases (174). A 43,000-Da glycoprotein (gp43) has been shown to be the major antigenic component of *P. brasiliensis*, recognized by 100% of patients' sera (175).

B. Pathogenicity

The *P. brasiliensis* organism binds to laminin, and the main receptor at the surface of yeast cells that react with this structural glycoprotein is gp43. Coating of yeast-phase cells with laminin enhanced fungal virulence, causing a more rapid onset and a more severe form of granulomatous disease (176).

Both α- and β-glucans have also been strongly implicated in the virulence of *P. brasiliensis*. Differences in virulent strains are considered to be due partly to the quantitative modification of the amount of glucan in the yeast cell wall (9,177). Both Y and M forms of *P. brasiliensis* express acidic glycoconjugates containing *N*-acetyl-neuraminic acid units synthesized de novo. The presence of sialic acids on the surface of *P. brasiliensis* yeast cells may protect the fungus against phagocytosis by macrophages (178).

C. Cell-Mediated Immunity

The gp43 component, mentioned above, is also the main component eliciting delayed hypersensitivity reactions in humans and sensitized guinea pigs. A crude antigenic preparation of *P. brasiliensis*, when specifically depleted of gp43 epitopes, no longer gives positive delayed hypersensitivity reactions (179).

It has been reported that cell-wall β-glucan can induce leucocyte migration and a granulomatous inflammatory reaction (180). *Paracoccidioides brasiliensis* β-glucan induces peritoneal macrophages to secrete tumour necrotic factor (TNF) in vitro. Differences in TNF levels in serum could be correlated with the β-glucan concentration in the cell wall of both virulent and avirulent strains of *P. brasiliensis*. Levels of TNF in mice challenged with an avirulent strain were significantly higher than those of mice challenged with a virulent strain (181). Tumor necrosis factor is necessary for the production of interferon-gamma, which can activate macrophages to secrete TNF and thus inhibit replication of *P. brasiliensis*.

Cell-wall components of *P. brasiliensis*, such as lipid and an alkali-insoluble fraction containing chitin and β-glucan (FI), were capable of effecting an inflammatory response in experimental animals; FI induced the accumulation of PMN during the early phase of this inflammatory response (182). It was dependent on the complement system, with the

ACP preferentially involved (183). Other studies also suggest the involvement of the classic complement pathway of activation (184).

VIII. *Sporothrix schenckii*

A. Structural Composition and Pathogenicity

Sporothrix schenckii is a dimorphic fungus giving, at room temperature, hyphal and conidial forms that convert to yeastlike cells at 37°C (185). Calcium has a stimulating effect on the germination of *S. schenckii* conidia, and it may well play a role in controlling the yeast-to-mycelium transition (186). An association between melanization and virulence has been noted for *S. schenckii*. Virulent isolates grew at 37°C and produced melanin (187). The glucans of *S. schenckii* cell walls are β-linked and are found, together with chitin, in similar amounts in yeast and mycelial forms. Thus there is no evidence that glucans influence the cell shape of *S. schenckii*. Levels of protein and lipid in the mycelial cell wall are higher than those reported for other mycotic organisms (15,188). The presence of sialic acids as surface components of *S. schenckii* has been suggested (189).

B. Immunochemistry and Immunology

Peptidorhamnomannan complexes occur as the readily soluble surface coat of *S. schenckii*. They contain *N*-linked high-molecular-weight polysaccharides and O-linked di, tri, tetra, and pentasaccharides. The amounts of O-glycosidically linked chains found in the yeast phase are higher than those found in the mycelial phase cells. Antigenicity in all cases is associated with terminal α-L-rhamnopyranosyl units. Acidic oligosaccharides containing rhamnose, α-glucuronic acid, and mannose residues constitute novel structures for *S. schenckii* (190). It has been suggested that peptidorhamnomannans or synthetic antigens bearing these epitopes should be used for the detection of specific antibodies to *S. schenckii* (191). The peptido portion of the rhamnomannan is important structurally, and it is also important as the presumed source of determinants capable of evoking cell-mediated immunity.

Common antigens have been demonstrated on the cell wall of both morphological phases of *S. schenckii* (192). *Sporothrix schenckii* cross-reacts with *Aspergillus fumigatus* and other fungi due to the shared presence of β-D-galactofuranosyl units (193). The surface antigens of *S. schenckii* bind heavily to concanavalin A (con A); the con A–binding layer on hyphae proved to be much thinner than that found in yeast cells (194). The surface antigens can activate complement through the ACP. Isolated rhamnomannans showed a stronger anticomplementary activity than did the corresponding peptidopolysaccharides (195).

IX. *Aspergillus*

A. Structural Composition

Aspergillus mycelial cell wall contains predominantly glucan, chitin, and GM (196). An alkali-soluble extract was obtained that displayed an x-ray diffraction pattern similar to (1–3)-α-glucan; this type of glucan has been found in several fungal species (197). *Aspergillus niger* contains nigeran, a glucan with alternating α-1,3 and α-1,4 linkages that is also found in *Aspergillus awamori* but not in *A. fumigatus* (198,199). The alkali-insoluble β-1,3-glucan of *A. niger* was found to be chitin-associated (200). Recently it has been shown that for *A. fumigatus*, the glucan appears to be linked to chitin in linkages involving both glucosamine and *N*-acetylglucosamine residues (201). In this it differs from *Aspergillus nidulans*, where deacetylated amino sugars do not play a significant role (202).

B. Immunochemistry and Immunology

Mycelial GM of *A. fumigatus* contains a core of 1,6-linked α-D-mannopyranosyl (man*p*) units with 1,5-interlinked β-D-galactofuranosyl (gal*f*) units as side chains joined by 1,6 linkages to the backbone (203). Analysis of alkali-extracted GMs from several species of *Aspergillus* showed similar structures, with only small quantitative differences (203). The gal*f* residues most likely account for cross-reactivity with the GM-II of dermatophytes (204). There is some evidence that a number of the oligogalactosyl side chains may contain α-D-gal*p*-linked units (205). The similar structure of oligomannoside side chains of *A. fumigatus* GM and *Candida* mannan offers a plausible explanation for the observed immunological cross-reactivity of the two species (204,205). The nature of *Aspergillus* GM has recently been reviewed (206). Immunoelectron microscopy work using *A. fumigatus* in thin section has shown that many of the highly reactive cellular antigens appear surface located in both conidia and mycelium (207,208). Antigens on *A. fumigatus* conidial and hyphal surfaces reacted identically with IgG and IgE antibodies from patients with allergie bronchopulmonary aspergillosis (ABPA) (209). It has been suggested that the degree of conservation of antigenic proteins is higher in the wall and membrane fractions of different growth phases and strains that it is in the cytosol (210).

Water extraction of *A. fumigatus* mycelium yielded a glycoprotein with immunological activity (211). Alkali extraction of *A. fumigatus* has yielded a glucan or glucan complex coisolated with a galactomannoprotein. This extract showed major components of apparent molecular mass between 60 and 68 kDa, which reacted with sera of patients with aspergillosis (201). Galactomannan exists on the surface of *A. fumigatus* cell wall, and it is found in a wide range of intra- and extracellular glycoproteins of *A. fumigatus* (212).

C. Cell-Mediated Immunity

Aspergillus fumigatus and *A. flavus* possess a far greater ability to germinate in the presence of alveolar macrophages than does *A. niger* (213,214). Resting conidia cannot be killed by PMNLs, which can kill swollen conidia. The former are relatively poor stimulators of the PMN leukocyte respiratory burst and degranulation. It has been postulated that this reactivity might result from greater expression or exposure of certain surface antigens (215). Suboptimal stimulation of degranulation and phagocytosis could contribute to the inability of neutrophils to kill resting conidia. It was proposed the PMN-released lactoferrin (the secondary granule marker) may contribute to antifungal activity at the conidial surface by competing for iron, which is an essential growth factor (216). The PMNs can be stimulated with lectinlike receptors such as those for β-glucans (217). However, it is unknown whether β-glucans or mannans on the cell wall are exposed on the surface of swollen conidia and whether they are capable of interacting with receptors on the PMN.

D. Adhesion Properties

Serum components such as fibrinogen can foster adherence of *Aspergillus* conidia to phagocytic cells. Fibrinogen receptors appear to be located exclusively on conidia and on mother cells of germ tubes (218). Cell receptors for fragment D of fibrinogen had apparent molecular masses of 54,58, and 140 to 150 kDa on SDS-PAGE and were proteinaceous in nature (219). *Aspergillus fumigatus* can bind to and degrade membrane components such as laminin. The authors suggested that *A. fumigatus* possesses mechanisms to bind and degrade some host proteins, allowing adherence of conidia to epithelium and subsequent invasion of surrounding tissue by hyphae (220). Production of a mutant strain of *A. fumigatus* reduced binding to host proteins by only 10%, indicating the minor involvement of this layer in cellular adhesion (221).

E. Complement

Aspergillus fumigatus is a potent activator of the complement system (222). Complement activation by resting conidia is mediated by the ACP while dependence on the classic pathway increased as the fungus matured into swollen conidia and then hyphae (223). The lack of participation of the classic pathway in complement activation by resting conidia may have important implications regarding their ability to effectively stimulate phagocytes.

Human complement component C3 and/or a C3 fragment(s) are bound by glycoproteins of apparent molecular mass of 54 and 58 kDa present on *A. fumigatus* conidial cell surface. Deposited C3 is rapidly degraded to lower-molecular-mass fragments. Evidence indicates that these fragments are produced as a result of proteolytic activity present in the outer conidial wall (224). The apparent conversion of most bound C3b to iC3b has been demonstrated with many *Aspergillus* species. However, *A. niger* and *A. nidulans* appear to promote further breakdown of opsonic C3 fragments to C3dg. Neither *A. fumigatus* nor *A. flavus* promotes iC3b breakdown to C3dg; therefore evasion of phagocytosis by conversion of bound C3 to nonopsonic fragments does not appear to be a pathogenic mechanism for these two species. However, highly pathogenic *A. fumigatus* and *A. flavus* bound fewer C3 molecules per unit of conidial surface area than did the less pathogenic species. It is possible that diminished C3 binding by these species may be related to pathogenicity (225). A role for complement in the phagocytosis of *A. fumigatus* by human PMN cells has been proposed (226). Optimal cell-cell interaction appears to be dependent on an active ACP (227).

X. *Dermatophytes*

A. Morphogenesis and Pathogenicity

In infected tissue, dermatophytes produce exclusively arthroconidia or parasitic conidia. Arthroconidiogenesis proceeds readily for *Trichophyton rubrum* and *Trichophyton mentagrophytes* grown at 37°C but not at 25°C (228,229). Relatively high temperatures are needed for induction—rather than the progression—of arthroconidiation in the dermatophytes, which is also supported by certain amino acids (230). Two-thirds of the isolated arthroconidial wall is chitinous in nature, which may help to explain these organisms' resistance to antifungal agents (231). It has been found that mycelial cell walls of dermatophytes have a high chitin content of approximately 30% (232). Germination of *T. mentagrophytes* is triggered by several amino acids and peptides, most effectively by L-leucine (233). The degree of pathogenicity of dermatophytes has been directly related to the production of proteinases, especially keratinase (234). Intracellular proteinase activity of *Microsporum canis* was found to be membrane-bound (235).

B. Antigenic Composition

Antisera to soluble extracts of *T. rubrum* localized antigens in the mycelial cell wall (235). Analysis by Bishop, Blank, Perry, and others of GM structures from five dermatophyte species established the basic composition of these heteropolysaccharides. Galactomannan antigens of the dermatophytes occur in two forms, based on the method of extraction from whole mycelium. Glycopeptides with trichophytin activity were solubilized in warm ethylene glycol (236). Hot alkali was used to solubilize polysaccharides of limited serological activity (237). The GM-I is only lightly glycosylated. There is evidence for linear sequences of 1,6-linked mannose residues with mannose or galactofuranose as single substituents (233). The GM-II is more heavily glycosylated and is more structurally complex than GM-I. It has a backbone of alternating 1,2- and 1,6-linked mannose residues with relatively more 1,2 linked mannose present than in GM-I. Galactofuranose residues exist as nonreducing termini and contribute greatly to the antigenic activity of these molecules. They are also responsible for the cross-reactivity with GM-II components of other species including *Aspergillus*, *Penicillium*, and *Cladosporium* (238). Antigenic glycopeptides of the dermatophytes are likely to contain GM-I and GM-II.

XI. CONCLUSIONS

The fungal cell wall possesses certain properties that help the organism to survive, frequently with detrimental effects on the human host. These factors include its adaptability to its surroundings and the interplay between the cell surface and the medium, hence the emphasis placed here on environmental conditions. Cell-wall biosynthesis, where the growing apical structure is plastic but the subapical wall must be rigid to withstand internal turgor pressure is relevant here (239). Also important is the dynamic state of the fungus associated with morphogenesis and the presence or absence of certain surface structures. Some of these have been shown to affect adhesive properties or to modulate the host response. Progress has been made in determining the relationship between structure and function of some of the many identified components of the fungal cell wall. However, the observation made by Wessels and Sietsma (197) is still valid. A complete understanding of function will require knowledge of exact positions, physical states, and interactions between various components identified after isolation from the wall.

ACKNOWLEDGMENTS

I am grateful to Pascale Bordon and Marie-Claude Facchinetti for their patience and expertise in typing this manuscript, and I acknowledge the valuable advice of Professor L. R. Travassos, Escola Paulista de Medicina, São Paulo, Brazil, in the preparation of this manuscript.

REFERENCES

1. Hector RF. Compounds active against cell walls of medically important fungi. Clin Microbiol Rev 1993;6:1–21.
2. Nickerson JW. Symposium on the biochemical bases of morphogenesis in fungi: IV. Molecular bases of form in yeasts. Bacteriol Rev 1963;27: 305–324.
3. Cabib E, Roberts R, Bowers B. Synthesis of the yeast cell wall and its regulation. Annu Rev Biochem 1982;52:763–793.
4. Sietsma JH, Wessels JGH. Cell wall assembly in fungal morphogenesis. In: Latgé JP, Boucias D, eds. Fungal Cell Wall and Immune Response. Berlin: Springer-Verlag, 1991.
5. Peberdy JF. Fungal cell walls—A review. In: Kuhn PJ, Trinci APJ, Jung MJ, et al, eds. Biochemistry of Cell Walls and Membranes in Fungi. Berlin: Springer-Verlag, 1990:5–30.
6. Bull AT. Inhibition of polysaccharases by melanin: Enzyme inhibition in relation to mycolysis. Arch Biochem Biophys 1970;137:345–356.
7. Farbiarz SR, de Carvalho TU, Alviano C, De Souza W. Inhibitory effect of melanin on the interaction of Fonsecaea pedrosoi with mammalian cells in vitro. J Med Vet Mycol 1992;30:265–273.
8. Alviano CS, Farbiarz SR, De Souza W, et al. Characterization of Fonsecaea pedrosoi melanin. J. Gen Microbiol 1991;137:837–844.
9. San Blas G, San Blas F. Paracoccidioides brasiliensis: Cell wall structure and virulence. A review. Mycopathology 1977;62:77–86.
10. Klimpel KR, Goldman WE. Cell walls from avirulent variants of Histoplasma capsulatum lack α-(1,3)-glucan. Infect Immun 1988;56:2997–3000.
11. Bartnicki-Garcia S, Lippman E. The bursting tendency of hyphal tips of fungi: Presumptive evidence for a delicate balance between wall synthesis and wall lysis in apical growth. J Gen Microbiol 1972;73:487–500.
12. Kanbe T, Li RK, Wadsworth E, et al. Evidence for expression of the C3d receptor of Candida albicans in vitro and in vivo obtained by immunofluorescence and immuno-electron microscopy. Infect Immun 1991;59: 1832–1838.
13. Kennedy MJ, Sandin RL. Influence of growth conditions on Candida albicans adhesion, hydrophobicity and cell wall ultrastructure. J Med Vet Mycol 1988;26:79–92.
14. Torosantucci A, Boccanera M, Casalinuovo I, et al. Differences in the anti-

genic expression of immunomodulatory mannoprotein constituents on yeast and mycelial forms of Candida albicans. J Gen Microbiol 1990;136: 1421–1428.

15. Reiss E. Molecular Immunology of Mycotic and Actinomycotic Infections. New York: Elsevier/North-Holland, 1986.
16. Pereira Crott LS, Lucisano Valim YM, Silva CL, Barbosa JE. The role of the complement system in the neutrophil functions stimulated in vitro by alkali-insoluble cell wall fraction of Paracoccidioides brasiliensis. J Med Vet Mycol 1993;31:17–27.
17. Horstmann RD. Tanget recognition failure by the nonspecific defense system: surface constituents of pathogens interfere with the alternative pathway of complement activation. Infect Immun 1992;60:721–727.
18. Cole GT, Hoch HC, eds. The Fungal Spore and Disease Initiation in Plants and Animals. New York: Plenum Press, 1991.
19. Kuhn PJ, Trinici APJ, Jung MJ, et al, eds. Biochemistry of Cell Walls and Membranes in Fungi. Berlin: Springer-Verlag, 1990.
20. Kurstak E, ed. Immunology of Fungal Diseases. New York: Marcel Dekker, 1989.
21. Bishop CT, Blank F, Gardner PE. The cell wall polysaccharides of Candida albicans: glucan, mannan and chitin. Can J Chem 1960;38:869–881.
22. Chattaway FW, Holmes MR, Barlow AJE. Cell wall composition of the mycelial and blastospore forms of Candida albicans. J Gen Microbiol 1968; 51:367–376.
23. Ruiz-Herrera J, Mormeneo S, Vanaclocha P, et al. Structural organization of the components of the cell wall from Candida albicans. Microbiology 1994;140:1513–1523.
24. Sanjuan R, Zueco J, Stock R, et al. Identification of glucan-manno-protein complexes in the cell wall of Candida albicans using a monoclonal antibody that reacts with a (1,6)-β-glucan epitope. Microbiology 1995;141:1545–1551.
25. Chattaway FW, Shenolikar S, O'Reilly J. Changes in the cell surface of the dimorphic forms of Candida albicans by treatment with hydrolytic enzymes. J Gen Microbiol 1976;95:335–347.
26. Gale EF. Nature and development of phenotypic resistance to amphotericin B in Candida albicans. Adv Microbiol Physiol 1986;27:277–320.
27. Obayashi T, Yoshida M, Tamura H, et al. Determination of plasma (1-3)-β-D-glucan: A new diagnostic aid to deep mycosis. J Med Vet Mycol 1992; 30:275–280.
28. Chaffin WL, Stocco DM. Cell wall proteins of Candida albicans. Can J Microbiol 1983;29:1438–1444.
29. Ponton J, Jones JM. Analysis of cell wall extracts of Candida albicans by sodium dodecyl sulfate-polyacrylamide gel electrophoresis and Western blot techniques. Infect Immun 1986;53:565–572.
30. Elorza MV, Marcilla A, Sentandreu R. Wall mannoproteins of the yeast and mycelial cells of Candida albicans: Nature of the glycosidic bonds and polydispersity of their mannan moieties. J Gen Microbiol 1988;134: 2393–2403.

31. Casanova M, Chaffin WL. Phosphate-containing proteins and glycoproteins of the cell wall of Candida albicans. Infect Immun 1991;59:808–813.
32. Trinel PA, Borg-von-Zepelin M, Lepage G, et al. Isolation and preliminary characterization of the 14- to 18-kilodalton Candida albicans antigen as a phospholipomannan containing β-1,2-linked oligomannosides. Infect Immun 1993;61:4398–4405.
33. Kemp G, Solotorovsky M. Localization of antigens in mechanically disrupted cells of certain species of the genera Candida and Torulopsis. J Immunol 1964;93:305–314.
34. Han Y, Cutler J. Antibody response that protects against disseminated candidiasis. Infect Immun 1995;63:2714–2719.
35. Tsuchiya T, Fukazawa Y, Kawakita S. A method for the rapid identification of genus Candida. Mycopathologia 1959;10:191–206.
36. Shibata N, Arai M, Haga E, et al. Structural identification of an epitope of antigenic factor 5 in mannans of Candida albicans NIH B-792 (serotype B) and J-1012 (serotype A) as β-1,2-linked oligomannosyl residues. Infect Immun 1992;60:4100–4110.
37. Shibata N, Hisamichi K, Kobayashi H, Suzuki S. Complete assignment of ^{1}H and ^{13}C nuclear magnetic resonance chemical shifts of β-1,2-linked manno-oligosaccharides isolated from the phosphomannan of the pathogenic yeast Candida albicans NIH B-792 strain. Arch Biochem Biophys 1993;302:113–117.
38. Kobayashi H, Matsuda K, Ikeda T, et al. Structures of cell wall mannans of pathogenic Candida tropicalis IFO 0199 and IFO 1647 yeast strains. Infect Immun 1994;62:615–622.
39. Shibata N, Kojima C, Satoh Y, et al. Structural study of a cell-wall mannan of Saccharomyces kluyveri IFO 1685 strain: Presence of a branched side chain and β-1,2-linkage. Eur J Biochem 1993;217:1–12.
40. Marques G, Garzon S, Strykowski H, Auger P. Cell walls of normal and lysozyme-damaged blastoconidia of Candida albicans: Localization of surface factor 4 antigen and vicinal-glycol staining. Infect Immun 1991;59:1312–1318.
41. Podzorski RP, Gray GR, Nelson RD. Different effects of Candida albicans on antigen-stimulated lymphoproliferation in vitro. J Immunol 1990;144:707–716.
42. Hayette MP, Strecker G, Faille C, et al. Presence of human antibodies reacting with Candida albicans O-linked oligomannosides revealed by using an enzyme-linked immunosorbent assay and neoglycolipids. J Clin Microbiol 1992;30:411–417.
43. Treseler CB, Maziarz RT, Levitz SM. Biological activity of interleukin-2 bound to Candida albicans. Infect Immun 1992;60:183–188.
44. Smail EH, Jones JM. Demonstration and solubilization of antigens expressed primarily on the surfaces of Candida albicans germ tubes. Infect Immun 1984;45:74–81.
45. Poulain D, Hopwood V, Vernes A. Antigenic variability of Candida albicans. Crit Rev Microbiol 1985;12:223–270.

46. Brawner DL, Cutler JE. Ultrastructural and biochemical studies of two dynamically expressed cell surface determinants on Candida albicans. Infect Immun 1986;51:327–336.
47. Hernando FL, Estevez JJ, Cabrian M, et al. Identification of Candida albicans cell wall antigens lost during subculture in synthetic media. J Med Vet Mycol 1993;31:227–237.
48. Kobayashi H, Takahashi S-I, Shibata N, et al. Structural modification of cell wall mannans of Candida albicans serotype A strains grown in yeast extract—Sabouraud liquid medium under acidic conditions. Infect Immun 1994;62:968–973.
49. Barturen B, Bikandi J, San Millan R, et al. Variability in expression of antigens responsible for serotype specificity in Candida albicans. Microbiology 1995;141:1535–1543.
50. De Barnardis F, Molinari A, Boccanera M, et al. Modulation of cell-surface associated mannoprotein antigen expression in experimental candidal vaginitis. Infect Immun 1994;62:509–519.
51. Glee PM, Sundstrom P, Hazen KC. Expression of surface hydrophobic proteins by Candida albicans in vivo. Infect Immun 1995;63:1373–1379.
52. Brawner DL, Cutler JE, Beatty WL. Caveats in the investigation of form-specific molecules of Candida albicans. Infect Immun 1990;58:378–383.
53. Poulain D. Candidoses: Bases moléculaires de l'adaptation parasitaire de protistes pathogènes opportunistes. Ann Parasitol Hum Comp 1990;(65, Suppl I):125–130.
54. Torosantucci A, Gomez MJ, Bromuro C, et al. Biochemical and antigenic characterization of mannoprotein constituents released from yeast and mycelial forms of Candida albicans. J Med Vet Mycol 1991;29:361–372.
55. Mencacci A, Torosantucci A, Spaccapelo R, et al. A mannoprotein constituent of Candida albicans that elicits different levels of delayed-type hypersensitivity, cytokine production and anti-candidal protection in mice. Infect Immun 1994;62:5353–5360.
56. Blasi E, Pitzurra L, Puliti M, et al. Early differential molecular response of a macrophage cell line to yeast and hyphal forms of Candida albicans. Infect Immun 1992;60:832–837.
57. Casanova M, Lopez-Ribot JL, Monteagudo C, et al. Identification of a 58-kilodalton cell surface fibrinogen-binding mannoprotein from Candida albicans. Infect Immun 1992;60:4221–4229.
58. Edwards JE Jr, Mayer CL, Filler SG, et al. Cell extracts of Candida albicans block adherence of the organisms to endothelial cells. Infect Immun 1992; 60:3087–3091.
59. Ollert MW, Calderone RA. A monoclonal antibody that defines a surface antigen on Candida albicans hyphae cross-reacts with yeast cell protoplasts. Infect Immun 1990;58:625–631.
60. Lopez-Ribot JL, Casanova M, Martinez JP, Sentandreu R. Characterization of cell wall proteins of yeast and hydrophobic mycelial cells of *Candida albicans*. Infect Immun 1991;59:2324–2332.

61. Marot-Leblond A, Robert R, Aubry J, et al. Identification and immunochemical characterization of a germ-tube specific antigen of Candida albicans. Fed of Europ Microbiol Soc Microbiol Immunol 1993;7:175–186.
62. Ponton J, Marot-Leblond A, Ezkurra P, et al. Characterization of Candida albicans cell wall antigens with monoclonal antibodies. Infect Immun 1993; 61:4842–4847.
63. Torosantucci A, Bromuro C, Gomez MJ, et al. Identification of a 65-kDa mannoprotein as a main target of human cell-mediated immune response to Candida albicans. J Infect Dis 1993;168:427–435.
64. Calderone R, Diamond R, Senet J-M, et al. Host cell-fungal cell interactions. J Med Vet Mycol 1994;32(suppl 1):151–168.
65. Yu L, Lee KK, Ens K, et al. Partial characterization of a Candida albicans fibrial adhesin. Infect Immun 1994;62:2834–2842.
66. Tronchin G, Poulain D, Vernes A. Cytochemical and ultrastructural studies of Candida albicans: III. Evidence for modifications of the cell wall coat during adherence to human buccal epithelial cells. Arch Microbiol 1994; 139:221–224.
67. Vargas K, Wertz PW, Drake D, et al. Differences in adhesion of Candida albicans 3153A cells exhibiting switch phenotypes to buccal epithelium and stratum corneum. Infect Immun 1994;62:1328–1335.
68. Bailey A, Wadsworth E, Calderone R. Adherence of Candida albicans to human buccal epithelial cells: Host-induced protein synthesis and signalling events. Infect Immun 1995;63:569–572.
69. Polacheck I, Autman A, Barth I, et al. Adherence of Candida albicans to epithelial cells: Studies using fluorescently labelled yeasts and flow cytometry. Microbiology 1995;141:1523–1533.
70. Kimura LH, Pearsall NN. Relationship between germination of Candida albicans and increased adherence to human buccal epithelial cells. Infect Immun 1980;28:464–468.
71. Hazen BW, Hazen KC. Dynamic expression of cell surface hydrophobicity during initial yeast cell growth and before germ tube formation of Candida albicans. Infect Immun 1988;56:2521–2525.
72. Cutler JE, Brawner DL, Hazen KC, Julita MA. Characteristics of Candida albicans adherence to mouse tissues. Infect Immun 1990;58:1902–1908.
73. Kennedy MJ, Volz PA, Edwards CA, Yancey RJ. Mechanisms of association of Candida albicans with intestinal mucosa. J Med Microbiol 1987;24: 333–341.
74. Hazen KC, Hazen BW. Hydrophobic surface protein masking by the opportunistic fungal pathogen Candida albicans. Infect Immun 1992;60: 1499–1508.
75. Hazen KC, Brawner DL, Riesselman MH, et al: Differential adherence of hydrophobic and hydrophilic Candida albicans yeast cells to mouse tissues. Infect Immun 1991;59:907–912.
76. Calderone RA, Braun PC. Adherence and receptor relationships of Candida albicans. Microbiol Rev 1991;55:1–20.

77. Douglas LJ. Adhesion of Candida albicans to host surfaces. FEMS Symp 1991;50:43–48.
78. Tosh FD, Douglas LJ. Characterization of a fucose-binding adhesin of Candida albicans. Infect Immun 1992;60:4734–4739.
79. Lehrer N, Segal E, Lis H, Gov Y. Effect of Candida albicans cell wall components on the adhesion of the fungus to human and murine vaginal mucosa. Mycopathology 1988;102:115–121.
80. Brassart D, Woltz A, Golliard M, Neeser JR. In vitro inhibition of adhesion of Candida albicans clinical isolates to human buccal epithelial cells by Fuc $\alpha 1 \rightarrow 2$ Galβ- bearing complex carbohydrates. Infect Immun 1992;59:1605–1613.
81. Sawyer RT, Garner RE, Hudson JA. Effect of lectins on hepatic clearance and killing of Candida albicans by the isolated perfused mouse liver. Infect Immun 1992;60:1041–1046.
82. Miyakawa Y, Kuribayashi T, Kagaya K, et al. Role of specific determinants in mannan of Candida albicans serotype A in adherence to human buccal epithelial cells. Infect Immun 1992;60:2493–2499.
83. Klotz SA. Fungal adherence to the vascular compartment: A critical step in the pathogenesis of disseminated candidiasis. Clin Infect Dis 1992;14:340–347.
84. Klotz SA, Hein RC, Smith RL, Rouse JB. The fibronectin adhesin of Candida albicans. Infect Immun 1994;62:4679–4681.
85. Lopez-Ribot JL, Casanova M, Monteagudo C, et al. Evidence for the presence of a high-affinity laminin receptor-like molecule on the surface of Candida albicans yeast cells. Infect Immun 1994;62:742–746.
86. Martinez JP, Lopez-Ribot JL, La Jean Chaffin W. Heterogeneous surface distribution of the fibrinogen-binding protein on Candida albicans. Infect Immun 1994;62:709–712.
87. Santoni G, Gismondi A, Hong Liu J, et al. Candida albicans expresses a fibronectin receptor antigenically related to $\alpha 5\beta 1$ integrin. Microbiology 1994;140:2971–2979.
88. Fukayama M, Calderone RA. Adherence of cell surface mutants of Candida albicans to buccal epithelial cells and analyses of the cell surface proteins of the mutants. Infect Immun 1991;59:1341–1345.
89. Edgerton M, Scannapieco FA, Reddy MS, Levine MJ. Human submandibular-sublingual saliva promotes adhesion of Candida albicans to polymethylmethacrylate. Infect Immun 1993;61:2644–2652.
90. Hoffman MP, Haidaris CG. Analysis of Candida albicans adhesion to salivary mucin. Infect Immun 1993;61:1940–1949.
91. Palma C, Serbousek D, Torosantucci A, et al. Identification of mannoprotein fraction from Candida albicans that enhances human polymorphonuclear leukocyte (PMNL) functions and stimulates lactoferrin in PMNL inhibition of candidal growth. J Infect Dis 1992;166:1103–1112.
92. Scaringi L, Marconi P, Boccanera M, et al. Cell wall components of Candida albicans as immunomodulators: Induction of natural killer and macrophage-

mediated peritoneal cell cytotoxicity in mice by mannoprotein and glucan fractions. J Gen Microbiol 1988;134:1265–1274.
93. Vecchiarelli A, Puliti M, Torosantucci A, et al. In vitro production of tumor necrosis factor by murine splenic macrophages stimulated with mannoprotein constituents of Candida albicans cell wall. Cell Immunol 1991;134: 65–76.
94. Thierry J. Personal communication.
95. Blasi E, Pitzurra L, Bartoli A, et al. Tumor necrosis factor as an autocrine and paracrine signal controlling the macrophage secretory response to Candida albicans. Infect Immun 1994;62:1199–1206.
96. Blasi E, Pitzurra L, Chimienti AR, et al. Differential susceptibility of yeast and hyphal forms of Candida albicans to proteolytic activity of macrophages. Infect Immun 1995;63:1253–1257.
97. Morelli R, Rosenberg LT. Role of complement during experimental Candida infection in mice. Infect Immun 1971;3:521–523.
98. Czop JK, Austen KF. Properties of glycans that activate the human alternative complement pathway and interact with the human monocyte beta-glucan receptor. J Immunol 1985;135:3388–3393.
99. Fukayama M, Wadsworth E, Calderone R. Expression of the C3d-binding protein (CR2) from Candida albicans during experimental candidiasis as measured by lymphoblastogenesis. Infect Immun 1992;60:8–12.
100. Linehan L, Wadsworth E, Calderone RA. Candida albicans C3d receptor, isolated by using monoclonal antibody. Infect Immun 1988;56:1981–1986.
101. Heidenrich F, Dierich MP. Candida albicans and Candida stellatoidea, in contrast to other Candida species, bind iC3b and C3d but not C3b. Infect Immun 1985;50:598–600.
102. Tronchin G, Bouchara JP, Annaix V, et al. Fungal cell adhesion molecules in Candida albicans. Eur J Epidemiol 1991;7:23–33.
103. Franzke S, Calderone RA, Schaller K. Isolation of avirulent clones of Candida albicans with reduced ability to recognize the CR2 ligand C3d. Infect Immun 1993;61:2662–2669.
104. Eigentler A, Schulz TF, Larcher C, et al. C3bi-binding protein on Candida albicans: Temperature-dependent expression and relationship to human complement receptor type 3. Infect Immun 1989;57:616–622.
105. Alaei S, Larcher C, Ebenbichler C, et al. Isolation and biochemical characterization of the iC3b receptor of Candida albicans. Infect Immun 1993;61: 1395–1399.
106. Gustafson KS, Vercellotti GM, Lorenz JS, Hostetter MK. The iC3b receptor on Candida albicans mediates adhesion in a glucose-dependant reaction. Comp Inflam 1989;6:339–340.
107. James PG, Cherniak R. Galactoxylomannans of Cryptococcus neoformans. Infect Immun 1992;60:1084–1088.
108. Cherniak R, Sundstrom JB. Polysaccharide antigens of the capsule of Cryptococcus neoformans. Infect Immun 1994;62:1507–1512.
109. Turner SH, Cherniak R, Reiss E. Fractionation and characterization of

galactoxylomannan from Cryptococcus neoformans. Carbohydr Res 1984; 125:343–349.
110. Cherniak R, Morris LC, Meyer SA, Mitchell TB. Glucuronoxylomannan of Cryptococcus neoformans obtained from patients with AIDS. Carbohydr Res 1993;249:405–413.
111. Cherniak R, Reiss E, Slodki ME, et al. Structure and antigenic activity of the capsular polysaccharide from Cryptococcus neoformans serotype A. Mol Immunol 1980;17:1025–1032.
112. Spiropulu C, Eppard RA, Otteson E, Kozel TR. Antigenic variation within serotypes of Cryptococcus neoformans detected by monoclonal antibodies specific for the capsular polysaccharide. Infect Immun 1989;57:3240–3242.
113. Belay T, Cherniak R, Shinoda T. Specificity of Cryptococcus neoformans factor sera determined by enzyme-linked immunosorbent assay and dot enzyme assay. Infect Immun 1993;61:2879–2885.
114. Cherniak R, Morris LC, Belay T, et al. Variation in the structure of glucoronoxylomannan in isolates from patients with recurrent cryptococcal meningitis. Infect Immun 1995;63:1899–1905.
115. Murphy JW, Mosley RL, Cherniak R, et al. Serological, electrophoretic, and biological properties of Cryptococcus neoformans antigens. Infect Immun 1988;56:424–431.
116. James PG, Cherniak R, Jones RG, et al. Cell-wall glucans of Cryptococcus neoformans CAP 67. Carbohydr Res 1990;198:23–38.
117. Kwon-Chung KJ, Wickes BL, Stockman L, et al. Virulence, serotype and molecular characteristics of environmental strains of Cryptococcus neoformans var gattii. Infect Immun 1992;60:1869–1874.
118. Ikeda R, Jacobson ES. Heterogeneity of phenol oxidases in Cryptococcus neoformans. Infect Immun 1992;60:3552–3555.
119. Jacobson ES, Jenkins ND, Todd JM. Relationship between superoxide dismutase and melanin in a pathogenic fungus. Infect Immun 1994;62: 4085–4086.
120. Mitchell TG, Friedman L. In vitro phagocytosis and intracellular fate of variously encapsulated strains of Cryptococcus neorformans. Infect Immun 1972;5:491–498.
121. Vartivarian SE, Anaissie EJ, Cowart RE, et al. Regulation of cryptococcal capsular polysaccharide by iron. J Infect Dis 1993;167:186–190.
122. Vartivarian SE, Cowart RE, Anaissie EJ, et al. Iron acquisition by Cryptococcus neoformans. J Med Vet Mycol 1995;33:151–156.
123. Merkel GJ, Cunningham RK. The interaction of Cryptococcus neoformans with primary rat lung cell cultures. J Med Vet Mycol 1992;30:115–121.
124. Merkel GJ, Scofield BA. Conditions affecting the adherence of Cryptococcus neoformans to rat glial and lung cells in vitro. J Med Vet Mycol 1993; 31:55–64.
125. Segal E, Lehrer N, Ofek I. Adherence of Candida albicans to human vaginal epithelial cells: Inhibition by amino sugars. Exp Cell Biol 1982;50:13–17.
126. Bulmer GS, Sans MD. Cryptococcus neoformans: III. Inhibition of phagocytosis. J Bacteriol 1968;95:5–8.

127. Kozel TR. Suppression of host resistance by antigens of Cryptococcus neoformans. In: Latgé JP, Boucias D, eds. Fungal Cell Wall and Immune Response. Heidelberg, Germany: Springer-Verlag, 1991:399–413.
128. Sundstrom JB, Cherniak R. T-cell-dependent and T-cell-independent mechanisms of tolerance to glucoronoxylomannan of Cryptococcus neoformans: Serotype A. Infect Immun 1993;61:1340–1345.
129. Collins HL, Bancroft GJ. Encapsulation of Cryptococcus neoformans impairs antigen-specific T-cell responses. Infect Immun 1991;59:3883–3888.
130. Cross CE, Bancroft GJ. Ingestion of acapsular Cryptococcus neoformans occurs via mannose and β-glucan receptors, resulting in cytokine production and increased phagocytosis of the encapsulated form. Infect Immun 1995;63:2604–2611.
131. Mody CH, Syme RM. Effect of polysaccharide capsule and methods of preparation on human lymphocyte proliferation in response to Cryptococcus neoformans. Infect Immun 1993;61:464–469.
132. Vartivarian SE, Reyes GH, Jacobson ES, et al. Localization of mannoprotein in Cryptococcus neoformans. J Bacteriol 1989;171:6850–6852.
133. Bindschadler DD, Bennett JE. Serology of human cryptococcosis. Ann Intern Med 1968;69:45–52.
134. Nabavi N, Murphy JW. Antibody-dependent natural killer cell–mediated growth inhibition of Cryptococcus neoformans. Infect Immun 1986;51: 556–562.
135. Jimenez-Lucho V, Ginsburg V, Krivan HC. Cryptococcus neoformans, Candida albicans, and other fungi bind specifically to the glycosphingolipid lactosylceramide (Galβ1–4 Glcβ1-1Cer), a possible adhesion receptor for yeasts. Infect Immun 1990;58:2085–2090.
136. Mukherjie J, Scharff MD, Casadevall A. Protective murine monoclonal antibodies to Cryptococcus neoformans. Infect Immun 1992;60:4534–4541.
137. Wilson MA, Kozel TR. Contribution of antibody in normal human serum to early deposition of C3 onto encapsulated and nonencapsulated Cryptococcus neoformans. Infect Immun 1992;60:754–761.
138. Keller RG, Pfrommer GST, Kozel TR. Occurrences, specificities and functions of ubiquitious antibodies in human serum that are reactive with the Cryptococcus neoformans cell wall. Infect Immun 1994;62:215–220.
139. Levitz SM, Tabuni A. Binding of Cryptococcus neoformans by human cultured macrophages: Requirements for multiple complement receptors and actin. J Clin Invest 1991;87:528–535.
140. Kozel TR, Wilson MA, Pfrommer GST, Schlageter AM. Activation and binding of opsonic fragments of C3 on encapsulated Cryptoccocus neoformans by using an alternative complement pathway reconstituted from six isolated proteins. Infect Immun 1989;57:1922–1927.
141. Cox RA, Larsh HW. Isolation of skin test-active preparations from yeast-phase cells of Blastomyces dermatitidis. Infect Immun 1974;10:42–47.
142. Klein BS, Sondel PM, Jones JM. WI-1, a novel 120-kilodalton surface protein on Blastomyces dermatitidis yeast cells, is a target antigen of cell mediated immunity in human blastomycosis. Infect Immun 1992;60:4291–4300.

143. Klein BS, Jones JM. Purification and characterization of the major antigen WI-1 from Blastomyces dermatitidis yeasts and immunological comparison with 'A' antigen. Infect Immun 1994;62:3890–3900.
144. Klein BS, Chaturvedi S, Hogan LS, et al. Altered expression of surface protein WI-1 in genetically related strains of Blastomyces dermatitidis that differ in virulence regulates recognition of yeasts by human macrophages. Infect Immun 1994;62:3536–3542.
145. Hogan LH, Klein BS. Altered expression of surface α-1,3-glucan in genetically related strains of Blastomyces dermatitidis that differ in virulence. Infect Immun 1994;62:3543–3546.
146. Schaffner A, Davis CE, Schaffner T, et al. In vitro susceptibility of fungi to killing by neutrophil granulocytes discriminates between primary pathogenicity and opportunism. J Clin Invest 1986;78:511–524.
147. Morrison CJ, Stevens DA. Mechanisms of fungal pathogenicity: Correlation of virulence in vivo, susceptibility to killing by polymorphonuclear neutrophils in vitro, and neutrophil superoxide anion induction among Blastomyces dermatitidis isolates. Infect Immun 1991;59:2744–2749.
148. Brummer E, Kurita N, Yoshida S, et al. A basis for resistance of Blastomyces dermatitidis killing by human neutrophils: Inefficient generation of myeloperoxidase system products. J Med Vet Mycol 1992;30:233–243.
149. Brummer E, Stevens DA. Opposite effects of human monocytes, macrophages, and polymorphonuclear neutrophils on replication of Blastomyces dermatitidis in vitro. Infect Immun 1982;36:297–303.
150. Brummer E, Kurita N, Yoshida S, et al. Fungistatic activity of human neutrophils against Histoplasma capsulatum: Correlation with phagocytosis. J Infect Dis 1991;164:158–162.
151. Cole GT, Pan S, Zhu S, Seshan KR. Cell wall-associated proteinases of Coccidioides immitis. In: Latgé JP, Boucias D, eds. The Fungal Cell Wall and Immune Response. Heidelberg, Germany: Springer-Verlag, 1991: 269–284.
152. Cole GT, Zhu S, Hsu L, et al. Isolation and expression of a gene which encodes a wall-associated proteinase of Coccidioides immitis. Infect Immun 1992;60:416–427.
153. Pappagianis D, Lindsey NJ, Smith CE, Saito MT. Antibodies in human coccidioidomycosis: Immunoelectrophoretic properties. Proc Soc Exp Biol Med 1965;118:188–122.
154. Collins MS, Pappagianis D, Yu J. Enzymatic solubilization of precipitin and complement fixing antigen from endospores, spherules and spherule fractions of Coccidioides immitis. In: Ajello L, ed. Coccidioidomycosis: Current Clinical and Diagnostic Status. Symposia Specialists, Miami, 1977: 429–444.
155. Cox RA, Sun SH, Dolan MJ, Harrison JL. Localization of the tube precipitin and complement fixation antigens of Coccidioides immitis by immunoelectron microscopy with murine monoclonal antibodies. Infect Immun 1992;60:3315–3324.

156. Smith CE, Saito MT, Simons SA. Pattern of 39,500 serologic tests in coccidioidomycosis. JAMA 1956;160:546–552.
157. Levine HB, Kong Y-CM, Smith CE. Immunization of mice to Coccidioides immitis: Dose, regimen and spherulation stage of killed spherule vaccines. J Immunol 1965;94:132–142.
158. Cox RA. Immunosuppression of cell wall antigens of Coccidioides immitis. Rev Infect Dis 1988;10:S415–S418.
159. Dugger KO, Galgiani JN, Ampel NM, et al. An immunoreactive apoglycoprotein purified from Coccidioides immitis. Infect Immun 1991;59: 2245–2251.
160. Cox RA, Dolan MJ, Magee DM, Galgiani JN. Production of a murine monoclonal antibody that recognizes an epitope specific to Coccidioioides immitis antigen 2. Infect Immun 1993;61:1895–1899.
161. Kirkland TN, Zhu S, Kruse D, et al. Coccidioides immitis fractions which are antigenic for immune T lymphocytes. Infect Immun 1991;59:3952–3961.
162. San Blas G, Carbonell LM. Chemical and ultra-structural studies on the cell walls of the yeastlike and mycelial forms of Histoplasma farciminosum. J Bacteriol 1974;119:602–611.
163. Reiss E, Mitchell WO, Stone SH, Hasenclever HF. Cellular immune activity of a galactomannan-protein complex from mycelia of Histoplasma capsulatum. Infect Immun 1974;10:802–809.
164. Azuma I, Kanetsuma F, Tanaka Y, et al. Chemical and immunological properties of galactomannans obtained from Histoplasma duboisii, Histoplasma capsulatum, Paracoccidioides brasiliensis, and Blastomyces dermatitidis. Mycopathol Mycol Appl 1974;54:111–125.
165. Gomez AM, Rhodes JC, Deepe JrGS. Antigenicity and immunogenicity of an extract from the cell wall and cell membrane of Histoplasma capsulatum yeast cells. Infect Immun 1991;59:330–336.
166. Gomez AM, Allendoerfer R, Deepe JrGS. Vaccination with recombinant heat shock protein 60 from Histoplasma capsulatum protects mice against pulmonary histoplasmosis. Infect Immun 1995;63:2587–2595.
167. Kaufman L, Kaplan W. Preparation of a fluorescent antibody specific for the yeast phase of Histoplasma capsulatum. J Bacteriol 1961;82:729–735.
168. Klimpel KR, Goldman WE. Cell walls from avirulent variants of Histoplasma capsulatum lack α-(1,3)-glucan. Infect Immun 1988;56:2997–3000.
169. Groppe Eissenberg L, West JL, et al. Infection of P388D1 macrophages and respiratory epithelial cells by Histoplasma capsulatum: Selection of avirulent variants and their potential role in persistent histoplasmosis. Infect Immun 1991;59:1639–1646.
170. Wu-Hsieh B, Howard DH. Inhibition of growth of Histoplasma capsulatum by lymphokine-stimulated macrophages. J Immunol 1984;132:2593–2597.
171. Gomez FJ, Gomez AM, Deepe GS Jr. Protective efficacy of a 62-kilodalton antigen, H1S-62, from the cell wall and cell membrane of Histoplasma capsulatum yeast cells. Infect Immun 1991;59:4459–4464.
172. Kanetsuna F, Carbonell LM, Azuma I, Yamamura Y. Biochemical studies

on the thermal dimorphism of Paracoccidioides brasiliensis. J Bacteriol 1972;110:208–218.

173. San Blas F, San Blas G. Paracoccidioides brasiliensis. In: Szaniszlo PJ. ed. Fungal Dimorphism. New York: Plenum Press, 1985:93–120.

174. Kanetsuna F, Carbonell LM, Moreno RE, Rodriguez J. Cell wall composition of the yeast and mycelial forms of Paracoccidioides brasiliensis. J Bacteriol 1969;97:1036–1041.

175. Puccia R, Takaoka DT, Travassos LR. 43 kilodalton glycoprotein from Paracoccidioides brasiliensis: Immunochemical reactions with sera from patients with paracoccidioidomycosis, histoplasmosis or Jorge Lobo's disease. J Clin Microbiol 1991;29:1610–1615.

176. Vicentini AP, Gesztesi JL, Franco MF, et al. Binding of Paracoccidioides brasiliensis to laminin through surface glycoprotein gp43 leads to enhancement of fungal pathogenesis. Infect Immun 1994;62:1465–1469.

177. Silva CL, Alves LMC, Figueiredo F. Involvement of cell wall glucans in the genesis and persistence of the inflammatory reaction caused by the fungus Paracoccidioides brasiliensis. Microbiology 1994;140:1189–1194.

178. Soares RMA, Alviano CS, Angluster J, Travassos LR. Identification of sialic acids on the cell surface of hyphae and yeast forms of the human pathogen Paracoccidioides brasiliensis. FEMS Microbiol Lett 1993;108: 312–34.

179. Rodrigues EG, Travassos LR. Nature of the reactive epitopes in Paracoccidioides brasiliensis polysaccharide antigen. J Med Vet Mycol 1994;32: 77–81.

180. Silva CL, Fazioli RA. Paracoccidioides brasieliensis polysaccharide having granuloma-inducing toxic and macrophage-stimulating activity. J Gen Microbiol 1985;131:1497–1501.

181. Figueiredo F, Alves LMC, Silva CL. Tumour necrosis factor production in vivo and in vitro in response to Paracoccidioides brasiliensis and the cell wall fraction thereof. Clin Exp Immunol 1993;93:189–194.

182. Alves LMC, Figueiredo F, Brandao Filho SL, et al. The role of fractions from Paracoccidioides brasiliensis in the genesis of inflammatory response. Mycopathology 1987;97:3–7.

183. Calich VLG, Kipnis TL, Mariano M, et al. The activation of the complement system by P. brasiliensis in vitro: Its opsonic effect and possible significance for an in vivo model of infection. Clin Immunol Immunopathol 1979;12: 20–30.

184. Munk ME, Kajdacsy-Balla A, Del Negro G, et al. Activation of human complement system in paracoccicioidomycosis. J Med Vet Mycol 1992;30: 317–321.

185. Howard DH. Dimorphisin of Sporotrichum schenckii. J Bacteriol 1961;81: 464–469.

186. Rodriguez-Del Valle N, Rodriguez-Medina JR. Calcium stimulates molecular and cellular events during the yeast-to-mycelium transition in Sporothrix sckenckii. J Med Vet Mycol 1993;31:43–53.

187. Dixon DM, Duncan RA, Hurd NJ. Use of a mouse model to evaluate clinical and environmental isolates of Sporothrix spp. from the largest US epidemic of sporotrichosis. J Clin Microbiol 1992;30:951–954.
188. Previato JO, Gorin PAJ, Haskins RH, Travassos LR. Soluble and insoluble glucans from different cell types of the human pathogen Sporothrix schenckii. Exp Mycol 1979;3:92–105.
189. Alviano, CS, Pereira, MEA, Souza W, et al. Sialic acids are surface components of Sporothrix schenckii yeast forms. FEMS Microbiol Lett 1982;15: 223–227.
190. Lopes-Alves LM, Mendonça-Previato L, Fournet B, et al. O-glycosidically linked oligosacharides from peptidorhamnomannans of Sporothrix schenckii. Glycocon J 1992;9:75–81.
191. Lopez-Alves L, Travassos LR, Previato JO, Mendonça-Previato L. Novel antigenic determinants from peptidorhamnommans of Sporothrix sckenkii. Glycobiology 1994;4:281–288.
192. Castillo MC, Tapia FJ, Arciniegas E. Ultrastructural localization of specified surface antigens in the dimorphic fungus Sporothrix schenckii. J Med Vet Mycol 1990;28:91–94.
193. Travassos LR, Lloyd KO. Sporothrix schenkii and related species of Ceratocystis. Microbiol Rev 1980;44:683–721.
194. Travassos LR, Souza W, Mendonça-Previato L, Lloyd KO. Location and biochemical nature of surface components reacting with concanavalin A in different cell types of Sporothrix schenckii. Exp Mycol 1977;1:293–305.
195. Aisengart JF. Ativaçao de via alternativa do complemento com polissacarideos e peptido polis sacarideos purificados de fungos, em especial de Sporothrix schenckii. Thesis for M.Sc., 1988 Sao Paulo, Brazil.
196. Azuma I, Kimura H, Hirao F, et al. Biochemical and immunological studies on Aspergillus: II. Immunological properties of protein and polysaccharide fractions obtained from Aspergillus fumigatus. Mycopathol Mycol Appl 1969;37:289–303.
197. Wessels JGH, Seitsma JH. Fungal cell walls: A survey. In: Tanner W, Loewns FA, eds. Encyclopedia of Plant Physiology: Plant Carbohydrates Vol 13B. Heidelberg, Germany: Springer-Verlag, 1981:352–394.
198. Johnson IR. The composition of the cell wall of Aspergillus niger. Biochem J 1965;96:651–658.
199. Bobbitt TF, Nordin JH, Roux M, et al. Distribution and conformation of crystalline nigeran in hyphal walls of Aspergillus niger and Aspergillus awamori. J Bacteriol 1977;132:691–703.
200. Stagg CM, Feather MS. The characterization of a chitin-associated D-glucan from the cell walls of Aspergillus niger. Biochim Biophys Acta 1973; 320:64–72.
201. Hearn VM, Sietsma JH. Chemical and immunological analysis of Aspergillus fumigatus cell wall. Microbiology 1994;140:789–795.
202. Mol PC, Vermeulen CA, Wessels JGH. Glucan-aminoglycan linkages in fungal walls. Acta Botanica Neerlandica 1988;37:17–21.

203. Barreto-Bergter EM, Gorin PA, Travassos LR. Cell constituents of mycelia and conidia of Aspergillus fumigatus. Carbohydr Res 1981;95:205–218.
204. Suzuki S, Suzuki M, Yokota K, et al. On the immunochemical and biochemical studies of fungi. XI: Cross-reaction of the polysaccharides of Aspergillus fumigatus, Candida albicans, Saccharomyces cerevisiae and Trichophyton rubrum against Candida albicans and Saccharomyces cerevisiae antisera. Jpn J Microbiol 1967;11:269–273.
205. Ste-Marie L, Senechal S, Bouchira M, et al. Production and characterization of monoclonal antibodies to cell wall antigens of Aspergillus fumigatus. Infect Immun 1990;58:2105–2114.
206. Latge JP, Paris S, Sarfati J, et al. Exoantigens of Aspergillus fumigatus: Serodiagnosis and virulence. In: Powell KA, Peberdy J, Renwick A, eds, Aspergillus. Plenum Press, 1994:321–340.
207. Hearn VM, Latgé JP, Prevost MC. Immunolocalisation of Aspergillus fumigatus mycelial antigens. J Med Vet Mycol 1991;29:73–81.
208. Reijula KE, Jurup VP, Fink JN. Ultrastructural demonstration of specific IgG and IgE antibodies binding to Aspergillus fumigatus from patients with aspergillosis. J Allerg Clin Immunol 1991;87:683–688.
209. Kurup VP, Reijula KE, Fink JN. Ultrastructural localization of Aspergillus fumigatus antigens reacting with specific antibodies in aspergillosis. Abst Am Soc Microbiol 1990:F51.
210. Puente P, Ovejero MC, Fernandez N, Leal F. Analysis of Aspergillus nidulans conidial antigens and their prevalence in other Aspergillus species. Infect Immun 1991;59:4478–4485.
211. Azuma I, Kimura H, Yamamura Y. Purification and characterization of an immunologically active glycoprotein from Aspergillus fumigatus. J Bacteriol 1968;96:272–273.
212. Stynen D, Sarfati J, Goris A, et al. Rat monoclonal antibodies against Aspergillus glactomannan. Infect Immun 1992;60:2237–2245.
213. Schaffner A, Douglas H, Braude AI, Davis CE. Killing of Aspergillus spores depends on the anatomical source of the macrophage. Infect Immun 1983; 42:1109–1115.
214. Kurup VP. Interaction of Aspergillus fumigatus spores and pulmonary alveolar macrophages of rabbits. Immunobiol 1984;166:53–61.
215. Levitz SM, Diamond RD. Mechanisms of resistance of Aspergillus fumigatus conidia to killing by neutrophils in vitro. J Infect Dis 1985;152:33–42.
216. Levitz SM, Farrel TP. Human neutrophil degranulation stimulated by Aspergillus fumigatus. J Leukocyte Biol 1990;47:170–175.
217. Ross GD, Cain JA, Myones BL, et al. Specificity of membrane complement receptor type three (CR3) for β-glucans. Complement 1987;4:61–65.
218. Coulot P, Bouchara JP, Renier G, et al. Specific interaction of Aspergillus fumigatus with fibrinogen and its role in cell adhesion. Infect Immun 1994; 62:2169–2177.
219. Annaix V, Bouchara JP, Larcher G, et al. Specific binding of human fibrinogen fragment D to Aspergillus fumigatus conidia. Infect Immun 1992;60: 1747–1755.

220. Bouchara JP, Tronchin G, Larcher G, et al. Aspergillus fumigatus interactions with host proteins: Fixation and degradation. J Mycol Med 1992;2: 43–48.
221. Than N, Monod M, Crestani B, et al. Rodletless mutants of Aspergillus fumigatus. Infect Immun 1994;62:4380–4388.
222. Marx JJ, Flaherty DK. Activation of the complement sequence by extracts of bacteria and fungi associated with hypersensitivity pneumonitis. J Allergy Clin Immunol 1976;57:328–334.
223. Kozel TR, Wilson MA, Farrell TP, Levitz SM. Activation of C3 and binding to Aspergillus fumigatus conidia and hyphae. Infect Immun 1989;57: 3412–3417.
224. Sturtevant JE, Latgé JP. Interactions between condia of Aspergillus fumigatus and human complement component C3. Infect Immun 1992;60: 1913–1918.
225. Henwick S, Hetherington SV, Patrick CC. Complement binding to Aspergillus conidia correlates with pathogenicity. J Lab Clin Med 1993;122:27–35.
226. Waldorf AR, Diamond RD. Neutrophil chemotactic responses induced by fresh and swollen Rhizopus oryzae spores and Aspergillus fumigatus conidia. Infect Immun 1985;48:458–463.
227. Sturtevant JE; Latgé JP. Participation of complement in the phagocytosis of the conidia of Aspergillus fumigatus by human polymorphonuclear cells. J Infect Dis 1992;166:580–586.
228. Miyaji M, Nishimura K. Studies on arthrospore of Trichophyton rubrum (I). Jpn J Med Mycol 1971;12:18–23.
229. Emyanitoff RG, Hashimoto T. The effects of temperature, incubation atmosphere, and medium composition on arthrospore formation in the fungus Trichophyton mentagrophytes. Can J Microbiol 1979;25:362–366.
230. Emyanitoff RG. Cytology and physiology of arthrospore formation in the dermatophyte Trichophyton mentagrophytes. Ph. D. dissertation, Chicago, 1978.
231. Pollack JH, Lange CF, Hashimoto T. Non fibrillar chitin associated with walls and septa of Trichophyton mentagrophytes arthrospores. J Bacteriol 1983;154:965–975.
232. Noguchi T, Kitazima Y, Nozawa Y, Ito Y. Isolation, composition and structure of cell walls of Trichophyton mentagrophytes. Arch Biochem Biophys 1971;146:506–512.
233. Hashimoto T, Wu CDR, Blumenthal HJ. Characterization of L-leucine-induced germination of Trichophyton mentagrophytes microconidia. J Bacteriol 1972;112:967–978.
234. Grappel SF, Blank F. Role of keratinases in dermatophytosis: I. Immune response of guinea pigs infected with Trichophyton mentagrophytes and guinea pigs immunized with keratinases. Dermatol 1972;145:245–255.
235. Holden CA, Hay RJ, Mac Donald DM. The antigenicity of Trichophyton rubrum: In situ studies by an immunoperoxidase technique in light and electron microscopy. Acta Derm Venerol (Stock) 1981;61:207–211.
236. Barker SA, Cruickshank CND, Morris JH, Wood SR. The isolation of tri-

chophytin glycopepetide and its structure in relation to the immediate and delayed reactions. Immunology 1962;5:627–632.
237. Bishop CT, Perry MB, Blank F, Cooper FP. The water-soluble polysaccharides of dermatophytes: IV. Galactomannans I from Trichophyton granulosum, Trichophyton interdigitale, Microsporum quinckeanum, Trichophyton rubrum, and Trichophyton schonleinii. Can J Chem 1965;42:2862–2871.
238. Grappel SF, Blank F, Bishop CT. Immunological studies on dermatophytes: IV. Chemical structures and serological reactivities of polysaccharides from Microsporum praecox, Trichophyton ferrugineum, Trichophyton sabouraudii, and Trichophyton tonsurans. J Bacteriol 1969;97:23–26.
239. Gooday G. Cell envelope diversity and dynamics in yeasts and filamentous fungi. J Appl Bacteriol 1993;suppl 74:12S–20S.

4

Determinants of Polymorphism

HUGO VANDEN BOSSCHE
Janssen Research Foundation
Beerse, Belgium

I. INTRODUCTION

The term *dimorphic fungi* is used in medical mycology mainly to describe fungi having two morphological forms—namely, a yeast and mycelial form. This term is also used in a manner that implies that the saprophytic phase is hyphal, whereas the tissue phase is a yeast (1). Examples of fungi that have hyphal phases under saprophytic conditions and exhibit predominantly yeast development in vivo include *Blastomyces dermatitidis*, *Histoplasma capsulatum*, *Paracoccidioides brasiliensis*, *Penicillium marneffei*, and *Sporothrix schenckii* (2).

The dimorphic nature of a member of the genus *Mucor*, *M. racemosus*, was first described by Louis Pasteur in his *Etudes sur la Bière* (3), and the mold-yeast dimorphism of *Mucor rouxii* was studied in great detail by Bartnicki-Garcia (see, e.g., Ref. 4). *Mucor* species are usually not pathogens (5), but some have been isolated from patients with zygomycosis (2). One of them, *Mucor circinnelloides*, is dimorphic (2). The normal habit of Mucorales is mycelial; the dimorphic Mucorales grow yeastlike only as long as morphogenetic effectors are present. When these effectors are eliminated, the fungus goes back to the mycelial form (6). Therefore it is not surprising that, in contrast with the fungi listed above, it is the hyphal form of *Mucor* species that is found associated with diseased tissue (5).

Candida albicans, the most common pathogenic fungus, exists in four different morphological forms: yeasts (blastospores), pseudohyphae, hyphae, and chlamydospores; it occurs as yeasts and mycelia in both commensal and pathogenic states (7).

Coccidioides immitis is a diphasic microorganism, characterized by distinct saprophytic and parasitic cycles (8,9). Anthroconidia produced by mycelia during the saprophytic cycle are air-dispersed and, if inhaled, can establish a respiratory infection. In the lung, the conidia undergo an extended growth phase and convert to spherules, which become multinucleate, undergo segmentation and endosporulation. A myriad of uninucleate endospores is then released (9). *Wangiella dermatitidis* (10) may grow as a yeast, characterized by periods of polarized growth resulting in budding single cells and, less frequently, as pseudohyphae. The organism may exist as true hyphae, characterized by apical growth and production of blastoconidia. Third, *W. dermatitidis* may form enlarged, thick-walled cells characterized by isotropic growth and often the production of internal septa. Thus, these three species exist in more than two morphological forms; nevertheless, they are classified as dimorphic fungi.

Although the term *dimorphism* is too well established to be changed, usage of the term *polymorphism* is more appropriate (11) and is used in this overview on the molecular basis of morphogenesis from yeasts to hyphae and from hyphae or conidia to yeasts.

II. FACTORS REGULATING MORPHOGENESIS

Morphogenesis in polymorphic fungi includes the following events (6,12):

1. generation of an environmental signal
2. signal reception and transduction of the signal received into a biochemical message
3. alteration(s) in the genomic expression of the cell
4. reorganization of the elements responsible for polarization of cell growth

A. Signals

For most polymorphic fungi, changes in oxidation-reduction potential, CO_2 tension, temperature, and nutritional factors trigger a switch in morphology. In vitro and in vivo, *P. brasiliensis* grows at 37°C in a yeastlike form, whereas a mycelial phase is produced at temperatures below 25°C (13). *Penicillium marneffei* grows in culture at 25°C on Sabouraud agar as a myclelial fungus. When growing at 37°C in vitro on the appropriate media or in vivo, it converts to cylindrical and ovoid yeastlike cells that multiply by fission rather than budding (14). *Blastomyces dermatitidis* and *H. capsulatum* show morphological dimorphism that is also dependent on temperature, growing in a mycelial form at 25°C and a yeast form at 37°C. No amino acid, carbohydrate, or growth factors are essential for the mycelial-to-yeast-phase transition of *B. dermatitidis* (2). However, studies by Medoff et al. (15) showed that, next to the temperature shift to 37°C, cysteine or other sulfhydryl-containing compounds (e.g., β-mercaptoethanol) are required to complete the mycelial-to-yeast-phase transition. According to these and other investigators, a sulfhydryl component is also required by *H. capsulatum* (15). Some investigators suggest that the yeast form of *P. brasiliensis* also requires sulfhydryl-containing compounds (15,16), whereas earlier studies demonstrated that the dimorphic transition of this organism depends exclusively on the temperature of incubation (17).

The parasitic yeastlike *S. schenckii* cells develop from hyphae or conidia both in vivo and in vitro at 37°C. Yeast-phase formation depends on environmental conditions such as temperature, CO_2 tension, and the presence of hexoses in the media. In some media, a temperature shift is not even essential for phase transition. Studies by Resto and Rodríguez-Del Valle (18) present evidence that unbudded yeast cells of *S. schenckii* synchronously reproduce by budding when incubated under aeration at 25°C in a basal glucose medium (pH 7.2) with kinetics of growth faster than those obtained under the same culture conditions at 35°C.

In the pathogenic fungi described so far, the phenotypic switching is between two polarized forms of growth, leading to hyphal apical extension and to yeast budding. Some pathogenic fungi exhibit a different type of polymorphism, which replaces polarized yeast or hyphal development with a nonpolarized isotropic mode of growth, forming characteristic sclerotic bodies (10,19). In cases of chromoblastomycosis, the sclerotic bodies formed from invading spores or hyphal elements are thick-walled and darkly pigmented structures containing intersecting vertical and horizontal septa (19). The tissue phases of the agents of chromoblastomycosis but also those of coccidioidomycosis are most associated with this type of vegetative growth. In coccidioidomycosis, this isotropic mode of growth of *Coccidioides immitis* results in the formation of spherules (9). The etiologic agents of phaeohyphomycosis grow in the host tissue as dematiaceous yeasts, hyphae, pseudohyphae, and/or swollen entities. Next, *W. dermatitidis* has also the capability to form isotropically enlarged, thick-walled multicellular bodies (10). In vitro, multicellar forms can be produced in strains of *W. dermatitidis*, *Fonsecaea pedrosoi*, *Phiolophora verrucosa*, and *Cladosporium carrionii* by incubating cultures of these dematiaceous fungi under acidic conditions (10,19). For example, in the case of *W. dermatitidis*, the introduction of logarithmically growing yeasts into synthetic media (devoid of any other organic supplements other than thiamine and glucose), acidified to pH 2.5, induces within a few days their quantitative conversion to the multicellular phenotype (10). Next to the acidic pH a low, but critical concentration (0.1 mM) of calcium ions was crucial for multicellular body development (10). Szaniszlo et al. (10) also found that 1- to 5-mM additions of Ca^{2+} to the same synthetic medium were able to reverse the effects of the acidic medium conditions. The authors suggest that a Ca^{2+}/proton exchange mechanism might be involved in the phenotypic switching.

Cells of *C. albicans* accumulate as unbudded singlets at stationary phase at 25°C in the amino acid–containing medium formulated by Lee et al. (20). When released into fresh medium at 37°C and pH 6.5, these cells synchronously form elongate pseudomycelia; when released into fresh medium at either 25°C, pH 6.5, or 37°C, pH 4.5, they will synchronously form buds (21). Thus, the temperature and pH of the external environment are important parameters. By affecting the morphological form in *C. albicans*, pH may also affect the ability of the fungus to adhere to host cells. A pH optimum of 7.3 and an environmental temperature at 37°C have been reported to allow maximal cell adherence in vitro (22).

N-Acetyl-D-glucosamine (GlcNAc), the precursor of chitin, is another germ tube inducer. For example, in a tris-hydroxymethyl-aminomethan-HCl–buffered GlcNAc medium supplemented with $MgSO_4$ and NaCl (pH 7.5), all *C. albicans* strains used formed germ tubes, but no further elongation was seen, even after 24 hr of incubation (23). However, when cells were incubated in a medium containing GlcNAc, yeast nitrogen base and proline true hyphae were formed by all 30 *C. albicans* strains tested (23). These results suggest that both GlcNAc and proline are favoring filamentous forms of growth in *C. albicans*.

As in several di- and polymorphic fungi (24), exogenous Ca^{2+} induces germ tube formation in *C. albicans* (25). However, similar to what has been described for *W. dermatitidis*, unrestricted calcium uptake resulted in inhibition of mycelial growth, indicating a critical role for calcium in the regulation of *C. albicans* morphogenesis (26).

Several other growth conditions that favor development of the hyphal form of *C. albicans* have been described (Refs. 7, 27, and 28 and references therein). Examples are $CO_2:O_2$ ratio ($\geq$2:1), inoculum size ($\leq 10^6$ yeasts/ml), amino acid mixtures, serum, low zinc concentration, Fe^{2+} salts, low glucose, and low sulfhydryl concentration.

Thus, there seems to be no unique inducer of polymorphism; various external signals seem to act in parallel. These external signals are then to be processed.

B. Signal Processing and Morphological Regulations

During recent years, our knowledge of polymorphic fungi has increased vastly, particularly in the details about the biochemistry, physiology, and cytology. Furthermore, the technologies of molecular biology provide us information on the genes that may regulate, or are regulated by, the morphogenetic transitions. However, all knowledge gathered so far suggest that fungal polymorphism is more complicated than previously believed. Nevertheless, a mathematical analysis of the cellular basis of fungal dimorphism suggests that the underlying principle is much simpler than anticipated, at least conceptually.

Bartnicki-Garcia et al. (29) postulate that morphology would be regulated by vesicle dynamics as defined by the ratio between the rate (V) of displacement of the distribution center (the vesicle supply centor, VSC) of wall building vesicles and the amount (N) of wall-destined vesicles released from the VSC per unit time. The critical factor in dimorphism would be the rate of displacement of VSC: a stationary or slow-moving VSC would give rise to spherical or ellipsoidal yeast cells, respectively; a fast-moving VSC would produce hyphal tubes. These investigators predict that the molecular basis of dimorphism resides in the molecules that comprise and/or regulate the mechanism for the displacement of the VSC(s) of the cell. They speculate that components of the cytoskeleton are candidates for the displacement of the biological equivalent of the VSC such as the Spitzenkörper (29).

Not only mathematical analysis pinpoints the role of vesicles in the mechanisms responsible for cell shape. Growth of the cell wall depends on the activity of the vesicular apparatus, which carries biosynthetic enzymes and the components that make it up (6). The best-characterized vesicles are the chitosomes that transport chitin synthase (30–32). Next to these microvesicles, macrovesicles have been found at the hyphal tip of all filamentous and polymorphic fungi. They are thought to represent the major vesicles for the intracellular transport of membrane-bound and extracellular enzymes and for new cell membrane. These macrovesicles contribute most of the new membrane for tip expansion; they may also transport preformed nonfibrillar matrix polysaccharides and glycoproteins to the cell surface (for review, see Ref. 32).

Spherical growth would involve a random mobilization of both macro- and microvesicles to the whole cell surface or to the site where budding is going on; without doubt, cylindrical growth involves guidance mechanisms of the vesicles to the hyphal apex.

1. *Components of the Cytoskeleton*

As already mentioned, components of the cytoskeleton—i.e., actin microfilaments and/or microtubules—are the most logical candidates for providing the elements of the guidance mechanisms. In *Saccharomyces cerevisiae* and *Saccharomyces uvarum* actin distribution and the changing arrangements of the actin dots during the cell cycle at least suggest that actin is involved in the localized deposition of cell wall materials and in the selective growth of the yeast bud (33,34). If actin localization is also involved in the zones of wall expansion in, for example, *C. albicans*, it can be expected that the distribution of actin will differ between a growing bud and a growing hypha. This has been demonstrated by Anderson and Soll (35): before evagination, actin granules were distributed throughout the cytoplasmic cortex in both budding and hypha-forming cells. Just before evagination, actin granules clustered at the site of evagination, then filled the early evagination in both budding and hypha-forming cells. With continued bud growth, the actin granules redistributed throughout the cytoplasmic cortex. In marked contrast, with continued hyphal growth, actin clusters appeared more pronounced at the apex. In hyphae actin fibers are directed toward the apex (35).

A progressive increase in the synthesis of actin mRNA was observed when *C. albicans* cells were induced to form germ tubes at 37°C by *N*-acetyl-D-glucosamine (36). Presence of the calmodulin inhibitor, trifluoperazine, or incubation of cells at 25°C, or replacing *N*-acetyl-D-glucosamine with glucose which inhibits germ tube formation, lowers actin mRNA synthesis. In vitro translation of total mRNA revealed an increase in the synthesis of actin during germ tube formation. Thus, these studies suggest that the expression of the actin gene is regulated during morphogenesis of *C. albicans* (36).

Not only actin- but also tubulin-based systems have been implicated in the transport of apical vesicles. Barton and Gull (37) studied variation in cytoplasmic microtubule organization between the yeast and hyphal forms of *C. albicans*. However, their studies suggest a role only for the cytoplasmic microtubules in the nuclear migration that occurs during hyphal growth. Furthermore, studies of Yokoyama et al. (38) have demonstrated that actin microfilaments are important in apical cell elongation of *C. albicans* hyphae, whereas the cytoplasmic microtubules are not essential.

Yeast actin assembly is sensitive to calcium, a tight association has been established between actin filaments and regions of cell-wall growth, and the *CDC24* gene (CDC = cell division cycle) product, involved in bud emergence in *S. cerevisiae*, is a calcium-binding protein (10,39).

2. *Calcium, Calmodulin, Protein Kinases*

Calcium and its carrier, calmodulin, are involved in the control of cytoskeletal assembly and activity (39,40). In *S. cerevisiae*, calmodulin concentrates at sites of cell growth and is implicated in polarized cell growth

(41). Disruption or deletion of the *S. cerevisiae* calmodulin gene (*CMD1*) results in a recessive-lethal mutation; thus, calmodulin is essential for the growth of yeast cells (42).

The gene encoding *C. albicans* calmodulin is also isolated and characterized (12). Amino acid sequence comparisons between calmodulin of *C. albicans*, *S. cerevisiae*, *Schizosaccharomyces pombe*, *Aspergillus nidulans*, *Achlya klebsiana*, and bovine brain show that *C. albicans* calmodulin is more closely related to the calmodulins of vertebrates and filamentous fungi than those of yeast (12). In *C. albicans* calmodulin is important in the regulation of yeast-hyphal morphogenesis:

a. *Candida albicans* yeast-hyphal morphogenesis is antagonized by the calmodulin inhibitors trifluoperazine (TFP) (36,43,44), chlorpromazine, and calmidazolium (RO24571) (44). Of interest is the observation that TFP inhibits germ tube/hypha formation but not the growth of the organism (43).
b. Germ tubes and hyphae have more calmodulin activity than yeast cells, irrespective of the germ tube–inducing condition used (43). This increased calmodulin activity during hyphal development (43) may be due to posttranscriptional regulation of calmodulin rather than mRNA accumulation (12).

N-Acetyl-D-glucosamine–induced germ tube formation in *C. albicans* at 37°C was accompanied by an increase in the rate of protein phosphorylation (43). Trifluoperazine and the Ca^{2+}-ionophore A23187, which inhibited germ tube formation, also reduced the rate of phosphorylation. This rate was also reduced when cells were incubated at 25°C, which favored yeast-phase growth (43). These studies suggest the involvement of Ca^{2+}-calmodulin-dependent protein kinases in germ tube formation.

Calcium ions play a role in the control of early molecular (RNA, protein, and DNA synthesis) and cellular processes that accompany the yeast-to-mycelium transition in *S. schenckii* (45). The optimal stimulatory concentration for this transition was determined to be 1.0 mM (44). However, this transition can also occur in the absence of extracellular Ca^{2+}. The studies of Colon-Colon and Rodriguez-del-Valle (46) suggest the involvement of the signal-transducing enzyme protein kinase C in the control of the yeast-to-mycelium transition in *S. schenkii* grown in the absence of extracellularly added calcium. These studies again suggest the involvement of protein kinases in the control of morphogenetic processes in fungal cells.

3. *Internal pH*

As discussed above, the pH of the external environment can affect the morphological form of *C. albicans*. Gow and colleagues investigated the importance of internal pH in dimorphism (28,47). They found that conditions leading to filamentous growth in *C. albicans* also lead to alkalinization of the cell cytoplasm to pH 8.0 or above. This change in pH was larger than that observed when cells resumed growth by budding and was not seen in strains unable to undergo dimorphism. Thus, intracellular alkalinization seems to be important for the morphogenesis of *C. albicans*.

Both in *S. cerevisiae* and *Dictyostelium discoideum*, intracellular alkalinization correlates with an activation of the proton translocating ATPase in their plasma membranes and is probably caused by it (48). The rise in internal pH in differentiating *C. albicans* is also associated with an increase in plasma membrane ATPase activity. The plasma membrane ATPase of fungi plays a central role in the physiology of these organisms. It drives the proton efflux, and the proton gradient generated by this enzyme is the driving force for nutrient uptake, the secretion of acids, the maintenance of K^+-levels and the regulation of intracellular pH (for reviews see Refs. 48 to 50; the properties of *C. albicans* plasma membrane ATPase are described in Refs. 51, 52, and 52a,b). This ATPase may be another key signal-transducing enzyme in the morphogenesis of fungal cells. It would be of interest to look for mutants that overexpress the proton-ATPase gene (*PMA1*) or of which the ATPase gene is disrupted. The latter cells should not grow; the former might grow as hyphae only.

Fonzi and colleagues identified a gene, *PHR1* (pH-responsive), that is regulated in response to the pH of the growth environment (12,53,54). *PHR1* mRNA is absent in *C. albicans* grown at pH 4.5, but abundant in cells grown at pH 6.5. Expression is independent of temperature, since the same response is seen with cells incubated at 25°C or at 37°C. Expression is also independent of the morphology of the cells, since comparable levels of expression are seen in yeast (25°C, pH 6.5) and hyphal cells (37°C, pH 6.5). Nevertheless, when *PHR1* is deleted on both chromosomes, the double mutant (CAS-8) is unable to form hyphal cells.

The *PHR1* gene was sequenced and the deduced amino acid sequence was compared to sequences in the Genbank database (53). The predicted 50-kDa protein encoded by the *PHR1* gene showed 56% amino acid identity with a membrane glycoprotein of *S. cerevisiae* gp 115 (55,56). This *Saccharomyces* glycoprotein is anchored to the membrane by glycosylphosphatidylinositol (GPI). In addition to the overall 70% amino acid similarity, *N*- and *C*-terminal hydrophobic domains and *N*- and *O*-linked glycosylation sites are also conserved between the *S. cerevisiae* and *C. albicans* proteins (53). This suggests that the *PHR1* protein may also be GPI-linked. Such linkage allows the entire protein to be exposed at the cell surface. Examples of GPI-anchored proteins are the variant surface glycoproteins whose sequential expression enables African trypanosomes to evade the host system (57,58) and cell adhesion proteins such as *S. cerevisiae* a-agglutinin (59). The role of *PHR1* protein is still not known. Fonzi et al. (53) speculate that its role in the process of hypha formation may be as a structural protein necessary for germ tube formation or may be involved in transducing the signal to form hyphae from the external environment. By analogy with the a-agglutinin of *S. cerevisiae*, it may also be involved in the adhesion of *C. albicans* to host cells, a process that is also influenced by the pH of the external environment (22).

4. *Chitin and Polymorphism*

Chitin, the β-1,4-linked polymer of *N*-acetylglucosamine, is the principal load-bearing and shape-giving component of fungal cells (32). In *P. brasiliensis*, chitin is a major component of the cell wall of both the yeast and mycelial form, although in different proportions: 34% in the yeast form and 13% in the mycelial form (60). In *W. dermatitidis*, the chitin content increases and deposition is delocalized during the transition from yeast to multicellular form (61). In the *C. albicans* cell wall, chitin is a minor component quantitatively (1–5% of the cell wall components), but, it plays a very important regulatory and structural role for growth and morphogenesis (62). Chitin synthesis is activated during germ tube formation so that three to five times more chitin is synthesized. It is interesting that other cell-wall components, such as mannan, alkali-plus acid-soluble glucan, and insoluble glucan remain almost unchanged during yeast-mycelium transition in *C. albicans*.

N-Acetylglucosamine activates chitin synthases (62) and, as already discussed above, it favors filamentous forms of growth in *C. albicans*. Therefore, the study of the regulation of chitin synthesis may yield information about the dimorphic transition in *C. albicans*.

In *S. cerevisiae* (63–66) three chitin synthase genes (*CHS1*, *CHS2*, *CHS3*–also called *CSD2*) have been cloned and characterized. Homologues of *CHS* detected in *W. dermatitidis* also fall into three classes (61). The *Saccharomyces CHS1* product may serve as a repair enzyme (66,67), while *CHS2* is required for maintaining normal cell morphology, division, and chitin localization (67). However, gene-disruption studies suggest that it is not responsible for the major part of cellular chitin synthesis (68). A third chitin synthase, which, unlike the *CHS1* and *CHS2* gene products, is not stimulated by proteases (e.g., trypsin), appears to be responsible for the bulk of chitin-synthesized in *S. cerevisiae* (68,69). It should be noted that more recent studies revealed that in the presence of the substrate UDP-*N*-acetyl-D-glucosamine, protease treatment also stimulated activity of CHS3 (the product of the *CHS3* gene) (69a).

Candida albicans homologues of the genes *CHS1* and *CHS2* have also been cloned and sequenced (70–72). The *Candida CHS1* and *CHS2* enzymes are probably both zymogens similar to the *S. cerevisiae CHS1* and *CHS2* enzymes (71). The *CSD2* homologue in *C. albicans* has been identified on low-stringency Southern blots by Gow (73) but has not yet been cloned. The sequence of the *Candida CHS1* is somewhat more similar to *S. cerevisiae CHS2* than to *CHS1*. But *C. albicans CHS1*, although expressed, did not correct the growth defects associated with *S. cerevisiae CHS2* deletion (71).

Candida albicans cells undergoing hyphal outgrowth displayed high levels of *CHS2* message but little *CHS1* message (71). However, gene disruption of the *Candida CHS2* did not result in a significant perturbation of dimorphism or the inhibition of hyphal growth (73,73a). Although next to *CHS2*, other genes are present in *C. albicans* and these genes should be further analyzed, it is possible that the differences observed in chitin synthesis between the yeast and hyphal forms are regulated by the morphogenetic transitions rather than that they play a role in the regulation of these transitions.

Chitin microfibrils are present in the segmentation wall of the parasitic *Coccidioides immitis* cells (9). An important morphological difference between the early and advanced stages of endosporulation of *Coccidioides immitis* is the disappearance of this segmentation wall. Cole et al. (9) examined the possibility that the chitinase, assumed to be secreted by the endospores, may be involved in the digestion of the segmentation apparatus during the phase of endosporulation. It was found that the trigger for activation of the chitinase is a slight drop in pH when the central vacuole of the maternal spherule ruptures (9). It is possible that the chitinase gene is one of the internal and/or external pH regulated genes such as those present in enteric bacteria (for review, see Ref. 74) and the *PHR1* gene identified in *C. albicans*.

5. *Glucans*

As already discussed, the dimorphic transition of *P. brasiliensis* seems to depend exclusively on the temperature of incubation. The only biochemical features that distinguish the yeast wall from the mycelial form in *P. brasiliensis* are as follows (for review, see Ref. 60):

a. The presence of the alkali-soluble, acid-insoluble α-1,3-glucan in the former and the alkali insoluble β-1,3-glucan in the latter. The α-1,3-glucan is not found in the mycelial form.
b. The activity of the intracellular protein disulfide reductase is at least five times higher in the yeast form. This enzyme is substantially deactivated in the mycelial phase (75).

It is possible to induce the expression of α-glucanase in *P. brasiliensis* by using α-1,3-glucan as the only source of carbon; the expression of the enzyme is lethal to the fungus (17). This correlates with the hypothesis that the survival of *P. brasiliensis* in tissue seems to depend on the presence of α-1,3-glucan in the outermost layer of the yeast cell wall (17).

It is of interest that in the yeast form of *B. dermatitidis* the glucose polymer is also organized as α-1,3-glucan (95%), the other 5% is β-1,3-glucan, whereas that of the mycelial form consisted of about 60% α-1,3-glucan and 40% β-1,3-glucan (76).

San-Blas (75,76) formulated a working hypothesis in which the role of glucans and the regulation of protein disulfide reductase are decisive in the establishment of the yeast or mycelium form of *P. brasiliensis*: in the yeast phase (growth at the 37°C), the β-glucan synthase must be depressed to a minimum and the enzyme may be in a zymogenic state (it is also possible that at this temperature the β-glucanase is active and the α-glucanase is inactive or not expressed, or that the conformation of the protein is changed to allow α-1,3-glucan synthesis only). Together with the changes in glucan synthase activity, a stimulation in protein disulfide reductase provokes the breakage of disulfide bonds in cell-wall proteins, favoring the round shape of the yeast form. In transferring to the mycelial phase (incubation temperature below 25°C), cytosolic neutral proteinases are strongly activated, causing the conversion of the inactive β-glucan synthase into an active enzyme. This coincides with an inactivation of the protein disulfide reductase to allow for the establishment of long protein chains, which can be accommodated in the mycelial cell wall. In the conversion of the hyphal form to the yeast form, the activity of the proteinases decreases, resulting in a low rate of β-glucan synthesis and increased synthesis of α-1,3-glucan. In the meantime the protein disulfide reductase should be inactivated. Further studies are needed to characterize the proteinases. It may be worthwhile to evaluate the role of heat-shock genes during the induction of the yeast phase. These genes may play an important role in adaptation to a new environment that polymorphic fungal pathogens, such as *P. brasiliensis* and *H. capsulatum*, encounter when they invade a human host.

6. *Heat-Shock Proteins*

In *S. cerevisiae*, a sudden temperature change generates considerable temporary alterations in the pattern of protein synthesis (for review, see Ref. 77). Upon a shift of *S. cerevisiae* from 23 to 37°C, of 500 proteins examined, more than 80 were transiently induced, 20 of which could be classified as major heat-shock proteins; with more than 300 proteins, the synthesis was reduced (77). Some of the heat-shock proteins probably serve to sequester damaged, denatured, or unproperly folded proteins, such as heat-shock protein 70 (hsp 70), or to protect key plasma membrane enzymes such as the plasma membrane proton-ATPase (78). The latter stress-protective function has been attribution to hsp 30 (78).

Heat-shock proteins play major roles in many cellular processes and have a unique role in several areas of cell biology, including the host-invader interplay (79). These proteins have been detected in many parasites—e.g., *Leishmania* spp., *Trypanosoma brucei*, *Trypanosoma cruzi*, *Plasmodium* spp., schistosomes, and pathogenic fungi such as *H. capsulatum* and *C. albicans*—when, at the time of infection, temperature increases (79).

Work done by Maresca et al. has shown that in *H. capsulatum* isolates, a close relationship exists between the level of heat-shock gene expression, level of thermosensitivity, and degree of pathogenicity (80,81). There is, of course, no doubt that temperature works not only as a signal for induction of the heat-shock phenomenon (adaptation) but also for triggering the phase transition. For example, Shearer et al. (82) were unable to separate the induction of increased synthesis of heat-shock protein from the mycelial-to-yeast phase transition; those temperatures which led to one phenomenon also resulted in the other.

Despite extensive research concerning the mechanisms that regulate activation of heat-shock gene expression and phase transition, there is still a relative paucity of information concerning the nature of the sensor capable of monitoring specific temperatures that activate (induce) heat-shock gene transcription and/or phase transition (79–81,83). For example, the intracellular pH is implicated as the trigger for the acquisition of thermotolerance in *S. cerevisiae* (84) and is associated with the temperature-induced yeast-mycelium transition in, for example, *C. albicans* (see Sec. II.B.3). Whether the intracellular pH is also implicated in the synthesis of heat-shock proteins by *C. albicans* and other pathogenic fungi, and whether heat-shock proteins are involved in this transition remain unanswered questions. Studies of Maresca et al. (80) suggest that membrane fluidity, regulated at least partly by the Δ^9-desaturase (product of the *Ole1* gene), plays a central role not only in regulating the activity of membrane-bound enzymes but also directly influences the expression of specific genes probably involved in mycelium-to-yeast transition (determining the degree of virulence of *H. capsulatum*) and/or heat-shock mRNA induction. These results offer an abundance of research possibilities.

7. *Sterols and Steroids*

Sterols are known to maintain optimal membrane fluidity and integrity; they modulate the activity of membrane-bound enzymes and are required for cellular proliferation and differentiation (for reviews, see Refs. 85–88). Ergosterol, the characteristic sterol in the higher fungi, is not only the sterol best suited to maintain membrane integrity and activity in fungi (85,86) but there is evidence that this 24-alkylsterol is involved in critical non-membrane-associated functions in the cell, and this at nanomolar concentrations (89). For example, data obtained by Kawasaki et al. (90) and Dahl et al. (91) suggest that hormonal levels of ergosterol participate in a signaling process associated with a transmethylase, protein kinase, and/or phosphatidylinositol kinase possibly involved in yeast cell-cycle control. Thus ergosterol can serve as a signal for membrane-associated metabolic events. As suggested by Bloch (92), ergosterol may therefore prove to be the most primitive of the steroid hormones. Unfortunately, most of the experimental support for the "steroid hormone" function of ergosterol is indirect and comes mostly from studies with *S. cerevisiae* mutants. The potential relationship between morphogenesis and ergosterol is intriguing but still open to speculation.

Studies of Kinsman et al. (93) indicate that 17β-estradiol promotes germination in *C. albicans*. Increased hydroxylation of the estrogen and pregnane steroids increases the ability of steroids to promote germination, as does the addition of luteinizing hormone (LH) to the culture medium (93). More recently, the effects of human chorionic gonadotropin (hCG) and human LH and hCG-like material from *Xanthomonas maltophilia* on *C. albicans* transition from yeast to the germ tube stage have also been described (94). These proteins stimulated transition at a concentration of 100 ng/ml and bound with high affinity to *C. albicans* blastospores (93–95). Both hLH and hCG caused a two- to fivefold stimulation of adenylate cyclase activity in *C. albicans* microsomes (96,97). This plasma membrane enzyme catalyzes the synthesis of 3′,5′-cyclic AMP (cAMP) from ATP; cAMP has been described as a regulator of morphogenesis in, e.g., *C. albicans* (76), *H. capsulatum* (76,81), *S. schenckii* (98) and *Mucor* spp. (5,76). Of particular interest are the studies reported by Caticha et al. (99). These investigators purified and characterized a protein from *C. albicans* blastospores that has certain tertiary structural similarities to hCG. They also proved that this *C. albicans* CG-like protein (CaCGLP) induced significant increase in the transition rate. The minimal effective concentration was 1 ng CaCGLP/ml. Thus this *C. albicans* protein is 100 times more potent than hCG in producing germ tubes. It should be noted that both CaCGLP and hCG were not able to induce transition in the absence of serum, suggesting that serum substances are needed in order to permit induction of germ tube formation.

Further characterization of the serum substances required and of CaCGLP may offer valuable information concerning the regulation of *C.*

albicans morphogenesis. Detailed analyses of *C. albicans* mutants and other fungal cells should permit the elucidation of the role of this endogenous transition-inducing substance during morphogenesis in polymorphic fungi.

Malloy et al. (100) describe the cloning and characterization of the gene encoding a high-affinity corticosteroid-binding protein (CBP). The functional role of CBP in *C. albicans* has not yet been elucidated, and whether it is involved in the pathogenicity of this organism remains to be established (100).

Much more is known on the estrogen-binding protein of *P. brasiliensis*. *Paracoccidioides brasiliensis* possesses a cytosolic protein that binds estradiol with high affinity and stereospecificity (101–102), and estradiol inhibits the mycelium to yeast transition of *P. brasiliensis* (for more information on *P. brasiliensis* and hormones, see Refs. 75, 101, and 103). This suppressive effect is dose-dependent and is not found with testosterone. An estradiol-binding protein has also been found in *C. albicans*, *C. glabrata* (104), and *Coccidioides immitis* (105,106) but not in *Candida krusei*, *Candida pseudotropicalis*, and *Candida parapsilosis* (104). Thus, many fungal pathogens seem to contain specific binding sites for mammalian hormones. Further research is certainly needed to better characterize the endogenous fungal ligands and to elucidate the role of the "hormonal system" in morphogenesis.

III. CONCLUSIONS

Numerous environmental factors have been reported to affect morphogenesis. During recent years our knowledge of signal processing has increased vastly and many hypotheses have been formulated in which the role, for example, of cell-wall components, calcium, calmodulin, internal pH, macro- and microvesicles, peptide and steroid hormone-binding proteins, and components of the cytoskeleton in the regulation of the morphogenic transitions is highlighted.

All these hypotheses offer an abundance of research possibilities. The expansion of genetic tools will certainly help us move more rapidly toward understanding the regulatory mechanisms that lead to phase transition. The study of these regulatory mechanisms may also yield information on the mechanisms that induce virulence in polymorphic pathogenic fungi.

REFERENCES

1. Szaniszlo PJ. An introduction to dimorphism among zoopathogenic fungi. In: Szaniszlo PJ, Harris JL, eds. Fungal dimorphism with emphasis on fungi pathogenic for humans. New York: Plenum Press, 1985:3–13.

2. Kwon-Chung KJ, Bennett JE. Medical Mycology. Philadelphia: Lea & Febiger, 1992.
3. Pasteur L. Etudes sur la Bière. Paris: Gauthier-Villars, 1876.
4. Bartnicki-Garcia S, Lippman E. Fungal morphogenesis: Cell wall construction in *Mucor rouxii*. Science 1969;165:302–304.
5. Orlowski M. *Mucor* dimorphism. Microbiol Rev 1991;55:234–258.
6. Ruiz-Herrera J. Dimorphism in *Mucor* species. In: Vanden Bossche H, Odds FC, Kerridge D, eds. Dimorphic Fungi in Biology and Medicine. New York: Plenum Press, 1993:257–265.
7. Odds FC. *Candida* and Candidosis. A Review and Bibliography. London: Baillière Tindall, 1988.
8. Cole GT, Sun SH. Arthroconidium—spherule—endospore transformation in *Coccidioides immitis*. In: Szaniszlo PJ, Harris JL, eds. Fungal Dimorphism with Emphasis on Fungi Pathogenic for Humans. New York: Plenum Press, 1985:281–333.
9. Cole GT, Kruse D, Seshan KR. Factors regulating morphogenesis in *Coccidioides immitis*. In: Vanden Bossche H, Odds FC, Kerridge D, eds. Dimorphic fungi in biology and medicine. New York: Plenum Press, 1993: 191–212.
10. Szaniszlo PJ, Mendoza L, Karuppayil SM. Clues about chromoblastomycotic and other dematiaceous fungal pathogens based on *Wangiella* as a model. In: Vanden Bossche H, Odds FC, Kerridge D, eds. Dimorphic Fungi in Biology and Medicine. New York: Plenum Press, 1993:241–255.
11. Kerridge D. Fungal dimorphism: a sideways look. In: Vanden Bossche H, Odds FC, Kerridge D, eds. Dimorphic Fungi in Biology and Medicine. New York: Plenum Press, 1993:3–10.
12. Birse C, Fonzi WA, Saporito S, Irwin M, Sypherd PS. Molecular genetics of dimorphism in *Candida albicans* In: Bennett JE, Hay RJ, Peterson PK, eds. New Strategies in Fungal Disease. Edinburgh: Churchill Livingstone, 1992:133–152.
13. Salazar ME, Restrepo A. Morphogenesis of the mycelium to yeast transformation in *Paracoccidioides brasiliensis*. Sabouraudia 1984;22:7–11.
14. Deng Z, Ribas JL, Gibson DW, Connor DH. Infections caused by *Penicillium marneffei* in China and Southeast Asia. Rev Infect Dis 1988;10: 640–652.
15. Medoff G, Painter A, Kobayashi G. Mycelial-to yeast phase transitions of the dimorphic fungi *Blastomyces dermatitidis* and *Paracoccidiodes brasiliensis*. J Bacteriol 1987;169:4055–4060.
16. Paris S, Duran-Gonzalez S, Mariat F. Nutritional studies on *Paracoccidioides brasiliensis*: The role of organic sulfur in dimorphism. Sabouraudia 1985;23:85–92.
17. San-Blas F, San-Blas G. *Paracoccidioides brasiliensis*. In: Szaniszlo PJ, Harris JL, eds. Fungal Dimorphism with Emphasis on Fungi Pathogenic for Humans. New York: Plenum Press, 1985:93–120.
18. Resto S, Rodríguez-Del-Valle. Yeast cell cycle of *Sporothrix schenckii*. J Med Vet Mycol 1988;26:13–24.

19. Cooper CR Jr. Phase transition in *Wangiella dermatitidis*: Identification of cell-division-cycle genes involved in yeast bud emergence. In: Vanden Bossche H, Odds FC, Kerridge D, eds. Dimorphic Fungi in Biology and Medicine. New York: Plenum Press, 1993:105–119.
20. Lee KL, Buckley HR, Campbell CC. An amino acid liquid synthetic medium for the development of mycelial and yeast forms of *Candida albicans*. Sabouraudia 1975;13:148–153.
21. Mitchell LH, Soll DR. Commitment to germ tube or bud formation during release from stationary phase in *Candida albicans*. Exp Cell Res 1979;120: 167–179.
22. King RD, Lee JC, Morris AL. Adherence of *Candida albicans* and other *Candida* species to mucosal epithelial cells. Infect Immun 1980;27:667–674.
23. Marichal P, Gorrens J, Van Cutsem J, Vanden Bossche H. Culture media for the study of the effects of azole derivatives on germ tube formation and hyphal growth of *C. albicans*. Mykosen 1986;29:76–81.
24. Gadd GM, Brunton AH. Calcium involvement in dimorphism of *Ophiostoma ulmi*, the Dutch elm disease fungus, and characterization of calcium uptake by yeast cells and germ tubes. J Gen Microbiol 1992;138:1561–1571.
25. Sabie FT, Gadd GM. Involvement of Ca^{2+}-calmodulin interaction in the yeast-mycelial (Y-M) transition of *Candida albicans*. Mycopathologia 1989; 108:47–54.
26. Holmes AR, Cannon RD, Shepherd MG. Effect of calcium ion uptake on *Candida albicans* morphology. FEMS Microbiol Lett 1991;61:187–193.
27. Odds FC. Morphogenesis in *Candida albicans*. CRC Crit Rev Microbiol 1985;12:45–93.
28. Gow NAR. Biochemical and biophysical aspects of dimorphism in *Candida albicans*. In: Torres-Rodríguez JM, ed. Proceedings of the Xth Congress of the International Society for Human and Animal Mycology—ISHAM. Barcelona: JR Prous Science Publishers, 1988:73–77.
29. Bartnicki-Garcia S, Gierz G. Mathematical analysis of the cellular basis of fungal dimorphism. In: Vanden Bossche H, Odds FC, Kerridge D, eds. Dimorphic Fungi in Biology and Medicine. New York: Plenum Press, 1993: 133–144.
30. Bracker CE, Ruiz-Herrera J, Bartnicki-Garcia S. Structure and transformation of chitin synthetase particles (chitosomes) during microfibril synthesis in vitro. Proc Natl Acad Sci USA 1976;73:4570–4574.
31. Bartnicki-Garcia S, Bracker CE. Unique properties of chitosomes. In: Nombela C, ed. Microbial Cell Wall Synthesis and Autolysis. Amsterdam: Elsevier, 1984:101–112.
32. Gow NAR. Control of extension of the hyphal apex. In: McGinnis MR, Borgers M, eds. Current Topics in Medical Mycology. Vol 3. New York: Springer-Verlag, 1989:109–152.
33. Kilmartin JV, Adams AEM. Structural rearrangements of tubulin and actin during the cell cycle of the yeast *Saccharomyces*. J Cell Biol 1984;98: 922–933.

34. Adams AEM, Pringle JR. Relationship of actin and tubulin distribution to bud growth in wild-type and morphogenetic-mutant *Saccharomyces cerevisiae*. J Cell Biol 1984;98:934–945.
35. Anderson JM, Soll DR. Differences in actin localization during bud and hypha formation in the yeast *Candida albicans*. J Gen Microbiol 1986;132: 2035–2047.
36. Paranjape V, Datta A. Overexpression of the actin gene is associated with the morphogenesis of *Candida albicans*. Biochem Biophys Res Commun 1991;179:423–427.
37. Barton R, Gull K. Variation in cytoplasmic microtubule organization and spindle length between the two forms of the dimorphic fungus *Candida albicans*. J Cell Science 1988;91:211–220.
38. Yokoyama K, Kaji H, Nishimura N, Miyaji M. The role of microfilaments and microtubules in apical growth and dimorphism of *Candida albicans*. J Gen Microbiol 1990;136:1067–1075.
39. Anraku Y, Ohia Y, Iida H. Cell cycle control by calcium and calmodulin in *Saccharomyces cerevisiae*. Biochim Biophys Acta 1991;1093:169–177.
40. Greer C, Schekman R. Calcium control of *Saccharomyces cerevisiae* actin assembly. Mol Cell Biol 1982;2:1279–1286.
41. Brockerhof SE, Davis TN. Calmodulin concentrates at regions of cell growth in *Saccharomyces cerevisiae*. J Cell Biol 1992;118:619–629.
42. Davis TN, Urdea MS, Masiarz FR, Thorner J. Isolation of the yeast calmodulin gene: Calmodulin is an essential protein. Cell 1986;47:423–431.
43. Paranjape V, Gupta Roy B, Datta A. Involvement of calcium, calmodulin and protein phosphorylation in morphogenesis of *Candida albicans*. J Gen Microbiol 1990;136:2149–2154.
44. Buchan ADB, Kelly VA, Kinsman OS, et al: Effect of trifluoperazine on growth, morphogenesis and pathogenicity of *Candida albicans*. J Med Vet Mycol 1993;31:427–433.
45. Rodríguez-Del Valle N, Rodríguez-Medina JR. Calcium stimulates molecular and cellular events during the yeast-to-mycelium transition in *Sporothrix schenckii*. J Med Vet Mycol 1993;31:43–53.
46. Colon-Colon W, Rodríguez-Del Valle N. Studies on phase transitions in *Sporothrix schenckii*: Possible involvement of protein kinase C. In: Vanden Bossche H, Odds FC, Kerridge D, eds. Dimorphic Fungi in Biology and Medicine. New York: Plenum Press, 1993:225–239.
47. Stewart E, Gow NAR, Bowen DV. Cytoplasmic alkalinization during germ tube formation in *Candida albicans*. J Gen Microbiol 1988;134:1079–1087.
48. Serrano R. Structure and function of proton translocating ATPase in plasma membranes of plants and fungi. Biochim Biophys Acta 1988;947:1–28.
49. Prasad R. The plasma membrane of *Candida albicans*: Its relevance to transport phenomenon. In: Prasad R, ed. *Candida albicans*: Cellular and Molecular Biology. Berlin: Springer-Verlag, 1991:108–127.
50. Scarborough GA. The *Neurospora crassa* plasma membrane H^+-ATPase. In: de Pont JJ, ed. Molecular Aspects of Transport Proteins. Amsterdam: Elsevier, 1992:117–134.

51. Hubbard MJ, Sullivan PA, Shepherd MG. The kinetics and divalent cation inhibition of plasma membrane ATPase in the yeast *Candida albicans*. J Biol Chem 1985;260:6782–6787.
52. Hubbard MJ, Surarit R, Sullivan PA, Shepherd MG. The isolation of plasma membrane and characterisation of the plasma membrane ATPase from the yeast *Candida albicans*. Eur J Biochem 1986;154:375–381.
52a. Monk BC, Niimi M, Shepherd MG. The *Candida albicans* plasma membrane and H^+-ATPase during yeast growth and germ tube formation. J Bacteriol 1993;175:5566–5574.
52b. Monk BC, Perlin DS. Fungal plasma membrane proton pumps as promising new antifungal targets. Crit Rev Microbiol 1994;20:209–223.
53. Fonzi WA, Saporito-Irwin S, Chen J-Y, Sypherd P. Genetic basis for dimorphism and pathogenicity in *Candida albicans*. In: Vanden Bossche H, Odds FC, Kerridge D, eds. Dimorphic Fungi in Biology and Medicine. New York: Plenum Press, 1993:37–50.
54. Saporito-Irwin S, Birse CE, Fonzi WA. Putative virulence factors of *Candida albicans*. XIIth Congress of the International Society for Human and Animal Mycology. Adelaide: March 13–18, 1994 (abstract No. S23.1).
55. Vai M, Gatti E, Lacanà E, Popolo L, Alberghina L. Isolation and deduced amino acid sequence of the gene encoding gp115, a yeast glycophospholipid-anchored protein containing a serine rich region. J Biol Chem 1991;266: 12242–12248.
56. Nuoffer C, Jeno P, Conzelmann A, Reizman H. Determinants for glycophospholipid anchoring of the *Saccharomyces cerevisiae* GAS1 protein to the plasma membrane. Mol Cell Biol 1991;11:27–37.
57. Holder AA, Boothroyd JC, Cross GAM. Trypanosome variant glycoprotein: The C-terminus of the protein is the location of antigenically cross reacting carbohydrate groups, of a putative membrane attachment sequence and the site of proteolytic processing. In: Vanden Bossche H, ed. The Host Invader Interplay. Amsterdam: Elsevier/North-Holland, 1980:249–252.
58. Ferguson MAJ, Haldar K, Cross GAM. *Trypanosoma brucei* variant surface glycoprotein has a sn-1,2-dimyristyl glycerol membrane anchor at its COOH-terminus. J Biol Chem 1985;260:4963–4968.
59. Roy A, Lu CF, Marykwas DL, et al. The AGA1 product is involved in cell surface attachment of *Saccharomyces cerevisiae* cell adhesion glycoprotein a-agglutin. Mol Cell Biol 1991;11:4196–4206.
60. San-Blas G. *Paracoccidioides brasiliensis*: cell wall glucans, pathogenicity, and dimorphism. In: McGinnis MR, ed. Current Topics in Medical Mycology. Vol 1. New York: Springer-Verlag, 1985:235–257.
61. Szaniszlo PJ, Momamy M. Chitin, chitin synthase and chitin synthase conserved region homologues in *Wangiella dermatitidis*. In: Maresca B, Kobayashi GS, Yamaguchi H, eds. Molecular Biology and Its Application to Medical Mycology. Berlin: Springer-Verlag, 1993:229–242.
62. Cassone A. Cell wall of pathogenic yeasts and implications for antimycotic therapy. Drug Exp Clin Res 1986;12:635–643.

63. Bulawa CE, Slater M, Cabib E, et al. The *S. cerevisiae* structural gene for chitin synthase is not required for chitin synthesis in vivo. Cell 1986;46: 213–225.
64. Sburlati A, Cabib E. Chitin synthase 2, a presumptive participant in septum formation in *Saccharomyces cerevisiae*. J Biol Chem 1986;261: 15147–15152.
65. Bulawa CE. CSD2, CSD3 and CSD4 genes required for chitin synthesis in yeast: the CSD2 gene product is related to chitin synthases and to developmentally regulated proteins in *Rhizobium* and *Xenopus*. Mol Cell Biol 1992; 12:1764–1776.
66. Cabib E, Silverman SJ, Sburlati A, Slater ML. Chitin synthesis in yeast (Saccharomyces cerevisiae). In: Kuhn PJ, Trinci APJ, Jung MJ, et al, eds. Biochemistry of Cell Wall and Membranes in Fungi. Berlin: Springer-Verlag, 1990:31–41.
67. Cabib E, Sburlati A, Bowers B, Silverman SJ. Chitin synthase I, an auxiliary enzyme for chitin synthesis. J Cell Biol 1989;108:1665–1672.
68. Bulawa CE, Osmonds BC. Chitin synthase I and chitin synthase II are not required for chitin synthesis in vivo in *Saccharomyces cerevisiae*. Proc Natl Acad Sci USA 1990;87:7424–7428.
69. Baymiller J, McCullough JE. Identification of a *Saccharomyces cerevisiae* mutation that allows cells to grow without chitin synthase 1 or 2. Curr Genet 1993;23:102–107.
69a. Choi W-J, Sburlati A, Cabib E. Chitin synthase 3 from yeast has zymogenic properties that depend on both CAL1 and CAL3 genes. Proc Natl Acad Sci USA 1994;91:4727–4730.
70. Au-Young J, Robbins PW. Isolation of a chitin synthase gene (CHS1) from *Candida albicans* by expression in *Saccharomyces cerevisiae*. Mol Microbiol 1990;4:197–207.
71. Chen-Wu JL, Zwicker J, Bowen AR, Robbins PW. Expression of chitin synthase genes during yeast and hyphal growth phases of *Candida albicans*. Mol Microbiol 1992;6:497–502.
72. Robbins PW, Bowen AR, Chen-Wu JL, et al. The multiple chitin synthase genes of *Candida albicans* and other pathogenic fungi—A review. In: Vanden Bossche H, Odds FC, Kerridge D, eds. Dimorphic Fungi in Biology and Medicine. New York: Plenum Press, 1993:51–59.
73. Gow NAR, Swoboda R, Bertram G, Gooday GW, Brown AJP. Key genes in the regulation of dimorphism of *Candida albicans*. In: Vanden Bossche H, Odds FC, Kerridge D, eds. Dimorphic fungi in biology and medicine. New York: Plenum Press, 1993:61–71.
73a. Gow NAR, Robbins PW, Lester JW, et al. A hyphal-specific chitin synthase gene (CHS2) is not essential for growth, dimorphism, or virulence of *Candida albicans*. Proc Natl Acad Sci USA 1994;91:6216–6220.
74. Slonczewski JL. pH-Regulated genes in enteric bacteria: Researchers are gaining insight into pathogenesis and other adaptations to environmental change. ASM News 1992;58:140–144.

75. San-Blas G, San-Blas F. Biochemical and physiological aspects in the dimorphism of *Paracoccidioides brasiliensis*. In: Vanden Bossche H, Odds FC, Kerridge D, eds. Dimorphic Fungi in Biology and Medicine. New York: Plenum Press, 1993:219–224.
76. San-Blas G, San-Blas F. Molecular aspects of fungal dimorphism. CRC Clin Rev Microbiol 1984;11:101–127.
77. Mager WH, Ferreira PM. Stress response of yeast. Biochem J 1993;290: 1–13.
78. Panaretou B, Piper PW. The plasma membrane of yeast acquires a novel heat-shock protein (hsp 30) and displays a decline in proton-pumping ATPase levels in response to both heat shock and the entry to stationary phase. Eur J Biochem 1992;206:635–640.
79. Maresca B, Carratú L. The biology of the heat shock response in parasites. Parasitol Today 1992;8:260–266.
80. Maresca B, Di Lallo G, Pardini CL, et al. Addition of unsaturated fatty acids down-modulates heat shock gene expression and produces attenuated strains in the fungus *Histoplasma capsulatum*. In: Maresca B, Kobayashi GS, Yamaguchi H, eds. Molecular Biology and Its Application to Medical Mycology. Berlin: Springer-Verlag, 1993:243–250.
81. Maresca B, Kobayashi GS. Dimorphism in *Histoplasma capsulatum*: A model for the study of cell differentiation in pathogenic fungi: Microbiol Rev 1989;53:186–209.
82. Shearer G, Birge CH, Yuckenberg PD, et al: Heat-shock proteins induced during the mycelial-to-yeast transitions of strains of *Histoplasma capsulatum*. J Gen Microbiol 1987;133:3375–3382.
83. Jeavons L, Hunt L, Hamilton A. Immunochemical studies of heat-shock protein 80 of *Histoplasma capsulatum*. J Med Vet Mycol 1994;32:47–57.
84. Coote PJ, Cole MB, Jones MV. Induction of increased thermotolerance in *Saccharomyces cerevisiae* may be triggered by a mechanism involving intracellular pH. J Gen Microbiol 1991;137:1701–1708.
85. Köller W. Antifungal agents with target sites in sterol functions and biosynthesis. In: Köller W, ed. Target Sites of Fungicide Action. Boca Raton: CRC Press, 1992:119–206.
86. Vanden Bossche H. Importance and role of sterols in fungal membranes. In: Kuhn PJ, Trinci APJ, Jung MJ, et al, eds. Biochemistry of Cell Walls and Membranes in Fungi. Berlin: Springer-Verlag, 1990:135–157.
87. Mishra P, Bolard J, Prasad R. Emerging role of lipids of *Candida albicans*, a pathogenic dimorphic yeast. Biochim Biophys Acta 1992;1127:1–14.
88. Vanden Bossche H, Marichal P. Is there a role for sterols and steroids in fungal growth and transition from yeast to hyphal-form and vice-versa? In: Vanden Bossche H, Odds FC, Kerridge D. eds. Dimorphic Fungi in Biology and Medicine. New York: Plenum Press, 1993:177–190.
89. Parks LW, Rodriguez RJ, Low C. An essential fungal growth factor derived from ergosterol, a new end product of sterol biosynthesis in fungi? Lipids 1986;21:89–91.

90. Kawasaki S, Ramgopal M, Chin J, Bloch K. Sterol control of the phosphatidylethanolamine-phosphatidylcholine conversion in the yeast mutant GL7. Proc Natl Acad Sci USA 1985;82:5715–5719.
91. Dahl C, Biemann H-P, Dahl J. A protein kinase antigenically related to pp60$^{V\text{-}SRC}$ possibly involved in yeast cell cycle control: positive in vivo regulation by sterol. Proc Natl Acad Sci USA 1987;84:4012–4016.
92. Bloch K. Lipid structure and function. In: Op den Kamp JAF, Roelofsen B, Wirtz KWA, eds. Lipids and Membranes: Past, Present and Future. Amsterdam: Elsevier, 1986:45–59.
93. Kinsman OS, Pitblado K, Coulson CJ. Effect of mammalian steroid hormones and luteinizing hormone on the germination of *Candida albicans* and implications for vaginal candidosis. Mycoses 1988;31:617–626.
94. Caticha O, Grover S, Winge D, Odell WD. Stimulation of *Candida albicans* transition by human chorionic gonadotropin and a bacterial protein. Endocr Res 1992;18:133–143.
95. Bramley TA, Menzies GS, Williams RJ, et al. Specific high affinity binding sites for human luteinizing hormone and human chorionic gonadotropin in *Candida species*. Biochim Biophys Res Commun 1990;167:1050–1056.
96. Williams RJ, Dickinson K, Kinsman OS, et al. Receptor-mediated elevation of adenylate cyclase by luteinizing hormone in *Candida albicans*. J Gen Microbiol 1990;136:2143–2148.
97. Bramley TA, Menzies GS, Williams RJ, et al. Luteinizing hormone (LH)-binding sites in *Candida albicans*: Comparison with mammalian corpus luteum receptor. J Endocrinol 1991;130:177–190.
98. San Blas G. Fungi pathogenic to humans: molecular aspects of dimorphism. In: Arora DK, Ajello L, Mukerji KG, eds. Handbook of Applied Mycology. Vol 2. Humans, Animals and Insects. New York: Marcel Dekker, 1991: 459–475.
99. Caticha O, Li Y, Griffin J, Winge D, Odell WD. Characterization of a human chorionic gonadotropin-like protein from *Candida albicans*. Endocrinology 1993;132:667–673.
100. Malloy PJ, Zhao X, Madani ND, Feldman D. Cloning and expression of the gene from *Candida albicans* that encodes a high-affinity corticosteroid-binding protein. Proc Natl Acad Sci USA 1993;90:1902–1906.
101. Loose DS, Stover EP, Restrepo A, et al. Estradiol binds to a receptor-like cytosol binding protein and initiates a biological response in *Paracoccidioides brasiliensis*. Proc Natl Acad Sci USA 1983;80:7659–7663.
102. Stover EP, Schör G, Clemans KV, et al. Estradiol-binding proteins from mycelial and yeast-form cultures of *Paracoccidioides brasiliensis*. Infect Immun 1986;51:199–203.
103. Restrepo A, Salazar ME, Cano LE, et al. Estrogens inhibit mycelium-to-yeast transformation in the fungus *Paracoccidioides brasiliensis*: Implications for resistance of females to paracoccidioidomycosis. Infect Immun 1984;46:346–353.

104. Powell PL, Freu CL, Drutz DJ. Identification of a 17β-estradiol binding protein in *Candida albicans* and *C. glabrata*. Exp Mycol 1984;8:304–313.
105. Powell BL, Drutz DJ, Huppert M, Sun SH. Relationship of progesterone- and estradiol-binding proteins in *Coccidioides immitis* to coccidioidal dissemination in pregnancy. Infect Immun 1983;40:478–485.
106. Powel BL, Drutz DJ. Identification of a high-affinity binder for estradiol and a low-affinity binder of testosterone in *Coccidioides immitis*. Infect Immun 1984;45:784–786.

5

Lesser-Known Fungi of Clinical Significance

LYNNE SIGLER
University of Alberta
Edmonton, Alberta, Canada

I. INTRODUCTION

With advances in modern medicine, which have improved life expectancy of severely ill patients, and with the ability of fungi to exploit almost any substrate, it is perhaps not surprising that a greater number of fungi would be found capable of causing infection today. Various recent review articles have documented the increasing diversity of fungi of clinical significance (1–8). Further evidence of the increasing numbers of potentially pathogenic fungi comes from a medical mycology text published in 1992 (9), in which approximately 200 taxa have been indexed as common or rare pathogens, compared to about 120 in the edition published 15 years earlier. As the list of etiologic agents grows longer, it places increased demands on the clinical laboratorian to demonstrate proficiency in the identification of fungi potentially capable of causing infection. While many fungi have been implicated in causing infection, albeit sometimes from only a single case, other fungi are isolated often enough from clinical specimens to be considered "suspicious" for potential pathogenicity. Critical assessment of some species reported as etiologic agents is difficult in cases where the fungus is inadequately described and illustrated and if the isolate has not been deposited in a culture collection where it can be accessed for review. Accurate identification of a fungus as an etiologic agent is important in patient management, since it allows access to the literature on clinical manifestations and treatment. Since identification of these lesser-known fungi is often a formidable challenge, this chapter provides keys (Figs. 1–4) to a number of fungi that are encountered infrequently, either as pathogens or contaminants, and provides brief descriptions of selected taxa. Dermatophytes, yeasts, systemic fungi, and the zygomycetes are not treated here, nor are details of clinical spectra and treatment provided. The keys provide a general guideline to the identification of a given isolate, but they do not include *all* fungi, nor do they provide all salient characteristics required for identification. Moreover, some of the choices are arbitrary and may not apply to all species of a genus. One of the first choices separates fungi by color of spores, whether light or dark, but the genera *Aspergillus* and *Scopulariopsis*, for example, contain both moniliaceous (light-colored spores) and dematiaceous (dark-colored spores) species.

II. LABORATORY DIAGNOSIS

A. Assessment of Significance

The isolation of a known opportunist such as *Sporothrix schenckii* or *Cryptococcus neoformans* is generally presumptive of infection, but fungi such as *Pseudallescheria boydii* or *Aspergillus fumigatus* may be isolated from respiratory infections without clinical evidence of infection. The diagnosis of a mycosis caused by a saprophytic fungus relies on several pieces of evidence. Foremost among them are the results of the direct examination and the clinical history. A positive direct examination provides conclusive evidence of fungal infection; however, it should be confirmed that the fungus is actually growing in tissue and not in necrotic debris. For the experienced laboratorian, structures observed in tissue provide an important clue to the etiology of the species involved. Determination of the species requires culture. Important features include (1) characteristics of the hyphae, whether narrow (2–5 μm in width) or broad (7–10 μm or more in width); regularly or sparsely septate; branched or unbranched; hyaline, yellow, or brown in color; or whether unusual in shape, showing swellings, areas of collapse or constrictions at the septa (pseudohyphae); (2) presence of budding cells; (3) other diagnostic features, including conidial structures, muriform cells (having longitudinal and transverse septa), and presence of grains or granules indicative of mycetoma. Other evidence useful to confirm significance of an isolated mold includes isolation of colonies of the same mold from several pieces of the specimen and isolation of the same mold from a repeat specimen. However, even repeat isolation of some common saprophytes from respiratory specimens may not be significant unless accompanied by a positive direct examination (9).

B. Culture

Most saprophytic molds are not fastidious and will grow on a variety of agar media. The most common medium in use is Sabouraud dextrose agar, but many of the opportunistic fungi sporulate better on media such as potato dextrose agar (PDA), cornmeal agar, or malt agar. Another useful sporulation medium is Pablum cereal agar (10,11). Some species are ascomycetes and special media (e.g., cornmeal or oatmeal-salts agars or nutritionally deficient media) (10,12) are needed to demonstrate the sexual stage, but these media are not usually used for primary isolation. Some species are sensitive to cylcoheximide, so a medium without cylcoheximide should always be included. The usual incubation temperature for isolation is from 25–30°C, but determination of temperature maxima can be a useful criterion is distinguishing among some species (e.g., *Exophiala jeanselmei* and *Wangiella dermatitidis*) and can also be useful in ruling out a particular isolate as a suspected pathogen if growth is completely inhibited at 35–37°C.

Both macroscopic and microscopic examination is important in the identification of the isolate. The colony should be examined for growth rate, color, texture, presence of diffusible pigment or unusual reverse coloration, and presence of exudate droplets, hyphal knots, ''bumps,'' or

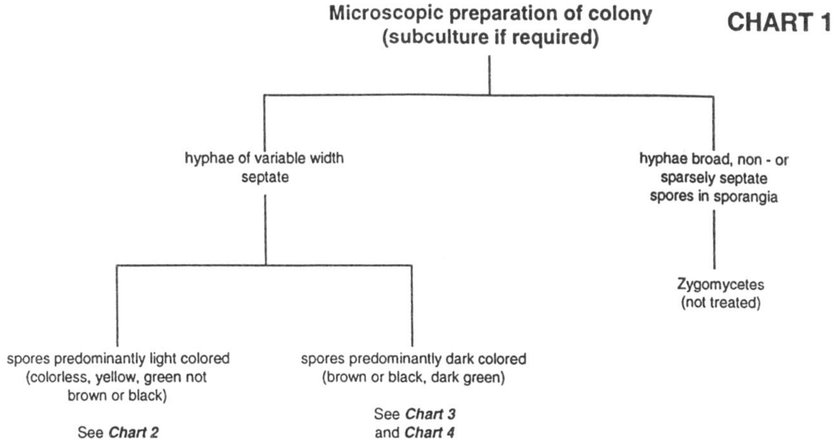

Figure 1 Key to the identification of some medically important fungi.

other features that may be indicative of developing fruiting bodies of a sexual stage or pycnidia of a coelomycete. The use of a dissecting microscope with basal illumination and magnification up to 60× is invaluable in examining colonies for structures such as fruiting bodies, hülle cells, sclerotia, or conidiomata submerged in the mycelium or in the agar (10,12,13). Both tease mounts and slide culture preparations are helpful in examining morphology, but the latter are particularly useful for assessing conidiogenesis in conidial fungi (10–13). Critical assessment of some microscopic features can be made only at high magnifications, i.e., under immersion oil, and using phase contrast or Nomarski optics.

It is beyond the scope of this chapter to provide a detailed description of how fungi form spores. The reader is referred to general mycological references (12,14) for this information.

Keys to the identification of selected species are presented in Figures 1–4. Descriptions are provided only for species that are numbered in the keys.

III. DESCRIPTIONS OF FUNGI

1. *Aureobasidium, Hormonema*

Aureobasidium pullulans (15) is a yeastlike hyphomycete common in damp indoor environments; it occurs on wood and painted surfaces, often staining the surface black, and on plastics, toiletry articles like soaps, and various other substrates.

a. *Significance* Documented human infections involve the skin and deeper tissues (spleen and liver abscesses); fungemia is also seen (3,9,16). A *Hormonema*-like fungus was reported from a case of mycetoma (17).

b. *Colonial* Initially cream to pale pink and mucoid (some isolates) or black and mucoid or dry with metallic sheen, becoming gray to black as pigmented hyphae develop. Relative abundance of the yeast form can be influenced by medium, with colonies often more yeast-like on PDA.

c. *Microscopic* Initial growth consists of budding cells, then light and dark hyphae form, giving rise to conidia simultaneously (synchronously) from conidiogenous cells, which are either integrated in the mycelium, terminal, or formed on short lateral branches. Dark hyphae may break apart to form pigmented swollen arthroconidia, which may also form secondary conidia.

d. *Differential* *Hormonema* includes species that produce conidia serially (one after the other) rather than simultaneously, as in *Aureobasi-*

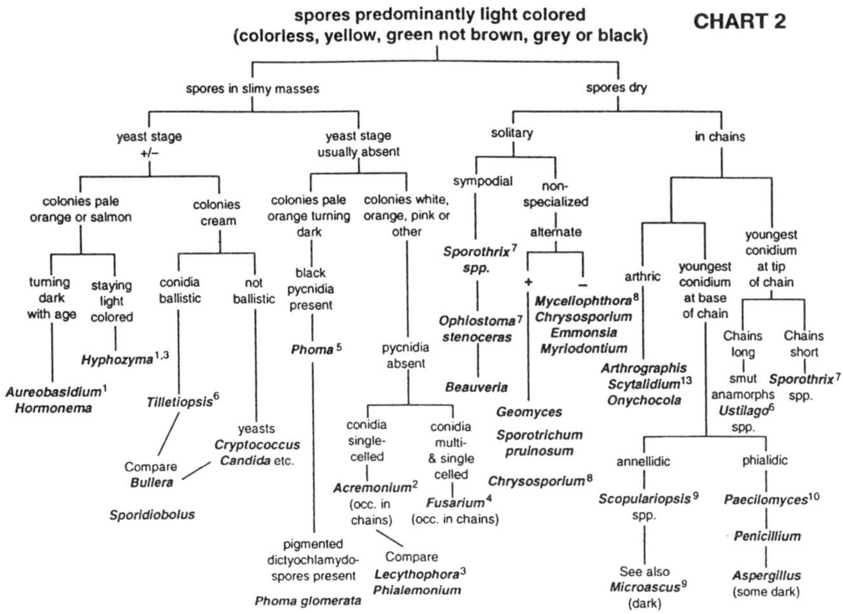

Figure 2 Key to the identification of some light-colored medically important fungi.

dium. These differences may be difficult to detect, but Dalmau plates (12) using PDA may be useful to observe these features. Early growth in *Hyphozyma* species (18) consists of budding cells, but colonies remain light orange or pale pink in color. The hyphal stage is similar to *Lecythophora*.

2. *Acremonium* Species (Formerly Called *Cephalosporium*)

a. Significance Cases of superficial (onychomycosis, mycotic keratitis) and invasive infections including pulmonary, meningitis, endocarditis, cerebritis, oesophagitis, osteomyelitis, and subcutaneous abscess are seen (9,13). Numerous species are known, but many reports fail to document the species involved.

A. *Acremonium strictum*

a. Colonial Initially pink and moist, gradually becoming more hyphal.

b. Microscopic Narrow hyphae forming simple, awl-shaped phialides. Conidia are narrow, cylindrical, and produced in slimy masses.

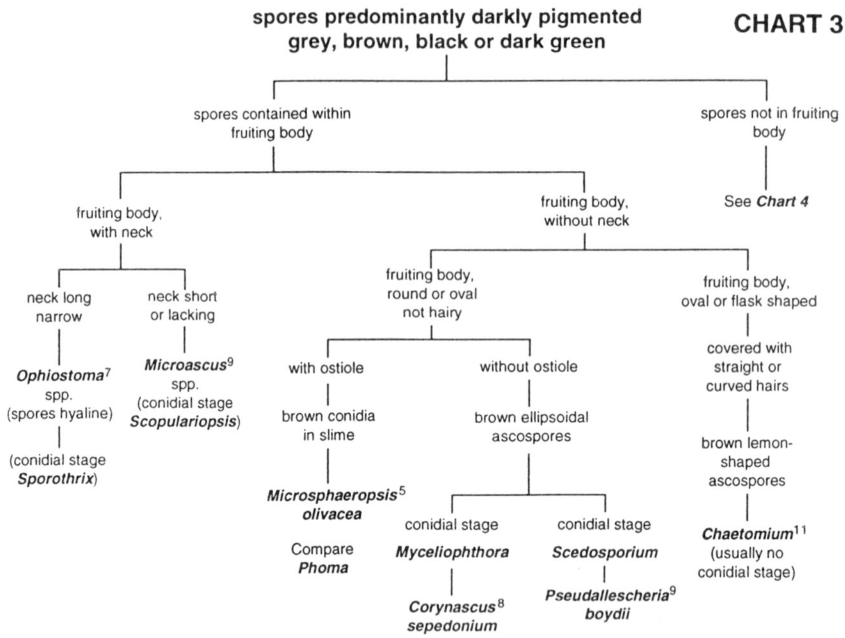

Figure 3 Key to the identification of some medically important fungi forming fruiting bodies.

c. *Differential* *Acremonium strictum* (15) is similar to *Lecythophora hoffmannii* (19), but its slender phialides are longer and better developed. Some species of *Fusarium* that fail to develop macroconidia (13,15) may be confused with species of *Acremonium*. However, *Fusarium* species grow more rapidly, usually reaching the perimeter of the petri dish within 7–10 days, and the hyphae and phialides are generally broader than those of *Acremonium* species.

3. *Lecythophora* and *Phialemonium*

Lecythophora (19) was reintroduced for some species, formerly placed in *Phialophora*, which form slimy conidia from peglike or reduced phialides (adelophialides) without a basal septum and usually lacking distinctive collarettes. Phialides may also be longer and slender and then resemble those of *Acremonium*. There are few microscopic differences between *L. hoffmannii* and *Phialemonium* species and the need for generic distinction may be questioned.

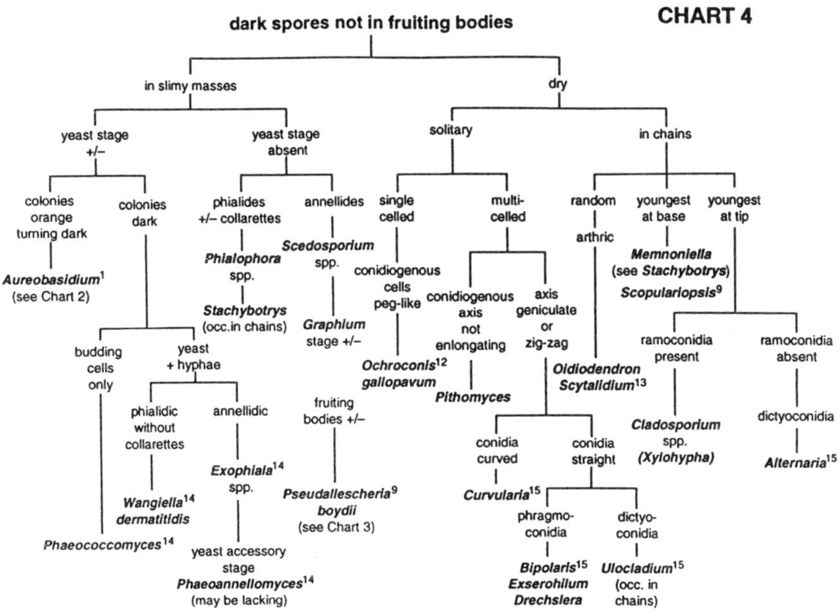

Figure 4 Key to the identification of some dark-colored medically important fungi.

a. *Significance* Skin lesions, subcutaneous abscesses, peritonitis, and endocarditis rarely reported (9,16,20).

A. *Lecythophora hoffmannii*

a. *Colonial* Salmon to bright orange, sometimes creamy white in degenerate strains, moist but becoming hairy with development of hyphae.

b. *Microscopic* Hyphae producing narrow, oval, or ellipsoidal to slightly curved conidia in slimy masses from short and stumpy (adelophialides) or longer phialides.

c. *Differential* *Hyphozyma* species (18) also form hyphae with short peglike conidiogenous cells or slender, scarcely differentiated phialides without distinctive collarettes.

B. *Phialemonium* species

a. *Colonial* Yellowish white, pale greenish, or grayish white in old cultures, depending upon species.

b. *Microscopic* Hyphae producing narrow, cylindrical, or curved (*Phialemonium curvatum*), ellipsoidal, curved, or obovate (egg-shaped)

(*Phialemonium dimorphosporum*) or obovate (*P. obovatum*) conidia from adelophialides or awl-shaped phialides (16,19,20).

4. *Fusarium* Species

Fusarium species (21) grow rapidly; colonies are initially white and cottony, often becoming pigmented rose or violet with age and developing mucoid areas when sporulating. Two types of conidia are produced: curved, multicellular macroconidia and unicellular microconidia. Some species produce thick-walled chlamydospores, which are solitary or in aggregates. Conidia are formed in slimy masses.

a. *Significance* *Fusarium* species are emerging pathogens of importance, causing superficial and invasive infections particularly in the neutropenic patient (1–5,7–9,13,22). They may be isolated from blood. *Fusarium solani*, *Fusarium oxysporum*, and *Fusarium moniliforme* are the commonest human pathogenic species.

A. ***Fusarium solani***

a. *Colonial* On potato dextrose agar, rapid-growing and cottony, becoming grayish white to blue-green or bluish brown, not orange. Slower growing than *F. oxysporum*.

b. *Microscopic* Microconidia are cylindrical to oval, produced from long phialides (monophialides) that may be borne on branched conidiophores (13,15,21). Macroconidia are abundant and thick-walled and have 1–5 septa. The apical cell is blunt and rounded and the basal cell is distinctly foot-shaped or notched. Chlamydospores are formed singly or in pairs.

c. *Differential* *Fusarium oxysporum* differs in having short, stout monophialides, and *F. moniliforme* differs in forming microconidia in chains or in heads, in lacking chlamydospores and in having sparse production of macroconidia in some isolates (13,15,21). *Fusarium proliferatum*, known so far only from a single case of disseminated disease, resembles *F. moniliforme* in forming microconidia in chains and sparse macroconidia but differs in having conidiogenous cells with two openings (polyphialides) (22).

5. *Phoma* Species

Species of *Phoma* (15,23) (compare *Microsphaeropsis*) form cellular, round or oval, dark-brown pycnidia (fruiting structures containing conidia). Many species are known, some of which can be identified only by association with particular host plants. *Phoma glomerata* (15,23) is an easily recognized species that has been associated with allergic responses and with human infection.

A. ***Phoma glomerata***

a. *Colonial* Colonies appear wet due to masses of conidia in slime, pale to reddish orange in hue, with black specks (pycnidia) in the wet areas, dark brown in hyphal areas.

b. *Microscopic* Conidia are borne from minute phialides that line the inner cavity of the pycnidium. Chains of brown dictyochlamydospores (brown, swollen structures having longitudinal and transverse septa) are common in the hyphae and may initially be mistaken for an *Alternaria*.

c. *Differential* *Microsphaeropsis olivacea* (23) is similar to *Phoma* in forming pycnidia, but conidia are brown rather than hyaline.

6. Basidiomycetous Yeastlike Fungi (Ustilaginales)

Tilletiopsis species and *Ustilago* species are not uncommon as contaminants from many kinds of specimens, including blood.

A. ***Tilletiopsis* species**

This genus accommodates anamorphic yeastlike basidiomycetous fungi that form ballistic conidia. Its higher taxonomic position is still in dispute; moreover, identification to species is difficult (24).

a. *Colonial* White, cream, pinkish cream, or yellowish colonies appear dry and smooth with fine nap of aerial hyphae.

b. *Microscopic* Hyphae septate, narrow, and often showing regions of lysis (some parts of hyphae take up stain whereas other parts do not). Ballistoconidia slightly curved with small blunt end formed from narrow hyphal projections or sterigmata. When ballistic conidia are present, the lid of the petri dish often appears cloudy.

B. ***Ustilago* species**

a. *Colonial* Similar to colonies of *Tilletiopsis* or appearing moist and yeastlike.

b. *Microscopic* Conidia form in chains with youngest at tip; hyphae narrow, septate, showing regions of lysis. Resembles *Hyalodendron*, a hyaline counterpart of *Cladosporium*, but hyphae are very narrow. Some species of *Sporothrix* that produce secondary conidia are also similar.

7. *Sporothrix* Species

The well-known pathogen *Sporothrix schenckii* is not described here (see Refs. 9 and 16). *Ophiostoma stenoceras* occurs on wood and wood products and in similar habitats to *S. schenckii.* Although *S. schenckii* has been suggested to be the anamorph of *O. stenoceras*, based on morphology and nucleic acids, no isolate of the dimorphic *S. schenckii* has been shown to produce a teleomorph.

A. ***Ophiostoma stenoceras* (anamorph *Sporothrix*)**

a. *Significance* Isolated infrequently from nail specimens and reported as possible agent of onychomycosis (10,25).

b. *Colonial* Colonies white, hyphal, may convert to yeast phase at 37°C.

c. *Microscopic* Forms rosettes of slender, ellipsoidal conidia at the apex of erect hyphae; darkly pigmented solitary conidia absent (10,25). If grown on a medium that promotes development of ascigerous states (low carbohydrate or medium containing cellulosic materials) (10,13), black perithecia having small round bases and long slender necks may form. Ascospores are hyaline and shaped like orange segments; they are released from an opening at the neck, where they accumulate in slimy masses.

d. *Differential* Colonies of *S. schenckii* become brown-pigmented in age due to production of darkly colored conidia directly on the sides of the hyphae.

B.* *Sporothrix cyanescens

a. *Significance* Isolated from skin and blood, and from respiratory secretions of several patients following renovations in a hospital but so far known only as a contaminant (26).

b. *Colonial* Colonies white, developing lavender pigmentation and red or blue diffusing pigment; sensitive to cycloheximide.

c. *Microscopic* Conidia borne sympodially from inflated conidiogenous cell or from denticles along the side of a narrow conidiophore. Conidia are borne in two series; primary conidia are ellipsoidal and they bear one to three secondary conidia (26).

8. Aleurioconidial Fungi

A number of fungi produce solitary, usually single-celled conidia that are called aleurioconidia because of their lytic method of dehiscence. Some species additionally produce chains of arthroconidia, which are separated by empty cells. Conidia of some *Chrysosporium* species resemble the microconidia of dermatophytes, whereas conidia of some other species are similar to those of the systemic pathogens (10).

A. *Chrysosporium* anamorph of *Aphanoascus fulvescens*

a. *Significance* Rarely causing dermatophytic-type lesions in humans and animals.

b. *Colonial* Velvety or granular, ivory, becoming buff with development of ascocarps, tolerant of cycloheximide and may demonstrate pH change on dermatophyte test medium.

c. *Microscopic* Pyriform aleuro conidia are produced at the ends or on the sides of stalks, and cylindrical to barrel-shaped alternate arthroconidia are formed within the length of the hypha (i.e., intercolary) (10). Most isolates form brown, globose ascocarps containing rough-walled ascospores.

d. *Differential* Differs from dermatophytes in larger size of single-celled conidia and production of ascocarps.

B. *Emmonsia parva (Chrysosporium parvum)*

a. *Significance* Causes pulmonary or disseminated infection known as adiaspiromycosis (9,27). Large, thick-walled adiaspores in tissue are diagnostic. Two varieties of the species are known (9,10,13).

b. *Colonial* Colonies yellowish-white, buff or tan, glabrous, woolly or powdery.

c. *Microscopic* Aleurioconidia are formed on the sides of the hyphae or at the ends of short unswollen or slightly swollen stalks; swollen ends sometimes produce two or three conidia on narrow denticles. Conidia are slightly flattened and often slightly broader than long. No conversion to yeast phase, but adiaspores are formed at maximum growth temperature (37°C for *E. crescens* and 40°C for *E. parva*).

d. *Differential* Differs from *Blastomyces dermatitidis* by failure to convert to yeast phase, by formation of thick-walled chlamydospores or adiaspores at maximum temperature, and by formation of more than one conidium on swollen stalk.

C. *Myceliophthora thermophila* (formerly *Chrysosporium thermophilum*)

a. *Significance* Recently reported from lung infection in a patient with leukemia (28).

b. *Colonial* A thermophilic mold growing rapidly at 37–45°C forming pink to buff, then cinnamon brown colonies; diffusing pigment produced.

c. *Microscopic* Yellowish to reddish-brown oval, rough-walled conidia formed on short stalks, which are often slightly swollen (10,28).

d. *Differential* Some species of *Myceliophthora* produce a sexual stage in *Corynascus* (15). Round fruiting bodies contain brown, lemon-shaped ascospores.

9. *Scopulariopsis* Species

Many species are known, but *Scopulariopsis brevicaulis* is the commonest as both a contaminant and pathogen (9,10,13). Rare reports document other species as etiologic agents, including dark-colored species connected to ascomycetous stages in *Microascus*.

A. ***Microascus cinereus*** **(anamorph** ***Scopulariopsis*****)**

a. *Significance* Rarely reported from nail, sinus, and lung. In sinus, characteristic fruiting bodies were seen (29).

b. *Colonial* Slow-growing, initially pale, becoming gray to black and granular.

c. *Microscopic* Conidia smooth and oval, slightly pointed at the tip and flattened at the base. Conidiogenous cells (annellides) borne singly on hyphae, or commonly in complex penicillate arrangement, forming conidia in chains with the youngest at the base of the chain. Fruiting bodies black, usually with small nipplelike protuberance, ascospores lens-shaped (almost flattened on one size and hemispherical on other side), pale reddish brown (30).

d. *Differential* *Microascus cirrosus*, also rarely known as a pathogen (31), differs in having fruiting bodies with short necks and ascospores that appear almost heart-shaped (30). *Pseudallescheria boydii* has round fruiting bodies without an opening and conidia are produced in slimy masses (9,13,16).

10. *Paecilomyces* Species

Paecilomyces variotii and *Paecilomyces lilacinus* are well-documented opportunists causing a variety of clinical syndromes including endocarditis and eye disease (9,13). Surgical procedures, prosthetic implants and inadequate sterilization of lenses are risk factors predisposing to infection.

a. *Colonial* Mostly in colors other than green to blue-green as found in *Penicillium*. *Paecilomyces variotii* is rapid-growing, greenish-brown, and powdery; *P. lilacinus* is slower-growing, reddish gray.

b. *Microscopic* Erect conidiophores bearing slender flask-shaped phialides in a whorl with ends of phialides pointing away from stalk (arranged divergently or spread out rather than close together or brushlike, as in *Penicillium*); phialides are sometimes borne on metulae. *Paecilomyces variotii* produces olivaceous brown conidia that are variable in size and shape and occur in long, tangled chains. It also forms solitary terminal or lateral conidia (9,13,15). *Paecilomyces lilacinus* produces phialides on rough walled conidiophores and conidia are small and pointed at each end (9,13,15).

11. *Chaetomium* Species

a. *Significance* A homothallic ascomycete occasionally isolated as contaminant; some species rarely involved in nail infection, peritonitis, subcutaneous infection, brain abscess, and disseminated disease (9,10,16,32).

A. ***Chaetomium globosum***

a. *Colonial* Growth rapid, filling petri dish within 7–10 days, colonies yellowish-green or yellowish-gray. Suspect *Chaetomium* when fast-growing fungus remains sterile on rich media.

b. *Microscopic* Fruits on media such as oatmeal salts or cornmeal agar, forming oval fruiting bodies (perithecia) that are covered with sterile, wavy, or undulate hairs. Ascospores are released through an opening at the tip and are brown and lemon-shaped (10,15,16,32).

c. *Differential* Many species are known but *Chaetomium globosum* is the commonest, occurring as both a contaminant and pathogen. *Chaetomium atrobrunneum* and *Chaetomium strumarium* are known from disseminated disease and localized infection involving the brain (32). These species differ from *C. globosum* in the smaller size of the ascocarps, the nature of the ascomatal hairs and their higher optimum growth temperatures (32).

12. *Ochroconis gallopavum* (Also Known as *Dactylaria gallopava*)

a. *Significance* This thermotolerant fungus causes epidemic disease of chickens and turkeys. In humans, it has been recovered from lesions of brain and skin and isolated from sputum, especially in coal mine workers (9,16).

b. *Colonial* Faster growing at 37°C than at 25°C, colonies reddish-brown, usually with diffusing reddish-brown pigment.

c. *Microscopic* One or two single-septate conidia are borne at the ends of peglike conidiogenous cells and released by fracture (rhexolysis) of a thin-walled cell (9).

13. *Scytalidium* Species

Scytalidium includes fungi that form arthroconidia by division of the hyphae into rectangular segments. Both light- and dark-colored species are included in the genus.

a. Significance *Scytalidium dimidiatum* and *Scytalidium hyalinum* cause dermatophytic-type infections of the nail, toe webs, and glabrous skin, especially in immigrants from parts of Africa, India, and the Caribbean (10,13,33). Subcutaneous and disseminated infections are rarely known (13,33).

A. ***Scytalidium dimidiatum*** **(synanamorph *Nattrassia mangiferae*, Formerly Known as *Hendersonula toruloidea*)**

a. Colonial Rapid-growing (filling petri dish in 7 days), black, ropy, black diffusing pigment, cycloheximide-sensitive.

b. Microscopic Hyphae variable in width (2.5–10 μm) and color, initially light-colored to dark brown, often surrounded by brown slime; hyphae break apart to form arthroconidia of varying width (2.5–7 μm or up to 16 μm). Some isolates produce pycnidia of the *Nattrassia* stage when grown on appropriate media. Two different forms are recognized by growth rates, abundance of arthroconidia, and production of pycnidia (13,33).

c. Differential *Scytalidium hyalinum* is similar in growth rate and cycloheximide sensitivity, but arthroconidia are hyaline, colonies are cream-colored, and they fail to develop pycnidia (13,33).

14. Black Yeastlike Fungi

This group includes several genera in which initial growth consists of yeastlike cells. The mechanism of development of the daughter cells varies among the genera.

A. ***Wangiella dermatitidis***

a. Significance Involved in a variety of infectious processes ranging from onychomycosis to subcutaneous and disseminated disease, with a tendency to involve the central nervous system (16,34).

b. Colonial Slow-growing, mucoid, and often stringy when manipulated, gray to black, becoming velvety with development of aerial mycelium. Most isolates grow at 40°C.

c. Microscopic Initial growth consists of oval budding cells, then developing hyphae that bear conidiogenous cells on the sides or at the tips of lateral branches (16,34,35). Conidiogenous cells produce conidia successively without apparent elongation of the tip of the cell and are often referred to as phialides without collarettes. Conidia are slimy and accumulate at the tip or slide down the side of the conidiogenous cell.

d. *Differential* The correct name for the fungus is still in dispute. It differs from *Exophiala jeanselmei* in having conidiogenous cells that do not usually elongate, in having a higher-growth temperature maximum (40°C), and in being unable to utilize potassium nitrate. Most species of *Phaeococcomyces* fail to develop hyphae.

B. ***Exophiala jeanselmei***

a. *Significance* Causes mycetoma and subcutaneous infection.

b. *Colonial* Slow-growing, initial yeast phase transitory in many isolates, pasty and gray to black, developing gray mycelium; temperature maximum near 37°C. Yeast phase may be enhanced on PDA.

c. *Microscopic* Initial growth consists of yeastlike cells; hyphal stage developing conidiogenous cells at the tip or on the sides of lateral branches; conidiogenous cells (annellides) elongating at the tip during successive production of conidia and becoming tapered; conidia borne in slimy masses (15,16,35). The yeast stage has been called *Phaeoannellomyces elegans* by some mycologists (16).

15. *Curvularia, Bipolaris, and Exserohilum* Species

a. *Significance* Rare to common as contaminants depending upon geographic area and increasingly important as agents of eye infection, sinusitis, and both subcutaneous and disseminated infection (9,16).

b. *Colonial* Rapid-growing, light gray, becoming dark gray to black as sporulation commences.

c. *Microscopic* Conidiophores erect, producing a solitary terminal conidium and then extending to form a zig-zag (geniculate) conidiogenous axis with solitary conidia produced in apical succession (sympodial). Conidia are large, multicellular, and thick-walled, with dark septa. Those of *Curvularia* are curved with the central cell larger, whereas those of *Exserohilum* and *Bipolaris* are straight (15,16,35). The latter genera include several medically important species formerly classified in *Drechslera*.

d. *Differential* Conidia of *Ulocladium* and *Alternaria* differ in having longitudinal and transverse septa (muriform or dictyoconidia) (15).

REFERENCES

1. Anaissie E, Bodey GP, Kantarjian H, et al. New spectrum of fungal infections with cancer. Rev Infect Dis 1989;11:369–378.
2. Anaissie EP, Bodey GP, Rinaldi MG. Emerging fungal pathogens. Eur J Clin Microbiol Infect Dis 1989;8:323–331.
3. Gradon JD, Timpone JG, Schnittman SM. Emergence of unusual opportunistic pathogens in AIDS: A review. Clin Infect Dis 1992;15:134–157.
4. Musial CA, Cokerill FR, Roberts GD. Fungal infections of the immunocompromised host: Clinical and laboratory aspects. Clin Microbiol Rev 1988;1: 349–364.
5. Padhye AA. Hyalohyphomycosis. In: Balows A, Hausler WJ Jr, Ohashi M, Turano A. et al, eds. Laboratory Diagnosis of Infectious Diseases. Principles and Practice: Vol I. Bacterial, Mycotic and Parasitic Diseases. New York: Springer-Verlag, 1988:654–662.
6. Perfect JR, Schell WA, Rinaldi MG. Uncommon invasive fungal pathogens in the acquired immunodeficiency syndrome. J Med Vet Mycol 1993;31: 175–179.
7. Vartivarian SE, Anaissie EJ, Bodey GP. Emerging fungal pathogens in immunocompromised patients: Classification, diagnosis, management. Clin Infect Dis 1993;17(suppl 2):S487–S491.
8. Weitzman I. Saprophytic molds as agents of cutaneous and subcutaneous infection in the immunocompromised host. Arch Dermatol 1988;122: 161–168.
9. Kwon-Chung KJ, Bennett, JE. Medical Mycology. Philadelphia: Lea & Febiger, 1992:1–866.
10. Kane J, Summerbell RC, Sigler L, et al. Handbook of Dermatophytes: A Clinical Guide and Laboratory Manual of Dermatophytes and Other Filamentous Fungi from Skin, Hair and Nails. Belmont, CA: Star Publishing, 1996. In press.
11. Sigler L. Preparing and mounting slide cultures. In: Isenberg HD, ed. Clinical Microbiology Procedures Handbook. Washington, DC: American Society of Microbiology 1992:6.12.1–6.12.4.
12. McGinnis MR. Laboratory Handbook of Medical Mycology. New York: Academic Press, 1980:1–661.
13. Kennedy MJ, Sigler L. Aspergillus, Fusarium, and other opportunistic moniliaceous fungi. In: Murray PR, Baron EJ, Pfaller MA, et al, eds. Manual of Clinical Microbiology, 6th ed. Washington, DC: American Society of Microbiology 1995:765–790.
14. Dixon DM, Fromtling RA. Morphology, taxonomy and classification of the fungi. In: Murray PR, Baron EJ, Pfaller MA, et al, ed. Manual of Clinical Microbiology, 6th ed. Washington, DC: American Society of Microbiology, 1995:699–708.
15. Domsch KH, Gams W, Anderson T-H. Compendium of Soil Fungi. Vols 1 & 2. Eching, Germany: IHW-Verlag 1980 (reprint 1993).

16. Schell WA, Pasarell L, Salkin IF, McGinnis MR. Bipolaris, Exophiala, Scedosporium, Sporothrix and other dematiaceous fungi. In: Murray PR et al, ed. Manual of Clinical Microbiology. 6th ed. Washington, DC: American Society of Microbiology, 1995:825–846.
17. de Hoog GS, Buiting A, Tan CS, et al. Diagnostic problems with imported cases of mycetoma in the Netherlands. Mycoses 1993;36:81–87.
18. de Hoog GS, Smith MTH. Hyphozyma a new genus of yeast-like Hyphomycetes. Ant v Leeuw 1981;47:339–352.
19. Gams W, McGinnis MR. Phialemonium, a new anamorphic genus intermediate between Phialophora and Acremonium. Mycologia 1983;75:977–987.
20. King D, Pasarell L, Dixon DM, et al. A phaeohyphomycotic cyst and peritonitis caused by Phialemonium species and a reevaluation of its taxonomy. J Clin Microbiol 1993;31:1804–1810.
21. Nelson PE, Toussoun TA, Marasas, WFO. Fusarium species: An Illustrated Manual of Identification. State College, PA: Pennsylvania State University Press, 1983:1–193.
22. Summerbell RC, Richardson SE, Kane J. Fusarium proliferatum as an agent of disseminated infection in an immunocompromised patient. J Clin Microbiol 1988;26:82–87.
23. Sutton BC. The Coelomycetes. Kew, England: Commonwealth Mycological Institute 1980:1–696.
24. Boekhout T. A revision of ballistoconidia-forming yeasts and fungi. Stud Mycol 1991;33:1–194.
25. Summerbell RC, Kane J, Krajden S, Duke EE. Medically important Sporothrix species and related ophiostomatoid fungi. In: Wingfield MJ, Seifert KA, Webber JF, eds. Ceratocystis and Ophiostoma, Taxonomy, Ecology and Pathogenicity, St.Paul, MN: APS Press, 1993:185–192.
26. Sigler L, Harris JL, Dixon DM, et al: Microbiology and potential virulence of Sporothrix cyanescens, a fungus rarely isolated from blood and skin. J Clin Microbiol 1990;28:1009–1015.
27. Echavarria E, Cano EL, Restrepo A. Disseminated adiaspiromycosis in a patient with AIDS. J Med Vet Mycol 1993;31:91–97.
28. Bourbeau P, McGough DA, Fraser H, et al. Fatal disseminated infection caused by Myceliophthora thermophila, a new agent of mycosis: Case history and laboratory characteristics. J Clin Microbiol 1992;30:3019–3023.
29. Lacey J. Microascus cinereus (Emile-Weil & Gaudin) Curzi: A human pathogen? Mycopathologia 1986;96:137–142.
30. Barron GL, Cain RF, Gilman JC. The genus Microascus. Can J Bot 1961; 39:1609–1631.
31. Krisher, KK, Holdridge NB, Mustafa MM, et al. Disseminated Microascus cirrosus infection in a pediatric bone marrow transplant patient. J Clin Microbiol 1995;33:735–737.
32. Abbott SP, Sigler L, McAleer R, et al. Fatal cerebral mycoses caused by the ascomycete Chaetomium strumarium. J Clin Microbiol 1995;33:2692–2698.
33. Moore MK. The infection of human skin and nail by Scytalidium species.

In: Borgers M, Hay R, Rinaldi MG, eds. Current Topics in Medical Mycology. New York: Springer-Verlag, 1992;1–42.
34. Matsumoto T, Matsuda T, McGinnis MR, Ajello L. Clinical and mycological spectra of Wangiella dermatitidis infections. Mycoses 1993;36:145–155.
35. Dixon DM, Polak-Wyss A. The medically important dematiaceous fungi and their identification. Mycoses 1990;34:1–18.

6

Ultrastructure of Fungi

MARCEL BORGERS
Janssen Research Foundation
Beerse, Belgium

I. INTRODUCTION

Advances made in the characterization of the detailed substructure of various yeasts and fungi have helped greatly to subdivide and classify different species and strains. The introduction of auxiliary methodologies such as cytochemistry, immunocytochemistry, and in situ hybridization to support descriptive ultrastructure has enabled us to document factors that govern virulence, mutant formation, morphogenetic transition of forms, invasiveness, and other aspects of pathogenicity, and host-fungal interactions.

The aim of this short review is to give an update on the ultrastructure of the main classes of medically important fungi—i.e., the filamentous and dimorphic fungi. In addition, the effects of antifungal treatment on the ultrastructure of these species are described.

The descriptive ultrastructure of yeasts and both dimorphic and filamentous fungi under in vitro culture conditions or in situ during infection of the host has been reported (1–3). Morphological characterization has been done using scanning electron microscopy (SEM) to display the surface structure, transmission electron microscopy (TEM) to reveal the internal subcellular organelles, and freeze-fracture electron microscopy to detail intramembranous molecular structures.

Complementary techniques to fill morphological "lacunes"—such as ultrastructural cytochemistry of enzymes, microanalysis of elements, autoradiography, specific and/or selective stains for carbohydrates, lipids, proteins, RNA, and DNA, and, last but not least, immunocytochemistry—have been essential to elucidate many basic questions and problems related to the structural identification and the interrelationships of subcellular entities (4).

II. FILAMENTOUS FUNGI

A. Dermatophytes

Filamentous fungi such as *Trichophyton rubrum*, *Trichophyton mentagrophytes*, and *Microsporum canis* can easily be fixed and prepared for electron microscopic examination, and all subcellular organelles are usually well displayed. The different subcellular compartments found in these fungi are largely the same as those of all other pathogenic fungi, including yeast as well as dimorphic and pleomorphic species. Easily recognized organelles in the septate hyphae are the relatively thin cell wall, plasma membrane, nuclei, round to oval-shaped mitochondria, Woronin bodies located at the septal pores, sparse profiles of endoplasmic reticulum, and numerous lipid bodies. Although varying from cell to cell, a prominent number of variously sized vacuoles are present in the cytoplasm. Their size usually increases with the age of the cells. In view of the fact that the enzymatic content comprises a large number of hydrolases, the vacuolar system may be considered a lysosomal (digestive) structure. The cytosol is filled with ribrosomes and varying amounts of glycogen.

With the exception of the cell wall, which is usually much thicker, the ultrastructure of dermatophytes found in infected skin is very similar to that found under culture conditions.

This is the case for fungi residing in and between the cells, constituting the stratum corneum, as well as those residing in the hair sheaths and shafts (5). A remarkable observation is that inflammatory cells, which infiltrate enmass the site of dermatophyte infection, are never seen in the process of engulfment of an infectious organism (6). A representative picture of *T. mentagrophytes*, in which all the substructures described above are visible, is given in Fig. 1. The ability of dermatophytes to invade the stratum corneum as well as the outer and inner hair structures is well demonstrated with SEM (Fig. 2).

B. *Aspergillus fumigatus*

Aspergillus fumigatus, is a filamentous mold whose substructures vary in number, shape, and size in relation to its developmental stage.

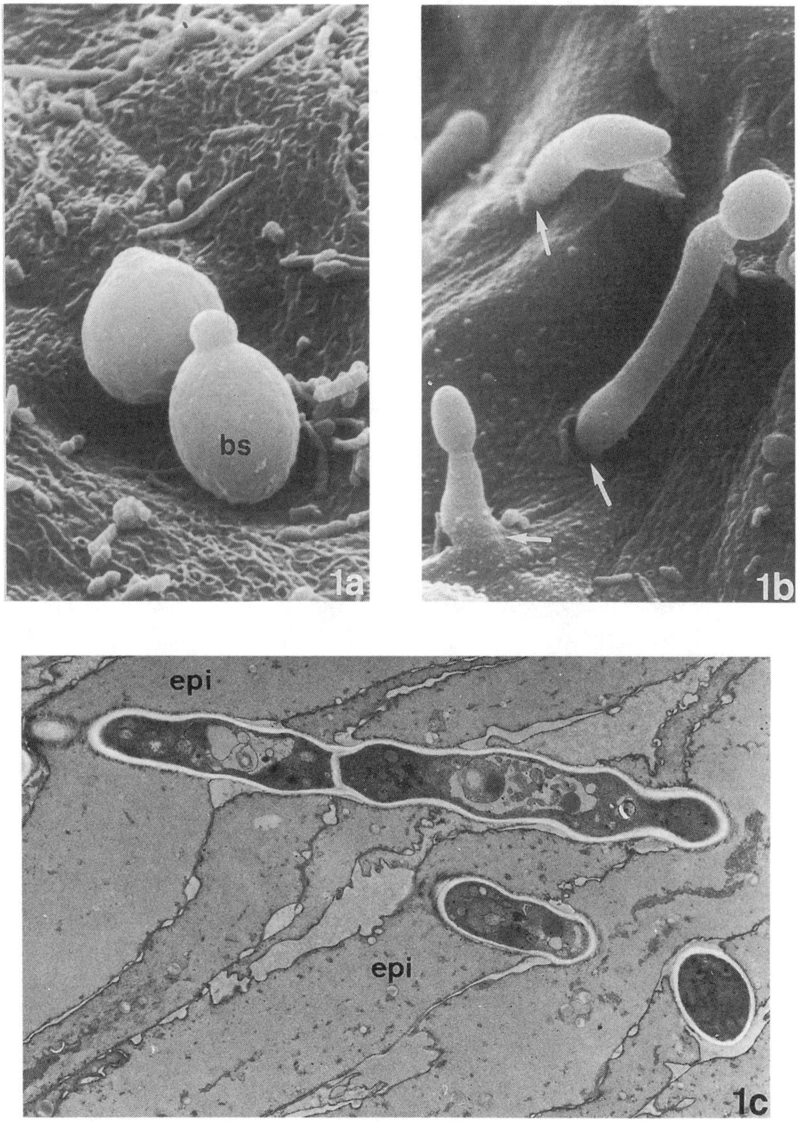

Figure 1 Vaginal candidiasis. a and b. Scanning electron microscopy (SEM) of the mucosal surface of the vagina infected with *Candida albicans* (a) 2 hr after infection with blastospores (bs) and (b) 24 hr later, when blastospores have transformed into hyphae that invade (arrows) the squamous epithelium. (a: ×5100; b: ×2300.) c. Transmission electron microscopy (TEM) showing hyphae penetrating through various layers consisting of squamous epithelial cells (epi). (×5440.)

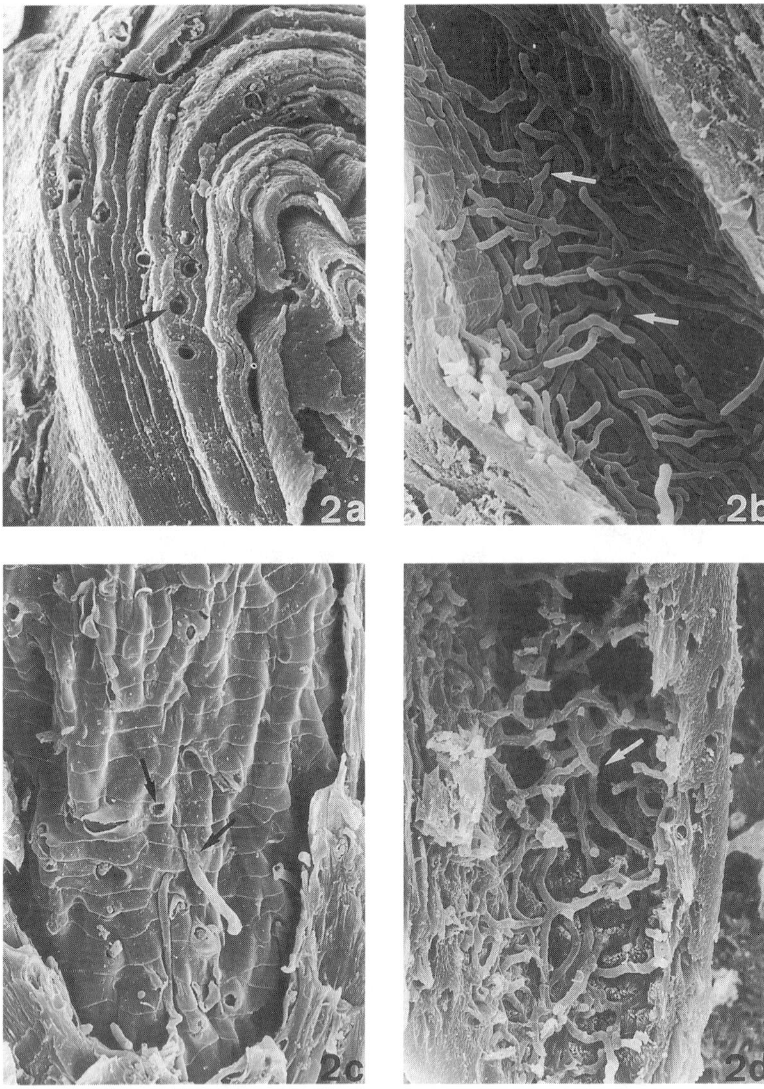

Figure 2 Scanning electron microscopy of *Trichophyton mentagrophytes* infection of guinea pig skin. Stratum corneum (a), hair sheath after removal of hair (b), surface of hair (c), and inner hair structure (d). Note many dermatophyte elements (arrows) penetrating the corneocytes and the hair sheaths and shafts. (a: ×1460; b: ×730; c: ×900; d: ×730.)

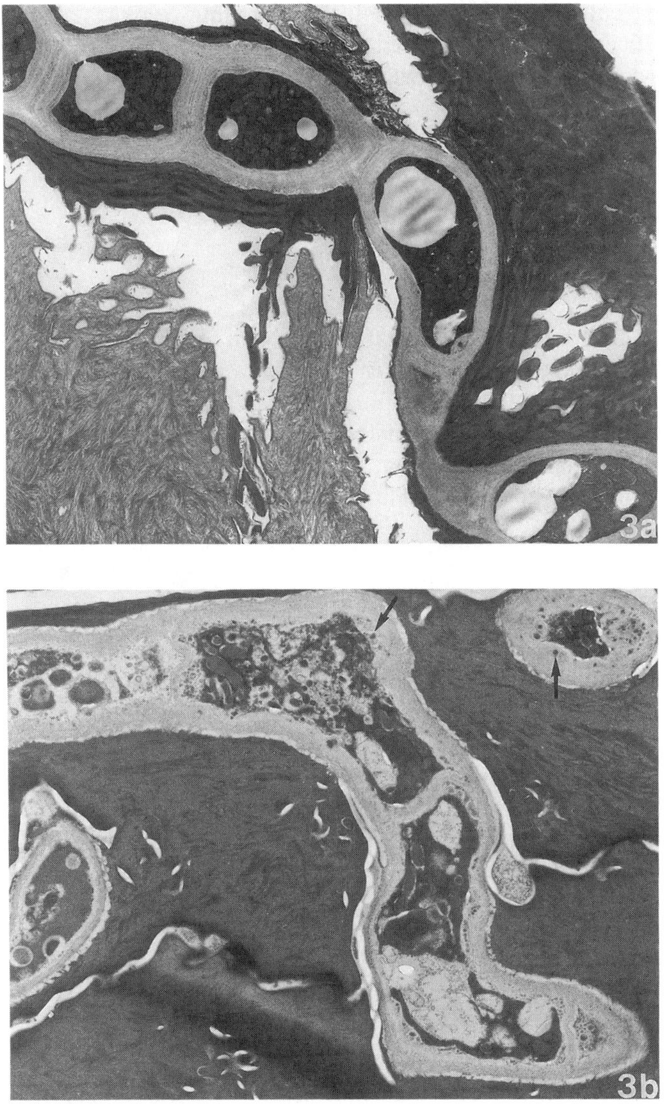

Figure 3 Transmission electron microscopy of *T. mentagrophytes* infection of guinea pig skin. a. In untreated skin, T. mentagrophytes is seen in the stratum corneum (×7830.) b. After 2 days itraconazole treatment. Note the thickened cell wall (cw), in which numerous phospholipid vesicles (arrows) have settled. Cytoplasmic organelles are in various stages of degeneration. (×8610.)

Young cultures consisting of long branching hyphae are thin-walled septate structures that contain many small nuclei, elongated mitochondria, and a cytosol that is filled with ribosomes and clusters of peripherally located glycogen. When grown to maturity, fully developed spore-bearing vesicles are formed (Fig. 3). The cell walls of the spores are laminated and much thicker than those of the originating segments. Hence the substructures are more difficult to discern.

III. DIMORPHIC FUNGI

The restricted permeation of fixatives through the thick cell wall of species such as *Candida albicans* and *Pityrosporum ovale* has hampered the identification of subcellular structures for a long time (3). Only recently, with the advent of microwave-assisted techniques, has this problem been largely solved in the sense that structures are rapidly immobilized and fixatives quickly reach the cell interior, resulting in a detailed visualization of all substructures.

A. *Candida albicans*

Candida albicans is polymorphic and grows as multipolarly budding yeasts, as pseudohyphae of elongated yeastlike cells, and as true septate hyphae (mycelium) (7). Both the true hyphae and pseudohyphae may regenerate the yeast phase by producing clusters of yeastlike blastospores. Morphogenetic and ultrastructural aspects have been reported extensively (1,4). The yeast cell wall is a laminated structure from 100 to 300 nm thick consisting five to eight layers of different density, depending on the culture conditions and the fixation procedure used.

Yeast cells have ovoid nuclei, round to elongated mitochondria containing linearly arranged cristae, ribosomes, sparse profiles of endoplasmic reticulum often connected with the nuclear membrane, and a vacuolar system. The cytoplasm is surrounded by an undulating cell membrane, which possesses tubular invaginations called lomasomes.

In budding cells, new cell material evaginates from a polar site and enlarges to a diameter less than that of the parent cell. The nucleus migrates into the neck region between parent and bud, where it divides and a septum is formed. Mitochondria and membranous strands are transported from the parent to the daughter cells. The septum is laid down centripetally in two stages: an electron-transparent, primary septum is followed by secondary deposition of material of higher electron density on each side of the primary septum. After separation, the primary and secondary septa remain as part of the mother cell wall and form a bud scar; the secondary septum alone forms the birth scar of the daughter cell.

During mycelial development, new cell material grows in an elongated form, the nucleus migrates into the neck of the germ tube, and a septum is formed in two stages, as in yeast. A transit of all organelles into the germ tube can be observed. Mitochondria elongate and sometimes reach a length of 10 μm.

Germ tube formation from yeast cells is accompanied by substantial rearrangement of the cell wall layers. The common finding is that the cell walls of germ tubes are thinner than those of parent yeast cells. This is also obvious under in vivo circumstances; thus a yeast can be distinguished from a transverse-cut mycelium in an electron microscopic section simply by the difference in wall thickness.

The pseudohyphal (pseudomycelial) morphology of *C. albicans* consists of elongated yeasts possessing complete septa. Individual cells range from 2 to 5 μm in diameter and reach 26 to 30 μm in length.

True hyphal (mycelial) cells of *C. albicans* are usually longer and thinner than yeast cells and measure from 0.8 to 1.3 μm in diameter. A perforated septum of 0.17–0.22 μm in width, with no evidence of Woronin bodies or septal plugs, separates the hyphal cells. The hyphal cell plasma membrane is significantly different from the yeast cell membrane and exhibits invaginations that are deeper and much more frequent.

Under some conditions, the hyphae or pseudohyphae of *C. albicans* produce chlamydospores. These are thick-walled, nondeciduous, intercalary or terminal asexual spores. Chlamydospores have a double- or triple-layered cell wall, which is much thicker than that of the yeast or mycelial cell and is continuous with that of the "suspensor" cell (1).

In infection, a transformation from the noninvasive or less invasive yeast form into the invasive hyphal form takes place, and like dermatophytes that penetrate the inner hair structures, *C. albicans* mycelium penetrates squamous epithelium such as the vaginal mucosa (Fig. 4).

B. *Cocciodioides immitis*

Coccidioides immitis exhibits a unique dimorphism characterized by the transition of arthroconidia into spherules. The arthroconidia are derived by disarticulation of a saprophytic mycelial phase consisting of septate hyphae. The arthroconidia are usually barrel-shaped, measuring 2.5 by 3–6 μm. The spherules, which become as large as 80 μm or more in diameter, develop by the isotropic enlargement of the arthroconidia and give rise to a self-perpetuating spherule-endospore phase.

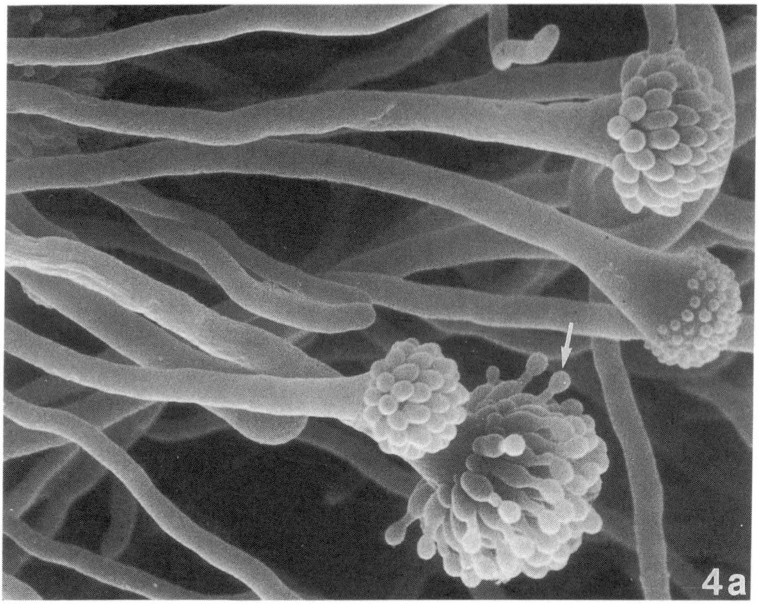

Figure 4 Aspergillus fumigatus in culture. a. Scanning electron microscopy of a culture showing the fungus in different stages of development. The mature form bears fully developed spores (arrow). (×1260.) b and c. Transmission electron microscopy of mature culture of *A. fumigatus* showing vesicles (ve) with sterigmata (st) and spores (sp). Untreated culture (a) and culture after exposure to 0.14 μg/ml of itraconazole (b). Note the complete degeneration of the vesicle (ve) and sterigmata (st). Only few spores (sp) remain morphologically unaltered. (b: ×3600; c: ×9075.)

Reproductive growth of the spherule-endospore phase in the host or in vitro is via liberation of endospores followed by their development into new endosporulating spherules. Detailed ultrastructure of *C. immitis* is given in the work of Sun et al. (8). Most arthroconidia contain two or three nuclei but may have as few as one or as many as eight. At first, cells of the spherule are multinucleate, but as cleavage continues, the number of nuclei per cell becomes diminished until each endospore has one or rarely two nuclei. Upon maturation, the spherule walls begin to rupture and endospores are released.

Electron microscopic studies demonstrate that the spherule wall is approximately 0.5 μm or more in thickness and is composed of at least two layers. Upon transition of spherules to mycelium, the outer electron-dense

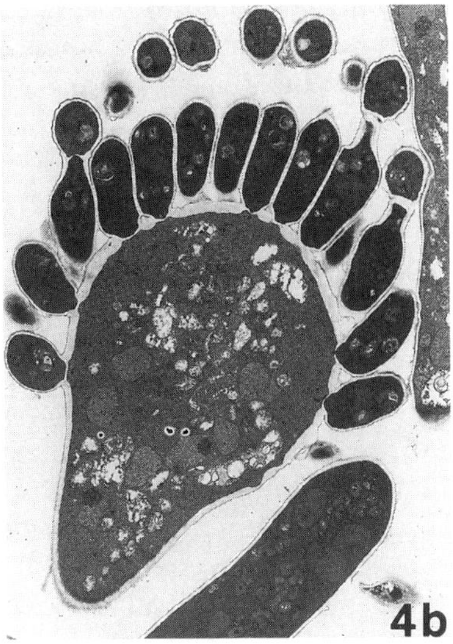

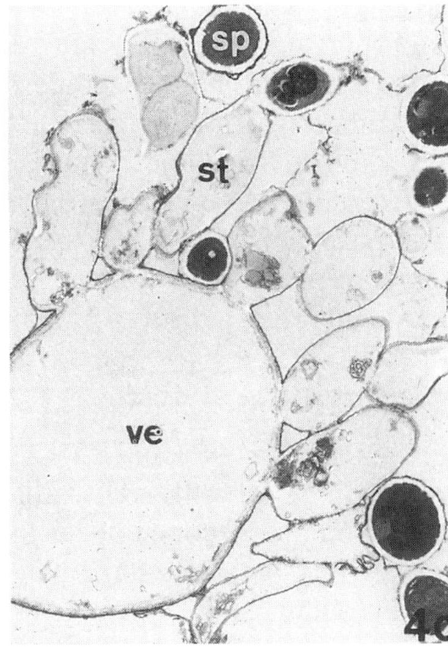

layer of the wall ruptures and the inner, less electron-dense portion becomes continuous with the wall of the germ tube. The new germ tube wall is 0.15 μm in thickness. Simple septa, septal pores, Woronin bodies, and septal pore plugs are characteristically seen in *C. immitis* mycelial cells.

C. *Paracoccidioides brasiliensis*

This dimorphic fungus is present in a saprophytic filamentous form and a parasitic form, which is that of a multiple budding yeast (9).

Blastoconidia are 2–3 μm in diameter and are directly associated with hyphae or borne singly on the tips of short conidiophores. Chlamydospores, ranging in size from 6.5–30 μm in diameter, are found on the hyphae.

Hyphae have cell dimensions of 0.8–2.4 μm by 6.4–29 μm. These cells are multinucleate and possess mesosomes, lomasomes, and numerous mitochondria whose long axes are parallel to those of the hyphal unit. Very often, the cytosol is filled with lipid globules and concentric lamellae or myelinlike structures. The cell walls of the hyphae are 80–150 nm in width and are composed of one to three discernible layers. The outermost layer is electron-dense and displays finely fibrillar material.

The parasitic morphology is that of a budding yeast and can be of two types. The first involves the production of narrow-necked buds, 2–10 μm in diameter, whereas the second involves cryptosporulation. In the latter, the chromatin is divided into chromidia, which function as potential spores. The chromidia become associated with the cell membrane and form numerous small buds, which encircle the mother cell. The cell wall is 0.2–0.6 μm thick and comprises from one to three layers (9).

The production of elongated buds with diameters greater than those of the hyphae indicates a yeast-mycelium transition. These multinucleate transitional cells have thinner cell walls than do mother yeast cells and also have perforated septa similar to those found in hyphae.

D. *Sporothrix schenckii*

Hyphae of *S. schenckii* are 1.5–3 μm in diameter, septate, and granular in appearance. Hyphal cell walls are thin (80–140 nm thick) and under the electron microscope appear to be bilayered. Pyriform to ovoid conidia arise laterally on the hyphae or from the conidiophore regions.

The yeast phase of *S. schenckii* ranges in shape from fusiform to spherical, but no cytoplasmic differences correlate with the different cell shapes. The yeast wall is bilayered and consists of an inner, electron-transparent layer and an outer, electron-dense layer (1).

Osmiophilic microfibrillar material is apparent at the outermost cell wall surface of yeastlike cells of *S. schenckii* but is much less apparent or even lacking at the outer cell walls of the corresponding mycelial phase.

Subcellular organelles of the cytoplasm are similar to those in other dimorphic organisms.

E. *Pityrosporum ovale*

Pityrosporum ovale cells in culture are characterized by a very thick, electron-dense cell wall that is closely apposed to the undulating plasma membrane. Due to its thick, impermeable wall structure, adequate visualization of intracellular substructures is more difficult in *P. ovale* than in the other dimorphic organisms. Characteristic for the ultrastructure of *P. ovale*, besides its wall, are the highly regular indentations of the plasma membrane, the virtual absence of a central vacuolar system, and the high amount of lipid globules in the cytosol.

Induction of the yeast-hyphae phase transition under in vitro conditions is possible by adding stratum corneum cells to *P. ovale* cultures (10). These cells resemble the short hyphae found in patients with pityriasis versicolor. Invasion of squamous cells by hyphae was seen only in patients with pityriasis versicolor, not under the above described in vitro condition. A characteristic cell wall, very similar to that of the yeasts as far as thickness and density is concerned, is present in the invading hyphae.

IV. ULTRASTRUCTURAL CHANGES AFTER ANTIFUNGAL TREATMENT

The correlates of antifungal treatment at the level of fungal ultrastructure are well documented for most antimycotic families, and this for both in vitro and in vivo circumstances (3).

The knowledge acquired during the last two decades on the ultrastructural correlates of antifungal action has contributed in a considerable way to the understanding of the mode of action of the principal antimycotic drugs, such as amphotericin B, griseofulvin, 5-fluorocytosine, azole derivatives, and allylamines. Depending on the nature and function of the attained target, a drug exerts fungicidal effects, morphologically expressed by subcellular necrosis and plasmalemmal breakdown or will be merely fungiastatic and act preferentially or uniquely against certain species. The morphological counterpart of a fungistatic effect is complex and varies from slight mitochondrial swelling, plasmalemmal proliferation, cell-wall thickening, deposition of abnormal membranous bodies in the cell wall, to a huge increase in cell volume with proliferation of peroxisomes and intracellular vacuolar extention (Figs. 1 and 4).

The subcellular target organelles and molecular target sites for antimycotic action have been established for most antifungal drugs. Polyenes like amphotericin B bind irreversibly to cell membranes, and the alteration in permeability of these structures precedes metabolic disruption and cell death. Ultrastructurally, all subcellular organelles deteriorate simultaneously, although cell wall changes are less obvious. Griseofulvin deteriorates spindle and cytoplasmic microtubules, thereby influencing cell division and outgrowth of hyphal tips. 5-Fluorocytosine (5-FC), once deaminated and phosphorylated, incorporates in RNA, which impairs protein synthesis. Another metabolite of 5-FC inhibits DNA synthesis. Nuclear degeneration and cytosol clumping of proteins are the predominant structural changes. Azole derivatives, through their interaction with cytochrome P450–dependent 14α-demethylase inhibit the biosynthesis of ergosterol and hence methylated sterols accumulate, thereby compromising ion homeostasis, normal growth, morphogenetic transformation and cell viability. Cell-wall and vacuolar alterations are typical for azole treatment (Figs. 1 and 4). Allylamines affect sterol synthesis in a manner similar to the azoles, although through interference with squalene expoxidase. Morphologically, the early changes to be observed at the cell periphery and the central vacuolar system (11) are very similar to those seen after azole treatment. The ability to induce cell necrosis after short exposure periods is, however, dissimilar between these antifungal compounds, at least for some dimorphic fungi and *Aspergillus* species.

REFERENCES

1. Garrison RG. Ultrastructural cytology of pathogenic fungi. In: Howard DH, ed. Fungi Pathogenic for Humans and Animals. New York: Marcel Dekker, 1983:229–321.
2. Szaniszlo PJ, Jacobs CW, Gers PA. Dimorphism: Morphological and biochemical aspects. In: Howard DH, ed. Fungi Pathogenic for Humans and Animals. New York: Marcel Dekker, 1983:323–463.
3. Borgers M. Ultrastructural correlates of antimycotic treatment. In: McGinnis MR, ed. Current Topics in Medical Mycology. Vol 2. New York: Springer-Verlag, 1988:1–39.
4. De Nollin S, Thoné F, Borgers M. Enzyme cytochemistry of Candida albicans. J Histochem Cytochem 1975;23:758–765.
5. Jansen T, Xhonneux B, Borgers M, et al. An investigation into the mechanism of action of itraconazole and terbinafine in experimental trichophytosis. Eur J Dermatol 1993;3:43–49.
6. Borgers M, Xhonneux B, Van Cutsem J. Oral itraconazole versus topical bifonazole treatment in experimental dermatophytosis. Mycoses 1993;36: 105–115.
7. Odds FC. Candida and Candidosis. Monograph. London: Bailliere Tindall, 1988:22–41.
8. Sun SH, Sekhon SS, Huppert M. Electron microscopic studies of saprobic and parasitic forms of Coccidioides immitis. Sabouraudia 1979;17:265–273.
9. San-Blas G. Paracoccidioides brasiliensis: Cell wall glucons, pathogenicity and dimorphism. In: McGinnis MR, ed. Current Topics in Medical Mycology. Vol 1. New York: Springer-Verlag, 1995:235–257.
10. Faergemann J. A new model for growth and filament production of Pityrosporium ovale on stratum corneum in vitro. J Invest Dermatol 1989;92: 117–119.
11. Meingassner JG, Sleytr U, Petranyi G. Morphological changes induced by naftifine, a new antifungal agent, in Trichophyton mentagrophytes. J Invest Dermatol 1981;77:444–451.

7

Cell-Mediated Immunity Mechanisms in Fungal Infections

ANTONIO CASSONE
Istituto Superiore di Sanità
Rome, Italy

I. INTRODUCTION

Although there is no doubt about the presence of valid immune responses aimed at prohibiting pathogenic fungi from infecting and causing disease in the normal human host, the relative efficacy and participation of the various arms of these responses is, for the most part, unknown or incompletely known. This largely depends on the difficulties of exactly interpreting clinical immunological data, where often the *cause* is not easily distinguished from the *consequence* or from a mere phenomenological effect. On the other hand, the results obtained from in vitro and ex vivo cellular or organ systems, as well as from animal experiments, are always difficult to extrapolate to the human clinical situation, given their artefactual nature as well as the low degree of similarity in the genetic background of, for instance, an inbred mouse to that of a "wild-type" human being!

Nonetheless, there are sound reasons to believe that cell-mediated immunity (CMI) plays an important, sometimes predominant role against many fungal infections in humans. Patients with primary or acquired T-cell immunodeficiency—for instance, those with the acquired immunodeficiency syndrome (AIDS), the landmark of which is the well-known deletion, first functional and then numerical, of $CD4^+$ T cells, an essential component of the CMI response—are exquisitely susceptible to a number of deep-seated or superficial fungal infections. Treatments involving therapeutic compounds with a well-demonstrated, strong effect on CMI responses (e.g., corticosteroids) have long been known as a major predisposing factor to fungal disease. Human pathogenic fungi have evolved a number of mechanisms (not dealt with in depth here) giving them the chance to escape from or attenuate the consequences of the immune response. In vivo growth under different forms (polymorphism), phenotypic switching, antigenic variation, and molecular mimicry are widespread among fungi. Some of these mechanisms affect antigens that are recognized targets of the CMI in a protected individual. Finally, the *association* between an altered CMI response and the onset or spread of fungal infection is in several cases rather tight and cannot be dismissed simply as fungus-procured immunosuppression.

This chapter gives examples of the importance of CMI in the fight against fungal pathogens; outlines how this essential host response must be finely tuned to avoid an exaggerated, host-harmful expression; and shows how CMI must be working in concert with other essential arms of the immune response in order to avoid infection or disease. In reviewing the subject, I assume that the reader is somewhat acquainted with basic immunology, in particular the terminology, definitions, and activities of T cells, MHC-restriction, macrophages, and cytokines (see below). The list of references at the end of this chapter includes basic immunology and mycology textbooks (1–4) and several reviews or recent papers that are recommended as further readings (5–19).

II. CONCEPTS AND DEFINITIONS

By definition, CMI covers a complex of acquired, adaptive immune responses by which antigen-specific T cells directly kill a pathogen or a pathogen-infected host cell and/or help cells of natural immunity (e.g., a macrophage or a polymorphonuclear leukocyte) to kill the ingested or noningested pathogen. In the former case, the effector cell is generally but not exclusively a $CD8^+$ *T-cytotoxic lymphocyte*, whereas in the latter case, $CD4^+$ *T-helper lymphocytes* are involved.

Central to this definition is that CMI responses are mediated by T cells and are directed against a foreign intracellular or extracellular parasite or even a host cell recognized as "foreign" or "parasitic," such as tumor or transplanted cells. Consequently, an antigen-specific CMI response can be transferred by cells (adoptively) from an immune to a nonimmune (naive) animal. The adoptive transfer is the classic operation by which the experimental immunologist demonstrates that an immune response is mediated by cells rather than by antibodies. Although evidence exists that adequately primed (and helped) T lymphocytes can kill a phagocytic cell bearing the internalized fungus or can directly attack the extracellular pathogen, by far the most numerous findings support a main role of CMI in providing help to phagocytic cells themselves in their intracellular or extracellular killing of fungal cells.

Accompanying CMI, though not necessarily related to protection, is the phenomen of *delayed-type hypersensitivity* (DTH) to fungal antigens, which is a classic $CD4^+$-mediated CMI response at the cutaneous level, of wide clinical utility. It consists of an erythematous/induration reaction seen 48 to 72 hr after intradermal inoculation of a suitable antigenic preparation of the infecting organism. As CMI, DTH is also transferred from an immunized animal (in this case also called sensitized) to a nonimmunized one by viable lymphoid cells and not by antibodies. It should be emphasized here that a DTH reaction is an initial example of an exaggerated CMI response at a local level, bringing about a limited but clearly evident inflammation and tissue destruction. It highlights a recurrent property of the immune response, in particular of the CMI response—that is, an apparently easy deviation from a beneficial effect to a harmful one. This will be reconsidered later on.

Both the cytotoxic and helper activities so characteristic of a CMI response are regulated by *cytokines*. These are polypeptide or glycoprotein molecules which, upon activation, are transiently produced by various cells of the organism, in particular those of the lymphomonocytic lineages. After binding to a receptor, the cytokines act on the same producing cells or their neighbors (*autocrine* or *paracrine* actions, respectively), and this action leads either to cell proliferation or differentiation to the acquisition or modulation of a new function (for instance, killing of the microbial target). Although cytokines are often called "hormonelike" factors, there are remarkable differences between them and the hormones. These latter have an *endocrine* activity (they affect distant cells or organs), are produced by one type of specialized cell, affect one or few target cells, and are rather unique in their action. What is typical of the cytokines, on the other hand, is their *redundant* and *pleiotropic network*. Thus, different cytokines may have the same effect on one kind of cell, and, conversely, any given cytokine may affect a multitude of different cells. However, most cytokines dealt with here in the context of CMI response—interleukin-2 (IL-2), interleukin-4 (IL-4), interleukin-5 (IL-5), and interferon-γ (IFN-γ)—are mostly or exclusively produced by T cells; for this reason, they are also referred to by the more restricted name *lymphokines*. A scheme outlining the properties of cytokines dominantly involved in CMI responses is presented in Table 1.

Table 1 Main Properties of Cytokines (Lymphokines) Most Commonly Involved in CMI Responses

Cytokines	Properties
IL-1β	Activation of natural immunoeffectors (neutrophil-macrophage) Activation of T cells Pyrogenicity, proinflammation and septic shock mediator
IL-2	T-cell proliferation Induction of highly cytolytic T and NK cells, highly interactive with fungal cells
IFN-γ	Activators of neutrophils and macrophages Enhancer of MHC-class II antigen expression Mediator of IL-2 activity and potentiator of NK activity
IL-4	Stimulation of B-cell response, in particular IgE formation Inhibition of macrophage activation Block of IL-2-induced T-cell activation Also produced by mast cells
IL-5	Stimulation of B-cell differentiation and immunoglobulin responses
IL-6	Many functions, among which are stimulation of B-cell growth and induction of IgG production; pyrogenicity, inflammation, septic shock mediator
IL-10	Induction of IgG production Inhibition of natural immunoeffector activation, with particular effect on antimicrobial and pro-inflammatory cytokines Suppresses IL-12 production by macrophages
IL-12	Regulation of NK and T-cell function Control of IFN-γ production Produced by phagocytic cells It has probably a pivotal role in Th1-Th2 polarization of CMI response through IFN-γ induction
TNF-α	Induction of inflammatory cytokine cascade (IL-1β, IL-6) Stimulation of neutrophils and macrophages Septic shock Direct cytotoxicity (tumor necrosis)

Source: From Refs. 1, 2, 5, 7, 8, 10, and 12.

III. METHODS TO ASSESS CMI RESPONSES

The experimental and clinical ways of assessing the existence (and efficiency) of a CMI response to a given fungal organism or antigen thereof logically follow from the foregoing. In vitro, this assessment usually involves the capacity of lymphoid cells from the sensitized subject to proliferate upon stimulation with the relevant fungal antigen, or, less commonly, to exert a cytotoxic activity against a sensitive cellular target. The lymphocyte proliferation is assayed by measuring DNA synthesis in lymphoid cells of lymphocyte-monocyte cultures from the peripheral blood or lymph node tissues, in particular spleen cells when the test is being performed in mice. In humans, the peripheral blood constitutes a convenient source of mononuclear cells/B lymphocytes as antigen-presenting cells and of T cells (these are 70–80% of the total lymphocyte population), among which the antigen stimulates the multiplication of the relevant antigen-specific T cell clones. Figure 1 shows an example of lymphocyte proliferation in the peripheral blood of HIV-negative (normal) or HIV-positive subjects (at different stages of the infection) in response to *Candida* antigen. For this proliferation to occur and as a consequence of it, lymphokines must be produced, and their direct titration, or the detection of their effects on macrophages and cytotoxicity generation, may also be a convenient way to assess the CMI response. For this purpose, a *migration-inhibition factor* (MIF) and *lymphotoxin* (LT) have been exploited, in particular the former, whose action consists in a retardation

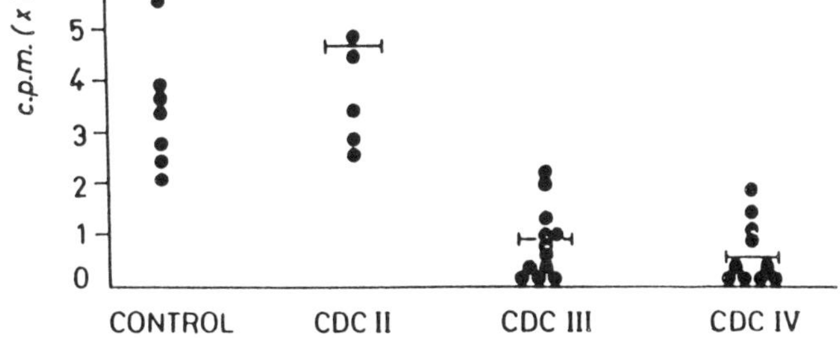

Figure 1 Proliferative responses of peripheral blood mononuclear cells (PBMC) from subjects uninfected or at different stages of HIV infection (CDC II–CDC IV, AIDS) to the stimulation with a *Candida* antigen. The proliferation is expressed as incorporation of radioactive thymidine into DNA, measured as counts per minute (cpm). Each dot represents a PBMC culture from a separate subject. The bar indicates the median value for each group of subjects (From Ref. 9.)

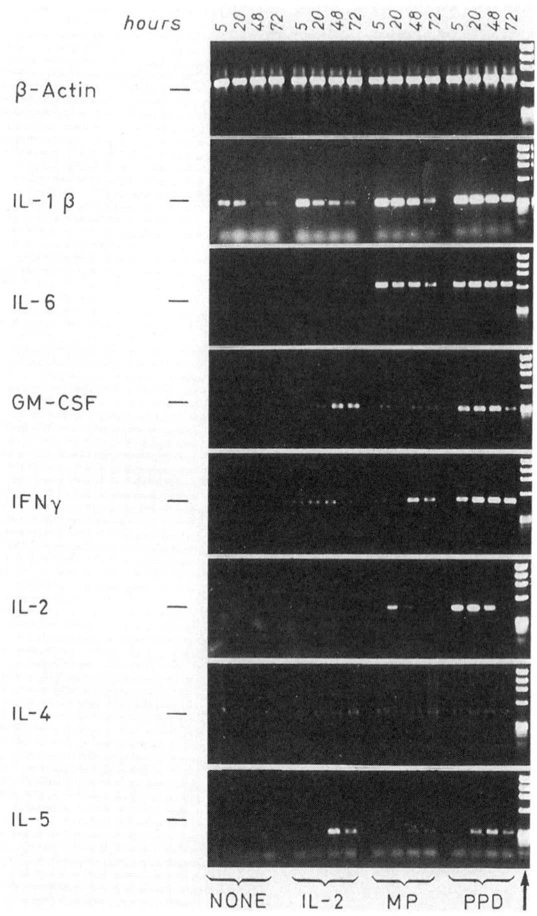

Figure 2 Expression of the message for various cytokines in PBMC cultures from a normal subject stimulated with two microbial antigens (PPD, protein purified derivative of *Mycobacterium tuberculosis;* MP, major mannoprotein antigen of *C. albicans*) or by a polyclonal activator (interleukin-2), or unstimulated. β-Actin is the control message. The mRNA is evaluated through reverse transcription and the cDNA amplified by PCR. Note the very low signal for Th-2 cytokines IL-4 and IL-5 in *Candida*-antigen-stimulated cells, in contrast to an abundant signal for Th-1 cytokines IFN-γ and IL-2. The arrow indicates the Mr standards. (Courtesy of A. La Sala, Laboratory of Bacteriology and Medical Mycology, I.S.S., Rome, Italy.)

or inhibition of macrophage migration. This is particularly useful, as it has been shown to strongly correlate with the skin test (see below). Although MIF assay is a suitable method to explore CMI in animals, its application in humans is hampered by the limited availability of a sufficient number of monocytic-macrophage cells from the peripheral blood. Although indirect methods may be used to increase the number of these cells, the system is somewhat cumbersome and has been displaced by the proliferation assay.

Of course, typical cytokines produced by proliferating T cells can be detected in these cultures, among which IFN-γ and IL-2 are widely assayed for. Both biological and immunoenzymatic methods have been developed, and both the actual cytokine or its message (mRNA) can be detected by Northern blot or the polymerase chain reaction (PCR) of its correspondent cDNA. Figure 2 gives an example of cytokine mRNAs detected by the latter technique in a CMI assay to a *Candida* antigen.

Among the in vivo assays, the skin tests represent a valid tool for detecting specific CMI responses to fungal antigens when care is exerted in distinguishing an immediate (a few minutes or hours) hypersensitivity reaction from the true, delayed (24–72 hr) response to the antigen. When suitably performed, the skin tests are better predictors of a functional CMI response; as such, they correlate much better than the in vitro test (lymphoproliferation, lymphokine assays) with progression of a fungal disease when CMI is altered, thus they are particularly valid clinical indicators. For instance, recent studies with AIDS patients have documented a much longer preservation of antigen recognition, an assayed by skin tests, with respect to the apparent early loss of CMI response to the same antigens in vitro. This persistence correlated with absence of opportunistic infections at CDC stages II and III of HIV infection.

IV. INVOLVEMENT OF CMI IN MYCOSES

In practically all diseases caused by the principal human pathogenic fungi, there is evidence that a more or less intense CMI reactivity is generated in the normal or simply colonized host, and that this is lost or greatly diminished when the host is affected by the disease. However, the true impact of CMI largely depends on the specific fungal infection and on the host and its tissues whenever the fungus is capable of causing a diversified set of pathologies.

In dermatophytosis, a number of clinical and experimental studies have demonstrated that, once the primary infection has healed, a potent CMI response (clearly visible through DTH) is generated in association with a degree of resistance to reinfection. During active infection, the DTH is no longer visible; instead, the host develops a strong "wheal-and-flare" response, or *immediate type hypersensitivity* (IgE-dependent), that plays a part in the clinical aspects of dermatophytosis. The inverse relationship between delayed and immediate-type responses to dermatophyte antigen is probably an example of the different involvement of Th-1 and Th-2 $CD4^+$ lymphocyte subsets, whereby the cytokines from Th-2 subset helping IgE antibody response contrast with the activity of Th-1 cytokines determining the CMI response. This is a recurrent theme of this chapter, as there are many applications of this recent, fundamental discovery.

Evidence for the development of a strong, positive CMI response and for its association with protection from fungal disease exists also in infections caused by *Histoplasma capsulatum*, *Cryptococcus neoformans*, *Blastomyces dermatitidis*, *Coccidioides immitis*, and *Candida albicans*. In the latter case, this is more evident with mucocutaneous or chronic rather than deep-seated, acute forms of the disease. In coccidiodomycosis, there is an inverse relationship between the intensity of the DTH response to *C. immitis* antigen and severity of disease; furthermore, a positive DTH response has a prognostic survival value in patients with the most serious disseminated forms of the disease. For histoplasmosis and cryptococcosis, there is also circumstantial evidence for an association between the severity of disease and lack or a low level of CMI response. The increased incidence and severity of these diseases in $CD4^+$-depleted AIDS patients adds to the clear results of past studies showing a correlation between disseminated, rapidly fatal forms of disease and anergy in skin tests or lymphoproliferation assays in vitro. Anergy to *B. dermatidis* antigen extract has also been associated with poor prognosis, especially when the lack of DTH response is paralleled by a high titer of complement-fixing antibody, stressing an apparent dichotomy between humoral and CMI responses in the course of disease.

V. CMI MECHANISMS: THE CENTRAL ROLES OF CYTOKINES AND T-HELPER CELL SUBSETS

Studies in humans relating predisposing factors, primary or acquired immunodeficiencies, and therapeutic interventions to the clinical parameters and outcome of fungal infections, generally offer only circumstantial insights into the correlation between immunological state and disease. More specifically, instead, studies with "ex vivo" models and experimental animals allow us to go deep into the mechanisms of CMI response and ask to what extent this response is truly relevant to the protection against disease, is neutral, or by itself aggravates the clinical events. As for other aspects of medical mycology, there are remarkable achievements in this area that depend mainly on the exciting recent progress in understanding the molecular and cellular basis of immunological processes and its widespread application to the field of infectious diseases in general. These developments are progressing rapidly and it can be anticipated that they will significantly advance our knowledge of the CMI's role in fungal diseases. In addition, they will probably provide a rationale for improved immunoprophylactic or therapeutic interventions. The use of recombinant DNA technology and sophisticate animal models (e.g., gene-knockout mice) will increasingly serve as useful tools for unraveling the fine mechanisms of immune response and pathogenesis of infections.

A. CD4$^+$ T Cells and Th Subsets

It has long been believed that CD4$^+$ cells play a major regulatory role in CMI whereas CD8$^+$ lymphocytes exert cytotoxic activity against parasite-infected cells. This is no longer valid, however, as both regulatory and cytotoxic roles can be played, in different biological situations, by both T-cell phenotypes. Of outstanding importance is the notion that CD4$^+$ lymphocytes can be subdivided into (at least) two sets, the Th-1 and Th-2 cells, which are endowed with distinct cytokine expression profiles and different roles in the protection against fungal diseases. This subdivision, which was first proposed for the L3T4 cells of the mouse, is now also accepted with some restrictions for the human CD4$^+$ cells (5,7,10,13). Concerning the functions of each subset, Th-1 appears to be mainly involved in CMI effector functions through the preferential expression of IL-2 and IFN-γ, whereas the Th-2 subset, through the expression of IL-4 and IL-5, would mostly provide help in antibody formation. Another CD4$^+$ cell subset (Th-0), capable of producing a mixed (both Th-1 and Th-2) cytokine profile exists, probably bearing special importance during the early "immature" stages of the immune response or following stimulation by particular antigens or immunization routes.

Importantly, Th-1 and Th-2 subsets do not represent separate roads of the immune response but rather are "cross-regulated" in that the cytokines of each subset (mostly, the IFN-γ for Th-1 and IL-4 for Th-2), while facilitating the expression of their own functions, strongly inhibit the growth and differentiation of the alternative CD4$^+$ Th subset. This provides a firm biological basis for the frequent observation of clinical immunologists, already mentioned, that antibody formation and DTH have an inverse relationship during the course of many chronic fungal infections, exactly as happens for parasitic infections.

Once established, the specific Th profile of CD4$^+$ cells following a given antigenic stimulation tends to be stabilized, so that, for instance, most of T-cell clones against the PPD antigen of *Mycobacterium tuberculosis* in infected but tuberculosis-free adults are Th-1, whereas most of the clones against an allergen remain Th-2 for life. Finally, the divergence of the two subsets is directly manifest through the action of each subset cytokine on "effector" function of the alternative subset. For instance, IFN-γ *activates* whereas IL-4 *depresses* the antifungal activity of the macrophage. What determines whether the Th-1 or Th-2 road should be taken is not exactly known. Among the various factors that have been suggested to be involved, there are the nature of the antigen and its initial processing, the form of antigen presentation and adjuvant, the initial cytokines produced and other soluble factors in the place of the first encounter with the antigen, and last but not least, the host itself, with its individual or familiar genetic background. Antigen presentation and processing might have a predominant role if further research corroborates the idea that IL-12, a cytokine produced by antigen-presenting cells (macrophages and B lymphocytes) is indeed a selective activator of the Th-1 pathway (11,12).

One of the best-studied example of the differential Th subset involvement in an experimental fungal infection is that provided by Bistoni et al. in a murine model of systemic candidiasis (reviewed in Ref. 14). A separate patterns of healing and nonhealing *Candida* infections, according to the Th type (Th-1 and Th-2, respectively) of the immune response following experimental infections with high- or low-virulence *C. albicans* strains, has been clearly demonstrated. The occurrence of a healing, protective pattern of immunization correlated with a predominant Th-1 $CD4^+$ response and was largely dependent on both the host genetics and physiological factors early in the course of infection. Importantly, the protective and nonprotective responses could be modified by antibodies or receptor antagonists of the relevant lymphokine. For instance, treatment with anti-IL-4 or IL-4-receptor or anti-IL-10 transformed a nonprotective to a protective pattern. Conversely, neutralization of IFN-γ transformed a protective pattern into its opposite, and this was mediated by IL-4 production. Finally, the healing pattern was accompanied by strong DTH development, which did not occur in the nonhealing pattern. An example of how the production of a typical Th-1 cytokine (IFN-γ) by fungal antigen or mitogen-stimulated murine splenocytes is affected by neutralization of the concomitant production of Th-2 cytokines is shown in Figure 3. Overall, these patterns are strikingly similar to the events described in the experimental cutaneous infection by *Leishmania major*, which remains a sort of prototypical, paradigmatic model of the separate, cross-regulated activities of Th-1 and Th-2 lymphocyte subsets (5,10).

It should be stressed here that, although a role of T cells in *mucocutaneous forms of candidiasis* has always been safely assumed, the evidence

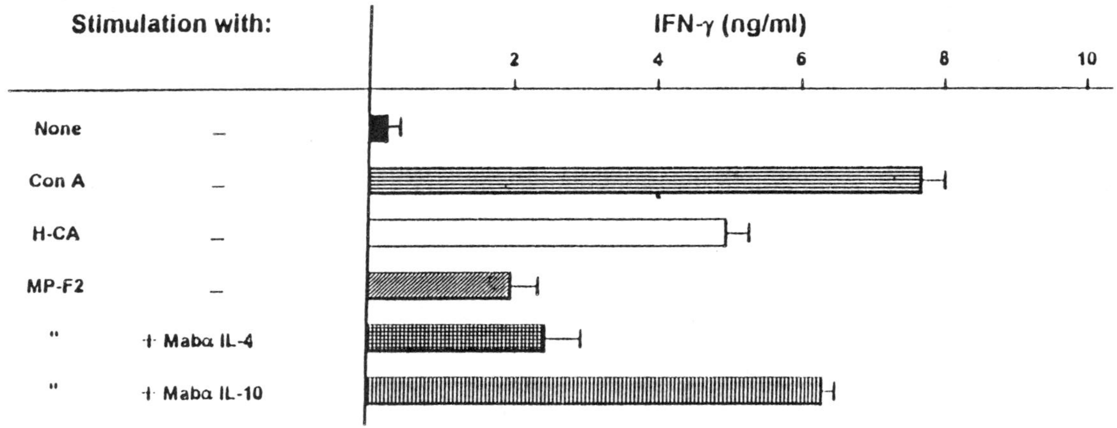

Figure 3 Production of IFN-γ by $CD4^+$ murine cells from the spleen of mice immunized with *C. albicans*, in response to a polyclonal activator concanavalin A (con A), or the relevant antigens (whole, heat-inactivated cells of *C. albicans*, H-CA, or its mannoprotein antigen MP-F2) in the absence or presence of antibodies neutralizing IL-4 or IL-10. (For technical detail, see Ref. 17.)

depicted in the studies by Bistoni's group in *systemic candidiasis* would apparently contrast with previous indications stemming from the natural resistance to systemic *Candida* challenge of congenitally athymic nude mice. A relevant issue is also the nature of the specific stimulation of the protective response in the model—that is, a chronic infection by a low-virulence strain of *C. albicans* (vaccine). Indeed, chronic protozoal infections have been the best models to dissect healing and nonhealing, Th-1- and Th2-mediated responses.

The importance of T cells for protecting mice from a lethal *C. albicans* challenge has recently been addressed by the use of a murine *Candida*-specific T-cell line. This line was able to confer a degree of protection in a disseminated model of candidiasis. Interestingly, the T-cell line was α/β TCR and $CD4^+$, but $CD8^-$. It would be important to assess the efficacy of T-cell clones, their cytokine patterns, and which specific *Candida* antigens are recognized by these clones. Meantime, if corroborated by further investigations, these data would provide strong confirmation to the supposed role of T cells in the development of adaptive immunity to systemic *Candida* challenge.

Evidence is mounting that the production of Th-1 cytokines IL-2 and IFN-γ also play a significant protective role in other fungal infections—for instance, in experimental cryptococcosis and histoplasmosis. In particular, it has been shown that clearance of *H. capsulatum* from mouse organs is dependent on the possession of an intact $CD4^+$ cell compartment. The role of these cells could be mediated by IFN-γ, which activates the macrophages to restrict the intracellular growth of the fungus (see also below). It is also emerging that IFN-γ production is upregulated or induced by IL-12, a cytokine produced mainly by macrophages and B cells but also, and interestingly, by neutrophils. Recent investigations suggest that IL-12 plays a pivotal role in inducing and orienting antiinfectious CMI (12). Figure 4 draws a plausible flow of events leading to the expression of CMI response mediated by Th-1 cells in fungal infections.

While the cellular and cytokine mechanisms leading to an effective (protective) CMI response in the above infections are being elucidated, it is discouraging to see that the identification of fungal antigens eliciting or targeting the CMI response lags very far behind, despite the fact that the nature and the way of processing any immunodominant antigen can play an important role in Th-1 subset activation. Moreover, antigen identification is essential to devise efficient diagnostic or immunoprophylactic treatments. Cell-surface glycoproteins are being intensely investigated in *Candida*, *Cryptococcus*, and *Histoplasma* as well.

A 65-kDa mannoprotein (MP65) has been purified from *C. albicans*; it is recognized as a major target of anticandidal CMI in humans. Another glycoprotein of similar molecular mass exists in *H. capsulatum* and is

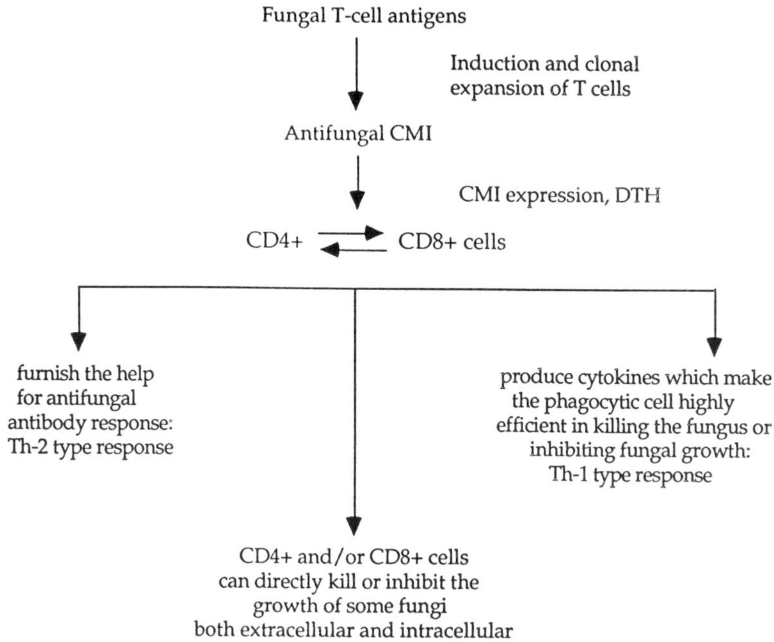

Figure 4 A scheme drawing a possible flow of events from antigen recognition to antifungal effector mechanism, as mediated by CMI activation. (For details, see the text.)

genetically related to a 60-KDa heat-shock protein (HSP60). The CMI response in vitro to MP65 generates a pattern of $CD4^+$ cells cytokines that is the one expected from the preferential expansion-activation of Th-1 cell subset, and an MP65 containing mannoprotein fraction of *C. albicans* induces a $CD4^+$ Th-1 cell development, accompanied by partial protection, in a murine model of candidiasis. Enolase, an enzyme of the glycolytic pathway, has also recently been advocated as a major target of CMI response in both experimental models and humans, but there is no evidence of a protective role of the CMI response to this antigen in candidiasis. Thus, the search for protection-relevant immune responses should be accompanied by the search for truly protective fungal antigens.

B. $CD4^+$ Cells and Antibodies: An Intriguing Issue

While it is clear enough that individuals infected by pathogenic fungi produce antibodies to immunodominant fungal antigens, the role played by these antibodies in the infection is difficult to assess; with the possible exception of the anti-capsular polysaccharide antibodies against *Cryptococcus neoformans*, it is often underestimated. Treatment of this topic is beyond the scope of this chapter. Nonetheless, it should be stressed here that CMI and antibody-mediated responses are not (or not always) mutually exclusive phenomena. They may rather coexist and interact favorably in the defense against mycoses. This may occur at least in those infections where the infecting organism is essentially extracellular that are, indeed, the majority in the field of mycotic diseases.

A key point here is that $CD4^+$ T-helper cells of Th-1 subset also intervene with their cytokines in modulating antibody responses, as exemplified by the memory $CD4^+$ cells (CD45RO), upon which most of the vigor and duration of a protective response to fungal antigens depends. Thus, IFN-γ, a classic Th-1, CMI-inductive cytokine is able to stimulate antibody isotype switching toward IgG2a, both in vitro and in vivo, and here again its action is competed for by IL-4 (13). Antibodies of IgG2a class are well-known for their protective, mostly opsonizing effects on extracellular pathogens including fungi. As already mentioned, IL-4 is a potent IgE switch inducer; thus the two most typical cytokines of the two different Th subsets (IL-4 and IFN-γ) not only dictate the pattern of CMI responses but also discriminate between antibodies by determining isotype–C_H related responses that are so different biologically. In this context, the observation is relevant that IgG antibodies against particular mannoprotein antigens are protective in a model of candidal vaginitis where strong CMI responses are elicited and strong clinical evidence supports a role for CMI in infection. A similar phenomenon has recently been observed in a model of disseminated candidiasis (15).

C. $CD8^+$ Cells

$CD8^+$ T are classically known to exert a protective role against tumor or virus-infected cells, but recent research show clearly that these lymphocytes are also involved in protection against infections by other microrganisms, including pathogenic fungi. $CD8^+$ T cells express cytolytic activities on *Candida*-infected bone marrow murine macrophages and produce remarkable quantities of IFN-γ, which, as previously noted, orient the CD4 Th-1 protective subset and activate the fungicidal macrophages. The lysis of the infected mononuclear phagocyte by $CD8^+$ T-cell releases a viable microrganism that can now either be more promptly killed or inhibited extracellularly or phagocytosed and killed by more efficient phagocytes. Since presentation of microbial antigen in the context of intracytoplasmic class I MHC is required for $CD8^+$ T-cell activation, it is not surprising that the CD8$^+$ T cells are mostly involved, perhaps as subsidiary or reserve to CD4$^+$ T cells, when the intracellular infectious agent is able to escape from the vacuole into the cytoplasm. This mechanism, which is largely employed by protozoal parasites, is probably of lesser importance with fungi, which only in some cases have a true, persistent intracellular growth (e.g., *Histoplasma capsulatum*).

Thus, it is probable that, in most fungal infections, the role of CD8$^+$ T cells is rather that of producing the macrophage-activating antimicrobial cytokines or inhibiting fungus growth directly. In the latter context, recent evidence suggests that CD8$^+$ (but also CD4$^+$) T lymphocytes, when suitably activated by IL-2, may directly inhibit the growth of *C. neoformans* and *C. albicans*. All T cells have indeed a striking capacity to form closely interactive conjugates with both *C. neoformans* and *C. albicans*. The relevance of these in vitro observations to the in vivo control of fungal infection by the direct activity of T cells remains to be established.

D. Natural Killer (NK) Cells

These large granular lymphocytes (TCR-CD3$^-$), which kill virus-infected or tumor targets in a non-MHC-restricted fashion, probably also have an impact in the defense against fungal infections. By their ability to intervene rapidly without prior antigen-specific sensitization, NK cells are, together with phagocytic cells, an ideal first defensive line. However, their precise role in antifungal defense, in connection or not with CMI responses, awaits further definition. Intact cells of *C. albicans* or some of their cell-wall constituents exert a strong activation of NK cells both in vitro and in vivo; one significant effect of this activation is the production by NK cell of cytokines such as TNF-α, IFN-γ, and GM-CSF. These exert their expected activating effects on macrophages and neutrophils, which engulf and kill the fungus, even extracellularly, much more efficiently than in the non-cytokine-activated state.

In addition, and perhaps more importantly, the IFN-γ produced by the NK cells might exert an impact on CMI-specific responses, as obviously descends from the role of this cytokine on Th-1–Th-2 divergence (see Secs. V.A and V.B). Although theoretically sound, no precise experimental evidence has been furnished that in fungal infections it is the IFN-γ produced by activated NK cells to orient the Th pattern. At any rate, the cytokine-producing ability of NK cells has been interpreted as probably explaining why B- and T-cell depleted scid mice are no more susceptible to experimental candidiasis than their normal littermates, as also happens with only nude (congenitally athymic) or T-cell depleted mice. However, the scid mice have also normal level of granulocytes, which are rather potent anticandidal effectors even when they are not cytokine-activated. Moreover, the depletion of NK cells with specific antisera has not led to an increased susceptibility to experimental infection. It has also been shown that the IFN-γ secreted by NK cells hardly affects the pathway of Th-1 subset activation in experimental candidiasis (although this may happen in other infections).

Interleukin-2-activated murine and human NK cells (LAK) have also been advocated by Mathews et al. to inhibit the growth of the hyphal form of *C. albicans*, which might be relevant in the context of *Candida* infections where the predominant tissue invasive form is the hyphal one. These forms of growth are tenaciously and extensively bound by human LAK cells in vitro (Fig. 5), but their true inhibitory effects, like those of T cells, await confirmation, with particular regard to the in vivo situation. The same conclusion holds true for other fungal pathogens such as *Aspergillus* and *Histoplasma*, for the control of which a role for NK cells has also been advocated. A more evident role for NK or T cells inhibiting the

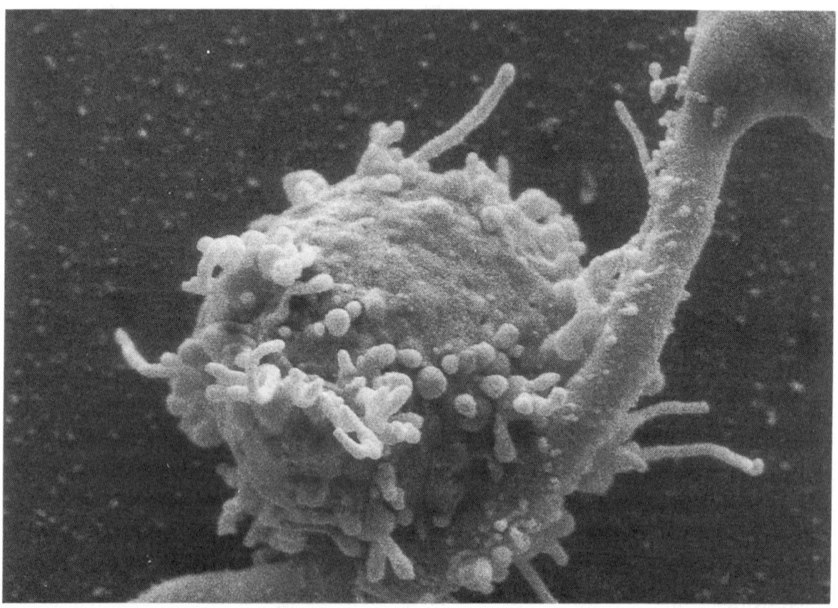

Figure 5 Interaction between a human LAK (interleukin-2-activated) cell and the germ tube of *C. albicans*, as seen by scanning electron microscopy. (×18,000.) (For technical details, see Ref. 18.)

growth or also killing *C. neoformans* has been demonstrated by the studies of Murphy, Levitz, and their collaborators, who showed that T cells may discharge lytic granules to kill *C. neoformans* in vitro (9). Notably, a main NK-activator is IL-12 which promotes the Th-1 differentiation pattern (12). Whether this implies that NK cells influence the adaptive immunity to fungi is being actively investigated.

VI. POSITIVE AND NEGATIVE EFFECT ON CMI AND CMI REGULATION IN THE ANTIFUNGAL DEFENSE

In order to display its potential protective role against a fungal infection, the CMI response must be finely tuned to avoid that the cytolytic potential of $CD8^+$ or even $CD4^+$ T cells or an exaggerated production of cytokines such as IL-6 or the tumor necrosis factor (TNF)-α could be detrimental for the host. In experimental models, an effective tuning depends, among other things, on the number of infecting cells. When this is low, the microbicidal function predominates and the lesion heals. But with a high number of infectious particles, it is likely that the continuous request for T-cell activation and cytokine production may bring on a more or less marked host tissue destruction, which attempts but may not guarantee microbial eradication.

Another special area of interest in the regulation of CMI is the recognized ability of fungal antigens, mostly polysaccaride in nature, to downregulate or suppress CMI itself. There are generalized examples showing whether and how fungal antigens may suppress the afferent and/or efferent arms of CMI induction response, but the mostly intensely studied cases concern anti-*Candida* or *Cryptococcus* CMI.

Particularly in the latter, Murphy and collaborators have demonstrated that a cascade of different-order suppressor cells (Ts) are induced in a murine model of cryptococcal infection by administration of a suitable polysaccharide antigen. This leads to inhibition of the anticryptococcal CMI, as measured by DTH, which, in turn, is causally related to the lack of cryptococcal cell eradication from the mouse body. The true suppressive factors may be either directly the Ts cells or soluble factors released by them and inhibiting macrophage phagocytosis. Little is known about the mechanism of suppression itself. A logical target of Ts cells would be the production of cytokines by the $CD4^+$ Th-1 subset. It has indeed been observed that some Ts actually inhibit the production of IFN-γ and IL-2, leaving intact the production of a typical Th-2 cytokine such as IL-5. The exact manner by which T suppressor cells downregulate cytokine production by Th-1 $CD4^+$ cells is a very interesting issue awaiting further investigations. Importantly, however, the cryptococcal antigen inducing the cascade of suppressor cells and factors in the mouse is analogous to that circulating in large quantities in the meningeal fluid and blood of the patients affected by cryptococcosis and is correlated with a poor prognosis. As said before, in various other fungal infections the CMI response is depressed by fungal antigens. Not always, however, the inhibited CMI, as assessed by DTH response correlates with lack of protection in vivo. This is the case for mannan-induced DTH suppression in candidiasis.

VII. PHAGOCYTIC CELLS AS MAJOR, FINAL EFFECTORS OF ANTIFUNGAL CMI

Although not disregarding the already mentioned contribution of the direct fungal killing or growth inhibition that can be expressed by suitably activated T cells or NK cells, doubtless a major role in the final fight against the aggressive fungal invader is played by the professional phagocytes, such as the polymorphonuclear granulocytes (neutrophil, PMNG) and, mostly, the macrophages (MP). Both cells are highly responsive to IFN-γ activation and both can kill fungal cells intracellularly or extracellularly. Macrophages are specially involved with intracellularly growing fungi like *Histoplasma*. Here, the MP represents the growth environment of the fungus as well as its most potent killer when suitably armed by an efficient, finely tuned CMI. Clearly, MP from different tissues and different hosts have different antifungal activities with respect to the different fungal targets. Human alveolar macrophages are, for instance, extremely potent anti-*Candida* effectors (and this probably explains why *Candida* pneumonia is so rare), even in T-cell-immunodepressed patients, whereas this is not true for MP from other body areas or for blood. Activated murine MP are fungicidal for *C. albicans* but only fungistatic for *H. capsulatum*, which is, however, killed by activated human MP.

The actual fungicidal properties of MP impinge on multiple, probably concurrent mechanisms, inclusive of the generation of reactive oxygen and nitrogen intermediates, iron limitation, antifungal peptides called *defensins*, and other peptide-proteinaceous substances generated in the strongly acid milieu of phagolysosomes. Interestingly, an acidic milieu in the phagosome is induced by IFN-γ treatment. Cytokine-activation of MP is often essential to mobilize all these mechanisms together, and cytokines other than IFN-γ may be involved.

Reactive oxygen intermediates have a documented role in the microbicidal activities of MP, but recent attention has been drawn to the powerful activity of nitrogen-reactive intermediates. NO•, the actual cytocidal substance, is generated by the enzyme nitric oxide (NO)-synthase. Its expression is induced by IFN-γ and apparently inhibited by IL-10, pointing again to a differential role of Th subsets cytokines in the tuning of antifungal macrophage activity. For optimal NO• synthesis by murine macrophages, synergistic induction by cytokines and microbial products themselves, such as the LPS of gram-negative bacteria, is often necessary. This synergism appears to be mediated by TNF-α production by the macrophage itself, which acts in an autocrine fashion to amplify NO• release by IFN-γ primed cells.

In vitro and partially also in vivo experiments have demonstrated a certain relationship between NO• production and antimicrobial effects. *C. neoformans*, *H. capsulatum*, and *C. albicans* are among those fungi that proved to be susceptible to inhibition or cytocidal effects of NO• radical, but since NO• has a very wide target spectrum, practically encompassing all kinds of cells, it is not surprising that it is active on all other pathogenic fungi and host tissues. Indeed, NO• is one of the smallest biologically active catabolites that can dramatically affect the host's tissues when its production is high and sustained for longer periods. To avoid this, several inhibitors come into play, among which the Th-2 cytokines IL-4 and IL-10, and the transforming growth factor-β (TGF-β) have a predominant role. If, after a burst, NO• production is not rapidly inhibited, immunopathological effects occur. Thus, excessive NO• synthesis is relevant in the hypotension that landmarks the septic shock and leads to the suppression of host immunity. This again stresses the recurrent idea of a fine tuning of the CMI response in order to achieve protection and how this tuning can be easily distorted during an infection.

Concerning the mechanisms of the cytocidal effect of NO•, some data point to the interaction of NO• with intracellular iron. Iron is essential for the fungus to survive in the macrophage, and a complex mechanism of transport (via transferrin) and accumulation (via ferritin) operates to ensure the right intramacrophagic iron levels. These are necessary for NO• production (as well as for oxygen-reactive intermediates). Interestingly, IFN-γ mediates upregulation of NO• as well as downregulating the transferrin receptor, with a net effect of iron intracellular pool deprivation. A clear example of the interplay between iron restriction and NO• production for the MP inhibition of *H. capsulatum* growth has recently been provided by Howard's group (9). It must be remembered here that all the experiments clearly demonstrating the NO• effects have been performed in the mouse macrophages. Human macrophages appear to be much more impermeable to the antimicrobial effects of NO•, and the role of this powerful gaseous compound in human fungal disease remains to be carefully studied.

VIII. ADAPTIVE CMI RESPONSES AND NATURAL, INNATE IMMUNITY

While the efferent side of the CMI-phagocyte flow of events is well established, recent evidence points to the importance of an afferent phagocytic NK cell–CMI response pathway (see also Sec. V above). The basic observations of this afferent pathway reside on the recognized capacity of macrophages and polymorphonuclear phagocytes to produce Th-1-orienting cytokine IL-12 and on the strong IFN-γ induction of the latter by NK cells. In addition, mast cells are good producers of IL-4, the key Th-2–promoting cytokine. If further evidence strengthens these notions, they will probably have a great impact on the interpretations of the key events in the initiation of antifungal CMI responses and their therapeutic exploitation and also for vaccine design. Suffice it to say here that PMN and macrophages are strongly activated by selective fungal components that are abundantly expressed on fungal cell wall (e.g., polysaccarides and their complexes with lipids) (16). This activation is rapid and results in abundant production of cytokines. The intervention of natural immunoeffectors largely precedes any sort of T-cell activation and may indeed be instrumental to that. The strong adjuvant effects of whole fungal cells (like those of many bacterial cells) in eliciting nonspecific anti-infectious and antitumor responses probably lie on the above cytokines. It is anticipated that a full understanding of the afferent limb of phagocyte-CMI connection might have important implications for the selection of vaccinating or immunomodulating antigens in fungal diseases.

IX. MUCOSAL AND CUTANEOUS CMI

Both mucosa and skin harbor numerous T cells, which supposedly play an important role in local immunity, as they are the first lymphocytes encountered by the pathogenic fungi in their settlement on or invasion of the mucosal or cutaneous surface. The number of T lymphocytes present in normal human skin of a healthy adult usually reaches approximately 4 billion. In the mouse, these T cells (generally CD8$^+$) have an increased proportion of those bearing a γ/δ T cell receptor (about 40%) but this is not verified in humans. The specific role of γ/δ-TCR bearing lymphocytes has not yet been clarified. Their increase in number after infection by several microorganisms points to a protective function, that may be rather nonspecific, as the γ/δ TCR lymphocytes, in contrast to the more common α-β TCR cells, possess a very limited antigenic repertoire. Once stimulated, these γ/δ TCR lymphocytes are cytotoxic and produce cytokines as IFN-γ and TNF-α which are particularly important in protective CMI.

One possibly relevant function of γ/δ T cells, coherent with their limited antigenic repertoire, is the recognition of heat-shock proteins (HSP). These are protein families largely homologous both in microorganism and host cells, which are synthesized in response to increase in temperatures, stress, or trauma of various origins, including infection itself. They are strongly antigenic and can induce autoimmune reactivity. It has been postulated that γ/δ-bearing TCR lymphocytes may respond to commonly shared epitopes of these highly conserved proteins of various microorganisms and also recognize autologous stressed cells. This may be the mode by which a "trauma signal" is sensed by the immune system (through the increased expression of a shock constituent) and a γ/δ T lymphocyte could be alerted for the elimination of the traumatizing agent together with the self-HSP-expressing traumatized cell.

Among the cells that are more easily recognized by the γ/δ T lymphocytes are just the keratinocytes, whose antigen stimulatory capacity is increased by heat shock or chemical stress. Interestingly, this recognition of "stressed" keratinocytes by the γ/δ T lymphocytes is non-MHC-restricted, at least not under the usual sense of antigen restriction. Thus, these intraepithelial γ/δ T lymphocytes could be the sentinels in such skin sites where only few offending microbes, expressing few antigens, may be found. In this function, relevant are the recent observations that γ/δ T cells recognize and directly bind simple, MHC-unconjugated microbial epitopes and are strongly activated by nonproteinaceous, even low-molecular-weight compounds. Phosphate-bound molecules are among these $\gamma\delta$-T-cell–recognized constituents, and it is immediately suggestive to consider the number of nonproteinaceous, phosphorylated saccharidic and/or lipidic molecules that are so abundantly present on fungal cell walls.

X. CONCLUSIONS AND PERSPECTIVES

The importance of CMI responses in fungal infections has been briefly summarized. Most of the evidence related to human infection is rather circumstantial; nonetheless, it is founded upon numerous clinical, immunological, and pathological observations and receives support from experimental animals studies. Although the role of the different CD4 Th subsets is an exciting clue and a useful, unifying scheme of clinical and experimental data interpretation, many other mechanisms consisting in different cytokines and cell receptors, with their multiple relevant interactions, as well as their direct influence on the phagocytic cells and on antibody response, are on the stage. From a medical viewpoint, the recent acquisitions on CMI relevance and mechanisms in fungal diseases are already paving the way for new prophylactic or therapeutic actions, especially in vaccine design and application or immunotherapy with cytokine-anticytokine compounds.

It seems now that, also for fungal diseases, we are not too far from the possibility of predicting and orienting a desirable immune response (previously totally empirical) and then maximizing the effects favorable to the host and minimizing the harmful ones. This requires, however, a very precise knowledge of the protective versus nonprotective immune mechanisms in any given infection. For some common and opportunistic fungal pathogens, such as *Candida* spp., the overall pictures may seem very complicated because of the number of different pathologies in which the fungus is involved, among which the distinction between superficial and deep-seated infections is basic as are acute or chronic settings, and also because of the underlying state of immunocompromise that is so relevant in these diseases.

As a general, empirical rule, it can be suggested that where the antibodies play a mainly protective role (as, for instance, in some forms of extracellular invasive diseases), it would be desirable to work with antigens and routes of administration that mostly rely upon facilitation of Th-2 subset cytokines, or even Th-1, according to the antibody isotype involved. In contrast, in most of superficial or chronic illnesses, where typical CMI-regulated effector functions are involved, the selection should be made to favor the vaccination eliciting Th-1 cytokines, even by indirect intervention on the mechanisms of natural immunity (see Sec. VIII).

The data discussed above also raise the possibility of influencing or reversing the negative aspects of the vaccination, natural immunization, or pathological episodes due to the expression of a given cytokine subset, by driving the opposite signals, even in the course of the infection itself, by means of cytokines or cytokine antagonists (antibodies or soluble receptors). In many fungal infections, an allergic reaction to inappropriate or contiguous antigen stimulation occurs, as, for instance, in some recurrent forms of vaginitis by *C. albicans* or dermatophytic infections. Cytokine or cytokine antagonists aimed at attenuating IgE synthesis by antagonizing the cytokines of the opposite patterns might prove of remarkable benefit.

In this context of the cytokine approach to fungal disease, it appears of utmost importance that future research in the field be oriented to identifying the major protective T-cell antigens and epitopes in fungal cells, the nature of the presenting cells, and the orientation exerted by natural immunoeffectors on cytokine production, the interplay of the various humoral factors, such as cytokines and antibodies, and the mechanisms that are biologically relevant in the control and, eventually, the eradication of pathogenic fungi from the whole body or from a restricted body area. Together with more appropriate antifungal chemotherapy, the cytokine approach, in the wide context described above, will probably play an important role in the therapy and prevention of fungal infections in the future.

REFERENCES

1. Paul WE. Fundamental Immunology, New York: Raven Press, 1991.
2. Roitt IM. Essential Immunology, Oxford, England: Blackwell, 1988.
3. Howard DH, ed. Fungi Pathogenic for Humans and Animals. Vols 1–3. New York: Marcel Dekker,
4. Murphy JW, Friedman J, Bendinelli M, eds. Fungal Infections and Immune Responses. New York: Plenum Press,
5. Sher A, Coffman RL. Regulation of immunity to parasites by T cells and T cell-derived cytokines. Annu Rev Immunol 1992;10:385–397.
6. Murphy JW. Immunity to fungi. Curr Opin Immunol 1990;2:360–367.
7. Powrie F, Coffman RL. Cytokine regulation of T cell function: Potential for therapeutic interventions. Immunol Today 1993;270:14.
8. Thomson A, ed. The Cytokine Handbook. London: Academic Press, 1991.
9. Fukazawa Y, et al. Mechanisms of cell-mediated immunity in fungal infections. J Med Vet Mycol 1994;32(suppl 1):123–132.
10. Mossman TR, Coffman RL. Annu Rev Immunol 1989;7:145–158.
11. Chehimi J, et al. IL-12 deficiency in HIV-infected patients. *J Exp Med* 1994; 179:1361–1366.
12. Scott P. IL-12: Initiation of cytokine for cell-mediated immunity. Science 1993;90:5879–5882.
13. Kauffmann SHE. Immunity to intracellular microbial pathogens. Immunol Today 1995;16:338–342.
14. Puccetti P et al. A Th1-Th2-like switch in candidiasis: New perspectives for therapy. Trends Microbiol 1995;3:237–240.
15. Cassone A, et al. Rats clearing a vaginal infection by Candida albicans acquire specific, antibody-mediated resistance to vaginal reinfection. Infect Immun 1995;63:2619–2624. Han and Cutler, ibidem, 1995.
16. Cassone A, et al. Cell wall constituents of C. albicans as biological response modifiers. CRC Crit Rev Microbiol 1987;15:87–102.
17. Mencacci et al., Infect Immun 1994;62:5353–5360.
18. Arancia et al., Infect Immun 1995;63:282–288.
19. Sieck TG, et al., Protection against murine disseminated caudiolian's mediated by a **Caudiole olbicaus**-specific T-cell line. Infect Immun 1993;61: 3540–3543.

8

Biochemical Mechanisms of Fungicidal Activity with Tissue Extracts

HISASHI TAKAHASHI, SHINICHI WATANABE, and KENICHIRO CHIKAKANE
School of Medicine
Teikyo University
Tokyo, Japan

MASATO KASHIMA
St. Marianna Medical College
Tokyo, Japan

I. INTRODUCTION

Plants have no migrating cells, such as leukocytes, as do animals to protect against invading microorganisms, but they have survived in the presence of other microorganisms because they protect themselves with so-called phytoalexins in their tissue. The evidence suggests the existence of some fungicidal substance, as found in plants as well as in animal tissue, that shields against the invasion of ordinary nonpathogenic microorganisms including fungi. We obtained crude extract of guinea pig skin and proved that there was a high candidacidal activity in it (1). We reported that some tissue-bound immunity (2), like phytoalexin in plants, was found in the skin of the guinea pig. The characterization of the substance was very difficult, and during the process of purification, we noticed that the substance was cationic. Similar cationic substances like skin extract seem to be ubiquitous in many tissues of animals and humans and engage in the host defenses. In this report, we introduce a battery of such substances from the literature and our own laboratory investigations.

Fungus infections exhibit an opportunistic nature and provide good models for the studies of "pathogenicity," because the term *pathogenicity* denotes the "invading capability of microorganisms by overcoming the host resistance.'' Although the substances toxic to microorganisms contained in the cells and tissues of the hosts and involved in the resistance to them vary across a wide range of chemicals, it seems likely that these are arranged in several categories, such as oxidative, cationic, enzymatic, and chelating substances. Among these, cationic substance is widespread in the host tissues and seems to be the major tissue-bound defense substance. The following is a review of this substance.

II. TISSUE-BOUND IMMUNITY OF VARIOUS TISSUES

A. Polymorphonuclear Leukocyte

1. Historical Perspective

Research by Mechinikoff (3) was the starting point on host defense. More than a century ago, he classified phagocytic cells into two groups: microphages (polymorphonuclear leukocytes, or PMNs) and macrophages (macrophage-monocytes) according to their size. These cells are provided with condensed microbicidal substances, and the understanding of these substances gives us the clue for the study of host defense. After phagocytosis, release of lysosomal substances into phagocytic vacuoles begins, and cidal substances are removed into phagolysosome together with digesting enzymes. Cohn and Hirsch (4) undertook the isolation of the cytoplasmic granules of PMNs in 1960. The mechanism of phagocytosis was then further studied morphologically (5) and electron microscopically (6). Lehrer and Cline (7) reported on the phagocytosis of *Candida albicans* by PMNs in 1969. Phagocytosis is also accompanied by extracellular release of lysosomal substances like secretions (6,8), which cause inflammation in surrounding tissue (9); among lysosomal substances, some cationic protein was identified (10,11) together with another substance (12), and further exploration (13,14) of this substance was conducted by Spitznagel (15–20) and Lehrer (21).

Polymorphonuclear cells are the condensed model of microbicidal substances, and many studies have been reported on killing substances such as lysozyme and myeloperoxidase (22); but as to the microbiocidal activity of cationic substance, the investigators mentioned above have tried mainly to understand the underlying mechanism.

2. Process of Phagocytosis of PMNs

According to Horn et al. (5), just after phagocytosis of the microorganism and particles by PMNs, phagosome is formed intracellularly, and two kinds of lysosome granules, azurophilic and specific, come into contact with phagosome and fuse to form phagolysosome. This process occurs within 3 min, and the phagosomal content becomes acidic (pH 4). According-ing to Bainton (8), two types of granules sequentially undergo intracellular secretion—that is, after 30 sec, about half of a specific granule is released, and by 3 min azurophil develops. By 10 min, phagolysosome is completed. Polymorphonuclear cells have a battery of killing substances—such as myeloperoxidase, lactoferrin, lysozyme, and cationic protein—together with many kinds of lytic enzymes in their granules. With regard to the oxygen-dependent microbicidal substances, Klebanoff and coworkers (22) reported precisely on their mode of action. Myeloperoxidase is heat-stable (80°C); it has an Ip above 10 and is most active at pH 5.0. Odeberg (23) studied the activity of this system and demonstrated a killing activity of 53% against *Candida* spp. in 17 normal subjects.

3. *Granular Release of PMNs*

Zucker-Franklin and Hirsch (6) reported on the extracellular release of granular material outside PMN cells concurrently with its intracellular release by forming phagolysosome; they proposed the term *exoplasmosis* for the former. In this regard, the PMN is a type of secretory cell; on the other hand, it is a phagocytic cell as well (24,25). The following are the modes of secretions proposed by these investigators:

a. *Regurgitation* When PMNs engulf some substance, like yeast cells, they release 25–30% of their lysosomal neutral peptidase and nonspecific collagenase into the surroundings subsequently, released neutral proteases bind to the α_1-antichymotripsin and α_2-macroglobulin of protease inhibitors.
b. *Lysis of PMNs.* Lysis by toxins, detergents, monosodium ureate, and silica causes PMN cells to release lysosomal substances.
c. *Reversed Endocytosis.* When cells are stimulated by immune reactants, such as IgG or activated complement, a large part of their lysosomal content is released.
d. *Release During Migration.* Even during the migration of cells, lysosomal release occurs.
e. *Secretion by Soluble Compounds.* Polymorphonuclear cells respond to C3 and release both azurophilic and specific granules. Concanavalin A and phorbol myristate acetate induce secretion of only specific granules, and the immune complex is a potent inducer of release.

Spitznagel and Chi (10) reported that *Escherichia coli* injected into rabbit skin gradually become stainable with anionic dye, Luxol fast blue and loses viability. They noticed that cationic substances have the ability to kill bacteria and fungi. In a series of studies (15–20), the substance was observed to be more basic than lysozyme. The electrophoretic patterns of rabbit neutrophil revealed seven fractions of cationic nature. These proteins migrate to the cathode ahead of the lysozyme. Their molecular weight ranges from 5000 to 12,000, and all bands are arginine-rich by amino acid analysis. Four of seven fractions exhibit bactericidal and fungicidal activities. These substances were called *cationic proteins*.

Zeya and Spitznagel (15) carried out the fractionation and characterization of guinea pig peritoneal PMNs using zone electrophoresis. They fractionated the extract into seven parts. Among them, bands I, II, and III caused heavy agglutination of bacteria in phosphate buffer, pH 6.2. The antibacterial fraction showed bactericidal activity against gram-positive and gram-negative organisms and *C. albicans*. The antibacterial activity of fraction 1 + II was 16, and of fraction III, 32 (diluted to obtain 50% growth inhibition).

Subsequently Lehrer (7,21,26,27) studied (in cooperation with Spitznagel) the microbicidal substance of PMNs, mainly against *Candida*. Lehrer's work (21) on the candidacidal potency of PMNs' from myeloperoxidase-deficient patients revealed remarkable activity in proving that there is a nonoxidative (21) second (26) mechanism for the killing of *Candida*. His colleagues, Ganz et al (28), characterized the substance in detail and called it Defensin. The substance consisted of three small (Mw <3500) antibiotic peptides (human neutrophil peptide HNP-1, HNP-2, and HNP-3). Defensins killed *Staphylococcus aureus*, *Pseudomonas aeruginosa*, and *E. coli* in vitro in nutrient-containing buffer and showed highly potent activity against *Cryptococcus neoformans* as well as against virus. The substance is localized in azurophil granule.

According to these investigators, the antimicrobial capabilities of the substance were as follows (29) (50 μg/ml, 2 hr, 10 mM phosphate buffer pH 7.4, 1% vol/vol trypticase soy broth for bacteria, the values decrease in bacterial population):

Cryptococcus neoformans	$\log_{10}$ 3.08
Escherichia coli	$\log_{10}$ 3.52
Pseudomonas aeruginosa	$\log_{10}$ 1.16
Staphylococcus auerus	$\log_{10}$ 1.65
Herpes simplex virus	$\log_{10}$ 2.62

The lysosomal PMN granule has killing substance other than cationic protein. Odeberg (23) noted the importance of the oxidative system as an actual killing substance, and that lactoferrin and lysozyme in PMN lysosome should not be overlooked.

B. Macrophage

Lysosomal granules of macrophage contain less peroxidase than PMNs. Arai et al. (30) reported that guinea pig PMNs phagocytoze and kill *C.*

albicans cells; by contrast, rabbit alveolar macrophages, also phagocytoze the yeast cell at the same rate, but cannot kill it. Recently, Petterson-Delafield and coworkers (31,32) reported the existence of cationic protein in rabbit alveolar macrophage but not in peritoneal macrophage. Selsted et al. (33) have further characterized peptides of rabbit alveolar macrophages MCP-1 and MCP-2. These peptides are highly microbicidal against *Candida parapsilosis*, *Bacillus subtiltis*, and *Escherichia coli* but less active against *Salmonella typhimurium*. Within 20 min, 1 μg/ml MCP-1 and MCP-2 kill 99.6 and 80% of *C. albicans* respectively.

C. Eosinophil Leukocyte

The role of eosinophil leukocyte still remains obscure. It increases in the peripheral blood in parasite infections and the so-called hypereosinophilic syndrome. The eosinophil granule is composed of three proteins: the major basic protein (MBP), neurotoxin, and cationic protein. According to Olsson et al. (34), it contains an arginine-rich basic protein of Mw 21,000 with 2.6 M Zn/mol protein. About 30% of the protein of the eosinophilic granule is in a cyrstalloid granule, but the granule has no bactericidal activity. The eosinophilic granule is similar to the lysosomal granule of PMNs because it contains cathepsin, libonuclease, arylsulfatase, and β-glucuronidase; MBP of guinea pig eosinophilic granule has no peroxidase activity. Human eosinophilic granule also contain MBP with an isoelectric point of pH 11.

Wasson et al. (35) measured the MBP blood level of the guinea pig by radioimmunoassay. The MBP level of normal guinea pig serum was 5 ng/ml, and it did not increase in response to infection with *Trichinella spiralis*. However, MBP on the parasite increased and the content in the muscle of an infected animal was also significantly elevated.

The serum level of human eosinophilic cationic protein correlates with the count of eosinophil leukocyte in peripheral blood. A patient with asthma revealed a low serum level of eosinophilic cationic protein (36).

In spite of the eosinophil leukocyte's high content of the cationic protein, the cell has no microbicidal activity. Only a few reports of the cell's activity against parasites have appeared:

1. Kierzenbaum and coworkers reported on the killing activity against *Trypanosoma cruzi* and of MBP; it was reported that 1×10^{-5}M against the blood-born form of *T. cruzi* (37).
2. Butterworth et al. reported the eosinophil-mediated antibody-dependent killing of shistosomules of *Schistosoma mansonii* (38) and direct damage of it by MBP (39).
3. Grove et al. reported activity against *Trichinella spiralis*. The rela-

tionship between eosinophil leukocyte and fungus infection is not clear (40).

D. Platelet

The major contribution of the platelet's antibacterial activity was reported by Donaldson et al. (41–44).

The platelet has no nucleus, but it is contractile and engulfs particles such as carbon powders, latex particles, collagen, and lipid by pseudopod formation.

The platelet has a dense body (ADP, ATP, serotonin, calcium) and granules (fibrinogen, lysosomal enzyme, platelet factor 4, platelet-mediated growth factor). The main function of the platelet is the protection of blood vessels from inside, and about 35,000/cm platelets are used for this purpose.

Platelet cationic protein, which has an Mw 30,000, increases vascular permeability (45). Platelet beta-lysin kills 80% of *Bacillus subtilis* within 2 min; the rat platelet has the highest killing activity. Since the characterization of platelet beta-lysin is not yet complete, the substance is not confirmed for its activity, but it is said that platelet beta-lysin acts to break down cell membrane, in contrast to lysozyme, which breaks down the cell wall.

Wincor et al. (46) reported that platelet function is disturbed in patients with diabetes mellitus; the predisposition to fungus infection especially to zygomycosis in a diabetic patient is suggested as the cause.

Benveneste et al. (47) reported on the rabbit platelet activation factor (PAF) in supernatant of IgE-sensitized rabbit basophils. Produced in a wide range of tissues of various kinds of animals, PAF activates not only platelet itself but also many other kinds of cells (PMN, lymphocyte, macrophage). It induces antimicrobial activity of myeloic cells (48) and may relate to host defense.

E. Epidermis

1. Protection by Epidermis

Epidermis is the outermost skin layer of the body and is likely to be exposed to invasion by microorganisms from the outside. The rigid horny layer is the first barrier against invasion. When microorganisms digest this layer with keratinase, they can easily invade the skin, but the invasion stops at the level of the granular layer in cases of superficial dermatomycoses and superficial cutaneous candidosis. Despite the existence of many kinds of bacteria and fungi, only a limited number of these microorganisms invade the horny layer, which may suggest that the horny layer is impregnated by some antimicrobial substance likely to originate in the deeper living layer of the epidermis. There may be some host-specificity factor in the impregnating substance, because host-parasite relationships are recognized in fungus infections,—for example, with *Trichophyton rubrum* (humans) *Microsporum canis* (canines), *Microsporun nanum* (swine), and so on. In the plant kingdom, host specificity is partly understood as follows:

Alternaria alternata

Pathotype	Host-Specific Toxin
1. Apple pathotype	AM-toxin
2. Citrus pathotype	AC-toxin
3. Japanese pear pathotype	AK-toxin
4. Strawberry pathotype	AF-toxin
5. Tobacco pathotype	AT-toxin
6. Tomato pathotype	AL-toxin

Alternaria alternata, pathogenic to tomato, contains AL toxin (49). The chemical structures of each host-specific toxin of *A. alternata* have already been elucidated. Other than host-specific toxins, plants contain phytoalexins as basic defense toxins. Phytoalexins are unspecifically toxic to the invading microorganism. The chemical structures of these phytoalexins have also been demonstrated. In animals, substances like phytoalexins have been attributed to fungicidal substances in serum (50–55), like the iron-chelating substance transferrin (56,57). Other reports have ascribed it to keratinase inhibitor in serum (58) or in the epidermis (59).

On this account, we conducted experiments to identify the fungicidal activity of crude epidermal extract and reported in 1981 on the high potency of candidacidal activity of guinea pig epidermal extract (1). This report appeared in English (2) in 1989.

2. Experimentation and Discussion

Heat-separated guinea pig epidermis was used. The microbicidal substance was extracted in accordance with the procedure for extracting PMNs outlined by Lehrer et al. (26). The extract is supposed to be cationic because the extraction is carried out in acidic conditions with citric acid (Fig. 1). The results of the experiment are shown in Tables 1 and 2. Candidacidal activity was measured by using *C. albicans* and *C. parapsilosis* as targets.

According to the tables, the crude epidermal extract is highly candidacidal, as 10 μg/ml of the substance killed 100% of *C. albicans* within 60 min. The substance killed *Candida* especially at a lower pH condition.

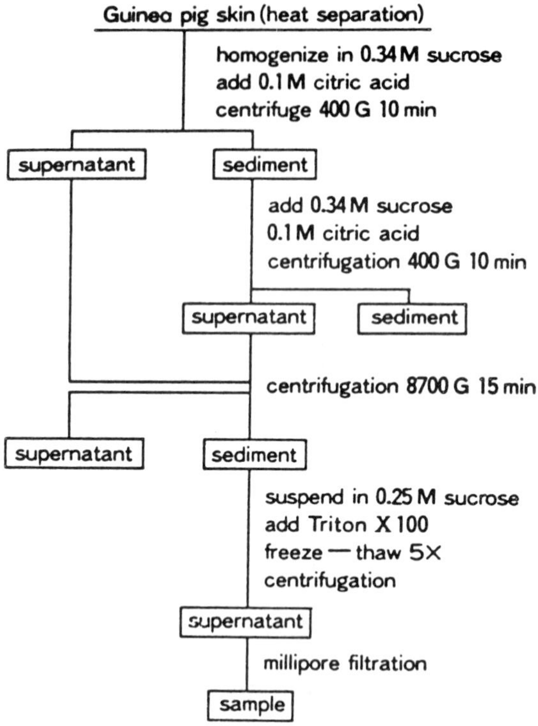

Figure 1 Process of extraction of epidermal sample solution from guinea pig skin. Epidermal extract from humans was obtained by the same process.

Table 1 Influence of Concentrations of Sample Solution on Candidacidal Rate (Guinea Pig Epidermis; Protein Concentration Measured by Method of Lowry)[a]

Protein concentration (μg/ml)	Candidacidal rate (%)
40	100
20	100
10	100
5	87
2.5	40.5
1.25	6.5
0.625	1
0.3125	0

[a] Citric acid buffer pH 4.5, 37°C, 1 hr.

Table 2 Time Course of the Candidacidal Process (Guinea Pig)[a]

Time (min)	Candidacidal rate (%)
15	94
30	100
60	100
120	100

[a] Citric acid buffer pH 4.5, sample solution 20 μg/ml.

By fractionation with Sephadex G100, the extract revealed two protein peaks coincident with the candidacidal peaks (Fig. 2).

Further purification of the sample solution by Kashima et al. (60) revealed that after Mono S column fractionation, the preparation had candidacidal activity as high as 0.2 μg/ml, which is somewhat reduced by additional purification with Mono S and Phenyl 5PW column (Fig. 3).

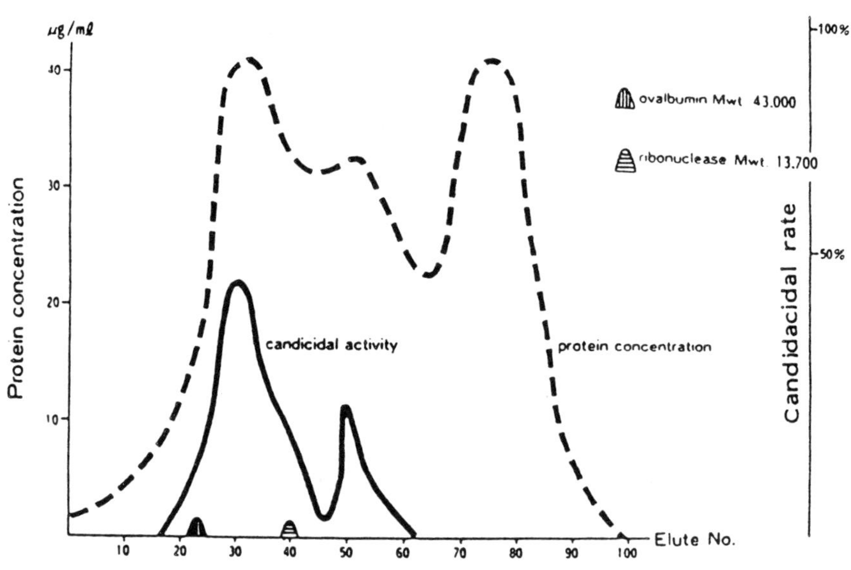

Candidacidal activities of fractionated sample solution.

Figure 2 Candidacidal activity of fractionated sample solution. (Crude epidermal extract of guinea pig, Cephadex G-100; candidacidal assay was conducted by trypan blue dye exclusion.)

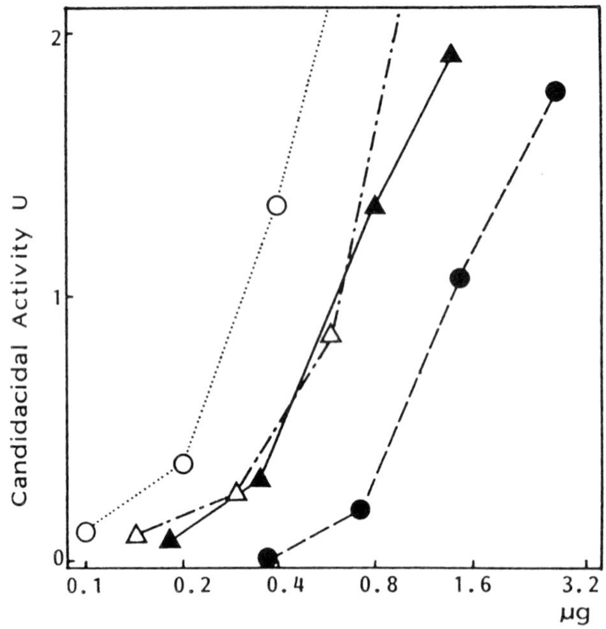

Figure 3 Change of candidacidal activity in each step of purification (human epidermal extract was applied on a Mono S column. Among 38 eluted fractions, the most potent fractions were further underwent Phenyl 5 PW column, and fr.7 and fr.9 were of the highest potencies; candidacidal assay was conducted by turbidimetry of A_{660}). Key: Closed circles, crude extract; open circles, Mono S fraction; closed triangles, Phe 5PW fr 7; open triangles, Phe 5PW fr 9.

Kashima (61) engaged in further characterization of a sample of human epidermis. Among many candidacidal fractions (Fig. 4), fractions Phe-I through Phe-V were most potent in activity; after the amino acid analysis, these fractions were coincident with H1 histone. Histones of H1 through H4 (in case of birds, H5 instead of H1) are basic substances that are lysine- and arginine-rich. According to Gabrielli (62), the possible role of histone is a component of nuclear content. However, it is highly basic, and H1 histone is especially lysin-rich and has the possibility of microbicidal activity when it is finally released into the granular and horny layers as an apoptotic product by the turnover of the keratinocyte. There is another kind of epidermal basic protein: Dale (63) extracted and purified the stratum corneum basic protein (SCBP) with Mw 50,000 and IP9-10. According to Bhatnagar and Freedberg (64), one of the epidermal basic proteins is Mw 12,800 and rich in lysine, glycine, alanine, and varine. Keratohyalin

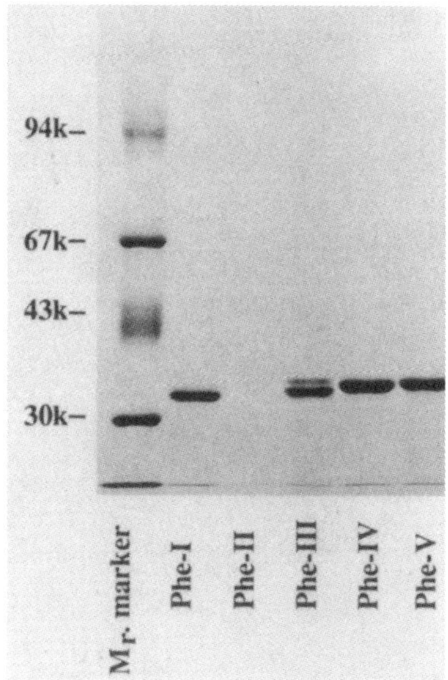

Figure 4 SDS-PAGE of the most potent human epidermal candidacidal protein by Mono S followed by Phenyl 5PW column purification (Coomassie brilliant blue R-250).

granules are of low molecular weight, Mw 10,000–18,000, and are characterized by high histidine content. One of these proteins revealed ribonuclease activity.

Candida treated with sample solution were surrounded by electron-dense material, which seems to be Zn-rich epidermal component (Fig. 5).

Bernstein (65) reported histidine-rich protein (HRP) in keratohyaline granules as macroaggregate. The HRP is Mw 30,000 and is similar to basic protein in stratum corneum of Mw 68,000. Reaven and Cox (66) reported that histidine may be responsible for the Zn-binding property of the transitional (granular layer–horny layer) zone and the keratohyaline granule. In vitro histochemical studies (67) have also demonstrated that the proteins in keratohyaline granules and cornified cell bind to Zn.

3. *Magainins*

In 1987, Zasloff (68) reported on the basic protein of *Xenopus laevis* (African clawed frog) skin and named it *magainin*. His idea is based on evidence that frogs may live in environments of poor hygienic conditions and can survive only by repelling microorganisms flourishing in such envi-

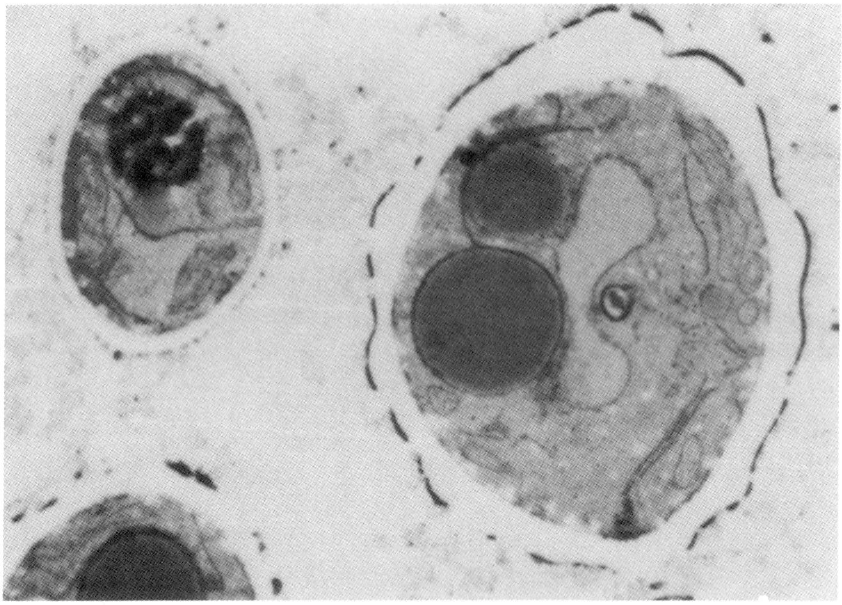

Figure 5 *Candida* cells treated with crude epidermal extract (cells are surrounded by electron-dense material).

ronmental settings. These self-defense substances may be especially dense in the skin, the outermost tissue of the body. The magainin peptides are composed of magainin 1 and 2. Both peptides are closely related, each contains 23 amino acids, and they differ in only two places. The killing activities of magainins are as follows: *Escherichia coli* (5 μg/ml), *Klebsiella pneumoniae* (10), *Staphylococcus epidermidis* (10), *Staphylococcus aureus* (50), *C. albicans* (80), *Pseudomonas aeruginosa* (100), *Serratia marcescens* (100), and *Proteus mirabilis* (>100).

Magainin peptides are bactericidal by disrupting the membranes of microorganisms.

F. Parotid Saliva

In 1984, Pollock and coworkers (69–71) reported on the candidacidal activity of human parotid saliva. The active substance is histidine-rich and can kill *Candida* at a concentration of 5 μg/ml. According to the investigators, the activity was not weakened even when the target cell was in the resting phase. The molecular weight of parotid salivary histidine-rich polypeptide is Mw 7500, and its activity is reduced by increased ionic strength in the buffer solution. The substance is basic and different from the extract of PMNs in arginine content: however, its mode of action may be similar to that of another basic microbicidal substance, inducing leakage of potassium at the site of membrane damage. Histidine-rich protein of the parotid killed 100% of *C. albicans* within 24 hr at a concentration of 5 μg/ml.

According to MacKay and coworkers (70), human parotid salivary histidine-rich polypeptide is bacteriostatic and bactericidal against *Streptococcus mutans* at concentrations of 250 μg/ml and killed 80% of *S. mutans* within 24 hr.

Characterization of the substance was carried out by MacKay and coworkers (71). According to their study, the substance was a histidine-rich polypeptide, and up to 14 bands were recognized by polyacrylamide gel electrophoresis. All bands migrated more rapidly to the cathode than purified human leukocyte cationic polypeptides. The substance contained at least 48% cationic residues, and half of them were histidine.

There are many opinions on the bactericidal substance of saliva, such as lysozyme, oral microfloral products, and peroxidase. Green (72) reported the activity of beta-lysin in 1966.

G. Thymus

Antimicrobial research on the activity of the thymus has been conducted for more than five decades. According to Skarnes et al. (73), as early as 1947, Bloom, Watson, and Cromartie obtained an anthracidal substance from calf thymus. Even at that time, the material was considered to be stable to heat and acid and basic due to the presence of large amounts of lysine. The substance was thought to be derived from histone. Skarnes reported that the sample from the thymus was pH 3.1, and that 5 μg/ml of thymus peptide inhibited *Staphylococcus* after 8 hr, as well as being interfered with by the addition of 0.5–1% NaCl, and acidic polymers such as hyaluronic acid and nucleic acid. The thymus peptide was active against gram-positive cocci but not active against gram-negative bacilli. It contained lysine, which represented nearly 35% of the total weight of the protein. Spitznagel studied the anthracidal activity of calf thymus by assaying its viability with fast green staining and obtained the result that 50 μg/ml of the sample reduced bacterial count from 5×10^6 within 60 min. The significance of thymus has been discussed from two points of view, classic and immunological. Thymus contains epithelial tissue, named Hassal's body, and among thymus tissue components, thymulin is metalloprotein with Zn-binding capacity. The role of the thymus in relation to cryptococcosis and aspergillosis has been discussed by Chen and Goldstein (75); Mankowski (76) reported that injection of thymus extract three times a day increased the host resistance against *C. albicans*.

H. Seminal Plasmin

Block (72) published a monograph on spermatogenesis in 1969. According to his report, replacement of sperm histone is an event in the course of sperm differentiation and comes as one of the last stages.

The basic proteins of sperm nuclei are classified into five substances: minoprotamin (salmon), stable protamines or basic keratins (mouse), intermediate protein (mussel), typical histones (frog), and relatively nonbasic proteins (crab). Salmin is protamin taken from ripe salmon sperm cells (77). The Mw is reported to be 2855–7000 and is quite basic owing to the guanidine group of arginine. Its mode of action is similar to that of polymyxin. It has a tendency to attach to the surface of microorganisms and is drawn more to gram-positives than to gram-negatives. Several reports have dealt with the bactericidal activity of human semen (78,79).

High contents of spermine and spermidine in animal tissues are found in the pancreas, prostate, and human semen. The major parts of polyamines in human semen are contained in seminal plasma rather than in spermatozoa, and they presumably originate from prostatic secretion (80). Protamine and other basic proteins are found in the spermatozoa of mollusks (81).

I. Others (Serum, Amnionic Fluid, Milk, Tears)

1. Serum

At the starting point of the history of the bactericidal substances, Nuttal (82) in 1888 reported that bactericidal humoral factors of pleural exudate, clotted blood and pericardial effusions of pigeon, sheep, rabbit, frog, and tortoise,—in terms of their killing activities against *Bacillus anthracis, Bacillus subtilis, Bacillus megatherium*, and *S. aureus*—could be classified into two types: thermolabile and thermostable. The former is inactivated by heating for 30 min at 56°C and was called alexin by Buchner (83). Bordet (84) also reported that *Vibrio cholerae* is killed by the microbiolytic activity of serum and that the active substance consists of two components—thermostable and thermolabile alexin. The latter plays only a complementary role.

Donaldson and Ters (41) reported on the thermostable substance in detail. They called it beta-lysin, of which there are four kinds in serum: lysozyme, platelet-derived substance, and two less defined components. Platelet-derived substance, plakin, was classified into two components:

the first substance killed gram-negative bacilli previously injured by complement and by entering through the hole formed by the injury. The second beta-lysin is the substance isolated from rabbit serum. It is a basic peptide of 17 amino acids. Beta-lysin killed gram-positives at concentrations of 5–50 μg/ml (90% MIC) and gram-negatives at concentrations of 299–350 μg/ml. According to the investigators, the mode of action is the disruption of cytochrome *c* oxidase. Beta-lysin adsorbs to Saitz filter disk and eluted from the disk with high concentrations of salt. The purified substance kills 80% of *Bacillus subtilis* within 2 min. The activity of platelet-derived beta-lysin vairies widely according to the animal species. Rat and rabbit revealed high activity, and humans, cattle, cats, swine, guinea pigs, and mice showed low activity. The substance was found to be absent in sweat, spinal fluid, and urine. Activation of platelet can be induced by trauma or by injections of glycogen or saline into the peritoneal cavity, subcutaneous injection of aluminum silicate, and diseases such as pneumonia and myocardial infarction. Enzymes such as neuraminidase cover the surface of the platelet and evoke the release of beta-lysin. Studies on beta-lysin have been published by Donaldson and coworkers (42–44,85–90). The activity of beta-lysin was enhanced by endotoxin (91,92) and the immune complex (42).

2. *Amnionic Fluid*

Amnionic fluid (93) has antibacterial activity ascribed to two kinds of substances of high and low molecular weight. The former is beta-lysin, with Zn-binding capacity, and the latter is an uncharacterized antibacterial substance of Mw <1000. The activity was lost after treatment with EDTA and restored by addition of Mg, Ca, or Zn. Among two kinds of active substance is similar to the beta-lysin of serum and different from the low-molecular-weight substance.

3. *Milk*

Gillin and coworkers (94) reported that despite the removal of IgA antibody, normal human milk did not decrease in giardiacidal activity but immobilized trophozoites, deprived them of motility, and lysed them. According to him, the activity was specific to human milk; cow's milk and goat's milk were devoid of activity. The activity was much decreased by heating or treating with a specific esterase inhibitor, which suggests that the substance seems to be different from those discussed above.

4. *Tears*

Human lacrimal secretions have microbicidal activity, and beta-lysin is though to exist in lacrimal secretion (95,96). Tears are rich in lysozyme;

however, it is microbiostatic, not microbicidal, whereas a more microbicidal substance prevents ophthalmic fungus infection.

J. Cationic Polypeptide of Other Sources

Self-defense mechanisms by cationic polypeptides seem to be so ubiquitous that many reports other than those involving humans can be collected. These polypeptides are found in every living thing, from bacteria to higher animals, and even in plants. Sahl (98) and Dempsey (99) surveyed bee venom mellitin, cecropin from cecropia moth, and nisin from *Streptococcus lactis*. Only the table from their review is referenced here (Table 3).

Vertebrates and insects attained the two peaks on the phylogenic scale from the standpoint of archeological biology. Vertebrates are provided with cellular and humoral immunological mechanisms; in contrast, insects are provided with the phagocytic mechanism and antibiotic substance formation. Insects produce lysozyme like vertebrates; and, other than lysozyme, some basic heat-stable substance of Ip 7.7, Mw 5000. By injection of *E. coli* into larva of *Bombyx mori* (silkworm), formation of the antibiotic substance is enhanced in the larva. The MICs (100) of the substance are as follows: *E. coli* (4 μg/ml), *P. aeruginosa, Streptococcus hemolytica* (16.0), and *B. subtilis* (>1000).

Table 3 Cationic Bactericidal Polypeptides of Various Origin

Bacterial origin			
Nisin	*Streptococcus lactis*	Mw 3500	
Pep 5	*Staphylococcus epidermidis*	3300	Ip 105
Bacteriocin IYS2	*Staphylococcus aureus*	5000	10.0
Bacteriocin C3 603	*Streptococcus mutans*	4800	10.0
GramicidinS	*Bacillus brevis*		
Fungal origin			
Hypelcin A	Fungi imperfecti		
Alamethicin			
Insect origin			
Cecropins	*Hyalophora cecropia*		
Melittin	Bee venom	2800	
Vertebrate origin			
Seminal plasmin			
Defensin			
Magainin			
MCPs			

The mode of action of these substances is the disruption of cell membrane of the target microorganism like colistin. The substance of the insect has some similarity to cationic polypeptide of vertebrates.

III. MODE OF ACTION OF CATIONIC POLYPEPTIDES

A series of studies on the mode of action of cationic polypeptides has been reported by Sahl and coworkers (98,101–105). They have dealt with staphylococcal basic polypeptide Pep 5 and experiments using an artificial membrane model, from which they concluded that the substance damages the cell membrane. On the other hand, some pharmacological studies have been based on the chemical standpoint of the cell membrane bilayer; on peptide-induced membrane permeation. According to the theory of these investigators, acidic phospholipid (phosphatidylglycerol, cardiolipin) and acid lipopolysaccharide of lipid bilayer of microbial cell membrane react with cationic polypeptides and can easily induce damage.

Recently, the mechanism of magainin-induced membrane damage was reported (106).

IV. CONCLUSIONS

In superficial candidosis and dermatophytosis, the causative organisms invade the horny layer, but never invade deeply into the granular layer and squamous cell layer. When the host dies, fungus invades deeper into the dermis and subdermal tissues. This means that there is some antimycotic substance in the deeper layers and also in the horny layer, because of all the fungi and bacteria with keratinase, only a small number can invade the horny layer. This may mean that some antimycotic physiological substance impregnates from a deeper layer to the horny layer. In case of granuloma trichophyticum, the fungus element invade deeper into the dermis and even metastasize to the internal organs through lymphatic and blood pathways, whereas it may be caused by the lack of the substance.

The main component of the substance we extracted from the epidermis was H1 histone, which may finally be released into the horny layer during the metamorphosis of the epidermis.

Naturally occurring antibiotic substances, found physiologically in tissues, seem to be widespread and exist in many tissues in a variety of hosts, from vertebrates to microorganisms. We dealt with these tissue-bound antibiotic substances. Of course, there are other substances engaged in host defense of tissues. The possible categories involved are:

1. Oxidative system, such as myeloperoxidase
2. Enzymatic system, such as lysozyme

3. Chelating system, such as transferrin and lactoferrin
4. Immunological system, such as perforin
5. However, the substances with high potency ability for host defense is the cationic system (e.g., defensin, magainin)

In this article, the last of these systems was discussed with reference to the literature. The cationic system has the following characteristics:

1. Heat stability
2. Adhesion to target cell surface
3. Chelating tendency of divalent metals
4. Activity tends to decrease in high-ionic-strength buffer

This is the first publication that systematically deals with the tissue-bound host-defense system.

REFERENCES

1. Takahashi H, Kaneko O, Chikakane K, et al. Candidacidal activities of guinea pig skin extracts. Proc Jpn Soc Invest Dermatol 1981;5:141–142.
2. Takahashi H, Chikakane K, Kaneko O, et al. Tissue bound immunity. In: McGinis MR, Borgers M, eds. Current Topics in Medical Mycology. Vol. 3. New York: Springer-Verlag, 1989:50–63.
3. Metchnikoff F. Leukocyte and phagocytosis. In: Mizunuma S, Kakisawa K, eds. Virchow's Arch Pathol Anat. Tokyo: Kodansha Scientific. 1979: 78.
4. Cohn ZA, Hirsch JG. The isolation and properties of the specific cytoplasmic granules of rabbit polymorphonuclear leukocytes. J Exp Med 1960; 110:983–1004.
5. Horn RG, Spicer SS, Wetzel BK. Phagocytosis of bacteria by heterophil leukocytes. Acid and alkaline phosphatase cytochemistry. Am J Pathol 1964;45:327–335.
6. Zucker-Franklin D, Hirsch JG. Electron microscope studies on the degranulation of rabbit peritoneal leukocyte. J Exp Med 1964;120:569–575.
7. Lehrer RI, Cline MJ. Interaction of Candida albicans with human leukocytes and serum. J Bacteriol 1969;98:996–1004.
8. Bainton DF. Sequential degranulation of the two types of polymorphonuclear leukocyte granules during phagocytosis of microorganisms. J Cell Biol 1973;58:249–264.
9. Janoff A, Schaefer S, Sherer J, Bean M. Mediators of inflammation in leukocyte lysosomes. II. Mechanism of action of lysosomal cationic protein upon vascular permeability in the rat. J Exp Med 1965;122:841–851.
10. Spitznagel JK, Chi HY. Cationic proteins and antibacterial properties of infected tissues and leukocytes. Am J Pathol 1963;43:697–711.
11. Janoff A, Zweifach BW. Production of inflammatory changes in the micro-

circulation by cationic proteins extracted from leukocytes lysosomes. J Exp Med 1964;120:747–764.
12. Pryzwansky KB, Martin LE, Spitznagel JK. Immunocytochemical localization of myeloperoxidase, lactoferrin, lysozyme and neutral proteases in human monocytes and neutrophilic granulocytes. J Reticuloendothelial Soc 1978;24:295–310.
13. Olsson I, Venge P. Cationic proteins of human granulocytes. II. Separation of the cationic proteins of the granules of leukemic myeloid cells. Blood 1974;44:235–246.
14. MacRae EK, Spitznagel JK. Ultrastructural localization of cationic proteins in cytoplasmic granules of chicken and rabbit polymorphonuclear leukocytes. J Cell Sci 1975;17:79–94.
15. Zeya HI, Spitznagel JK. Antibacterial and enzymic basic proteins from leukocyte lysosomes: Separation and identification. Science 1963;142: 1085–7.
16. Zeya HI, Spitznagel JK. Cationic proteins of polymorphonuclear leukocyte lysosomes. I. Resolution of antibacterial and enzymatic activities. J Bacteriol 1966;91:750–754.
17. Zeya HI, Spitznagel JK. Antimicrobial specificity of leukocyte lysosomal proteins. Science 1966;154:1049–1051.
18. Zeya HI, Spitznagel JK. Arginine-rich proteins of polymorphonuclear leukocyte lysosomes. Antimicrobial specificity and biochemical heterogeneity. J Exp Med 1968;127:927–941.
19. Zeya HI, Spitznagel JK. Cationic proteins bearing granules of polymorphonuclear leukocytes: Separation from enzyme-rich granule. Science 1969; 163:1069–1071.
20. Zeya HI, Spitznagel JK. Characterization of cationic protein-bearing granules of polymorphonuclear leukocytes. Lab Invest 1971;24:229–236.
21. Lehrer RI, Ladra KM, Hake RB. Nonoxidative fungicidal mechanisms of mammalian granulocytes: Demonstration of components with candidacidal activity in human, rabbit, and guinea pig leukocytes. Infect Immun 1975; 11:1226–1234.
22. Klebanoff SJ, Clem WH, Luebke RG. The peroxidase-thiocyabate-hydrogen peroxide antimicrobial system. Biochim Biophys Acta 1966;117: 63–72.
23. Odeberg H, Olsson I. Microbiocidal mechanisms of human granulocytes, synergistic effects of granulocyte elastase and myeloperoxidase of chymotrypsin-like cationic protein. Infect Immun 1976;14:1276–1283.
24. Leffel MS, Spitznagel JK. Intracellular and extracellular degranulation of human polymorphonuclear azurophil and specific granules induced by immune complexes. Infect Immun 1974;10:1241–1249.
25. Linkoeping LBE, Goeteborg LE, Linkoeping OIS. Endocytosis and Exocytis in Host Defense. Basel: S. Karger, 1981:130–147.
26. Lehrer RI. Functional aspect of a second mechanism of candidacidal activity by human neutrophils. J Clin Invest 1972;51:2566–2572.

27. Lehrer RI. The fungicidal activity of human leukocytes. In: Williams RC, Fundenberg HH, eds. Phagocytic Mechanisms in Health and Disease. New York: International Medical Book Corp. 1972:151–166.
28. Ganz T, Selsted ME, Szkarek D, Harwig SSL, Daher K, Bainton DF, Lehrer RI. Defensins, natural peptide antibiotics of human neutrophils. J Clin Invest 1985;76:1427–1435.
29. Rice WG, Ganz T, Kinkade JM, et al. Defensin-rich granules of human neutrophils. Blood 1987;70:757–765.
30. Arai T, Mikami Y, Yokoyama K. Phagocytosis of Candida albicans by rabbit alveolar macrophages and guinea pig neutrophils. Sabouraudia 1977; 15:171–177.
31. Patterson-Delafield J, Szklarek D, Martinez RJ, Lehrer RI. Microbiocidal cationic proteins of rabbit alveolar macrophages: Amino acid composition and functional attributes. Infect Immun 1981;31:723–731.
32. Patterson-Delafield J, Martinez RJ, Lehrer RI. Microbiocidal cationic proteins in rabbit alveolar macrophages: A Potential host defense mechanism. Infect Immun 1980;30:180–192.
33. Selsted ME, Brown DM, DeLange RJ, Lehrer RI. Primary structure of MCP-1 and MCP-2, natural peptide antibiotics of rabbit lung macrophages. J Biochem Chem 1983;258:14485–14489.
34. Olsson I, Venge P, Spitznagel JK, Lehrer RI. Arginine-rich cationic proteins of human eosinophil granules. Lab Invest 1977;36:493–500.
35. Wassom DL, Loegering DA, Gleich GJ. Measurement of guinea pig eosinophil major basic protein by radioimmunoassay. Molecular Immunol 1979; 16:711–719.
36. Venge P, Zetterstroem O, Dahl R, et al. Low levels of eosinophilic cationic proteins in patients with asthona. Lancet 1977;20:373–375.
37. Kierszenbaum F, Ackerman SJ, Gleich GJ. Destruction of bloodstream forms of Trypanosoma cruzei by eosinophil granule major basic protein. Am J Trop Med Hyg 1981;30:775–779.
38. Butterworth AE, David JR, Franks D, et al. Antibody-dependent eosinophil-mediated damage to ^{51}Cr-labeled schistosomula of schistosoma mansoni: damage by purieid eosinophils. J Exp Med 1977;145:136–150.
39. Butterworth AE, Wassom DL, Gleich GJ, Loegering DA, David JR. Damage to schistosomula of Schistosoma mansoni induced directly by eosinophil major basic protein. J Immunol 1979;122:221–229.
40. Grove DI, Mahmoud AAF, Warren KS. Eosinophils and resistance to Trichinella spiralis. J Exp Med 1977;145:755–759.
41. Donaldson DH, Ters JG. Beta-lysin of platelet origin. Bacteriol Rev 1977; 41:501–513.
42. Donaldson DM, Roberts RR, Larsen HS, Tew JG. Interrelationship between serum beta-lysin, lysozyme and the antibody-complement system in killing Escherichia coli. Infect Immun 1974;10:657–666.
43. Matheson A, Donaldson DM. Alteration in the morphology of Bacillus subtilis after exposure to beta-lysin and ultraviolet light. J Bacteriol 1968;95: 1892–1902.

44. Matheson A, Donaldson DM. Effect of beta-lysin on isolated cell walls and protoplast of Bacillus subtilis. J Bacteriol 1970;101:314–317.
45. Nachman RL, Weksler B, Ferris B. Characterization of human platelet vascular permeability-enhancing activity. J Clin Invest 1972;51:549–556.
46. Winocour PD, Halushka PV, Colwell JA. The Platelets. New York: Academic Press, 1985:341–366.
47. Benveniste J, Henson PM, Cochrane CG. Leukocyte-dependent histamine release from rabbit platelets, the role of IgE, basophils and a platelet-activating factor. J Exp Med 1972;136:1356–1377.
48. Jago R, Jacox RF. Cellular source and character of heat stable bactericidal property associated with rabbit and rat platelets. J Exp Med 1961;113:701–709.
49. Nishimura S, Kohmoto K, Otani H, et al. Pathological and epidermiological aspects of Alternaria arternata infection depending on a host-specific toxin. In: Asada Y, Bushnell WR et al, eds. Plant Infection, Heidelberg: Springer-Verlag, 1982:199–214.
50. Ayres S, Anderson NP. Inhibition of fungi in cultures by blood serum form patients with phytid eruptions. Arch Dermatol Syphilol 1940;42:426–437.
51. Lorincz AL, Priestley JO, Jacobs PH. Evidence for a humoral mechanism which prevents growth of dermatophytes. J Invest Dermatol 1958;31:15–17.
52. Jessner M, Hoffman H. Der Einfluss des Serums allergischer auf Trichophyon Pilze. Arch Dermatol Syphilol 1923;145:187–192.
53. Per MI, Braude R. Contribution a la question de la valeur diagnostique et therapeutique de la trichophytine au cours de la dermatomycose a la lumiere des connaisances contemporaines sur l'allergic specifique et l'immunile. Acta Derm Venerol 1928;9:1–8.
54. Carlisle DH, Inouye JC, King RD, Jones HE. Significance of serum dermatophyte inhibitory factor in dermatophytosis. J Invest Dermatol 1974;63:239–241.
55. Louria DB, Brayton RG. A substance in blood lethal for Candida albicans. Nature 1964;201:309.
56. Bezkorovainy A. Antimicrobial properties of iron-binding proteins. In: Phillips M, Baetz A, eds. Diet and Resistance to Disease. New York: Plenum Press, 1981:139–154.
57. Martin CM, Jandle JH, Finland M. Enhancement of acute bacterial infection in rat and mice by iron and their inhibition by human transferrin. J Infect Dis 1963;112:158–163.
58. Yu RJ, Grappel SF, Blank F. Inhibition of keratinase by alpha$_2$-macroglobulin. Experientia 1972;28:886.
59. Wakimoto A, Sagawa Y, Higuchi M, Takiuchi I. On the extracellular low molecular keratinase inhibitor extracted from human epidermis (in Japanese, with English legends and summary). Jpn J Med Mycol 1953;24:128–132.
60. Kashima M, Takahashi H, Shimozuma M, Epstein W, Fukuyama K. Candidacidal activities of epidermal proteins, partially purified from rat epidermis. Infect Immun 1989;57:186–190.

61. Kashima M. H1 Histone contribute to candidacidal activities of human epidermal extract. J Dermatol (Tokyo) 1991;18:695–706.
62. Gabrielli F. Human histone variants. In: Hnilca LS, ed. Histones and other basic nuclear proteins. Boca Raton, Florida: CRC Press, 1989:3–16.
63. Dale BA. Purification and characterization of a basic protein from the stratum corneum of mammalian epidermis. Biochim Biophys Acta 1977;491: 193–204.
64. Bhatnagar GM, Freedberg IM. Biochemical and immunological analysis of basic protein from newborn rat epidermis. Biochem 1977;16:4856–4862.
65. Bernstein IA. The proteins of keratohyalin. In: Goldsmith LA, ed. Biochemistry and Physiology of the Skin. New York. Oxford Univ Press 1983: 170–183.
66. Reaven EP, Cox AJ. The histochemical localization of histidine in the human epidermis and its relationship to zinc binding. J Histochem Cytochem 1963;11:782–790.
67. Ito Y, Horie N, Fukuyama K. Enzymatic activities of metal binding protein (MBP) in rat epidermis. J Invest Dermatol 1983;80:353.
68. Zasloff M. Magainins, a class of antimicrobial peptides from Xenopus skin: Isolation, characterization of two active forms, and partial cDNA sequence of precursor. Proc Natl Acad Sci USA 1987;84:5449–5453.
69. Pollock JJ, Denepitiya L, MacKay BJ, Iacono VJ. Fungistatic and fungicidal activity of human parotid salivary histidine-rich polypeptides on Candida albicans. Infect Immun 1984;44:702–707.
70. MacKay BJ, Denepitya L, Ianco VJ, et al. Growth inhibitory and bactericidal effects of human parotid salivary histidine-rich polypeptides on Streptococcus mutans. Infect Immun 1984;44:695–701.
71. MacKay BJ, Pollock JJ, Ianco VJ, Baum BJ. Isolation of milligram quantities of group of histidine-rich polypeptide from human parotid saliva. Infect Immun 1984;44:688–694.
72. Green GE. Properties of a salivary bacteriolysin and comparison with serum beta lysin. J Dental Res 1966;45:882–889.
73. Skarnes RC, Watson DW. Characterization of an antibacterial peptide from calf thymus. Proc Soc Exp Biol Med 1956;93:267–269.
74. Dardenne M, Pleau JM, Calenda A, et al. Recent developments in thymulin (FTS-Zn), biochemistry and molecular biology. In: Goldstein G, Bach J, Wigzell H, eds. Immune Regulation by Characterized Polypeptides. New York: Alan R Liss, 1986:259–270.
75. Chen J, Goldstein AL. Thymosins and other thymic hormones. In: Torrence PF, ed. Biological Response Modifiers, Orlando, Florida: Academic Press, 1985:121–137.
76. Mankowski ZT. Influence of cell-free thymus extracts on the course of experimental Candida albicans infection in mice. Mycopathol Mycol 1968; 36:247–256.
77. Brock TD. The effect of salmine on bacteria. Can J Microbiol 1958;4:65–71.
78. Gurevitch J, Rozansky R, Weber D, et al. The role of spermine in the

inhibition of Staphylococcus aureus by human semen. J Clin Pathol 1951; 4:360–365.
79. Razin S, Rozansky R. The responsibility of the antibacterial action of human semen. J Lab Clin Med 1957;49:877–881.
80. Harrison GA. Spermine in human tissues. Biochem J 1931;25:1885–1892.
81. Subirana JA, Cozcolluela C, Palau J, Unzeta M. Protamines and other basic proteins from spermatozoa of molluscus. Biochim Biophys Acta 1973;317: 364–379.
82. Nuttal G. Experimente ueber bakterienfeindlichen Einfluss des thierischen Koerpers. Z Hyg 1888;4:353–394.
83. Buchner H. Ueber die Bakterientoetende Wirkung des Zellfreien Blutserums. Z Bacteriol Parasitenkunde 1889;5:817–823.
84. Bordet J. Les leukocytes et les proprietes actives du serum chez les vaccines. Ann Pasteur 1895;9:462–506.
85. Amano T, Kato K, Shimizu R. Studies on the role of plakin. Med J Osaka Univ 1952;3:293–311.
86. Amano T, Tamatani Y, Kato K, et al. Studies on the role of plakin VIII. The mechanism of activation by serum. Med J Osaka Univ 1957;7:829–832.
87. Donaldson DM, Jensen RS, Jensen BM, Matheson A. Serological relationships among beta-lysin, plakin and leukin. J Bacteriol 1964;88:1049–1055.
88. Donaldson DM, Tew JG. Differentiation of muramidase and beta-lysin. Proc Soc Exp Biol Med 1966;122:46–49.
89. Donaldson DM, Tew JG. Beta-lysin of platelet origin. Bacteriol Rev 1977; 41:501–513.
90. Matheson A, Jensen RS, Donaldson DM. Serologic relationships between beta-lysins of different species. J Immunol 1966;96:885–891.
91. Hill AW, Shears AL, Hibbitt KG. Increased antibacterial activity against Escherichia coli in bovine serum after the induction of endotoxin tolerance. Infect Immun 1976;14:257–265.
92. Czuprynski CJ, Balish E. Killing of Listeria monocytogenes by conventional and germ free rat sera. Infect Immun 1981;33:348–354.
93. Scane TMN, Kawkins DF. Antibacterial activity in human amniotic fluid: Relationship to zinc and phosphate. Br J Obstet Gynecol 1984;91:342–348.
94. Dillin FD, Reiner DS, Wang C. Killing of giardia lambria trophozoites by normal human milk. J Cell Biochem 1983;23:47–56.
95. Janssen PT, Muytjens HL, Bijsterreld P. Nonlysozyme antibacterial factor in human teras. Invest Ophthalmol Vis Sci 1984;25:1156–1160.
96. Bron AJ, Seal DV. The defenses of the ocular surface. Trans Ophthalmol Soc UK 1986;105:18–25.
97. Ford LC, DeLange RJ, Petty RW. Identification of a nonlysosomal bactericidal factor (beta lysin) in human tears and aqueous humor. Am J Ophthalmol 1976;81:30–33.
98. Sahl H-G. Bactericidal cationic peptides involved in bacterial antagonism and host defense. Microbiol Sci 1985;2:212–217.
99. Dempsy CE. The action of melittin on membranes. Biochim Biophy Acta 1990;1031:143–161.

100. Kikuchi M. Antibiotic activity of haemolymph of Bombyx mori. In: Mizuno D, ed. Mechanism of host-defence. Tokyo: Univ of Tokyo Press. 1980: 19–39.
101. Sahl H-G, Brandis H. Efflux of low Mw substances from the cytoplasm of sensitive cells caused by the staphylococcin-like agent Pep 5. FEMS Microbiol Lett 1983;16:75–79.
102. Sahl H-G, Hahn C, Brandis H. Interaction of staphylococin-like peptide Pep 5 with cell walls and isolated cell wall components of gram-positive bacteria. Zbl Bakteriol Hyg 1985;A260:197–205.
103. Sahl H-G, Korael M, Grossgarten M, Brandis H. Action of the staphylococcin-like peptide Pep 5 on gram positive bacteria and cytoplasmic membrane vesicles. In: Jeljaszewicz J, ed. The Staphylococci, Zbl Bakteriol Supple 14. Stuttgart: Gustav Fisher Verlag. 1985:323–325.
104. Sahl H-G. Influence of stapholococcin-like peptide Pep 5 on membrane potential of bacterial cells and cytoplasmic membrane vesicles. J Bacteriol 1985;162:833–836.
105. Sahl H-G, Grossgarten M, Widger WR, et al. Structural similarities of the staphylococcin-like peptide Pep 5 to the antibiotic nisin. Antimicrob Agents Chemother 1985;27:836–840.
106. Cruciani RA, Baker JL, Durell SR, et al. Magainin 2, a natural antibiotic from frog skin, form ion channel in lipid bilayer membranes. Eur J Pharmacol 1992;226:287–296.

9

Cutaneous Defense Mechanisms Against Fungi

DAVID K. WAGNER
Medical College of Wisconsin
Milwaukee, Wisconsin

PETER G. SOHNLE
Medical College of Wisconsin
and Milwaukee Veterans Affairs Medical Center
Milwaukee, Wisconsin

I. INTRODUCTION AND OVERVIEW

This chapter covers mechanisms of cutaneous defense against superficial fungal infections such as cutaneous candidiasis, dermatophytosis, tinea versicolor, and some related mycoses. These infections are confined to the epidermis and cutaneous appendages, in contrast to the subcutaneous mycoses and cutaneous infections associated with deep mycoses, which are covered elsewhere. The review provided here is to describe the individual infections and predispositions to them, immunological and nonimmunological cutaneous defenses and mechanisms of host-defense defects in patients with chronic superficial fungal infections.

II. TYPES OF CUTANEOUS FUNGAL INFECTIONS AND PREDISPOSITIONS TO THEM

A. Cutaneous Candidiasis

Cutaneous candidiasis is an acute or chronic infection that is generally caused by the yeast *Candida albicans*. This organism is generally considered to be part of the normal flora of the gastrointestinal tract rather than that of the skin, although it can be found on the skin on occasion. Acute cutaneous candidiasis often presents as intertrigo and may produce intense erythema, edema, creamy exudate, and satellite pustules. In other cases the infection may be more chronic, particularly in the interdigital spaces of the feet, where there can be a thick white layer of infected stratum corneum overlying the epidermis. *Candida albicans* can also infect the periungual skin and the nail itself, producing the typical swelling and redness of candidal paronychia.

Chronic mucocutaneous candidiasis is an uncommon disorder characterized by persistent and recurrent infections of the mucous membranes, skin, and nails by *C. albicans*. These superficial infections last for years unless they are properly treated; however, deep candidal infections are very rare in this condition (1). Epidermal neutrophilic microabscesses, which are common in acute cutaneous candidiasis, are rare in the lesions of chronic mucocutaneous candidiasis. Nail involvement can be severe in this condition, with marked thickening, distortion, and fragmentation of the nails and chronic swelling of the distal phalanx.

There are a number of other disorders that are associated with the syndrome of chronic mucocutaneous candidiasis (reviewed in Refs. 2 and 3). Most prominent of these are the endocrinopathies, especially hypoadrenalism, hypoparathyroidism, hypothyroidism, ovarian insufficiency, pernicious anemia, and diabetes mellitus. Other manifestations of the syndrome include alopecia totalis, vitiligo, malabsorption, chronic hepatitis, dysplasia of the dental enamel, congenital thymic dysplasia, thymomas, and other kinds of infections. The latter include chronic dermatophytosis, recurrent bacterial infections, and occasional opportunistic infections such as cryptococcosis, histoplasmosis, and *Pneumocystis* pneumonia. Chronic mucocutaneous candidiasis is probably a group of syndromes with a variety of predisposing or secondary abnormalities in host defense function. Most common is a deficiency of cell-mediated immune responses against *Candida* antigens, as discussed below, although abnormalities in chemotaxis or phagocytic cell function have also been reported (4–8). On the other hand, humoral immunity and the complement system generally have been found to be normal in these patients (2,3,9–11).

Cutaneous candidiasis most frequently occurs when there are warm, moist conditions such as in skin folds, under the diapers of newborns, and also in tropical climates or during the summer months. Such drugs as broad-spectrum antibiotics, corticosteroids, cytotoxic agents, and oral contraceptives all predispose the treated patients to various forms of candidiasis. Diabetes mellitus (12) and infection with HIV (13–15) are both strongly associated with superficial candidiasis, although disseminated candidiasis is unusual in these conditions. Chronic mucocutaneous candidiasis may be inherited in some cases, with about 25% of these patients having relatives with this disease (16,17).

B. Dermatophytosis

Dermatophytosis is the infection of keratinized structures—including the nails, hair shafts, and stratum corneum of the skin—by a group of fungi termed the dermatophytes. The three genera of dermatophytes, *Trichophyton*, *Epidermophyton*, and *Microsporum*, together contain over 40 species that can be classified as anthropophilic, zoophilic, or geophilic. Anthropophilic species are better adapted to humans and tend to produce less inflammatory and more chronic infections than do members of the other two groups. Dermatophytes are probably not part of the normal human skin flora (18), so that this group of organisms is different from the agents of cutaneous candidiasis and tinea versicolor, in which the causative organisms are normal inhabitants of humans. Dermatophytosis is generally classified according to body site, using the word *tinea* followed by a term for the particular body site.

Scytalidium dimidiatum (Hendersonula toruloidea) and *Scytalidium hyalinum* are opportunistic organisms that can produce conditions clinically mimicking those caused by the usual dermatophyte species (19). These two organisms appear to be antigenically distinct from the dermatophytes (20). Some cases have apparently been acquired within the United States, but most come from endemic areas in other parts of the world. It is important to identify these pathogens by culturing infected skin, because these infections do not respond to conventional antifungal therapy.

Even in severely immunocompromised patients, dermatophytes rarely invade the deep tissues or produce systemic infections. On infrequent occasions, however, granulomas, draining sinuses, or actual abscesses can be produced by these organisms (21). As discussed below, competition for iron by serum proteins such as transferrin may preclude the dermatophytic fungi from invading deep tissues in most patients, even if they are immunosuppressed.

Local cutaneous factors appear to be very important in determining the outcome of an exposure to the dermatophytic fungi. For example, the warm, moist conditions in the swampy areas of Vietnam were felt to be responsible in part for the high incidence of dermatophytosis in combat troops there (22). Also, occlusion appears to be very important in enhancing susceptibility to experimental dermatophyte infections in humans and animals (22–27). Occlusion has been postulated to increase hydration of the underlying skin and also to increase the emission of carbon dioxide, which could favor dermatophyte growth (28).

A variety of medical conditions appear to predispose patients to chronic dermatophytosis. In relatively normal patients, most cases of dermatophytosis that persist for long periods are caused by *T. rubrum*. However, other dermatophytes can cause chronic infections in patients with some underlying disease, such as collagen vascular disease, systemic corticosteroid therapy, or Cushing's disease, hematologic malignancy, chronic mucocutaneous candidiasis, diabetes mellitus, or atopy (29–32). Advanced age has also been related to an increased incidence of dermatophytosis (33,34), and these infections are often asymptomatic (35). Disorders of keratinization and underlying peripheral vascular disease have also been found to be associated with chronic dermatophytosis (29). As discussed below, this condition seems to be related to a higher than expected rate of atopy in the affected patients. In addition, there is some evidence that chronic dermatophytosis, or at least susceptibility to this condition, may occur as an inherited trait (36). The best example is tinea imbricata, where predisposition to the infection has been demonstrated to be transmitted as an autosomal recessive trait (37).

C. Tinea Versicolor

Tinea versicolor is a chronic superficial fungal infection of the skin that generally affects the trunk or proximal parts of the extremities. It is caused by a yeastlike, lipid-requiring organism known as *Malassezia furfur* (*Pityrosporum orbiculare*). Although this infection can persist for years unless treated appropriately, the major symptoms associated with it are cosmetic. Electron microscopic studies of tinea versicolor have demonstrated that the organisms actually invade the cornified cells of the stratum corneum, producing a true intracellular infection (38). *Malessezia furfur* has also been postulated to play a role in certain other diseases, including atopic dermatitis, seborrheic dermatitis, psoriasis, and reticulate papillomatosis (39–42).

Warm climates definitely seem to be associated with an increased incidence of tinea versicolor (43). Since some conjugal cases of tinea versicolor do occur (44), there may be some degree of infectivity of the responsible organism. This infection has been reported to be more frequent in steroid-treated patients, those with Cushing's disease, those undergoing immunosuppression for renal transplantation, and in persons who are severely malnourished (32,45,46). Genetic susceptibility has also been postulated for tinea versicolor in that infections in relatives occur at a higher than expected rate (44,47,48).

D. Malassezia Folliculitis

This entity resembles to some extent acne vulgaris, the macronodular lesions of disseminated candidiasis in immunosuppressed patients, and the candidal papular folliculitis of heroin addicts (49). It may also be confused with graft-versus-host disease in bone marrow transplant recipients (50). Like tinea versicolor, *Malassezia* folliculitis is caused by *M. furfur* and tends to infect the same areas—the upper shoulders, back, and chest. However, the lesions begin as an inflammation of the hair follicles and are generally quite pruritic. The contents of the infected hair follicles include keratinaceous material, amorphous cellular debris, inflammatory cells, and the yeast forms (but not the hyphal forms) of the infecting organisms (51,52).

Malassezia folliculitis may develop in immunosuppressed patients (49–51,53) but this condition is also quite common in patients with presumably normal immunological function (54). Experimental infections with *Malassezia* suggest that certain patients, such as those with seborrheic dermatitis, have a predisposition to this condition (55).

E. Miscellaneous Superficial Fungal Infections

Tinea nigra is a superficial fungal infection of the palms that is generally caused by *Phaeoannellomyces werneckii* (*Exophiala werneckii*). The lesions are generally dark-colored, non-scaling macules. They are usually asymptomatic but can be confused with melanomas and perhaps result in unnecessary surgery (56). Tinea nigra is most often seen in tropical or semitropical areas of Central and South America, Africa, and Asia, although some cases do occur in North America. White piedra is an asymptomatic fungal infection of the hair shafts that is caused by *Trichosporon beigeli*. This infection produces light-colored, soft nodules on the hair shafts and may cause the involved hairs to break. Otherwise the condition appears to be asymptomatic, although the causative fungus can produce serious infections in immunocompromised patients. Cutaneous trichosporonosis and *Trichosporon* onychomycosis have also been reported (57,58). Black piedra is similar to white piedra in that it is a nodular, generally asymptomatic fungal infection of the hair shafts. The causative organism is *Piedraia hortae*, and the condition most commonly affects the scalp hair.

Tinea nigra and both black and white piedra are caused by fungi that are frequently found in the environment. These conditions all seem to be more frequent in warm climates, perhaps because the organisms may be more common there. In addition, *T. beigelii*, the cause of white piedra, colonizes the skin in a relatively small proportion of hospitalized patients (59).

III. NONIMMUNOLOGICAL CUTANEOUS DEFENSES

A. Structure of the Skin

The physical structure of the skin represents a form of defense against fungal pathogens. The skin surface is relatively inhospitable to fungal growth because of exposure to ultraviolet light, low moisture conditions, and competition from the normal bacterial flora of this site. The stratum corneum is made up of keratin, which most microorganisms cannot use for nutrition. *Candida albicans* and the dermatophytes, however, produce keratinases, which facilitate their growth in the stratum corneum (60–62). Also, this site of infection may protect the infecting organisms from direct contact with at least some of the effector cells of the immune system. Whereas neutrophils and small numbers of lymphocytes may enter the epidermis, the major infiltrates of cell-mediated immune responses are generally confined to the dermis.

B. Keratinization and Epidermal Proliferation

The process of keratinization, by which the stratum corneum is continually renewed, may also present a form of defense against organisms infecting this site. The basal epidermal cells, or keratinocytes, are responsible for continued growth of the epidermis and undergo continued cell divisions, which move the resulting daughter cells outward toward the surface. As they mature, these cells lose their nuclei and become flattened to form the keratinized cells. This process results in continuous shedding of the stratum corneum, potentially removing organisms residing there. In the periphery of annular dermatophytosis, keratinocytes have been found to divide at an increased rate (63). Immunological factors appear to enhance the process of keratinization, so that rates of transit of epidermal cells toward the stratum corneum are increased (64). Epidermal proliferation appears to be quite important in the defense against superficial fungal infections (63–67).

C. Antifungal Substances

Lipids extracted from adult hair contain saturated fatty acids that can significantly inhibit the growth of *Microsporum audouini*, a common cause of hair and scalp infections (68). Whereas the sebum of adults may not be significantly more fungistatic than that of children, older individuals appear to produce quantitatively more of this material than do children (69). In addition, fungicidal proteins have been isolated from normal epidermis and could play some role in the defense against cutaneous fungal infections (70).

D. Unsaturated Transferrin

In contrast to *C. albicans*, *M. furfur*, and *T. beigelii*, the dermatophytic fungi appear to be relatively incapable of infecting deep tissues, even in severely immunosuppressed patients. Therefore, infections with these organisms are generally confined to the dead, keratinized layers. This phenomenon has been related to presence in the dermis of unsaturated transferrin, which may prevent growth of the organisms in the deeper layers of the skin by competition for iron (71).

IV. THE INFLAMMATORY RESPONSE

A. Relationship Between Inflammation and Chronicity

Dermatologists have long been aware of the inverse relationship between the degree of inflammation produced by a particular fungal organism and the chronicity of that infection. *Malassezia furfur* and the anthropophilic dermatophytes *T. rubrum* and *M. audouini* generally produce little inflammation in their cutaneous lesions and frequently cause infections that persist for long periods. In contrast, many of the zoophilic or geophilic dermatophytes produce highly inflammatory infections that are usually self-limited. These observations suggest that the local inflammatory processes are indeed involved in the defense against this group of pathogens.

B. Chemotactic Mechanisms

In spite of the fact that some superficial fungal infections are highly inflammatory, the site of infection is generally a very superficial one in the stratum corneum. One can observe a variety of gross changes in the infected skin, including scaling, vesicles, pustules, annular dermatitis, and severe inflammatory reactions (kerions). Microscopically, the lesions are characterized initially by an accumulation of neutrophils in the infected skin, followed later by epidermal proliferation and a mononuclear cell infiltrate in the dermis.

The mechanism by which neutrophils are attracted into skin infected by fungi has received some attention. *Trichophyton rubrum* and *T. mentagrophytes* have both been shown to be capable of activating complement by the alternative pathway to produce chemotactic activity for neutrophils (72,73). *Candida albicans* and *M. furfur* have also been shown to activate complement by this pathway (74,75). *Trichophyton mentagrophytes* and *C. albicans* also produce low-molecular-weight chemotactic factors analogous to those made by growing bacteria (76,77). *Trichophyton rubrum* extracts have been shown to destroy chemotactic activity generated from serum (78), perhaps explaining why infection with this organism usually results in minimally inflammatory lesions. Finally, as discussed more fully below, keratinocytes can generate chemotactic cytokines that could also be responsible for some of the inflammation in the lesions of cutaneous fungal infections.

C. Antifungal Mechanisms of Phagocytic Cells

Both neutrophils and monocytes/macrophages appear to be important in the defense against fungal infections, including cutaneous mycoses. Neutrophils can directly attack pathogens, using a variety of microbicidal processes (reviewed in Refs. 79 and 80). Some of these processes depend upon microbicidal oxidants, including superoxide, hydrogen peroxide, hypochlorous acid, and monochloramine (81,82). Otherwise, the killing mechanisms may involve granule microbicidal substances, including cathepsin G (83), the defensins (84,85), bactericidal/permeability-increasing protein (86), lactoferrin (87), lysozyme (88), elastase (89), azuricidin (90,91), and a number of other proteins (92–94). Most of these substances are capable of killing the organisms, although lactoferrin may have both microbistatic and microbicidal effects (95). The neutrophil's oxidative mechanisms are capable of killing *Trichophyton spp*. in vitro (96), suggesting that they could have a role in the defense against dermatophytosis. Macrophages have an additional antimicrobial mechanism whereby they can use production of nitric oxide to inhibit growth of ingested fungal pathogens, such as *Cryptococcus neoformans* (97). It is possible that this mechanism might also be active against the organisms causing superficial fungal infections.

There is some recent evidence that neutrophils may have significant growth-inhibitory activity in addition to their microbicidal processes. These cells contain large amounts of a calcium- and zinc-binding protein, called calprotectin, that has potent microbistatic activity against *C. albicans* and other fungi (98–100). This protein appears to be released into inflammatory exudates as neutrophils die at sites of infection (101). This mechanism could supplement other host defenses in the infected skin by controlling growth of *C. albicans* or other fungi there.

V. THE CUTANEOUS IMMUNE SYSTEM

A. Potential Role in Superficial Fungal Infections

Since cutaneous fungal infections are more frequent and more severe in patients with immunological defects, it would appear that immune responses to fungal antigens must play an important role in the host defense against these infections. Immunological host defense mechanisms in normal hosts seem to be effective even when the infections are limited to superficial locations such as the stratum corneum. Thus, the epidermis of the skin represents much more than a passive barrier against entry of infecting organisms; it also acts as an immunological organ that has some unique elements. Cutaneous immune reactions are undertaken by a variety of cell types, including epidermal Langerhans cells, keratinocytes, T lymphocytes, and microvascular endothelial cells. The mechanisms employed are complex, involving a network of fixed or mobile cells interacting either by trafficking of the cells themselves from one site to another or by the production of cytokines that influence the function of other cells.

B. Cells with Immunological Potential in the Skin

1. Epidermal Langerhans Cells

Langerhans cells, which were first discovered in 1868 by Paul Langerhans, make up approximately 2–5% of the total epidermal cell population (102). They appear to represent part of a population of potent immunostimulatory cells, known as dendritic cells, that are present in various tissues and develop from bone marrow stem cells (103). Cytokines such as granulocyte-macrophage colony stimulating factor (GM-CSF) and tumor necrosis factor-α (TNF-α) influence development of Langerhans cells from their precursors (104). Epidermal Langerhans cells have a pronounced dendritic shape and contain rod-shaped organelles of varying length and position, called "Birkbeck's granules," first described in 1961 (105). These granules appear to have a role in antigen processing (106). Langerhans cells in the epidermis express a variety of antigenic markers on their surface, including cluster-of-differentiation antigen 1a (CD-1a), CD-45, human leukocyte antigen (HLA), class I and II antigens, the S-100 antigen, vimentin, and a number of others (reviewed in Ref. 107).

The observation of apposition between Langerhans cells and T lymphocytes in contact-allergic reactions suggested that Langerhans cells might function as antigen-presenting cells for T-lymphocyte activation (108). In this regard, phagocytosis of antigens by Langerhans cells has been demonstrated (109). After the interaction with a foreign antigen, these cells have been shown to migrate to regional lymph nodes, where they interact with T lymphocytes (103). The effect of stimulation of Langerhans cells is to produce enlargement and sheetlike processes (or veils) and loss of Birkbeck granules (110). Langerhans cells in this form are essentially indistinguishable from other dendritic cells. Electron microscopy studies have revealed that cells resembling either typical epidermal Langerhans cells or the stimulated form of these cells can be demonstrated in peripheral blood (111). The fate of Langerhans cells after stimulation of T lymphocytes is unclear. They may serve as targets of natural killer cells (or cytotoxic T cells) and be destroyed after stimulating T lymphocytes. On the other hand the observation that up to 1% of thoracic duct cells are dendritic cells would seem to suggest survival and recirculation of these cells (103).

The dermis contains a population of potent antigen-presenting cells that have been termed dermal dendritic cells. They are motile, express high levels of class II MHC antigens on their cytoplasmic dendritic processes, and lack the usual antigens of B lymphocytes, T lymphocytes, Langerhans cells, and natural killer cells (112). These cells may either be different from epidermal Langerhans cells or they may represent an immature form of these cells (103). In either case, they probably are important in the initiation of certain immunological responses in the skin, particularly those involving antigens present in the dermis. However, their role in the afferent phase of immune responses against antigens entering the epidermis is unclear at this time.

2. *Keratinocytes*

Keratinocytes represent the major cell type in the epidermis. In addition to their role in producing epidermal barriers and protective proliferative responses, they are important in cutaneous immune reactions. These cells produce soluble mediators that are capable of upregulating and downregulating immune responses; they also express cell surface products that mediate interactions with other cell types.

Keratinocytes produce a variety of cytokines, including interleukin-1 (IL-1), IL-6, IL-7, IL-8, interferon-α (IFN-α), monocyte chemotaxis and activating factor (MCAF), GM-CSF, and TNF-α (113–115). These cells also generate products of arachidonic acid metabolism that may influence inflammatory reactions in the skin and whose synthesis appears to be enhanced by IL-1 produced by the keratinocytes themselves (116). One of these products, prostaglandin E_2(PGE_2), increases vascular permeability and could promote the influx of inflammatory cells into the skin. Prostaglandin E_2, however, is primarily involved in downregulating immune responses, including T- and B-cell proliferation and suppression of IL-1 production by phagocytes (107,117).

In addition to the production of soluble factors, keratinocytes also express important cell-surface molecules such as major histocompatibility complex (MHC) antigens and adhesion molecules. Class I MHC antigens are expressed constitutively on keratinocytes and could represent a target for $CD8^+$ cytotoxic T-lymphocytes (107). Class II MHC antigen expression can be induced on keratinocytes, although they are still unable to process native protein antigens. Class II antigen expression in these cells may serve as targets for class II restricted cytotoxic T lymphocytes (118). Intercellular adhesion molecule 1 (ICAM-1) and leukocyte function–associated antigen 3 (LFA-3) are two other cell-surface molecules expressed by keratinocytes (119,120).

3. *Epidermal T Lymphocytes*

As discussed above, the mononuclear infiltrates characteristic of cell-mediated immune responses in the skin are generally confined to the dermis. However, the normal epidermis does contain a small population of T lymphocytes, constituting less than 5% of all of these cells in the skin (121). Two possibilities exist for the generation of sensitized T lymphocytes in the epidermis: (a) through antigenic stimulation of other, resting T lymphocytes at this site and (b) through attraction of already sensitized T lymphocytes by chemotactic cytokines, including members of the IL-8 family produced by keratinocytes.

4. *Microvascular Endothelial Cells*

Microvascular endothelial cells are located near the cutaneous microenvironment where the immunological reactions described above occur. Endothelial cells are known to be active participants in a variety of functions, including wound healing, angiogenesis, production of clotting factors, and maintenance of vascular tone. Their role in immunological events is not entirely clear, although there is increasing evidence for their participation in this area. These cells produce a number of factors that are capable of inducing inflammation and recruiting leukocytes, including IL-1, IL-6, IL-8, G-CSF, macrophage-colony stimulating factor (M-CSF), and the chemotactic factor MCAF (122). Adhesion molecules produced by microvascular endothelial cells include ICAM-1, vascular adhesion molecule 1 (VCAM-1), P-selectin, E-selectin, and several others (122). The expression of these molecules on the cell surface can be modulated by cytokines.

C. Interactions of Cutaneous Cells

1. *Langerhans Cells and T Lymphocytes*

An appropriate physical interaction between Langerhans cells and T lymphocytes is essential to allow for successful T-lymphocyte activation and clonal expansion. The contact between Langerhans cells and the receptor for antigen on T lymphocytes is dependent on class II MHC (123). The physical interaction has been shown by electron microscopy to be of two types: (a) a direct physical interaction between surface fibrillar components of the microvilli and protrusions of both cell types and (b) close apposition of wide areas between the cell membranes of the two cell types, apparently to maintain adhesiveness (124). The adhesion molecules LFA-3 and ICAM-1 are expressed on Langerhans cells, whereas the corresponding molecules CD-2 and LFA-1 are expressed on T-lymphocytes

(125). The LFA-1 is a member of the integrin family of adhesion-promoting proteins, while LFA-3, ICAM-1, and CD2 are members of the immunoglobulin superfamily. Interaction of LFA-3 with CD-2 and ICAM-1 with LFA-1 may enhance T-lymphocyte activation either by providing unique costimulatory signals or by augmenting T-lymphocyte–Langerhans cell interaction (110). Following cellular activation, the expression of all four adhesion molecules has been shown to be increased (125).

In addition to antigen/MHC and adhesion interaction, a second signal, such as IL-1, is required for optimal antigen-specific T-lymphocyte clonal expansion. The second signal is probably delivered to the T lymphocyte through the adhesion molecules described above (125,126). These molecules therefore act not only for physical adhesion, but also for delivery of stimulatory signals. Langerhans cells themselves can produce IL-1 as well as other cytokines such as IL-6 and TNF-α (107,113,127). A recent study indicates that the Langerhans cell–derived IL-1β may play a critical role as the second signal for T-lymphocyte activation (127).

2. *Keratinocytes and Langerhans Cells*

Keratinocytes interact with Langerhans cells through the production of cytokines and by direct contact. Interleukin-7 produced by keratinocytes appears to promote the survival and growth of Langerhans cells (115). Keratinocytes have also recently been shown to adhere to these cells directly through E-cadherin expressed on the Langerhans cell surface (128).

3. *Keratinocytes and Inflammatory Cells*

Keratinocytes may enhance inflammation through the production of cytokines such as IL-8, which is chemotactic for both neutrophils and lymphocytes (113,129). Also, MCAF, which is chemotactic for monocytes, is produced by keratinocytes in response to IFN-γ (114). Entry into the epidermis and attachment there of dermal T lymphocytes may be mediated by interactions of ICAM-1 and LFA-3 on keratinocytes with the corresponding adhesion molecules LFA-1 and CD-2 on the T lymphocytes (118–120).

4. *Microvascular Endothelial Cells and Lymphocytes*

Whereas microvascular endothelial cells have been shown to produce numerous cytokines and adhesion molecules, their specific role in inflammatory events is not clear. Of the adhesion molecules produced, however, P-selectin has been shown to mediate binding of T lymphocytes and natural killer cells (130) and may play an important role in immunological trafficking. Cytokine-activated microvascular endothelial cells in the dermis may mediate adhesion of memory T lymphocytes through adhesion molecules such as ICAM-1, VCAM-1, and E-selectin (122) and therefore help these cells migrate back from the draining lymph nodes to the involved cutaneous site.

D. Initiation and Expression of Cutaneous Immune Responses

A working hypothesis has been proposed for the mechanisms and pathways involved in the production of immune responses originating in the skin (131). In this scheme, foreign antigens entering the epidermis change the secretion by keratinocytes of soluble mediators of both the inflammatory and immune responses. Langerhans cells then take up the antigens and process them so that the antigenic fragment is complexed to MHC-encoded antigens. Within a short time, these antigen-processing Langerhans cells leave the epidermis, enter the dermal lymphatics, and migrate as veiled cells to the draining lymph nodes. Here they present the antigen-MHC complex on their surface to the proper receptors on resting T-lymphocytes and elicit an antigen-specific response in these cells. The resulting T-lymphocyte blasts then migrate back to the dermis of the damaged skin by homing to cytokine-activated microvascular endothelial cells in the area. At this site the T lymphocytes can be further stimulated by other antigen-presenting cells to undergo clonal expansion and generation of effector cells that can help to eliminate the pathogenic microorganisms.

VI. IMMUNE RESPONSES TO FUNGAL ANTIGENS

A. Cutaneous Candidiasis

Intradermal inoculation with viable *C. albicans* blastospores in mice has been shown to elicit cell-mediated immune responses to several different antigens of this organism (132). Experimental cutaneous candidiasis also sensitizes the infected animals, so that a second infection is cleared more rapidly than is the initial one in both guinea pigs (133) and mice (134). Clearance of the organisms in these experimental infections appears to be mediated at least in part by a vigorous epidermal proliferative response associated with cell-mediated immune responses to the antigens of the organisms (133,135). On the other hand, a certain degree of epidermal proliferation occurs in the infected skin of immunosuppressed mice, suggesting that other factors are also involved (136).

Titers of antibody against *C. albicans* in human patients with chronic mucocutaneous candidiasis have generally been found to be high (8–10,137–139). Whereas an occasional patient with this condition manifests some abnormality in antibody production, most seem to have intact humoral immunity to *C. albicans* (2). Patients with the hyper-IgE syndrome often have chronic superficial *C. albicans* infections along with elevated levels of IgE antibodies to this organism (141,142). Most normal humans have evidence of cell-mediated immunity to *C. albicans* as demonstrated by skin testing (143,144), in vitro lymphocyte stimulation (145,146), and lymphokine production (146,147). In contrast, patients with chronic mucocutaneous candidiasis often demonstrate significant immunological defects in cell-mediated immune responses to *C. albicans* antigens, as discussed below.

B. Dermatophytosis

Work with experimental dermatophytosis in animals has generally demonstrated that some kind of immunity, either local or systemic, results from a preceding infection (148,151). The findings in humans generally parallel those in animals, although the immunity may be only local in nature (65,152). This immunity may not be complete and is probably less than that found in animals (22,153).

Humoral immunity has been demonstrated in human dermatophytosis using a variety of techniques (154–157). Both immediate hypersensitivity to dermatophyte antigens and a higher than expected incidence of atopy have been found in patients with dermatophytosis (29,158–160). Whether chronic dermatophytosis stimulates IgE production or this condition tends to develop in persons who are already atopic has been the subject of some speculation (161). Frequently these patients have immediate but not delayed hypersensitivity to trichophytin (162–166).

Delayed-hypersensitivity responses to intradermal injections of trichophytin are fairly common in the normal human population (167–169). Several studies have demonstrated that experimental dermatophyte infections in animals do result in cell-mediated immunity to the antigens of the infecting organism (170–173). In addition, maximal erythema in the infected skin of animals appears to correlate with the development of cell-mediated immunity (170,173). In one model system, delayed hypersensitivity reactions in the infected skin appeared to promote clearance of the infection by increasing the rate of desquamation of the stratum corneum (62). The importance of cell-mediated immunity to trichophytin has been demonstrated using experimental infections in humans to show that persons with positive delayed trichophytin skin tests were more resistant to inoculation with *T. mentagrophytes* than were those with negative skin tests (174).

C. Tinea Versicolor

A number of studies have demonstrated that serum antibody to *M. furfur* is present in a large percentage of normal persons who do not show evidence of infection with this organism (137,175–178). Humoral responses to *Malassezia* in patients with tinea versicolor were found to be either slightly elevated as compared to controls in one study (137) or to be approximately equivalent in another (177). In *Malassezia* folliculitis, IgG antibodies against this organism were shown to be markedly higher in the patients than in normal subjects (178). Antibody to *Trichosporon* antigens has been found to be present not only in patients with invasive infections but also in uninfected controls (179). As demonstrated by lymphocyte transformation tests and lymphokine assays, cell-mediated immunity to *Malassezia* antigens is present in a majority of uninfected human subjects as well as those with tinea versicolor (180).

VII. MECHANISMS OF IMMUNOLOGICAL DEFECTS

A. Cutaneous Candidiasis

In human patients with chronic mucocutaneous candidiasis, defects in cell-mediated immunity are the most common immunological abnormalities found (2,3,9,10,16). These abnormalities fall into three general groups: (a) anergy to all antigens tested, (b) unresponsiveness to *Candida* antigens only, and (c) normal responses to all antigens, including those from *Candida*. In one study, 10 of 26 patients appeared to have normal cell-mediated immunity to *Candida* antigens (10). However, other patients appear to have significant abnormalities in lymphocyte function, with some having complete anergy to a battery of recall antigens and negative in vitro lymphocyte proliferation responses to mitogens and all antigens (3).

Some of the immunological defects in patient with chronic mucocutaneous candidiasis appear to be associated with serum inhibitors (10,181–184). In some cases the defects disappear after antifungal therapy (184–186). Several studies have demonstrated that parenteral administration of viable *C. albicans* yeast cells or extracts of this organism to experimental animals can result in suppression of cell-mediated immunity (187–190). Carbohydrate antigens from *C. albicans*, primarily mannans, have been shown to persist in the serum of patients with chronic mucocutaneous candidiasis and suppress lymphocyte proliferation responses of cells from control subjects (191). Defective handling of mannan by monocytes from patients with chronic mucocutaneous candidiasis has been postulated as the reason why this substance accumulates in the serum of these patients (192). Mannan-derived oligosaccharides from *C. albicans* can inhibit in vitro lymphocyte proliferation induced by *Candida* antigens (193). Therefore, catabolism of mannan in vivo may generate immunoinhibitory oligosaccharides that cause the defects in cell-mediated immunity in some patients with chronic mucocutaneous candidiasis. However, other patients with this syndrome probably have immunological abnormalities due to other mechanisms, and still others have no demonstrable immunological abnormalities at all and may be susceptible to chronic superficial *C. albicans* infections for other reasons.

B. Dermatophytosis

Suppression of lymphocyte blastogenic responses associated with potentially immunosuppressive serum factors has been demonstrated in acute *T. mentagrophytes* infections produced experimentally in animals (194,195). Studies in humans also suggest that serum factors may be involved in the suppression of cell-mediated immunity to fungal antigens in patients with chronic dermatophytosis (196–198). A mannan component of *T. rubrum* has been shown to be immunosuppressive of in vitro lymphocyte function (199). This substance appears to bind preferentially to monocytes (200). It has also been suggested that the lack of inflammation in *T. rubrum* infections may be due to dermatophyte-derived lymphocyte inhibitory factors acting locally rather than systemically (201).

Local antagonism between immediate and delayed hypersensitivity is another possible mechanism of immunosuppression in dermatophytosis (160). Most patients with chronic dermatophytosis have relatively normal cell-mediated immunity to nonspecific mitogens and antigens other than trichophytin (162,163,202,203), indicating that they are relatively intact immunologically. Subjects with immediate hypersensitivity to trichophytin have been found to be more easily infected experimentally with *T. mentagrophytes* than are those without this type of response (174). Also, production of an immediate skin-test response to trichophytin by passive transfer has been shown to block delayed reactions in patients who previously had only the delayed response (204). In some patients, positive delayed hypersensitivity reactions to trichophytin could be uncovered by suppression of immediate reactions to this antigen using injections of antihistamines into the site (67). Therefore, it is possible that in some patients with chronic dermatophytosis, an IgE response may inhibit the development of protective cell-mediated immune responses to dermatophyte antigens.

C. Tinea Versicolor

Most patients with tinea versicolor have normal proportions of B and T lymphocytes and subsets of T lymphocytes (205) and appropriate lymphocyte transformation responses against nonspecific mitogens and unrelated antigens (180,205). The cells infiltrating the infected skin of patients with tinea versicolor and *Malassezia* folliculitis have been characterized as predominantly helper/inducer rather than suppressor/cytotoxic cells by staining with monoclonal antibodies (178,205). Tinea versicolor patients have been found to have weaker lymphokine responses and a modest but statistically significant reduction in lymphocyte transformation responses to *Malassezia* antigens as compared to uninfected subjects (180); the diminished blastogenic response appears to be related to a decrease in the number of cells initially responding to this antigen (206). In addition, *M. furfur* appears to be less antigenic than is *C. albicans* (207). Therefore, two possible reasons for the minimal inflammation in tinea versicolor and the extreme chronicity of this condition are a reduction in the number of antigen-responsive cells in these patients to *Malassezia* antigens and a relative lack of antigenic material in the organism itself.

VIII. SUMMARY AND CONCLUSIONS

Predispositions to superficial fungal infections include warmth and moisture, natural or iatrogenic immunosuppression, and perhaps some degree of inherited susceptibility. Some of these infections elicit a greater inflammatory response than others, and the noninflammatory ones are generally more chronic. The immune system is involved in the defense against these cutaneous fungal infections, with cell-mediated immunity appearing to be particularly important. The mechanisms involved in generating immunological reactions in the skin are complex, with epidermal Langerhans cells, lymphocytes, and the keratinocytes themselves all playing important roles. A variety of defects in the immunological responses to these infections have been described. In some cases the defects may be preexistent, whereas in others the infection itself may interfere with protective cell-mediated immune responses against the organisms. A number of different mechanisms may underlie these immunological defects and lead to the development of chronic superficial fungal infections in individual patients.

REFERENCES

1. Kauffman CA, Shea MJ, Frame PT. Invasive fungal infections in patients with chronic mucocutaneous candidiasis. Arch Intern Med 1981;141: 1076–1078.
2. Filler SG, Edwards JE Jr. Chronic mucocutaneous. In: Murphy JW, Friedman H, Bendinelli M, eds. Fungal Infections and Immune Responses. New York: Plenum Press, 1993:117–133.
3. Kirkpatrick CH, Sohnle PG. Chronic mucocutaneous candidiasis. In: Safai B, Good RA, eds. Immunodermatology. New York: Plenum Press, 1981: 495–514.

4. Snyderman R, Altman LC, Frankel A, Blaese RKM. Defective mononuclear leukocyte chemotaxis: A previously unrecognized immune dysfunction. Ann Intern Med 1973;78:509–513.
5. Rycroft RJG, Valdimarsson H, Bannister LH, Wells RS. Chronic mucocutaneous candidiasis of late onset, thymoma and myopathy: A report of four cases. Clin Exp Dermatol 1976;1:59–74.
6. Van der Meer JWM, Leijh PCJ, Van den Barselaar M, Van Furth R. Functions of phagocytic cells in chronic mucocutaneous candidiasis. Br Med J 1978;1:147–148.
7. Yamazaki M, Yasui K, Kawaii H, et al. A monocyte disorder in siblings with chronic candidiasis. Am J Dis Child 1984;138:192–196.
8. Mobacken H, Lindholm L, Olling S. Deficient neutrophil function in a patient with chronic mucocutaneous candidiasis, thymoma and myasthenia gravis. Acta Derm Venereol 1977;57:335–339.
9. Kirkpatrick CH, Rich RR, Bennett JE. Chronic mucocutaneous: model building in cellular immunity. Ann Intern Med 1971;74:955–978.
10. Valdimarsson H, Higgs JM, Wells RS, et al. Immune abnormalities associated with chronic mucocutaneous. Cell Immunol 1973;6:348–361.
11. Kirkpatrick CH. Host defense against fungal infections. Am J Med 1984; 77(suppl 4D):1–12.
12. Montes LF. Candidiasis. In: Moschella SL, Hurley HJ, eds. Dermatology. 3d ed. Philadelphia: Saunders, 1992:913–923.
13. Crosby DL, Berger TG, Woosley JT, Resnick SD. Dermatophytosis mimicking Kaposi's sarcoma in human immunodeficiency virus disease. Dermatologica 1991;182:135–137.
14. Prose NS. Cutaneous manifestations of pediatric HIV infection. Pediatr Dermatol 1992;9:326–328.
15. Lowinger-Seoane M, Torres-Rodriguez JM, Madrenys-Brunet N, et al. Extensive dermatophytoses caused by Trichophyton mentagrophytes and Microsporum canis in a patient with AIDS. Mycopathology 1992;120:143–146.
16. Herrod HG. Chronic mucocutaneous candidiasis in childhood and complications of non-Candida infection: a report of the pediatric immunodeficiency study group. J Pediatr 1990;116:377–382.
17. Hermans PE, Ulrich JA, Markowitz H. Chronic mucocutaneous candidiasis as a surface expression of deep-seated abnormalities. Am J Med 1969;47: 503–519.
18. Cornbleet T. Cultures from the skin of apparently normal feet. Arch Dermatol 1926;13:670–671.
19. Elewski BE, Greer DL. Hendersonula toruloidea and Scytalidium hyalinum: Review and update. Arch Dermatol 1991;127:1041–1044.
20. Moore MK, Hay RJ. Circulating antibodies and antigenic cross-reactivity in Hendersonula toruloidea and Scytalidium hyalinum infections. Br J Dermatol 1986;115:435–445.
21. Faergemann J, Gisslen H, Dahlberg E, et al. Trichophyton rubrum abscesses in immunocompromised patients. Acta Derm Venereol 1989;69: 244–247.

22. Blank H, Taplin D, Zaias N. Cutaneous Trichophyton mentagrophytes infections in Vietnam. Arch Dermatol 1969;99:135–144.
23. Knight AG. A review of experimental human fungus infections. J Invest Dermatol 1972;59:354–358.
24. Baer RL, Rosenthal SA, Furnari D. Survival of dermatophytes applied on the feet. J Invest Dermatol 1955;24:619–622.
25. Strauss JS, Kligman AM. An experimental study of tinea pedis and onychomycosis of the foot. Arch Dermatol 1957;76:70–79.
26. Tagami H, Watanabe S, Ofugi S. Trichophytin contact sensitivity in guinea pigs with experimental dermatophytosis induced by a new inoculation method. J Invest Dermatol 1973;61:237–241.
27. Greenberg JH, King RD, Krebs S, Field R. A quantitative dermatophyte infection model in the guinea pig: A parallel to the quantitated human infection model. J Invest Dermatol 1976;67:704–708.
28. King RD, Cunico RL, Maibach HI, et al. The effect of occlusion on carbon dioxide emission from human skin. Acta Derm Venereol 1978;58:135–138.
29. Hay RJ. Chronic dermatophyte infections: I. Clinical and mycological features. Br J Dermatol 1982;106:1–7.
30. Nelson M, McNiece KJ. Recurrent Cushing's syndrome with Trichophyton rubrum infection. Arch Dermatol 1959;80:700–704.
31. Canizares O, Shatin H, Kellert AJ. Cushing's syndrome and dermatomycosis. Arch Dermatol 1959;80:705–712.
32. Findling JW, Tyrrell JN, Aron DC, et al. Fungal infections in Cushing's syndrome. Ann Intern Med 1981;95:392.
33. Gilchrest BA. Some gerontologic considerations in the practice of dermatology. Arch Dermatol 1979;155:1343–1346.
34. Peachey RDG, English MP. An outbreak of Trichophyton rubrum infection in a geriatric hospital. Br J Dermatol 1974;4:389–398.
35. Tindall JP, Smith JG. Skin lesions of the aged and their association with internal changes. JAMA 1963;186:1039–1042.
36. Hay RJ. Genetic susceptibility to dermatophytosis. Eur J Epidemiol 1992; 8:346–349.
37. Serjeantson S, Lawrence G. Autosomal recessive inheritance of susceptibility to tinea imbricata. Lancet 1977;1:13–15.
38. Montes LF. Systemic abnormalities and the intracellular site of infections of the stratum corneum. JAMA 1970;213:1469–1472.
39. Faergemann J, Maibach HI. The Pityrosporon yeasts—Their role as pathogens. Int J Dermatol 1984;23:463–465.
40. Bergbrant IM, Johansson S, Robbins D, et al. An immunological study in patients with seborrhoeic dermatitis. Clin Exp Dermatol 1991;16:331–338.
41. Shuster S. The etiology of dandruff and the mode of action of therapeutic agents. Br J Dermatol 1984;111:235–242.
42. Nordvall SL, Lindgren L, Johansson SGO, et al. IgE antibodies to Pityrosporum orbiculare and Staphylococcus aureus in patients with very high serum total IgE. Clin Exp Immunol 1992;22:756–761.

43. Marples MJ. The incidence of certain skin diseases in Western Samoa: A preliminary study. Trans R Soc Med Hyg 1950;44:319–332.
44. Roberts SOB. Pityriasis versicolor: A clinical and mycological investigation. Br J Dermatol 1969;81:315–326.
45. Boardman CR, Malkinson FD. Tinea versicolor in steroid-treated patients. Arch Dermatol 1962;85:84–92.
46. Koranda FC, Dehmel EM, Kahn G, Penn I. Cutaneous complications in immunosuppressed renal homograft recipients. JAMA 1974;229:419–424.
47. Burke RC. Tinea versicolor: Susceptibility factors and experimental infection in human beings. J Invest Dermatol 1961;36:389–401.
48. Hafez M, El-Shamy S. Genetic susceptibility in pityriasis versicolor. Dermatologica 1985;171:86–88.
49. Klotz SA. Malassezia furfur. Infect Dis Clin North Am 1989;3:53–64.
50. Bufill JA, Lum LA, Caya JG, et al. Pityrosporum folliculitis after bone marrow transplantation—Clinical observations in five patients. Ann Intern Med 1988;108:560–563.
51. Klotz SA, Drutz DJ, Huppert M, Johnson JE. Pityrosporum folliculitis: Its potential for confusion with skin lesions of systemic candidiasis. Arch Intern Med 1982;142:2126–2129.
52. Potter BS, Burgoon CF Jr, Johnson WC. Pityrosporum folliculitis—Report of seven cases and review of the Pityrosporum organism relative to cutaneous disease. Arch Dermatol 1973;107:388–391.
53. Yohn JJ, Lucas J, Camisa C. Malassezia folliculitis in immunocompromised patients. Cutis 1985;35:536–538.
54. Back O, Faergemann J, Hornqvist R. Pityrosporum folliculitis: A common disease of the young and middle-aged. J Am Acad Dermatol 1985;12:56–61.
55. Goodfield MJD, Saihan EM, Crowley J. Experimental folliculitis with Pityrosporum orbiculare: The influence of host response. Acta Derm Venereol 1987;67:445–447.
56. Palmer SR, Bass JW, Mandojana R, Wittler RR. Tinea nigra palmaris and plantaris: A black fungus producing black spots on the palms and soles. Pediatr Infect Dis J 1989;8:48–50.
57. Kamalan A, Senthamilselvi G, Ajithadas K, Thambiah AS. Cutaneous trichosporosis. Mycopathology 1988;101:167–175.
58. Fusaro RM, Miller NG. Onychomycosis caused by Trichosporon beigelii. J Am Acad Dermatol 1984;11:747–749.
59. Rose HD, Kurup VP. Colonization of hospitalized patients with yeast-like organisms. Sabouraudia 1977;15:251–256.
60. Negi M, Tsuboi R, Matsui T, Ogawa H. Isolation and characterization of proteinase from Candida albicans: Substrate specificity. J Invest Dermatol 1984;83:32–36.
61. Takiuchi I, Higuchi D, Sei Y, Koga M. Isolation of an extracellular proteinase (keratinase) from Microsporum canis. Sabouraudia 1982;20:281–288.
62. Yu RJ, Harmon SR, Blank F. Isolation and purification of an extracellular keratinase of Trichophyton mentagrophytes. J Bacteriol 1968;96:1435–1436.

63. Berk SH, Penneys NS, Weinstein GD. Epidermal activity in annular dermatophytosis. Arch Dermatol 1976;112:485–488.
64. Lepper AWD, Anger HS. Experimental bovine Trichophyton verrucosum infection: Comparison of the rate of epidermal cell proliferation and keratinization in non-infected and reinoculated cattle. Res Vet Sci 1976;20:117–121.
65. Kligman AM. The pathogenesis of tinea capitis due to Microsporum audouini and Microsporum canis. J Invest Dermatol 1952;18:231–246.
66. Sohnle PG, Kirkpatrick CH. Epidermal proliferation in the defense against experimental cutaneous candidiasis. J Invest Dermatol 1978;70:130–133.
67. Jones HE, Reinhardt JH, Rinaldi MG. Immunologic susceptibility to chronic dermatophytosis. Arch Dermatol 1974;110:213–220.
68. Rothman S, Smiljanic A, Shapiro AL, Weitkamp AW. The spontaneous cure of tinea capitis in puberty. J Invest Dermatol 1947;8:81–98.
69. Kligman AM, Ginsberg D. Immunity of the adult scalp to infection with Microsporum audouini. J Invest Dermatol 1950;14:345–356.
70. Kashima M, Takahashi H, Shimozuma M, et al. Candidacidal activities of proteins partially purified from rat epidermis. Infect Immun 1989;57: 186–190.
71. King RD, Khan HA, Foye JC, et al. Transferrin, iron, and dermatophytes: I. Serum dermatophyte inhibitory component definitively identified as unsaturated transferrin. J Lab Clin Med 1975;86:204–212.
72. Davies RR, Zaini F. Trichophyton rubrum and the chemotaxis of polymorphonuclear leucocytes. Sabouraudia 1984;22:65–71.
73. Swan JW, Dahl MV, Coppo PA, Hammerschmidt DE. Complement activation by Trichophyton rubrum. J Invest Dermatol 1983;80:156–158.
74. Ray TL, Wuepper KD. Activation of the alternative (properdin) pathway of complement by Candida albicans and related species. J Invest Dermatol 1976;67:700–703.
75. Sohnle PG, Collins-Lech C. Activation of complement by Pityrosporum orbiculare. J Invest Dermatol 1983;80:93–97.
76. Tagami H, Natsume N, Aoshima T, et al. Analysis of transepidermal leucocyte chemotaxis in experimental dermatophytosis in guinea pigs. Arch Dermatol Res 1982;273:205–217.
77. Cutler JE. Chemotactic factor produced by Candida albicans. Infect Immun 1977;18:568–573.
78. Davies RR, Zaini F. Enzymatic activities of Trichophyton rubrum and the chemotaxis of polymorphonuclear leucocytes. Sabouraudia 1984;22: 235–241.
79. Root RK, Cohen MS. The microbicidal mechanisms of human neutrophils and eosinophils. Rev Infect Dis 1981;3:565–598.
80. Thomas EL, Lehrer RI, Rest RF. Human neutrophil antimicrobial activity. Rev Infect Dis 1988;10(suppl 2):S450–S456.
81. Test ST, Lampert MB, Ossanna PJ, et al. Generation of nitrogen-chlorine oxidants by human phagocytes. J Clin Invest 1984;74:1341–1349.
82. Grisham MB, Jefferson MM, Melton DF, Thomas EL. Chlorination of exogenous amines by isolated neutrophils: Ammonia dependent bactericidal,

cytotoxic, and cytolytic activities of the chloramines. J Biol Chem 258: 10404–10413.
83. Drazin RE, Lehrer RI. Fungicidal properties of a chymotrypsin-like cationic protein from human neutrophils: adsorption to Candida parapsilosis. Infect Immun 1977;17:382–388.
84. Ganz T, Selsted ME, Szklarek D, et al. Defensins: Natural peptide antibiotics of human neutrophils. J Clin Invest 1985;76:1427–1435.
85. Selsted ME, Harwig SS, Ganz T, et al. Primary structures of three human neutrophil defensins. J Clin Invest 1985;76:1436–1439.
86. Weiss J, Elsbach P, Olsson I, Odeberg H. Purification and characterization of a potent bactericidal and membrane active protein from the granules of human polymorphonuclear leukocytes. J Biol Chem 1978;253:2664–2672.
87. Arnold RR, Brewer M, Gauthier JJ. Bactericidal activity of human lactoferrin: Sensitivity of a variety of microorganisms. Infect Immun 1980;23: 893–898.
88. Collins MS, Pappagianis D. Inhibition by lysozyme of growth of the spherule phase of Coccioides immitis in vitro. Infect Immun 1974;10:616–623.
89. Odeberg H, Olsson I. Microbicidal mechanisms of human granulocytes: Synergistic effects of granulocyte elastase and myeloperoxidase or chymotrypsin-like cationic protein. Infect Immun 1976;14:1276–1283.
90. Gabay JE, Heiple JM, Cohn ZA, Nathan CF. Subcellular location and properties of bactericidal factors from human neutrophils. J Exp Med 1986; 1407–1421.
91. Campanelli D, Detmers PA, Nathan CF, Gabay JE. Azuricidin and a homologous serine protease from neutrophils: Differential antimicrobial and proteolytic properties. J Clin Invest 1990;85:904–915.
92. Hirsch JG. Phagocytin: a bactericidal substance from polymorphonuclear leucocytes. J Exp Med 1956;103:589–611.
93. Skarnes RC, Watson DW. Characterization of leukin: An antibacterial factor from leucocytes active against gram-positive pathogens. J Exp Med 1956;104:829–845.
94. Modrzakowski MC, Cooney MH, Martin LE, Spitznagel JK. Bactericidal activity of fractionated granule contents from human polymorphonuclear leukocytes. Infect Immun 1979;23:587–591.
95. Arnold RR, Russell JE, Champion WJ, Gauthier JJ. Bactericidal activity of human lactoferrin: Influence of physical conditions and metabolic state of the target microorganism. Infect Immun 1981;32:655–660.
96. Calderon RA, Hay RJ. Fungicidal activity of human neutrophils and monocytes on dermatophytic fungi, Trichophyton quinckeanum and Trichophyton rubrum. Immunology 1987;61:289–295.
97. Alspaugh JA, Granger DL. Inhibition of Cryptococcus neoformans replication by nitrogen oxides supports the role of these molecules as effectors of macrophage-mediated cytostasis. Infect Immun 1991;59:2291–2296.
98. McNamara MP, Wiessner JH, Collins-Lech C, et al. Neutrophil death as a defense mechanism against Candida albicans infections. Lancet 1988;2: 1163–1165.

99. Steinbakk M, Naess-Andresen CF, Lingass E, et al. Antimicrobial actions of calcium binding leucocyte L1 protein, calprotectin. Lancet 1990;336: 763–765.
100. Murthy ARK, Lehrer RI, Harwig SSL, Miyasaki KT. In vitro candidastatic properties of the human neutrophil calprotectin complex. J Immunol 1993; 151:6291–6301.
101. Sohnle PG, Collins-Lech C, Wiessner JH. The zinc-reversible antimicrobial activity of neutrophil lysates and abscess fluid supernatants. J Infect Dis 1991;164:137–142.
102. Parker F. Skin diseases. In: Wyngaarden JB, Smith LD, eds. Cecil Textbook of Medicine. 18th ed. Philadelphia: Saunders, 1988:2300–2353.
103. Bergstresser PR, Cruz PD Jr, Niederkorn JY, Takashima A. Third International Workshop on Langerhans cells: Discussion overview. J Invest Dermatol 1992;99:1S–4S.
104. Caux C, Dezutter-Dambuyant C, Schmitt D, Banchereau J. GM-CSF and TNF-α cooperate in the generation of dendritic Langerhans cells. Nature 1992;360:258–261.
105. Birbeck MS, Breathnach AS, Everall JD. An electron microscope study of basal melanocytes and high-level clear cells (Langerhans cells) in vitiligo. J Invest Dermatol 1961;37:51–64.
106. Stossel H, Koch F, Kampgen E, et al. Disappearance of certain acidic organelles (endosomes and Langerhans cell granules) accompanies loss of antigen processing capacity upon culture of epidermal Langerhans cells. J Exp Med 1990;172:1471–1482.
107. Stingl G, Hauser C, Wolff K. The epidermis: An immunologic microenvironment. In: Fitzpatrick TB, Eisen AZ, Wolff K, et al, eds. Dermatology in General Medicine. 4th ed. New York: McGraw-Hill, 1993:172–197.
108. Silverberg I. Apposition of mononuclear cells to Langerhans cells in contact allergic reactions. Acta Derm Venereol 1973;53:1–12.
109. Sousa CR, Stahl PD, Austyn JM. Phagocytosis of antigens by Langerhans cells in vitro. J Exp Med 1993;178:509–519.
110. Johnson JG, Jenkins MK. Co-stimulatory functions of antigen-presenting cells. J Invest Dermatol 1992;99:62S–65S.
111. Knight SC, Stagg A, Hill S, et al. Development and function of dendritic cells in health and diseases. J Invest Dermatol 1992;99:33S–38S.
112. Nestle FO, Zheng XG, Thompson CB, et al. Characterization of dermal dendritic cells obtained from normal human skin reveals phenotypic and functionally distinct subsets. J Immunol 1993;151:6535–6545.
113. Matsue H, Cruz PD Jr, Bergstresser PR, Takashima A. Cytokine expression by epidermal cell subpopulations. J Invest Dermatol 1992;99:42S–45S.
114. Barker JNWN, Jones ML, Swenson CL, et al. Monocyte chemotaxis and activating factor production by keratinocytes in response to IFN-γ. J Immunol 1991;146:1192–1197.
115. Matsue H, Bergstresser PR, Takashima A. Keratinocyte-derived IL-7 serves as a growth factor for dendritic epidermal T cells in mice. J Immunol 1993;151:6012–6019.

116. Pentland AP, Mahoney MG. Keratinocyte prostaglandin synthesis is enhanced by IL-1. J Invest Dermatol 1990;94:43–46.
117. Goodwin JS. Prostaglandin regulation of mitogenesis. Cell Immunol 1980; 52:239–240.
118. Gaspari A, Katz SI. Induction and functional characterization of class II MHC (Ia) antigens on murine keratinocytes. J Immunol 1988;140: 2956–2963.
119. Dustin ML, Singer KH, Tuck DT, Springer TA. Adhesion of T lymphoblasts to epidermal keratinocytes is regulated by interferon γ and is mediated by intercellular adhesion molecule 1 (ICAM-1). J Exp Med 1988;167: 1323–1340.
120. DePanfilis GD, Manara GC, Ferrari C, Torresani C. Adhesion molecules on the plasma membrane of epidermal cells: III. Keratinocytes and Langerhans cells constitutively express the lymphocyte functional-associated antigen 3. J Invest Dermatol 1991;96:512–517.
121. Bos JD, Teunissen MBM, Cairo I, et al. T-cell receptor $\gamma\delta$ bearing cells in normal human skin. J Invest Dermatol 1990;94:37–42.
122. Swerlick RA, Lawley TJ. Role of microvascular endothelial cells in inflammation. J Invest Dermatol 1993;100:111S–115S.
123. Aiba S, Katz SI. The ability of cultured Langerhans cells to process and present protein antigens is MHC-dependent. J Immunol 1991;146: 2479–2487.
124. Concha M, Vidal A, Garces G, et al. Physical interaction between Langerhans cells and T-lymphocytes during antigen presentation in vitro. J Invest Dermatol 1993;100:429–434.
125. Teunissen MBM. Functional role of adhesion molecules LFA-3 and ICAM-1 on cultured human epidermal Langerhans cells in antigen-specific T-cell activation. J Invest Dermatol 1992;99:77S–79S.
126. Simon JC, Cruz PD Jr, Tigelaar RE, et al. Adhesion molecules CD11a, CD18, and ICAM-1 on human epidermal Langerhans cells serve a functional role in the activation of alloreactive T cells. J Invest Dermatol 1991;96: 148–151.
127. Enk AH, Angeloni VL, Udey MC, Katz SI. An essential role for Langerhans cell-derived IL-1β in the initiation of primary immune response in skin. J Immunol 1993;150:3698–3704.
128. Tang A, Amagai M, Granger LG, et al. Adhesion of epidermal Langerhans cells to keratinocytes mediated by E-cadherin. Nature 1993;361: 82–85.
129. Barker JNWN, Jones ML, Mitra RS, et al. Modulation of keratinocyte-derived interleukin-8 which is chemotactic for neutrophils and T lymphocytes. Am J Pathol 1991;139:869–876.
130. Moore KL, Thompson LF. P-selectin (CD-62) binds to subpopulations of human memory T lymphocytes and natural killer cells. Biochem Biophys Res Commun 1992;186:173–181.
131. Stingl G. The skin: initiation and target site of immune responses. Recent Results Cancer Res 1993;128:45–57.

132. Moser SA, Domer JE, Mather FJ. Experimental murine candidiasis: Cell-mediated immunity after cutaneous challenge. Infect Immun 1980;27:140–149.
133. Sohnle PG, Frank MM, Kirkpatrick CH. Mechanisms involved in elimination of organisms from experimental cutaneous Candida albicans infection in guinea pigs. J Immunol 1976;117:523–530.
134. Wilson BD, Sohnle PG. Participation of neutrophils and cell-mediated immunity in the defense against experimental cutaneous candidiasis in mice. Am J Pathol 1986;123:241–249.
135. Sohnle PG, Kirkpatrick CH. Epidermal proliferation in the defense against cutaneous candidiasis. J Invest Derm 1978;70:130–133.
136. Sohnle PG, Hahn BL. Epidermal proliferation and the neutrophilic infiltrates of experimental cutaneous candidiasis in mice. Arch Dermatol Res 1989;281:279–283.
137. DaMert GJ, Kirkpatrick CH, Sohnle PG. Comparison of antibody responses in chronic mucocutaneous candidiasis and tinea versicolor. Arch Allergy Immunol 1980;63:97–104.
138. Axelsen NH, Kirkpatrick CH, Buckley RH. Precipitins to Candida albicans in chronic mucocutaneous candidiasis studied by crossed immunoelectrophoresis with intermediate gels. Clin Exp Immunol 1974;17:385–394.
139. Takeya K, Nomoto K, Matsumoto T, et al. Chronic mucocutaneous candidiasis accompanied by enhanced antibody production. Clin Exp Immunol 1976;25:497–500.
140. Chappler RR, Maibach HI, Conant MKA, Aly R. Mucocutaneous candidiasis or mucocutaneous microbiosis. JAMA 1978;239:428–429.
141. Berger M, Kirkpatrick CH, Goldsmith PK, Gallin JI. IgE antibodies to Staphylococcus aureus and Candida albicans in patients with the syndrome of hyperimmunoglobulin E and recurrent infections. J Immunol 1980;125:2437–2443.
142. Schmitt C, Ballet JJ. Serum IgE and IgG antibodies to tetanus toxoid and candidin in immunodeficient children with the hyper-IgE syndrome. J Clin Immunol 1983;3:178–183.
143. Ferguson AC, Kershnar HE, Collin WK, Stiehm ER. Correlation of cutaneous hypersensitivity with lymphocyte response to Candida albicans. Am J Clin Pathol 1977;68:499–504.
144. Shannon DC, Johnson G, Rosen FS, Austen KF. Cellular reactivity to Candida albicans antigen. N Engl J Med 1966;275:690–693.
145. Gettner SMM, Mackenzie DWR. Responses of human peripheral lymphocytes to soluble and insoluble antigens of Candida albicans. J Med Microbiol 1981;14:333–340.
146. Bice DE, Lopez M, Rothschild H, Salvaggio J. Comparison of Candida delayed hypersensitivity skin test size with lymphocyte transformation, migration inhibitory factor production and antibody titer. Int Arch Allergy Appl Immunol 1974;47:54–62.
147. Sohnle PG, Collins-Lech C, Huhta KE. Kinetics of lymphokine production by lymphocytes from elderly humans. Gerontology 1983;29:169–175.

148. Greenbaum SS. Immunity in ringworm infections: I. Active acquired immunity with a note on complement fixation tests in superficial ringworm infections. Arch Dermatol 1924;10:279–288.
149. DeLamater ED, Benham RW. Experimental studies with the dermatophytes: II. Immunity and hypersensitivity produced in laboratory animals. J Invest Dermatol 1938;1:469–488.
150. Bonk AF, Friedman L, Derbes VJ. Experimental dermatophytosis. J Invest Dermatol 1962;39:281–286.
151. Poulain D, Tronchin G, Vernes A, et al. Experimental study of resistance to infection by Trichophyton mentagrophytes: Demonstration of memory skin cells. J Invest Dermatol 1980;74:205–209.
152. Jones HE, Reinhardt JH, Rinaldi MG. Acquired immunity to the dermatophytes. Arch Dermatol 1974;109:840–847.
153. Grappel SF, Bishop CT, Blank F. 1974, Immunology of dermatophytes and dermatophytosis. Bacteriol Rev 1974;38:222–250.
154. Grappel SF, Blank F, Bishop CT. Circulating antibodies in human favus. Dermatologica 1971;143:271–276.
155. Grappel SF, Blank F, Bishop CT. Circulating antibodies in dermatophytosis. Dermatologica 1972;144:1–11.
156. Papini M, Simonetti S. Humoral immunofluorescent antibodies in subjects with dermatophytosis. Mykosen 1985;28:419–429.
157. Kaaman T, von Stedingk LV, von Stedingk M, Wasserman J. ELISA-determined serological reactivity against purified trichophytin in dermatophytosis. Acta Derm Venereol 61:313–317.
158. Jillson OF, Huppert M. The immediate wheal and 24–48 hour tuberculin type edematous reactions to trichophytin. J Invest Dermatol 1949;12: 179–185.
159. Jones HE, Reinhardt JH, Rinaldi MG. A clinical, mycological, and immunological survey for dermatophytosis. Arch Dermatol 1973;108:61–65.
160. Jones HE. Immune response and host resistance of humans to dermatophyte infections. J Am Acad Dermatol 1993;28:S12–S18.
161. Jones HE. The atopic-dermatophytosis syndrome. Acta Derm Venereol (Suppl) 1980;92:81–85.
162. Hanifin JM, Ray LF, Lobitz WC. Immunological reactivity in dermatophytosis. Br J Dermatol 1974;90:1–8.
163. Hunziker N, Brun R. Lack of delayed reaction in presence of cell-mediated immunity in trichophytin hypersensitivity. Arch Dermatol 1980;116: 1266–1268.
164. Hay RJ. Failure of treatment in chronic dermatophyte infections. Postgrad Med J 1979;55:608–610.
165. Kaaman T. The clinical significance of cutaneous reactions to trichophytin in dermatophytosis. Acta Derm Venereol 1978;58:139–143.
166. Espiritu BR, Szpindor-Watson A, Zeitz HJ, Thomas LL. IgE-mediated sensitivity to Trichophyton rubrum in a patient with chronic dermatophytosis and Cushing's syndrome. J Allergy Clin Immunol 1988;81:847–851.

167. Wood SR, Cruickshank CND. The relationship between trichophytin sensitivity and fungal infection. Br J Dermatol 1962;74:329–335.
168. Grossman J, Baum J, Gluckman J, Fusner J, Condemi JJ. The effect of aging and acute illness on delayed hypersensitivity. J Allergy Clin Immunol 1975;55:268–275.
169. Palmer DL, Reed WP. Delayed hypersensitivity skin testing: I. Response rates in a hospitalized population. J Infect Dis 1974;130:132–137.
170. Krebs S, Greenberg J, Jesrani K. Temporal correlation of lymphocyte blastogenesis, skin test responses, and erythema during dermatophyte infections. Clin Exp Immunol 1977;27:526–530.
171. Cruickshank CN D, Trotter MD, Wood SR. Studies on trichophytin sensitivity. J Invest Dermatol 1960;35:219–223.
172. Green F, Balish E. Trichophyton mentagrophytes dermatophytosis in germfree guinea pigs. J Invest Dermatol 1980;75:476–480.
173. Lepper AWD. Experimental bovine Trichophyton verrucosum infection: The cellular responses in primary lesions of the skin resulting from surface or intradermal inoculation. Res Vet Sci 1974;16:287–298.
174. Jones HE, Reinhardt JH, Rinaldi MG. 1974, Model dermatophytosis in naturally-infected subjects. Arch Dermatol 1974;110:369–374.
175. Alexander S. Loss of hair and dandruff. Br J Dermatol 1967;79:549–552.
176. Sohnle PG, Collins-Lech C, Huhta KE. Class-specific antibodies in young and aged humans against organisms producing superficial fungal infections. Br J Dermatol 1983;108:69–76.
177. Faergemann J. Antibodies to Pityrosporum orbiculare in patients with tinea versicolor and controls of various ages. J Invest Dermatol 1983;80:133–135.
178. Faergemann J, Johansson S, Back O, Scheynius A. An immunologic and cultural study of Pityrosporum folliculitis. J Am Acad Dermatol 1986;14: 429–433.
179. Matthews RC, Burnie JP, Fox A, et al. Immunoblot analysis of the serological response in invasive Trichosporon beigelii and Blastoschizomyces capitus infections. J Clin Microbiol 1986;23:395–397.
180. Sohnle PG, Collins-Lech C. Cell-mediated immunity to Pityrosporum orbiculare in tinea versicolor. J Clin Invest 1978;62:45–53.
181. Kirkpatrick CH, Windhorst DB. Mucocutaneous candidiasis and thymoma. Am J Med 1979;66:939–945.
182. Burford-Mason AP, Matthews RC, Williams JRB. Transient abrogation of immunosuppression in a patient with chronic mucocutaneous candidiasis following vaccination with Candida albicans. J Infect 1987;14:147–157.
183. Lehner TJ, Wilton MA, Ivanyi L. Immunodeficiencies in chronic mucocutaneous candidiasis. Immunology 1972;22:775–787.
184. Twomey JT, Waddel CC, Krantz S, et al. Chronic mucocutaneous candidiasis with macrophage dysfunction, a plasma inhibitor and coexistent aplastic anemia. J Lab Clin Med 1975;85:968–977.
185. Kirkpatrick CH, Smith TK. Chronic mucocutaneous candidiasis: Immunologic and antibiotic therapy. Ann Intern Med 1974;80:310–320.

186. Drouhet E, Dupont B. Chronic mucocutaneous candidiasis and other superficial and systemic mycoses successfully treated with ketoconazole. Rev Infect Dis 1980;2:606–619.
187. Rogers TJ, Balish E. Effect of systemic candidiasis on blastogenesis of lymphocytes from germfree and conventional rats. Infect Immun 1978;20: 142–150.
188. Rogers TJ, Balish E. Suppression of lymphocyte blastogenesis by Candida albicans. Clin Immunol Immunopathol 1978;10:298–305.
189. Rivas V, Rogers TJ. Studies on the cellular nature of Candida albicans-induced suppression. J Immunol 1983;130:376–379.
190. Carrow EW, Domer JE. Immunoregulation in experimental murine candidiasis: Specific suppression induced by Candida albicans cell wall glycoprotein. Infect Immun 1985;49:172–181.
191. Fischer AJ, Ballet JJ, Griscelli C. Specific inhibition of the in vitro Candida induced lymphocyte proliferation by polysaccharide antigens present in the serum of patients with chronic mucocutaneous candidiasis. J Clin Invest 1987;62:1005–1013.
192. Fischer AJ, Pichat L, Audinot M, Griscelli C. Defective handling of mannan by monocytes in patients with chronic mucocutaneous candidiasis resulting in a specific cellular unresponsiveness. Clin Exp Immunol 1982;47:653–660.
193. Podzorski RP, Gray GR, Nelson RD. Different effects of native Candida albicans mannan and mannan-derived oligosaccharides on antigen-stimulated lymphoproliferation in vitro. J Immunol 1990;707–716.
194. Green F, Balish E. Suppression of in vitro lymphocyte transformation during an experimental dermatophyte infection. Infect Immun 1979;26: 554–562.
195. Calderon RA. Immunoregulation of dermatophytosis. CRC Crit Rev Microbiol 1989;16:339–368.
196. Walters BAJ, Chick JED, Halliday WJ. Cell-mediated immunity and serum blocking factors in patients with chronic dermatophyte infections. Int Arch Allergy Appl Immunol 1974;46:849–857.
197. Calderon RA, Hay RJ, Shennan GI. Circulating antigens and antibodies in human and mouse dermatophytosis: Use of monoclonal antibody to phosphorylcholine-like epitopes. J Gen Microbiol 1987;133:2699–2705.
198. Sherwin WK, Ross TH, Rosenthal CM, Petrozzi JW. An immunosuppressive serum factor in widespread cutaneous dermatophytosis. Arch Dermatol 1979;115:600–604.
199. Blake JS, Dahl MV, Herron MJ, Nelson RD. An immunoinhibitory cell wall glycoprotein (mannan) from Trichophyton rubrum. J Invest Dermatol 1991;96:657–661.
200. Grando SA, Hostager BS, Herron MJ, et al. Binding of Trichophyton rubrum mannan to human monocytes in vitro. J Invest Dermatol 1992;98: 876–880.
201. McGregor JM, Hamilton AJ, Hay RJ. Possible mechanisms of immune modulation in chronic dermatophytoses: an in vitro study. Br J Dermatol 1992; 127:233–238.

202. Hay RJ, Shennan G. Chronic dermatophyte infections: II. Antibody and cell-mediated immune responses. Br J Dermatol 1982;106:191–198.
203. Sorensen G, Jones HE. Immediate and delayed hypersensitivity in chronic dermatophytosis. Arch Dermatol 1976;112:40–42.
204. Marcussen PV. Relationship of the urticarial to the inflammatory reaction to trichophytin. Arch Dermatol 1937;36:494–514.
205. Scheynius A, Faergemann J, Forsum U, Sjoberg O. Phenotypic characterization in situ of inflammatory cells in pityriasis (tinea) versicolor. Acta Derm Venereol 1984;64:473–479.
206. Sohnle PG, Collins-Lech C. Analysis of the lymphocyte transformation response to Pityrosporum orbiculare in patients with tinea versicolor. Clin Exp Immunol 1982;49:559–564.
207. Sohnle PG, Collins-Lech C. Relative antigenicity of P. orbiculare and C. albicans. J Invest Dermatol 1980;75:279–283.

10

Fungal Enzymes Related to the Pathogenesis of Mycoses

HIDEOKI OGAWA and RYOJI TSUBOI
Juntendo University School of Medicine
Tokyo, Japan

I. INTRODUCTION

Considerable progress has been made in investigating the factors that contribute to the pathogenicity of fungi. Phenotypic variability, adherence to host tissues, toxins, and enzymes have been listed as candidates for virulence factors (1–4). Since the cell and basement membranes of host tissues are made up of lipids and proteins, destruction of these structures by physical and biochemical means is expected to be essential for fungal invasion. Substantial evidence is available to document that pathogenic fungi secrete various hydrolytic enzymes such as proteinase, lipase, and phospholipase (1,3–5). Extracellular hydrolytic enzymes may contribute to the invasiveness and proliferation of fungi by causing damage to the host cells and supplying degraded materials as nutrients for the organisms.

We describe here a series of our experiments concerning hydrolytic enzymes isolated from various species of pathogenic fungi and briefly review the relevant reports.

II. PROTEINASE

Among the fungal enzymes, proteinase has been listed as a likely pathogenic factor. Proteinases from various pathogenic fungi have been purified and characterized, as shown in Table 1. Since extracellular carboxyl proteinase from *Candida albicans* has been extensively discussed (5,24,25), our attention focuses mainly on the proteinase from *C. albicans*, with furthcr reference to those from dermatophytes and other rare species.

A. Proteinase from *Candida albicans*

Candida albicans invades the skin superficially, occasionally extending to the visceral organs and thereby causing severe systemic candidiasis. Two different theories concerning the invasion of the fungus into human

Table 1 Characteristics of Proteinases Purified from Pathogenic Fungi

Species	Reported by	Molecular size (kDa)	pH optimum	Isoelectric point	Type of proteinase
Candida albicans	Remold et al., 1968 (6)	40.0	3.2		Carboxyl
	Ruchel et al., 1981 (7)	45.0	3.9	4.4	Carboxyl
	Negi et al., 1984 (8)	42.0	4.0	4.0	Carboxyl
	Kaminishi et al., 1986 (9)	46.0	4.0	4.2	Carboxyl
Candida parapsilosis	Ruchel et al., 1986 (10)	33.0	4.3	5.3	Carboxyl
Trichophyton rubrum	Asahi et al., 1985 (11)	44.0	8.0	7.8	Serine
	Sanyal et al., 1985 (12)	34.7	9.0		Serine
	Apodaca et al., 1989 (13)	27.0	8.0		Serine
Trichophyton mentagrophytes	Yu et al., 1968 (14)	48.0	7.0		Serine
	Day et al., 1968 (15)	34.3	9.5		Serine
	Tsuboi et al., 1987 (16)	38.0	4.5	3.9	Serine
Microsporum canis	Takiuchi et al., 1982 (17)	45.0	7.5		Serine
Microsporum gypseum	Takiuchi et al., 1977 (18)	18.0	7.8		Cysteine
Sporothrix schenckii	Tsuboi et al., 1987 (19)	36.5	6.0	4.8	Serine
		39.0	3.5	3.8	Carboxyl
Hendersonula toruloidea	Rojanavanich et al., 1990 (20)	34.0	9.0	8.4	Serine
Scopulariopsis brevicaulis	Malviya et al., 1992 (21)	40–45	7.8		Serine
		24–29	7.8		Serine
Aspergillus fumigatus	Reichard et al., 1990 (22)	32.0	9.5	7.9	Serine
Aspergillus flavus	Rhodes et al., 1990 (23)	23.0	8.0	7.6	Metallo

skin have been suggested. The first theory is that the organism invades only the intercellular space of horny cells and acquires nutritive substances from soluble protein. The second theory states that it penetrates the membrane of horny cells and digests insoluble keratin proteins by releasing some form of proteolytic enzyme. With the electron microscope, we observed affected human skin of candidial intertrigo and found that portions of marginal band of the horny cell had disappeared (Fig. 1) (26), suggesting that some kind of proteolytic enzyme is produced extracellularly to digest insoluble keratin proteins.

In the biochemical studies on proteolysis caused by *C. albicans*, Staib (27) initially and subsequently Remold et al. (6) and Rüchel (7) reported the production of a proteolytic enzyme from *C. albicans* when cultivated in medium supplemented with bovine serum albumin (BSA). However, they did not mention a relationship between the production of the enzyme and the pathogenicity of cutaneous candidiasis. Therefore, we attempted to isolate a keratinolytic proteinase from a culture filtrate containing insol-

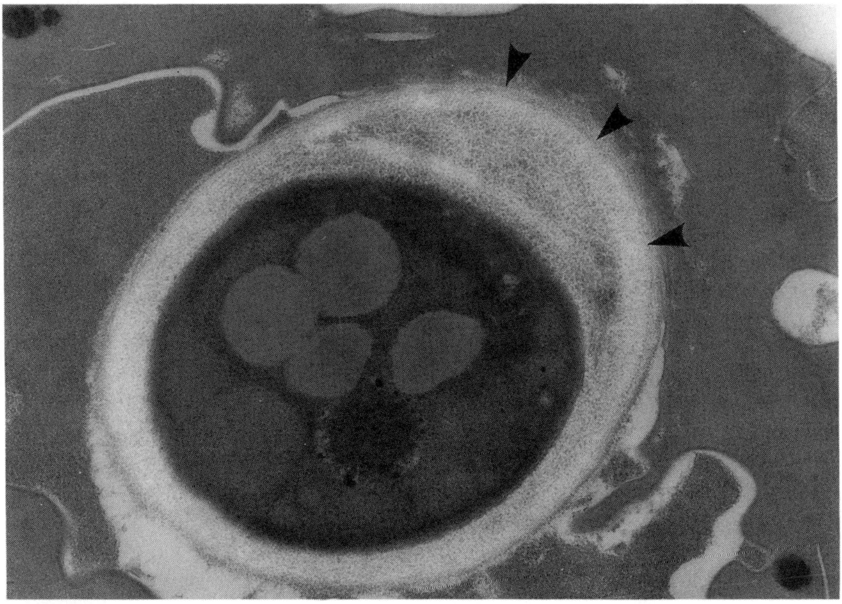

Figure 1 Electron microscopic features of candidial intertrigo (26). The arrows indicate those portions of the marginal band of the horny cell that have disappeared.

uble fractions of human stratum corneum as the sole nitrogen source, as such was thought to be similar to the conditions in vivo (28). Proteolytic enzyme was induced from stratum corneum-containing medium but not from Sabouraud dextrose medium, a medium frequently used in laboratories. A possible explanation for this phenomenon might be that as Sabouraud dextrose broth already contains sufficient nutrients; the secretion of proteinase is therefore not necessary. For the induction of proteinase, the absence of amino acids and the presence of insoluble or soluble proteins were required. Further investigation suggested that proteinase production was stimulated by the presence of peptides of eight or more amino acid residues and was repressed by low-molecular-weight nitrogen components (29). Proteinase production was correlated with cell growth in stratum corneum-containing medium but was not observed from media containing hoof or human hair (Fig. 2) (28). Concerning the induction of proteinase from human nail-containing medium, it called for a longer incubation period. These phenomena are similar to clinical observations where *C. albicans* affects stratum corneum but rarely nail and never hair.

Subsequently we purified this enzyme by DEAE-Cellulose and Sephacryl S-200 column chromatography (8). The molecular size of the purified enzyme was 42 kDa and the isoelectic point was 4.5. It had an optimum

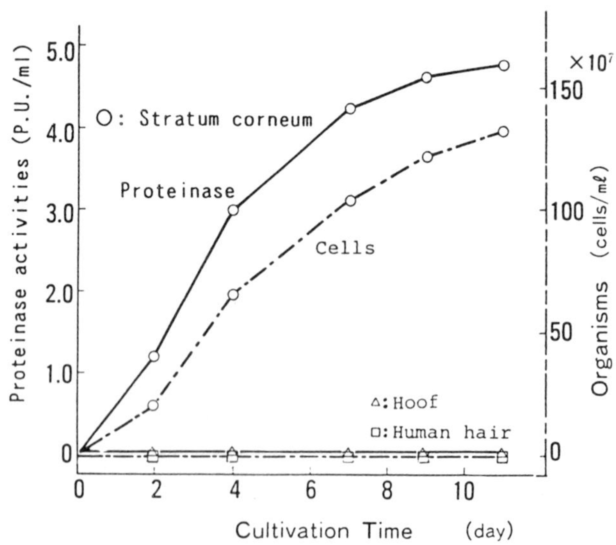

Figure 2 Correlation of proteinase activity and cell growth in various media (28). Key: ○ = human stratum corneum; △ = hoof; □ = human hair.

pH at 4.0, and the inhibitor profiles suggested that this enzyme belongs to the carboxyl proteinase group. Pepstatin, a low-molecular-size carboxyl proteinase inhibitor, was the strongest inhibitor for the purified proteinase. Comparison of the biochemical properties of the keratinolytic proteinase and other proteinases from *C. albicans* listed in Table 1 suggested that these are all the same enzyme. The proteinase digested BSA, ovalbumin, and hemoglobin as well as insoluble keratin proteins (8), suggesting that the term *proteinase* is a preferable to *keratinase*, as it has a broad substrate specificity. The proteinase was reported to digest the membranous fraction of stratum corneum (8), collagen (8,9), laminin (30), fibronectin (30), cystatin A (31), endothelin-1 (32), the Fc portion of immunoglobulin G (33) and complement C3 (33).

From the viewpoint of therapy, we investigated the antifungal effect of pepstatin on the growth of *C. albicans* (Fig. 3) (34). Among the four

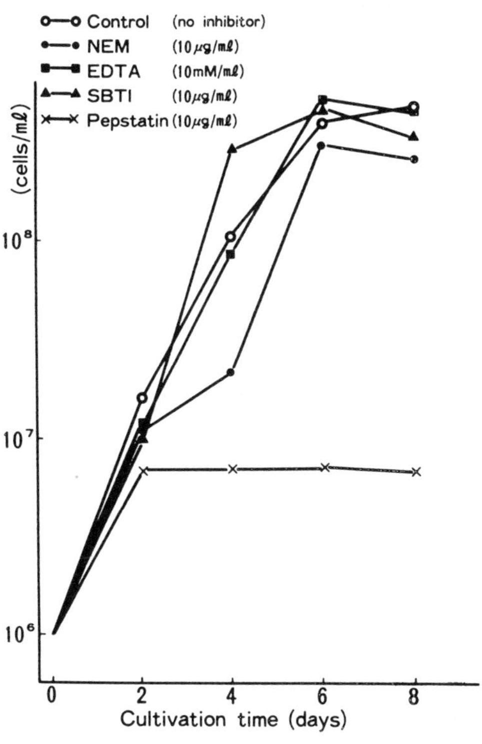

Figure 3 Inhibitory effect of various proteinase inhibitors on the growth of *C. albicans* (34).

types of proteinase inhibitors, only pepstatin inhibited the cell growth of *C. albicans* in stratum corneum-supplemented medium. The antifungal effect of pepstatin was found to be considerably stronger than that of clotrimazole in this condition. These phenomena confirmed that this is a key enzyme for fungal growth in this medium.

It is well known that the pH of normal skin surface is weakly acidic, which coincides with the optimal pH of the *C. albicans* proteinase. However, there is a wide range of pH environments in the human body, including the neutral pH of serum. Germaine and Tellefson (35) previously denied the role of extracellular proteinase in saliva-supplemented medium because of the neutral pH of saliva. Meanwhile, Samaranayake et al. (36) reported an increased concentration of acetate from sucrose- and glucose-supplemented media. In order to verify how *C. albicans* multiplies under a wide range of pH conditions with the use of an acidic proteinase, the correlation with the culture medium pH, extracellular proteinase activity, and fungal growth were investigated using unbuffered, variable pH media (Fig. 4) (37). As the cultivation period progressed, the medium pH decreased gradually to approximately pH 4 and then rapidly increased to approximately pH 7. A rapid increase in proteinase activity and cell growth was observed when the medium pH was approximately 4. The

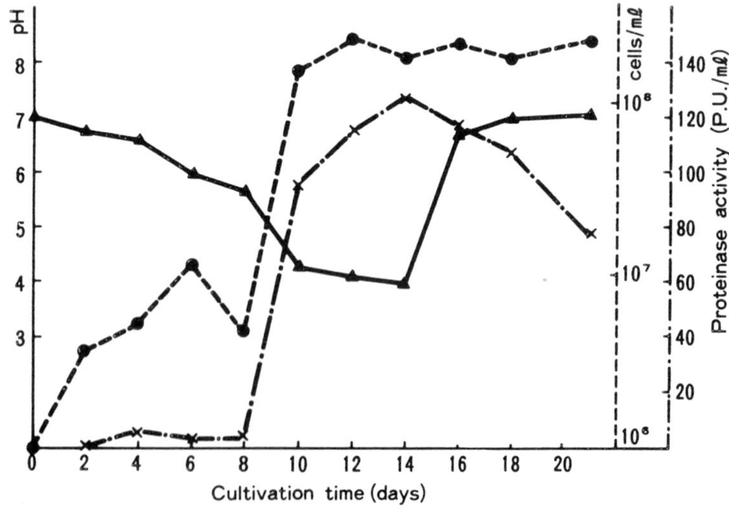

Figure 4 Relation between the change of medium pH, proteinase activity, and cell growth during cultivation (initial pH: 7.0) (37). Key: ▲ = pH; × = proteinase activity; ● = cells/ml.

lowering of the medium pH was attributed to the production of organic acids from carbon sources and the increase to the ammonia production from the degraded stratum corneum. It is known that the budding tips of yeast show a lower acidic pH than the subapical portions (38). These data suggest that *C. albicans* is able to acidify the microenvironmental pH, which simultaneously stimulates proteinase production and cell growth.

Evidence that extracellular carboxyl proteinase is an important pathogenic factor has been accumulating over the past 10 years. Such evidence is briefly summarized below:

1. The enzyme is secreted by the majority of *C. albicans* and to a lesser extent by *C. tropicalis* and *C. parapsilosis*, while *C. Kefyr*, *C. krusei*, *C. glabrata*, and *C. guiliermondii* rarely secrete the proteinase. This order correlates with the relative ranking of lethality in animal models (1).
2. *C. albicans* strains with a significantly high proteolytic activity showed strong lethality for mice (39–41) and high invasiveness to the chorioallantoic membrane of developing chicks (42). Cassone et al. (43) reported that *C. albicans* isolated from patients with vaginitis showed higher proteinase secretion than those from carriers.
3. Proteinase antigens were detected around yeasts in infected animal tissues (44), in murine macrophages after phagocytosis (45), and on the surface of adhering blastospores and invading filamentous cells of *C. albicans* (46).
4. Circulating antibody against the proteinase was detected in patients with candidiasis and in infected animals (44).
5. The proteinase production is related to adherence with the host cells (46). *C. albicans* isolates that adhered most strongly to endothelial cells had the highest relative proteinase activity and showed higher tissue colonization (47). Ray and Payne (48) showed that the proteinase may participate with *C. albicans* in the cavitation process of the corneocyte surface.
6. Pepstatin, an inhibitor of the proteinase, blocked the cavitation process (48) and adherence of *C. albicans* to cultured human epidermal keratinocytes (49).

At a scientific meeting in 1993, *C. albicans* proteinase was called secreted aspartyl proteinase (SAP). The techniques of gene cloning have recently revealed the nucleotide sequence of *C. albicans* proteinase. At least seven SAP genes from *C. albicans* (50–55), one gene from *C. tropicalis* (56), and two genes from *C. parapsilosis* (57,58) have been reported (Table 2). The predicted amino acid sequences of SAP had approximately

Table 2 Genes Encoding Secreted Aspartyl Proteinases (SAP) in *Candida* Species

Genes	Strains	Reported by
SAP1	*C. albicans* (ATCC 10231)	Hube et al., 1991 (50)
SAP2	*C. albicans* (ATCC 10261)	Wright et al., 1992 (51)
	C. albicans A (TIMM2726#114)	Mukai et al., 1992 (52)
SAP3	*C. albicans* (WO-1)	White et al., 1993 (53)
SAP4	*C. albicans* (WO-1)	Miyasaki et al., 1994 (54)
SAP5	*C. albicans* (C74)	Monod et al., 1994 (55)
SAP6	*C. albicans* (C74)	Monod et al., 1994 (55)
SAP7	*C. albicans* (C74)	Monod et al., 1994 (55)
SAPT1	*C. tropicalis* (ATCC750)	Togni et al., 1991 (56)
SAPP1	*C. parapsilosis* (CHUV E-18)	De Viragh et al., 1993 (57)
SAPP2	*C. parapsilosis* (CHUV E-18)	Fusek et al., 1993 (58)

60 to 80% homology to each other and had signal sequences for secretion. The low homology of the genes was initially thought to be due to strain differences; however, multiple copies of the genes were later identified in a single strain (53,59). Heterogeneity of the secreted proteinases, judged from the reactivities with the monoclonal antibodies, suggests the existence of a larger number of SAP genes than those that have been reported so far (60).

The fact that several genes encode similar but different proteinases suggests that the encoded proteinases have a distinct function and regulation mechanism. *SAP1* and *SAP3* were expressed during phenotypic switching between the white and opaque forms of the organisms (60). The *SAP2* mRNA was expressed as the dominant transcript in the yeast form of various strains. Such expressions were observed during the logarithmic growth phase in acidic pH media supplemented with BSA (60). The expression of the closely related *SAP4–6* genes was observed only at neutral pH during serum-induced yeast to hyphal transition (59,60).

The next target for research regarding the proteinase will be the gene disruption in a pathogenic strain of *C. albicans*. A lethality assay in mice with such a strain will strongly support the role of the proteinase as a pathogenic factor. However, the existence of multiple copies of SAP genes in a strain suggests that the disruption of one gene is not enough to stop the secretion of the proteinases. Published (61) and unpublished data suggest that a strain that lacks one gene of ASP does not show any significant difference with regard to lethality in mice when compared with the lethality of a wild strain.

B. Proteinases from Other Species

Dermatophytes invade hair, nail, and skin, causing superficial mycoses. Lesions are generally restricted to the nonliving cornified layers. Keratinolysis by proteinases (keratinases) has been considered an important pathogenic factor. Some extracellular proteinases have been isolated and characterized from species of *Trichophyton* and *Microsporum* (Table 1). Most of these proteinases were induced from medium supplemented with defatted hair as the sole nitrogen source; however, these proteinases have enzyme activity only at neutral or alkaline pH. It is doubtful whether they work as virulence factors, since normal human skin surface has a weakly acidic pH. For these reasons we attempted to isolate an extracellular proteinase with enzyme activity at acidic pH from a clinical isolate of *Trichophyton mentagrophytes* (16,62). Proteolytic activity was observed as a sharp peak in acidic pH and as a broad peak in neutral and alkaline pH (62). Since neutral proteinases have previously been isolated, purification of an acidic proteinase was performed (16). Our purified proteinase had an approximate molecular size of 40 kDa, an optimal pH at 4.5 for keratin, and an isoelectric point at pH 3.9. Inhibitor profiles suggested that this enzyme belongs to the serine proteinase group in spite of its acidic optimal pH. Natural substrate reactivity demonstrated that this enzyme digests hemoglobin, collagen, and albumin as well as keratins. The existence of more than two extracellular proteinases suggested the cooperative work of these enzymes.

Subsequently, we observed that *Trichophyton rubrum* also produces two proteinases that have maximal activities at pH 4.5 and 8.0. Cultivation of *T. rubrum* in albumin-supplemented medium showed an interesting phenomenon (Fig. 5) (63). At the beginning of cultivation, high proteolytic activity at acidic pH was observed, and as the cultivation progressed, the pH of the culture medium ascended to neutral pH, which induced alkaline proteolytic activity and reduced acidic proteolytic activity. By using two different types of proteinases, the organisms were able to achieve maximal growth in various pHs. Recently, proteolytic activities at neutral pH of *T. mentagrophytes* isolates were reported to be higher than those of *T. rubrum* isolates (64), suggesting that differences in the clinical manifestations caused by the two species may correlate with the proteinase activities of the organisms.

Two extracellular proteinases were also isolated from the yeast form of *Sporothrix schenckii*, a causative organism of sporotrichosis (19). Proteinase I, a serine proteinase, had an optimal pH of 6.0, and its activity was strongly inhibited by chymostatin. Proteinase II, a carboxyl proteinase, had an optimal pH of 3.5, and its activity was strongly inhibited by pepstatin. We investigated the inhibitory effects of either or both of the

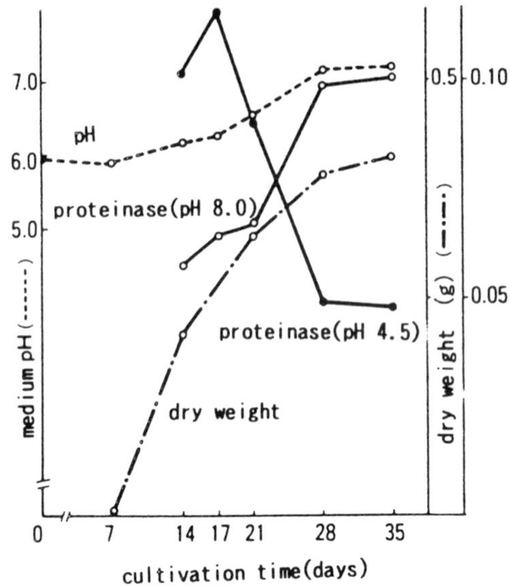

Figure 5 Relation between the change of medium pH, Proteinase activity and cell growth during cultivation (63). Key: ---○-- = pH; —●— = proteinase activity at pH 4.5; —○— = proteinase activity at pH 8.0; --○-- = cell growth by dry weight.

proteinase inhibitors on cell growth in albumin-supplemented medium (65). Table 3 shows a summary of the results. The addition of pepstatin or chymostatin to the culture medium reduced the inhibitor-sensitive proteinase production and stimulated the induction of another proteinase supplementary, which resulted in unaffected cell growth. The addition of both

Table 3 Antifungal Effect of Proteinase Inhibitors on Cell Growth (65)

Proteinase inhibitors	None	Pepstatin	Chymostatin	Pepstatin Chymostatin
Proteinase II activity (optimal pH 3.5)	↑	↓	↑↑	↓
Proteinase I activity (optimal pH 6.0)	↑	↑↑	↓	↓
Cell growth	↑	↑	↑	↓↓

inhibitors strongly inhibited fungal growth, suggesting that these enzymes are cooperatively crucial to cell growth in this medium.

III. LIPASE AND PHOSPHOLIPASE

Lipolysis appears to be very important for organisms to obtain nutrients. Although lipase from *Candida cylindracea* has been well characterized and cloned (66–68), isolation of lipases from *C. albicans* and *Malassezia furfur* has not been reported.

Malassezia furfur and its yeast forms, *Pityrosporum ovale* and *orbiculare*, are very common residents of the lipid-rich surfaces of the human skin. A source of lipid is essential for the cultivation of *M. furfur*, which suggests the existence of a lipase. We characterized the properties of a lipase from *P. ovale* and *P. orbiculare* and investigated the correlation of lipase activity and cell growth (69). Lipase activity was assayed by a colorimetric method using α-naphthyl palmitate as a substrate. Liquid growth medium for the induction of lipase included Tween 80 and glucose. Lipase activities were observed mainly in the insoluble fractions of the organisms, with no enzyme activity in the extracellular fractions. Lipase activity was maximal at pH 5.0 and strongly activated by the addition of sodium taurocholate. Rapid logarithmic cell growth during the first 2–4 days of cultivation was well correlated with lipase activity.

A lipase from *C. albicans* was induced from carbohydrate-restricted media (unpublished data). Extracellular lipase activities were detected from culture medium containing yeast nitrogen base (YNB) and Tween 80 but not from Sabouraud medium even in the presence of Tween 80. Cell growth and lipase production in YNB-Tween 80 medium were closely correlated and increased dependent on the concentration of Tween 80 in the medium. These results suggest that Tween 80 worked as a substrate for extracellular lipase but not as a detergent. The optimum pH of this enzyme was 5.5. Enzyme activity was not inhibited by the addition of an esterase inhibitor, ebelactone B, while sodium taurocholate increased enzyme activity twofold. Further study demonstrated that this enzyme was a monoacylglycerol hydrolase (not a lipase in the strict sense of the word).

We subsequently measured the lipase activity of 85 clinical isolates of *Candida* species. *Candida albicans*, *C. tropicalis* and *C. parapsilosis* had a tendency to show higher activity per milliliter medium than *C. kefyr*, *C. krusei*, *C. glabrata*, and *C. guilliermondii* (unpublished data).

C. albicans possesses various enzymes that are related to the metabolism of phospholipids, such as phospholipases, lysophospholipase, and lysophospholipase-transacylase (70–72). Samaranayake et al. (73)

screened the phospholipase activity of 41 *Candida* isolates and showed that 79% of the *C. albicans* isolates were phospholipase producers, whereas none of the *C. tropicalis*, *C. glabrata*, or *C. parapsilosis* isolates produced the enzyme. In another study, Barrett-Bee et al. (74) measured the amount of phospholipase activity in different isolates of *C. albicans* and found a correlation between phospholipase activity, pathogenicity, and adherence to epithelial cells. Pugh and Cawson (75) demonstrated the cytochemical localization of phospholipase in inoculated blastospores and developing hyphae in chick chorioallantoic membranes. Although the physiological meaning of the secretion of the hydrolytic enzymes related to phospholipid metabolism is not well understood, they are strong candidates for pathogenesis-related enzymes.

IV. OTHER ENZYMES

Various kinds of fungal enzymes related to metabolic processes have been isolated from *C. albicans* and extensively characterized (1). Examples of such are enzymes associated with carbohydrate metabolism (e.g., glucosidase, glucose-6-phosphate dehydrogenase), aminosugar metabolism, polysaccharide metabolism (e.g., chitinase, glucanase), and sterol metabolism (1). However, there have been few reports describing the correlation between these enzymes and fungal pathogenicity. During the process of searching for an inducible α-amylase from *C. albicans*, we recently observed that α-maltase (α-D-glucosidase) was induced from maltose-containing medium (76). The addition of a small amount of glucose rapidly suppressed the cell-associated maltase activity. Maltase activities of clinical isolates of *Candida* species were well correlated with fungal growth and the relative pathogenicity ranking of each species in vivo. Further studies focusing on virulence factors should be performed, since fungal enzymes related to metabolic processes have until now been investigated only as tools for biotyping.

V. CONCLUSIONS

The pathogenicity of fungi is determined by the integration of multiple parameters. It is becoming evident, as mentioned above, that fungal enzymes, especially hydrolytic enzymes, constitute one of the pathogenic factors. Hydrolytic enzymes may be produced to damage host tissues and obtain nutritive substances from degraded materials. The pathogenic role of inducible hydrolytic enzymes is expected to be more important in mycoses of the localized sites. Nutrients for fungal growth in skin and mucosa are more restricted than those in serum. In order to demonstrate definitive evidence that hydrolytic enzymes are involved as a pathogenic factor, further investigations should be continued mainly in *C. albicans*, a major pathogenic fungus. The technique of gene disruption will tell us whether a strain lacking SAP gene loses its pathogenicity in *in vitro* and *in vivo* assays.

As a final point to this commentary, we would like to emphasize that targeting of the method with reference to the biological behavior of the molecule *in vivo* is crucial to the strategy for identifying a pathogenic factor.

ACKNOWLEDGMENTS

The authors wish to acknowledge the following members in our laboratory for their significant contributions to the studies presented here: Dr. M. Hattori, Dr. M. Negi, Dr. K. Matsuda, Dr. I. J. Ko, Dr. T. Sanada, Dr. V. Rojanavanich, Dr. K. Sekiguchi, Dr. Y. Ran, Dr. T. Yoshiike, Dr. H. Komatsuzaki, and Dr. K. Bramono.

REFERENCES

1. Odds FC. Candida and candidosis, 2d ed. London: Baillière Tindall, 1988.
2. Calderone RA. Host-parasite relationships in candidosis. Mycoses 1989; 32(suppl 2):12–17.
3. Ghannoum MA, Abu-Elteen KH. Pathogenicity determinants of Candida. Mycoses 1990;33:265–282.
4. Culter JE. Putative virulence factors of Candida albicans. Annu Rev Microbiol 1991;45:187–218.
5. Ogrydziak DM. Yeast extracellular proteases. Crit Rev Biotechnol 1993;13: 1–55.
6. Remold H, Fasold H, Staib F. Purification and characterization of a proteolytic enzyme from Candida albicans. Biochim Biophys Acta 1968;167:399–406.
7. Ruchel R. Properties of a purified proteinase from the yeast *Candida albicans*. Biochim Biophys Acta 1981;659:99–113.
8. Negi M, Tsuboi R, Matsui T, Ogawa H. Isolation and characterization of proteinase from Candida albicans. J Invest Dermatol 1984;83:32–36.
9. Kaminishi H, Hagihara Y, Hayashi S, Cho T. Isolation and characterization of collagenolytic enzyme produced by Candida albicans. Infect Immun 1986; 53:312–316.
10. Rüchel R, Boning B, Borg M. Characterization of a secretory proteinase of Candida parapsilosis and evidence for the absence of the enzyme during infection in vitro. Infect Immun 1986;53:411–419.
11. Asahi MR, Lindquist K, Fukuyama K, et al. Purification and characterization of major extracellular proteinases from Trichophyton rubrum. Biochem J 1985;232:139–144.
12. Sanyal AK, Das SK, Banerjee AB. Purification and partial characterization

of an exocellular proteinase from Trichophyton rubrum. Sabouraudia 1985; 23:165–178.
13. Apodaca G, McKerrow JH. Purification and characterization of a 27,000-Mr exocellular proteinase from Trichophyton rubrum. Infect Immun 1989; 57:3072–3080.
14. Yu R, Harmon SR, Blank F. Isolation and purification of an extracellular keratinase of Trichophyton mentagrophytes. J Bacteriol 1968;96:1435–1436.
15. Day WC, Tonic P, Stratman SL, et al. Isolation and properties of an extracellular protease of Trichophyton granulosum. Biochim Biophys Acta 1968;167: 597–606.
16. Tsuboi R, Ko IJ, Takamori K, Ogawa H. Isolation of a keratinolytic proteinase from Trichophyton mentagrophytes with enzymatic activity at acidic pH. Infect Immun 1989;57:3479–3483.
17. Takiuchi I, Higuchi D, Sei Y, Koga M. Isolation of an extracellular proteinase (keratinase) from Microsporum canis. Sabouraudia 1982;20:281–288.
18. Takiuchi I, Higuchi D. Isolation, purification and biochemical properties of keratinase elaborated from Microsporum gypseum. Jpn J Dermatol 1977;87: 305–309.
19. Tsuboi R, Sanada T, Takamori K, Ogawa H. Isolation and properties of extracellular proteinases from Sporothrix schenckii. J Bacteriol 1987;169: 4104–4109.
20. Rojanavanich V, Yoshiike T, Tsuboi R, et al. Purification and characterization of an extracellular proteinase from Hendersonula toruloidea. Infect Immun 1990;58:2856–2861.
21. Malviya HK, Rajak RC, Hasija SK. Purification and partial characterization of two extracellular keratinases of Scopulariopsis brevicaulis. Mycopathologia 1992;119:161–165.
22. Reichard U, Buttner S, Eiffert H, et al. Purification and characterization of an extracellular serine proteinase from Aspergillus fumigatus and its detection in tissue. J Med Microbiol 1990;33:243–251.
23. Rhodes JC, Amlung TW, Miller MS. Isolation and characterization of an elastinolytic proteinase from Aspergillus flavus. Infect Immun 1990;58: 2529–2534.
24. Odds FC. Candida albicans proteinase as a virulence factor in the pathogenesis of Candida infections. Zbl Bakt Hyg 1985;A260:539–542.
25. Ray TL, Payne CD, Morrow BJ. Candida albicans acid proteinase: Characterization and role in candidiasis. Adv Exp Med Biol 1991;306:173–183.
26. Tsuboi R, Kurita Y, Iwahara K, et al. The biological role of keratinolytic proteinase and its inhibitor on the growth of Candida albicans. In: Ogawa H, Lazarus GS, Hopsu-Havu VK, eds. The Biological Role of Proteinases and Their Inhibitors in Skin. Tokyo: University of Tokyo Press, 1985: 161–173.
27. Staib F. Serum proteins as nitrogen source for yeast-like fungi. Sabouraudia 1965;4:187–193.
28. Hattori M, Yoshiura K, Negi M, Ogawa H. Keratinolytic proteinase produced by Candida albicans. Sabouraudia 1984;22:175–183.

29. Lerner CG, Goldman RC. Stimuli that induce production of Candida albicans aspartyl proteinase. J Gen Microbiol 1993;139:1643–1651.
30. Ray TL, Payne CD. Degradation of basement membrane matrix proteins laminin, fibronectin and type IV collagen by Candida acid proteinase. J Invest Dermatol 1991;96:606A.
31. Tsushima H, Mine H, Kawakami Y, et al. Candida albicans aspartic proteinase cleaves and inactivates human epidermal cysteine proteinase inhibitor, cystatin A. Microbiology 1994;140:167–171.
32. Tsushima H, Mine H. Cleavage of human big endothelin-1 by Candida albicans aspartic proteinase. FEMS Immun Med Microbiol 1995;11:69–72.
33. Kaminishi H, Miyaguchi H, Tamaki T, et al. Degradation of humoral host defense by Candida albicans proteinase. Infect Immun 1995;63:984–988.
34. Tsuboi R, Kurita Y, Negi M, Ogawa H. A specific inhibitor of keratinolytic proteinase (KPase) from Candida albicans could inhibit the cell growth of C. albicans. J Invest Dermatol 1985;85:438–440.
35. Germaine GR, Tellefson LM. Effect of pH and human saliva on protease production by Candida albicans. Infect Immun 1981;31:323–326.
36. Samaranayake LP, Geddes DAM, Weetman DA, MacFarlane TW. Growth and acid production of Candida albicans in carbohydrate supplemented media. Microbios 1983;37:105–115.
37. Tsuboi R, Matsuda K, Ko IJ, Ogawa H. Correlation between culture medium pH, extracellular proteinase activity, and cell growth of Candida albicans in insoluble stratum corneum-supplemented media. Arch Dermatol Res 1989; 281:3442–3455.
38. Turian G. Low pH in fungal bud initials. Experientia 1981;37:1278–1279.
39. MacDonald F, Odds FC. Virulence for mice of a proteinase-secreting strain of Candida albicans and a proteinase-deficient mutant. J Gen Microbiol 1983; 129:431–438.
40. Kwon-Chung KJ, Lehaman D, Good C, Magee PT. Genetic evidence for role of extracellular proteinase in virulence of Candida albicans. Infect Immun 1985;49:571–575.
41. Kondoh Y, Shimizu K, Tanaka K. Proteinase production and pathogenicity of Candida albicans: II. Virulence for mice of C. albicans strains of different proteinase activity. Microbiol Immunol 1987;31:1061–1069.
42. Shimizu K, Kondoh Y, Tanaka K. Proteinase production and pathogenicity of Candida albicans: I. Invasion into chorioallantoic membrane by C. albicans strains of different proteinase activity. Microbiol Immunol 1987;31: 1045–1060.
43. Cassone A, Bernardis FD, Mondello F, et al. Evidence for a correlation between proteinase secretion and vulvovaginal candidosis. J Infect Dis 1987; 156:777–783.
44. MacDonald F, Odds FC. Inducible proteinase of Candida albicans in diagnostic serology and in the pathogenesis of systemic candidosis. J Med Microbiol 1980;13:423–435.
45. Borg M, Rüchel R. Demonstration of fungal proteinase during phagocytosis of Candida albicans and Candida tropicalis. J Med Vet Mycol 1990;28:3–14.

46. Borg M, Rüchel R. Expression of extracellular acid proteinase by proteolytic Candida spp. during experimental infection of oral mucosa. Infect Immun 1988;56:626–631.
47. Ghannoum MA, Abu-Elteen K. Correlative relationship between proteinase production, adherence and pathogenicity of various strains of Candida albicans. J Med Vet Mycol 1986;24:407–413.
48. Ray TL, Payne CD. Scanning electron microscopy of epidermal adherence and cavitation in murine candidiasis: A role for Candida acid proteinase. Infect Immun 1988;56:1942–1949.
49. Ollert MW, Söhnchen R, Korting HC, et al. Mechanisms of adherence of Candida albicans to cultured human epidermal keratinocytes. Infect Immun 1993;61:4560–4568.
50. Hube B, Turver CJ, Odds FC, et al. Sequence of the Candida albicans gene encoding the secretory aspartate proteinase. J Med Vet Mycol 1991;29: 129–132.
51. Wright RJ, Came A, Hieber AD, et al. A second gene for a secreted aspartate proteinase in Candida albicans. J Bacteriol 1992;174:7848–7853.
52. Mukai H, Takeda O, Asada K, et al. cDNA cloning of an aspartic proteinase secreted by Candida albicans. Microbiol Immunol 1992;36:1207–1216.
53. White TC, Miyasaki SH, Agabian N. Three distinct secreted aspartyl proteinases in Candida albicans. J Bacteriol 1993;175:6136–6133.
54. Miyasaki SH, White TC, Agabian N. A fourth secreted aspartyl proteinase gene (SAP4) and a CARE2 repetitive element are located upstream of the SAP1 gene in Candida albicans. J Bacteriol 1994;176:1702–1710.
55. Monod M, Togni G, Hube B, Sanglard D. Multiplicity of genes encoding secreted aspartic proteinases in Candida species. Mol Microbiol 1994;13: 357–368.
56. Togni G, Sanglard D, Falchetto R, Monod M. Isolation and nucleotide sequence of the extracellular acid protease gene (ACP) from the yeast Candida tropicalis. FEBS Lett 1991;286:181–185.
57. De Viragh PA, Sanglard D, Togni G, et al. Cloning and sequencing of two Candida parapsilosis genes encoding acid proteinases. J Gen Microbiol 1993; 139:335–342.
58. Fusek M, Smith EA, Monod M, Foundling SI. Candida parapsilosis expresses and secretes two aspartic proteinases. FEBS Lett 1993;327:108–112.
59. Hube B, Monod M, Schofield DA, et al. Expression of seven members of the gene family encoding secretory aspartyl proteinases in Candida albicans. Mol Microbiol 1994;14:87–99.
60. Morrison CJ, Hurst SF, Bragg SL, et al. Heterogeneity of the purified extracellular aspartyl proteinase from Candida albicans: Characterization with monoclonal antibodies and N-terminal amino acid sequence analysis. Infect Immun 1993;61:2030–2036.
61. Togni G, Sanglard D, Monod M. Acid proteinase secreted by Candida tropicalis: Virulence in mice of a proteinase negative mutant. J Med Vet Mycol 1994;32:257–265.

62. Tsuboi R, Ko IJ, Matsuda K, Ogawa H. A new keratinolytic proteinase from clinical isolates of Trichophyton mentagrophytes. J Dermatol 1987;14: 506–508.
63. Sekiguchi K, Nishiyama C, Morishima T, et al. Relation between movement of acid or alkaline proteinase from Trichophyton rubrum and the growth of fungus, pH in medium. Jpn J Dermatol 1990;100:215–217.
64. Samdani AJ, Dykes PJ, Marks R. The proteolytic activity of strains of T. mentagrophytes and T. rubrum isolated from tinea pedis and tinea unguium infections. J Med Vet Mycol 1995;33:167–170.
65. Tsuboi R, Sanada T, Ogawa H. Influence of culture medium pH and proteinase inhibitors on extracellular proteinase activity and cell growth of Sporothrix schenckii. J Clin Microbiol 1988;26:1431–1433.
66. Brahimi-Horn M-C, Guglielmino ML, Elling L, Sparrow LG. The esterase profile of a lipase from Candida cylindracea. Biochim Biophys Acta 1990; 1042:51–54.
67. Kawaguchi Y, Honda H, Taniguchi-Morimura J, Iwasaki S. The codon CUG is read as serine in an asporogenic yeast Candida cylindracea. Nature 1989; 341:164–167.
68. Longhi S, Fusetti F, Grandori R, et al. Cloning and nucleotide sequences of two lipase genes from Candida cylindracea. Biochim Biophys Acta 1992; 1131:227–232.
69. Ran Y, Yoshiike T, Ogawa H. Lipase of Malassezia furfur: Some properties and their relationship to cell growth. J Med Vet Mycol 1993;31:77–85.
70. Bannno Y, Yamada T, Nozawa Y. Secreted phospholipase of the dimorphic fungus, Candida albicans; Separation of three enzymes and some biological properties. Sabouraudia 1985;23:47–54.
71. Mago N, Khuller GK. Subcellular localization of enzymes of phospholipid metabolism in Candida albicans. J Med Vet Mycol 1990;28:355–362.
72. Takahashi M, Banno Y, Shikano Y, et al. Purification and characterization of lysophospholipase-transacylase of pathogenic fungus Candida albicans. Biochim Biophys Acta 1991;1082:161–169.
73. Samaranayake LP, Raeside JM, MacFarlane TW. Factors affecting the phospholipase activity of Candida species in vitro. Sabouraudia 1984;22:201–207.
74. Barrett-Bee K, Hayes Y, Wilson RG, Ryleey JF. A comparison of phospholipipase activity, cellular adherence and pathogenicity of yeasts. J Gen Microbiol 1985;131:1217–1221.
75. Pugh D, Cawson RA. The cytochemical localization of phospholipase in Candida albicans infecting the chick chorio-allantoic membrane. Sabouraudia 1977;15:29–35.
76. Bramono K, Tsuboi R, Ogawa H. A carbohydrate-degrading enzyme from Candida albicans: Correlation between α-glucosidase activity and fungal growth. Mycoses 1995;38:349–353.

11

Immunomodulation in Superficial Fungal Infections

RODERICK JAMES HAY
St. John's Institute of Dermatology
Guy's Hospital
London, England

I. INTRODUCTION

The mechanisms of host resistance to fungi that infect the epidermis are different from those involved in defense against mycoses affecting internal sites (1). This is not due, as originally thought, to the absence of cells involved in immunological surveillance or effector action. Rather, specific afferent and efferent pathways for immunologically mediated responses have evolved in the epidermis. Uptake and immunological processing of foreign antigens is largely performed by modified dendritic cells, Langerhans cells, and other cells within the dermis and epidermis. One of the major discoveries of recent years has been the growing understanding of the role of keratinocytes in immunological activities. For instance, they are activated to express class II antigens and release cytokines as well as other inflammatory mediators such as the tumor necrosis factors (TNF) and interleukin-1 (IL-1) and IL-8. They also produce and express other substances involved in the development of an inflammatory responses, including adhesion molecules such as ICAM-1. The immunological surveillance system of the skin is inextricably linked with other elements of the immunological system, such as B and T lymphocytes and neutrophils. The importance of the changes which develop in response to a foreign antigen is that the epidermis is "switched on," a feature that helps localize the need for effector cells at one particular site and also makes it possible to reactivate the system at some later time.

One of the other observed features of the interaction between certain fungi, such as *Pityrosporum* yeasts, and the skin is tolerance of surface commensals. It is therefore necessary to reconcile the existence of a sophisticated epidermal immunological reception system with an apparent lack of response, under "normal" conditions, to foreign antigenic materials, including microbes, on the superficial epidermis and within hair follicles. It is also not clear how effector responses are developed in the epidermis. Certain effector mechanisms such as the migration of polymorphonuclear leukocytes into an area or cytokine-regulated increased epidermal cell turnover may act to remove foreign substances such as microorganisms from the skin surface. The efficiency of such mechanisms in countering skin infection is difficult to assess. Likewise, responses may vary from site to site on the skin surface. It is, therefore, possible that there are some areas on the skin where immunological defense is less effective than it is in others. In other words, inefficiency in effector action may allow persistence of microorganisms. Other possibilities include the alteration of the immunological response by an intrinsic host mechanism or by organisms. An understanding of these processes is necessary in order to explain the phenomenon of commensalism, the persistence of certain skin infections—such as plantar *Trichophyton rubrum* and human papillomavirus infections—and, on the other hand, the vigorous inflammatory response that develops in response to certain dermatophyte infections.

In approaching this problem, the immunological response to infections by ringworm fungi, the dermatophytoses, is discussed, as these pathogens encompass a range of different clinical and host-inflammatory responses. At one end of this spectrum of responsiveness are dermatophyte infections, which are self-limited, elicit an inflammatory reaction, and generally respond to minimal therapy without recurring (2). Zoophilic dermatophyte infections in humans are often highly inflammatory, and resolution is followed by lasting immunity. Second infections with the cattle ringworm, *Trichophyton verrucosum*, are rare (3). By contrast, human anthropophilic dermatophytoses are seen to be persistent and are often noninflammatory; they may also persist despite otherwise effective therapy (4). Relapse after treatment is also frequent. Examples include *T. rubrum* infections of the feet and hands, *Trichophyton tonsurans* in the scalp (5), and tinea imbricata due to *Trichophyton concentricum* (6), an extensive type of tinea corporis in remote areas of the humid tropics such as the West Pacific. Chronic dermatophytosis due to these species is common and is believed to have contributed to the increase in numbers of cases of dermatophyte infections in many countries. In certain occupational groups persistent dermatophyte infections are equally problematic. In the United Kingdom's coal mining industry, 30–35% of miners have chronic foot infections that lead to moderate disability. It is apparent that this situation has scarcely changed over the past 20 years, despite coordinated approaches to the control of infection (7).

II. INFECTION BY DERMATOPHYTES: THE "NORMAL" PROCESS

Dermatophytic fungi generally do not penetrate further than the granular layer of the stratum corneum. The first phase of invasion follows the process of adherence between the fungal cell and the keratinocyte (8). This has been shown to be a finite process during which arthrospores are attached to keratinocytes over a period of 2–3 hr before germination. The process is accompanied by changes such as swelling of arthrospores. In practice, adhesion may well involve other elements as well, particularly keratinocyte-to-keratinocyte adhesion, as this is the most likely vehicle for transmission via desquamated skin fragments. Germination follows this process of adherence; again, it can be followed in vitro and has been shown to depend on ambient conditions such as humidity (9). Penetration of the dermatophytes through the outer keratinocyte layer is followed by invasion of the outer stratum corneum. In experimentally infected mice, this process is confronted within 4–6 hr by the mobilization of neutrophils, which congregate at the site of infection (10). In human skin biopsies, neutrophil accumulation is seen where fungi penetrate the hair follicle, but it is less common in the interfollicular epidermis (11). The reasons for this are not clear, but the lack of neutrophil accumulation may reduce the possibility of early elimination of organisms during a vulnerable phase of skin infection.

Human dermatophyte infections can be classified as acute or chronic; acute infections in humans are often caused by zoophilic fungi and chronic infections by anthropophilic organisms. In their natural host, zoophilic infections may also elicit no pronounced inflammatory response. Host defense against dermatophytes depends on both immune and nonimmune mechanisms. The principal modes of defense involve binding of unsaturated transferrin to fungal cells, migration of polymorphonuclear leukocytes into the area of infection, and T-lymphocyte activation as well as increased epidermal cell turnover (2,12–14). Little attention has focused on the nonspecific mechanisms of defense against dermatophytosis. Generally the fungi are inhibited in a number of different ways. The unsaturated transferrin inhibits the growth of dermatophytes by a direct mechanism involving binding to the fungal membrane (12). The speed of growth of the epidermis is also increased in human dermatophytosis; a similar phenomenon has been shown in experimental candidosis in guinea pigs (14) and experimental dermatophytosis in mice. In these experimental infections, increased epidermal proliferation occurs early in the infection—within 48 hr in mice—or, in other words, before classic immunological activation can have occurred (10). There is an acceleration of the proliferative response in the guinea pig system after 10 days, suggesting that at this stage there is some amplification of the proliferative response. In addition, the production of medium-chain fatty acids in sebum is thought to inhibit dermatophytic fungi, a phenomenon that can be demonstrated in vitro.

Killing of dermatophytes by both murine and human neutrophils and macrophages can be demonstrated (15). The former are important components of the histological response to hair follicle invasion in humans and animals. Human polymorphonuclear cells (PMNs) have been shown to destroy up to 60% of *T. rubrum* and *T. quinckeanum* germlings within 2 hr; macrophages are less efficient in causing fungal death. Little synergy can be demonstrated between these two cell types in dermatophyte killing (15). The effects of PMNs have been reproduced by an in vitro system using lactoperoxidase, hydrogen peroxidase, and potassium iodide and can be abrogated with catalase, superoxide dismutase, and histidine, which are known scavengers of hydrogen peroxide, superoxide anion, and singlet oxygen respectively (16). Killing can proceed even in the absence of ingestion of fungal hyphae by neutrophils. The existence of a second type of phagocyte-mediated defense, as occurs with *Candida* via the elaboration of "killer" peptides, has not been found in dermatophytosis. Neutrophils are attracted to the site of infection both by production of epidermally derived chemotactic factors such as leukotriene derivatives and also by certain dermatophyte cell wall or cytoplasmic antigens, which activate the alternate pathway of complement (13).

In experimental murine and human infections, T lymphocytes appear to play the major role in host defense. During primary infection in mice, there is evidence of activation of both B and T lymphocytes in peripheral draining lymph nodes (17). However, immunity to infection can be transferred to unexposed animals from previously infected mice with T lymphocytes bearing the Thy-1 but not Ly-2.2 phenotype (18). Transfer of serum containing antibody from infected mice will also not confer resistance on recipients. In humans, there is a similar correlation between inflammatory responses, T-lymphocyte blastogenesis, and recovery. Once again, the development of delayed-type hypersensitivity, positive skin tests to trichophytin, and lymphocyte transformation to fungal antigen occur at the same time as the clinical response (19,20). There is also epidemiological evidence that after recovery from inflammatory ringworm, second infections are infrequent (3). All this suggests that mechanisms for the elimination of infections such as dermatophytosis are present and potentially effective. It is also apparent, though, that a superficial fungal infection is not always followed by recovery.

III. THE CHRONICALLY INFECTED PATIENT: POSSIBLE EXPLANATIONS

A large number of superficial fungal infections, from pityriasis versicolor to plantar dermatophytosis due to *T. rubrum*, are persistent and seldom show a natural tendency to recovery. They are also notoriously susceptible to relapse. Previous studies have occasionally revealed a number of underlying diseases in patients with superficial infections such as dermatophytosis, notably hereditary palmoplantar keratoderma and Raynaud's phenomenon (21). In the case of keratoderma, increased epidermal thickness and alterations in cell turnover rates, rather than a specific defect in immunological function, are thought to predispose to chronic infection. By contrast, a high proportion of patients with *T. rubrum* infections, over 40% in some surveys, have been found to be atopic on personal or family history (22). Chronically infected patients are also likely to develop IgE class antibodies to dermatophytes and immediate-type sensitivity (23). It has also been shown that this occurs with *T. rubrum* infections in other sites, such as the groin. It is not clear though whether this chronic infection among atopics occurs because of some defect in T-cell responsiveness seen in these individuals or whether the production of specific IgE and consequent release of mediators such as histamine affect the expression of an effective immunological response (24). Diversion of the immune response down a T2 pathway may be a further explanation of chronicity. It is also known that patients with disorders of immunity such as chronic mucocutaneous candidosis (CMC) are particularly susceptible to widespread intractable dermatophytosis as well as candidosis; persons infected with human immunodeficiency virus (HIV) may also have chronic ringworm (25). These observations suggest that patients with impairment of immunological defense mechanisms, in particular those affecting T-lymphocyte function, are prone to chronic infection. Despite this, and with the exception of atopy, underlying disease or abnormalities affecting immune function are not seen in the vast majority of patients with dermatophytosis (4).

Patients with persistent foot infections (*T. rubrum*) or tinea corporis (*T. concentricum*) have been reported to show reduced lymphocyte blastogenesis or leukocyte migration inhibition to dermatophyte antigen (20,26). In chronic infections caused by *T. rubrum* compared to those infections due to *T. mentagrophytes*, for instance, there may be weak lymphocyte transformation responses and inflammatory reactions; relapse or persistence of infection are also common. Delayed-type hypersensitivity demonstrated by intradermal trichophytin tests may be absent in many patients with *T. rubrum* or *T. concentricum* infection.

There is evidence that, in many cases, the immunomodulation that appears to underlie some of these changes may be caused by the organisms themselves. In addition to producing enzymes, oligosaccharides from glycoproteins present in dermatophytes are able to interfere with both T- and B-lymphocyte activation (27). This is a reversible process in vitro, but preexposure of lymphocytes to dermatophyte inhibitory factor (DIF) will prevent proliferation of T cells in response to mitogens such as phytohaemaggutinin (PHA) as well as dermatophyte antigens (28). In extensive or chronic dermatophytosis, circulating antigen can be identified in serum (29). Dermatophytes may therefore produce substances that can affect the expression of immune responses. Are such mechanisms operative in naturally acquired infections?

There have been a few instances where patients with persistent dermatophytosis had defective in vitro lymphocyte blastogenesis to T-cell mitogens and dermatophyte antigen and this was reversed either by substituting heterologous (fetal calf) for autologous serum or after successful antifungal treatment (30). A similar finding is seen with neutrophil responses. This suggests that an inhibitory factor or factors may be present in serum (31). Dermatophyte antigen has been identified in such infected serum employing an immunoradiometric assay with the mouse antidermatophyte IgM monoclonal TQ-1 (29). The TQ-1 antibody reacts with phosphoryl-choline (PC), and immunoreactivity can be abrogated by pretreatment with PC. Phosphoryl-choline hapten is found in other parasites, including filaria, and also affects expression of immune responses in these infections. Another, probably different factor has also been identified. This is a glycoprotein that causes reversible inhibition of lymphocyte blastogenesis at certain concentrations. Exposure of patients' lymphocytes to dermatophyte extracts inhibits antigen- or mitogen-elicited blastogenesis; this can be reversed by washing the cells (28). Interestingly not all lymphocyte functions are affected, and cells will still express HLA-DR after exposure to dermatophyte extracts. The nature of this substance in dermatophytes is not entirely understood, although it is possible that it is an oligosaccharide component.

Further evidence that dermatophyte components interfere with normal expression of immunity can be found in experiments designed to study the effect of dermatophyte components in experimental infections. Antigen derived from *Trichophyton* species increases susceptibility of Balb/c mice to dermatophyte infection and interferes with T-cell-mediated immunity (17). It is most active if administered with adjuvant such as alum, suggesting that sustained release is important in producing its effect. The possibility that dermatophytes interfere with the process of immunological activation in human skin is also supported by observations on the presence of activity markers such as adhesion molecules in biopsies from chronically infected patients. Normally, immunophenotypic techniques can demonstrate the presence of large numbers of effector lymphocytes in the vicinity of the infection (32). Work has now shown that the dermal infiltrate mainly contain cells that were Leu2a-positive (namely, T-helper cells) (33). Conversely, few expressed CD-8 (T-suppressor markers). HLA-DR was strongly expressed, and most biopsies showed Langerhans cells using a variety of different cell markers. Despite the presence of an infiltrate, the adhesion molecules, ICAM-1, were poorly expressed in the epidermis. This may reflect suppression of the production of this substance in the epidermis despite intact cell-mediated immunity. Suppression of this aspect of immune activation by DIF produced by dermatophytes in situ is a possible explanation, which may account for the success of dermatophytes such as *T. rubrum* in causing persistent infections. It still remains to be seen whether this explains the difference in responsiveness seen with zoophilic dermatophytes.

Dermatophytes may also affect immune responses in other ways. For instance, *T. rubrum* produces a catalase that may affect the outcome of phagocyte-mediated defense (18). Other fungi may produce secreted superoxide dismutases, which play a similar role, although the presence of such a mechanism among dermatophytes is not known.

Immunomodulation either by substances produced by the organisms themselves or by alterations in the normal immune responses in the host appear to be possible in dermatophytosis. Whether these are the factors that account for chronicity of infection has yet to be established, but there is sufficient evidence to suggest that they may play an important role in some infections.

IV. IMMUNOMODULATION AND OTHER SUPERFICIAL FUNGI

With infections due to *Candida albicans*, the picture is more confusing, as two main groups of immunologically predisposed subjects are affected by this opportunistic pathogen—those with abnormalities of neutrophil or T lymphocyte function. Individuals in the latter category, including patients with chronic mucocutaneous candidosis (CMC) and AIDS, usually have chronic cutaneous or oropharyngeal rather than systemic infections. There is some clinical evidence to show that in CMC, immunological defects may resolve with removal of the organism (34). One explanation, as with dermatophytosis, would be the alteration of the normal pathways of immunological responses; suppressor lymphocytes have been identified in such patients, and *Candida* polysaccharides have been shown to generate T-suppressor cells (35). In addition, with *C. albicans*, antigens that mediate immunosuppressive responses have been identified. For instance, a glycoprotein extracted with ethylene-diamine suppresses transformation of murine splenic lymphocytes to a range of mitogens, and cell-wall mannan can elicit a similar response that is concentration-dependent (36). Once again, as with dermatophytosis, oligosaccharides can be shown to affect blastogenesis in this way (37). Antigen-mediated regulatory mechanisms seen with dermatophytes are therefore likely to be shared by other human fungal pathogens. Similar work with *Pityrosporum* yeasts has not been carried out as yet.

REFERENCES

1. Tagami H, Kudoh K, Takematsu H. Inflammation and immunity in dermatophytosis. Dermatologica 1989;179(suppl 1):1–8.
2. Sohnle PG. Dermatophytosis. In: Cox RA, ed: Immunology of the Fungal Diseases. New York: CRC Press, 1989:1–27.
3. Hall FR. Ringworm contract from cattle in western New York State. Arch Dermatol 1962;94:35–37.
4. Hay RJ. Chronic dermatophyte infections: I. Clinical and mycological features. Br J Dermatol 1982;106:1–9.
5. Rasmussen JE, Ahmed AR. Trichophytin reactions in children with tinea capitis. Arch Dermatol 1978;114:371–372.
6. Hay RJ. tinea imbricata. In: Current Topics in Medical Mycology. New York: Springer-Verlag, 1987;2:55–72.
7. Hope YM, Clayton YM, Hay RJ, et al: Foot infection in coal miners: A reassessment. Br J Dermatol 1985;112:405–413.
8. Zurita J, Hay RJ. The adherence of dermatophyte microcondidia and arthroconidia to human keratinocytes in vitro. J Invest Dermatol 1987;89:529–534.
9. Aljabre SHM, Richardson MD, Scott EM, et al. Adherence of arthroconidia and germlings of anthropophilic and zoophilic varieties of Trichophyton mentagrophytes to human corneocytes as an early event in the pathogenesis of dermatophytosis. Clin Exper Dermatol 1993;18:231–236.
10. Hay RJ, Calderon RA, Mackenzie CD. Experimental dermatophytosis in mice: Correlation between light and electron microscopic changes in primary, secondary, and chronic infection. Br J Exp Pathol 1988;69:703–716.
11. Graham JH, Barroso-Tobilia C. Dermatophytosis. In: Baker RD, ed: The Pathologic Anatomy of the Mycoses. Berlin: Springer-Verlag, 1971:211–235.

12. King RD, Khan HA, Foye JC. Transferrin, iron and dermatophytes: 1. Serum dermatophyte inhibitory component definitely identified as unsaturated transferrin. J Lab Clin Med 1975;86:204–212.
13. Davies RR, Zaini F. Drugs affecting Trichophyton rubrum induced neutrophil chemotaxis in vitro. Clin Exper Dermatol 1988;13:228–231.
14. Green F, Lee KW, Balish E. Chronic T. mentagrophytes dermatophytosis of guinea pig skin grafts on nude mice. J Invest Dermatol 1982;79:125–131.
15. Calderon RA, Hay RJ. Fungicidal activity of human neutrophils and monocytes in dermatophyte fungi, Trichophyton quinckeanum and Trichophyton rubrum. Immunology 1984;61:289–296.
16. Calderon RA, Shennan GI. Susceptibility of Trichophyton quinckeanum and T. rubrum. Immunology 1987;61:283–288.
17. Calderon RA, Hay RJ. Cell-mediated immunity in experimental murine dermatophytosis: I. T-suppressor activity elicited in dermatophyte infections caused by T. quinckeanum. Immunology 1984;53:457–464.
18. Calderon RA, Hay RJ. Cell-mediated immunity in experimental murine dermatophytosis: II. Aoptive transfer of immunity to dermatophyte infections. Immunology 1984;53:465–472.
19. Jones HE, Reinhardt JH, Rinaldi MG. Acquired immunity to dermatophytosis. Arch Dermatol 1974;109:840–848.
20. Jones HE, Reinhardt JH, Rinaldi MG. Model dermatophytosis in naturally infected subjects. Arch Dermatol 1974;110:369–374.
21. Elmros T, Liden S. Hereditary palmoplantar keratoderma: Incidence of dermatophyte infections and the results of topical treatment with retinoic acid. Acta Dermatol 1983;63:254–257.
22. Jones HE, Reinhardt JH, Rinaldi MG. A clinical, mycological and immunological survey of dermatophytosis. Arch Dermatol 1973;108:61–68.
23. Kaaman T, von Stedingk LV, von Stedingk M. ELISA-determined serological reactivity against purified trichophytin in dermatophytosis. Acta Derm Venereol 1981;61:313–317.
24. Wang SR, Zweiman B. Histamine suppression of human lymphocyte response to mitogens. Cell Immunol 1978;36:28–31.
25. Torssander J, Karlsson A, Morfeldt-Mason L. Dermatophytosis and HIV infection—Study in homosexual men. Acta Derm Venereol 1988;68:53–59.
26. Hay RJ, Shennan GI. Chronic dermatophyte infections: II. Antibody and cell-mediated immune responses. Br J Dermatol 1982;106:191–198.
27. Blake JS, Dahl MV, Herron MJ, Nelson RD. An immunoinhibitory cell wall glycoprotein (mannan) from Trichophyton rubrum. J Invest Dermatol 1991; 96:657–661.
28. McGregor JM, Hamilton AJ, Hay RJ. Possible mechanisms of immune modulation in chronic dermatophytoses: An in vitro study. Br J Dermatol 1992; 127:233–238.
29. Calderon RA, Hay RJ, Shennan GI. Circulating antigens and antibodies to phosphorylcholine-like epitopes. J Gen Microbiol 1987;133:2699–2705.
30. Mayou SC, Calderon RA, Goodfellow A, Hay RJ. Deep (subcutaneous) der-

matophyte infection presenting with unilateral lymphoedema. Clin Exper Dermatol 1987;12:355–358.

31. Allen DE, Snyderman R, Meadows L. Generalized Microsporum audouinii infection and depressed cellular immunity associated with a missing plasma factor required for lymphocyte blastogenesis. Am J Med 1977;63:991–1000.
32. Brasch J, Sterry W. Immunophenotypical characterization of inflammatory cellular infiltrates in tinea. Acta Derm Venereol 1992;72:345–347.
33. Schectman RC, Allen MH, McGregor JM, Hay RJ. Skin inflammation in chronic dermatophyte infections caused by Trichophyton rubrum—Lack of epidermal expression of ICAM-1. J Med Vet Mycol 1993;31:459–462.
34. Valdimarsson H, Higgs JM, Wells RS, et al. Immune abnormalities associated with chronic mucocutaneous candidiasis. Cell Immunol 1973;6:348–361.
35. Piccolella E, Lombardi G, Morelli R. Generation of suppressor cells in vitro by Candida albicans. J Immunol 1981;126:2151–2155.
36. Carrow EW, Domer JE. Immunoregulation in experimental murine candidiasis-specific suppression induced by Candida albicans cell wall gluycoprotein. Infect Immun 1985;49:172–181.
37. Nelson RD, Shibata N, Podzorski RP, Herron MJ. Candida mannan: Chemistry, suppression of cell-mediated immunity and possible mechanisms of action. Clin Microbiol Rev 1991;4:1–19.

12

Immune and Chemical Responses to Paracoccidioidomycosis

GIOCONDA SAN-BLAS and FELIPE SAN-BLAS
Centro de Microbiología y Biología Celular
Instituto Venezolano de Investigaciones Científicas (IVIC)
Caracas, Venezuela

I. INTRODUCTION

Paracoccidioidomycosis (PCM) is the most frequent systemic mycosis in Latin America, where it is geographically confined. Humans are apparently the only hosts susceptible to natural infection by its etiological agent, *Paracoccidioides brasiliensis* (1). The fungus propagates as a yeast (Y) at body temperature and as mycelium (M) at lower temperatures (Fig. 1) (2). It usually reaches the human host via the respiratory route, giving rise to the different clinical forms of PCM, i.e., the acute or subacute form (juvenile type) and the chronic form (adult type) (1). Active disease is traced mainly to male adults, while infection (measured as a positive skin reaction to paracoccidioidin) is equally prevalent in both sexes in endemic areas, with a much higher frequency than active disease (3). Cases of PCM in patients with acquired immunodeficiency syndrome (AIDS) have been reported (4). In endemic countries, diagnostic evaluation for PCM should be done in AIDS patients with fungal invasion.

To establish the true prevalence of PCM (the disease as well as the infection), clinical diagnosis and serological tests help greatly in establishing an unequivocal diagnosis. The former requires the demonstration of characteristic multiple budding yeast cells in biological fluids or tissue sections; the latter requires the existence of specific antigens for reliable

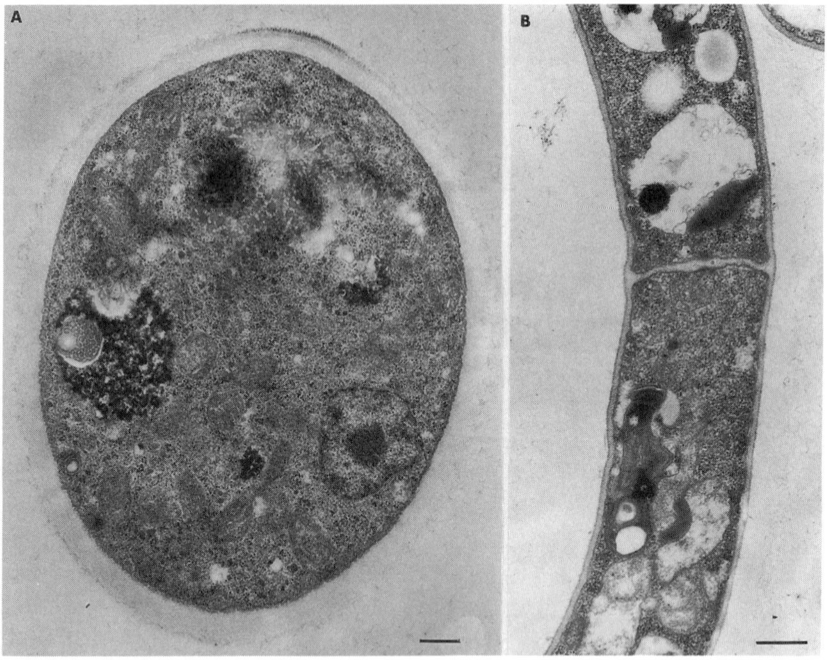

Figure 1 Electron microscopy of *P. brasiliensis*: (A) Y phase; (B) M phase. Bar: 50 nm.

results. As for treatment, several drugs have been used with variable success in PCM patients, and alternatives are discussed below.

II. IMMUNOLOGICAL ASPECTS OF PARACOCCIDIOIDOMYCOSIS

A. Serodiagnosis

According to their origin, *P. brasiliensis* antigens have been classified as (a) exocellular (metabolic) antigens; (b) intracellular (somatic or cytoplasmic) antigens; and (c) cell wall antigens (5). The latter are mainly composed of galactomannan, not only in *P. brasiliensis* but also in other pathogenic fungi (6). They are immunologically related; therefore they are of limited usefulness for skin and serological testing and have not been studied further.

1. Exocellular Antigens

The only serological test of high specificity that can currently be used alone for the diagnosis of PCM is the immunodiffusion test (7). This is so because of the isolation of a specific glycoprotein antigen called gp43 (43 kDa molecular weight) from concentrated dialysed supernatant fluids of yeast cultures (8). It is a relatively heat-stable glycoprotein (Fig. 2) with proteinase activity (caseinolytic and collagenolytic) (9).

Treatment of gp43 with endo-β-*N*-acetyl-glucosaminidase H (endo H; EC group 3.2.2) produces a nonglycosylated protein of 38 kDa molecular weight (EH38) (Fig. 2), for which it is presumed that most of the carbohydrate chains are *N*-linked to the peptide core, probably conforming a glycoprotein belonging to the high-mannose type. The presence of β-galactopyranosyl residues as non-reducing end units is suggested by binding to the peanut lectin but not to the *Griffonia simplicifolia* lectin, which recognizes the α-anomeric form of galactose. The β-galactopyranosyl residues might be partly located in *O*-linked chains, which are not susceptible to Endo H or *N*-glycanase actions, since EH38 reacts, though very weakly, with concanavalin A and peanut agglutinin (10). *O*-Linked chains must be minor structures since β-elimination does not produce a molecule smaller than 38 kDa (10) (Fig. 2). *N*-Deglycosylation does not prevent secretion of gp43, since treatment with tunicamycin makes *P. brasiliensis*

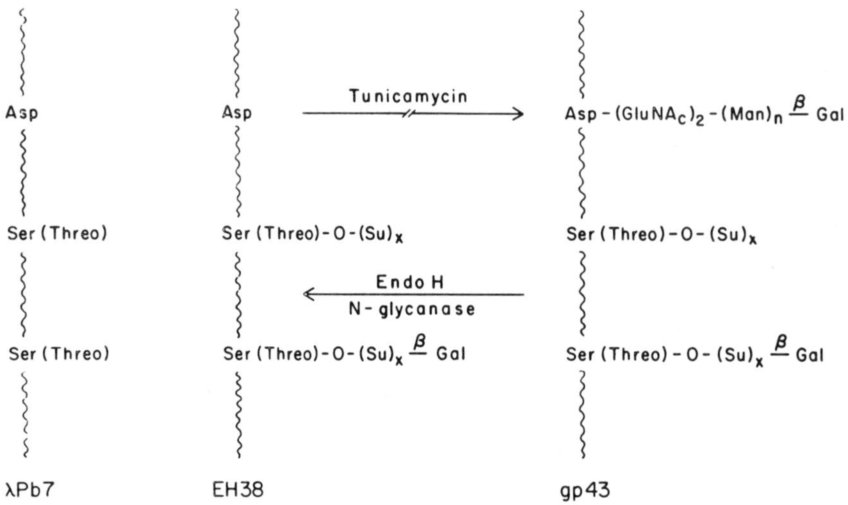

Figure 2 Structure of *P. brasiliensis*–specific antigen gp43, deduced from results in Refs. 10–12. Asparagine (Asp), serine (Ser) and threonine (Threo) are amino acids belonging to the peptide chain of the molecule. Abbreviations: GluNAc = *N*-acetyl glucosamine; Man = mannose; Gal = galactose; β = linkage configuration; Su = undetermined sugar; $\times$ <5 sugar residues; n = 25–30 sugar residues.

excrete a 38-kDa protein identical to EH38 (10). Moreover, clone λPb7 (isolated after the construction of *P. brasiliensis* genomic libraries in bacteriophage λgt11) expressed a recombinant polypeptide specifically recognized by sera from patients with PCM and which immunoprecipitated the gp43 antigen (11). Therefore, it follows that peptide epitopes and not carbohydrate moieties are responsible for the highly specific reactions of gp43 (11,12). Puccia and Travassos (12) concluded that gp43 is highly specific for serodiagnosis of PCM if immunodiffusion or immunoprecipitation is used as the technique of choice, since reaction goes through the specific peptide epitope. But in using ELISA, cross-reactivity is observed with other systemic mycoses through the carbohydrate epitopes of the molecule (12). This lack of specificity when the antigen is fixed on ELISA plates can be minimized only by using the deglycosylated form of the antigen (EH38) or by adding galactose to the reaction system. The different behavior of gp43 according to the test can be interpreted by suggesting that gp43 is presented in different conformations when bound to plastic substrates or in solution, since exposure of carbohydrate epitopes recognizable by antibodies from heterologous sera requires binding to the ELISA plates, while peptide epitopes reactive with the PCM sera are expressed in the gp43 molecule either in solution or immobilized on enzyme-linked immunosorbent assay (ELISA) plates or nitrocellulose paper.

Recently, the dot immunoblotting assay (12a) and a monoclonal antibodies assay (12b), both using gp43 as antigen, were developed. The first was tested with sera from patients with PCM, histoplasmosis, Jorge Lobo's disease, aspergillosis, candidiasis, and cryptococcosis and from healthy subjects. Native gp43 gave positive results with all sera from PCM patients and 31% of sera from those with Jorge Lobo's disease. Patients undergoing antimycotic treatment showed a decreased titer for antibodies in their sera. No false-positive reactions were obtained for assays in which gp43 was treated with sodium metaperiodate, showing a specificity and sensitivity of 100%. The method is recommended for seroepidemiological investigations, being inexpensive, rapid, and easily visualized (12a). The second assay (12b) relies on the production of four monoclonal antibodies (17C, 21A, 21F, and 32B) raised against gp43 and detection of specific human anti-gp43 immunoglobulin G in patients with PCM by a capture enzyme immunoassay. Anti-gp43 was detected at 500 pg/ml, recognizing two different epitopes. Specific antibodies in the sera from PCM patients were detected at dilutions as high as 1:819,200, greatly improving ELISA assays. The sensitivity for PCM was 100%, with 96.7% specificity.

Figueroa et al. (13) used a modification of an immunosuppressive technique directed against immunodominant epitopes to raise species-specific monoclonal antibodies against *P. brasiliensis*. Four of them (P4, 7E2, 7B9, and 2E2) showed no cross-reactivity with the other fungal antigens, monoclonal antibody P4 showing the strongest recognition of *P. brasiliensis* by means of a linear epitope in a glycoprotein of molecular weight 70–75 kDa.

Using Western blotting, it was shown that anti-*P. brasiliensis* IgG reacted with four exocellular major components of 70, 52, 43, and 20 kDa, obtained from strain B339 (14,15). The 43-kDa glycoprotein was the predominant IgG recognized by 100% of the patients' sera, while the 70-kDa glycoprotein was recognized by 96% of the sera, its titer decreasing in patients under treatment. Both glycoproteins were considered as markers for PCM (7).

2. *Cytoplasmic Antigens*

In other experiments using strain Linder 2511 of *P. brasiliensis* (14), intracellular (somatic) antigen was prepared. Of the several bands obtained in the Western blot, antigens of molecular weights 58, 57, 21, and 16 kDa were specific for *P. brasiliensis*. They were not identified in other fungal species such as *Aspergillus niger*, *A. nidulans*, *A. flavus*, *Candida albicans*, and *Blastomyces dermatitidis*, nor were they recognized with aspergillosis, candidiasis, or histoplasmosis sera. Instead, the 48- and 45-kDa antigens of *C. albicans*, *B. dermatitidis*, and *A. fumigatus* were recognized by PCM sera but not in *P. brasiliensis* extracts by sera from patients with other mycoses. Therefore they were considered specific for PCM. However, variability in the presence and intensity of these bands according to the strains was later reported (15).

B. Humoral Immunity

Patients with PCM have a hyperactive humoral immunity, with increased levels of serum IgG, IgE, and IgA (16). This increment in antibody production is partly related to the virulence of the fungal strain, inasmuch as intermediate and slightly virulent isolates induce weak IgG antibody production, whereas the most virulent isolates induce stronger specific humoral responses (17). Hypergammaglobulinemia is also induced by the alkali-insoluble fraction and β-glucan present in *P. brasiliensis* cell wall (18).

Ferreira-da-Cruz et al. (19) measured the serological responses of 66 patients by double immunodiffusion, using metabolic antigen from a pool of strains, they showed that (a) a decrease in antibody titers in all patients is associated with clinical improvement and (b) detection of antibodies to

P. brasiliensis by double immunodiffusion does not necessarily indicate active disease. Also, sheep red blood cells, treated with glutaraldehyde and sensitized with gp43, were used to detect antibodies to *P. brasiliensis* by passive hemagglutination (PHA) (19a). In PCM patients, PHA titers were higher than 1/800, while in healthy persons and patients with other mycoses, titers were below 1/100, suggesting that at a cutoff of 1/200, the specificity was 100%.

In another report (20), sera from 39 patients contained IgG-, IgA-, and IgM-specific antibodies to the 43-kDa exoantigen. By the fourth month of chemotherapy, there was a decay of IgG, IgA, and IgM antibody titers to this antigen, correlating with clinical improvement. Therefore, these authors suggest that changes in antibody titers may be useful indicators of the extent of active disease and valuable for determining the prognosis of the infection. Immunoblot tests in sera from patients with the acute and chronic forms of PCM (21) produced a reactivity profile of IgG, but not of IgM or IgA, similar for both types of patients, gp43 being recognized by all the sera.

Using an experimental murine model of PCM, Singer-Vermes et al. (21a) found that susceptible mice displayed high numbers of colony-forming units (CFU) together with high antibody titers and depressed delayed-type hypersensitivity (DTH) response after 16 weeks of infection, results that were reversed in resistant animals. These results mimicked those found in human PCM in multifocal and severe forms of the disease.

C. Cellular Immunity

Polymorphonuclear neutrophils (PMNs) and macrophages become involved in lesions within days after infection, but PMNs and resident macrophages do not appear to be fungicidal for *P. brasiliensis* in vitro (22) unless activated with γ-interferon or lymphokines (23). This fungicidal activity is blocked by inhibitors of protein synthesis such as cycloheximide, therefore suggesting a requirement for de novo protein synthesis in the activation of the microbicidal activity of macrophages.

The PMNs from PCM patients have a digestive deficiency against sonicated or autoclaved *P. brasiliensis* (24). Whether this is due to the possible release of cell-wall material during either of these treatments is not elaborated upon by the authors. This effect is not mediated by serum factors, since neither sera from PCM patients blocked digestive abilities of PMN from healthy individuals against *P. brasiliensis* nor did sera from healthy donors enhance the digestive capacities of PMNs from patients. The complement system plays an important role in the early phases of PMN accumulation in response to inflammatory stimuli which, in the case of *P. brasiliensis*, are induced by its insoluble cell-wall fraction (24a).

The defective cellular immune response of alveolar macrophages against *P. brasiliensis* might be the result of poor stimulation of the T-lymphocyte population, probably related to a decrease in the major histocompatibility complex class II (MHC-II) (24b). *P. brasiliensis* stimulated T-cell expansion, interleukin-2 production, and differentiation into cytotoxic T cells when *P. brasiliensis* lysates were confronted with cord blood T cells. Involved in this response were *P. brasiliensis* proteins of 100,000 and <1000 kDa (24c). T-cells may regulate B-cell activity in PCM through the γ/δ subset of the T-cell receptor (24d).

As for the immunological characteristics of patients, Mota et al. (25) reported abnormalities in lymphocyte mononuclear subpopulations in patients from Brazil, and Bava et al. (26), in Argentina, reported that half of the patients were lymphopenic, with a low number of $CD4^+$ T lymphocytes and low CD4/CD8 ratios. In them, in vitro production of interferon and tumor necrosis factor induced by interleukin-2 was significantly lower than in normal subjects, results that led the authors to suggest that the defect in blood lymphocyte populations and in the ability to produce regulatory cytokines was of a quantitative rather than a qualitative type.

T lymphocytes (mainly T-helper cells) in PCM are distributed either in a localized pattern related to epithelioid granulomas or in a diffuse arrangement, predominantly around the blood vessels (27). In patients, the great majority of cells at the site of skin tests with paracoccidioidin were T-cells (48%) with a T-helper phenotype (CD45 RO-positive cells), 25% were macrophages (CD68-positive cells), and very few were B lymphocytes (CD20-positive cells), consistent with a DHT pattern (27a). Natural killer cells are increased in number though decreased in cytotoxic activity in PCM patients, either chronic or acute, a result that suggests a defect both in target-cell recognition and binding (28).

Sensitivity to *P. brasiliensis* antigen (sonically treated culture of yeast cells) was transferred by immune dialysable leukocyte extracts (DLE) to normal recipient hamsters (29). Immune and nonimmune DLE maintained a positive cell-mediated immune response in hamsters infected with *P. brasiliensis* (30), animals that developed less extensive infection, with a significantly lower number of fungi in the lesions. These results look promising for immunotherapy.

III. CHEMICAL RESPONSES TO PARACOCCIDIOIDOMYCOSIS

The chemical armamentarium to treat PCM has been enriched slowly throughout the years. By 1940, sulfapyridine and other sulfamide derivatives were used in the treatment of PCM. The introduction of polyene antibiotics in the 1950s and of azoles in the 1970s and '80s have led to more successful treatments (31). Studies of the in vitro effectiveness of antifungal drugs against *P. brasiliensis* have correlated with in vivo efficacy, a goal not always achieved when testing antifungal susceptibilities in vitro.

A. Sulfamides and Derivatives

The sulfamides and derivatives are bacteriostatic drugs with limited use in mycology, almost exclusively in PCM. They must be administered for an indefinite period of time, not less than 2 years (31). Adequate responses are obtained in approximately 70% of the patients subjected to continuous and prolonged therapy, whereas relapses occur in about 10% of the cases, presumably because of fungal resistance acquired during the course of inadequate treatment or by infection with a sulfonamide-resistant strain (32). Even with all these limitations, sulfas are still drugs of choice, the reasons being mainly good tolerance, good gastrointestinal absorption, low toxicity, and particularly, low cost for patients who come almost exclusively from the impoverished rural areas of Latin America.

Traditional sulfamide treatment of PCM seems to have been surpassed in its therapeutic success by TMP/SMX (a fixed combination of trimethoprim and sulfamethoxazole), used because of the synergistic effect of both drugs against *P. brasiliensis*. Treatment of chronic PCM in 22 male patients (33) consisted in one tablet of cotrimazine (820 mg sulfadiazine + 180 mg trimethoprim per tablet) orally every 12 hr for 6 months, followed by a maintenance treatment of 500 mg sulfadoxine twice a week. The only failure occurred in a patient with serum sulfadiazine levels below 40 μg/ml; therefore the authors recommend maintenance of serum sulfadiazine above this level.

In vitro susceptibility testing of *P. brasiliensis* to sulfonamides was checked on 60 clinical isolates of the fungus. At a concentration of 50 μg/ml, 51.6% of the isolates were inhibited, while 6–8% of the strains grew abundantly in the presence of high levels of sulfonamides (200 μg/ml). Because the majority of the isolates were obtained before therapy, the authors suggested that de novo resistance existed in a small number of isolates. Furthermore, acquired resistance also was shown in the difference in susceptibility of the original and the relapse isolates obtained from one patient (32).

Sulfonamide derivatives and trimethoprim have mechanisms of action involving the metabolism of folic acid, the former by competitive inhibition of *p*-amino benzoic acid incorporation into the folic acid molecule, and the latter by blocking the conversion of dihydrofolic acid to its tetrahydro- structure by inhibition of the enzyme dihydrofolate reductase. Inhibitors of folic acid synthesis are then bacteriostatic because bacteria synthesize their own folic acid, which is required as an essential cofactor in their metabolism. Cells of higher organisms are not able to synthesize it and must obtain it from outside, this being the reason for the selective action of sulfonamides and trimethoprim on bacteria. Their action on *P. brasiliensis* has not been well documented, although their mechanisms may be the same as those described for bacteria.

B. Membrane-Disturbing Antibiotics

1. Physical Disturbance of the Membrane (Polyene Antibiotics)

Of the polyene antibiotics, amphotericin B has been extensively used in the treatment of PCM since 1958, being administered exclusively by the parenteral route in doses of 0.5 to 1 mg/kg body weight to a maximum of 50 mg for the adult and 25 mg for children, applied three to four times a week for 3 to 4 months and rarely for longer periods (28). However, the drug has significant nephrotoxicity, for which patients must be monitored continuously in order to suspend treatment when abnormal values of creatinine and blood urea are detected (31).

In vitro susceptibility of *P. brasiliensis* to amphotericin B was studied with three isolates from different sources (34). All of them were similarly susceptible to the drug (0.05 to 0.18 μg/ml). A synergistic effect was observed when amphotericin B was tested in conjunction with ketoconazole, whereas an antagonism was detected between it and rifampin.

Polyenes form complexes with ergosterol in the fungal plasma membrane, leading to the formation of pores from which K^+ leakage occurs, probably accompanied by lipid peroxidation and alteration in the activity of fungal plasma membrane ATPases (35).

2. Disturbance on Ergosterol Synthesis of the Membrane (Azoles)

One of the first azoles launched as a therapeutic agent against mycoses was miconazole. *P. brasiliensis* is very sensitive to it and, in fact, PCM is the only systemic mycosis that can be treated with oral miconazole (36). Ketoconazole has also been successfully used in the treatment of PCM, even with patients who had previously failed to respond to other drugs. In a multicenter study, 75 patients were treated by six investigators with ketoconazole (200 mg) given once or twice daily for a median treatment period of 10 weeks (range of 3 to 55 weeks). Of these 75 patients, 79% were judged to be in remission, 16% were markedly improved, 4% were moderately improved, and a single patient was unchanged after treatment (36). Among 14 patients followed up after achieving remission, relapses were observed in 2 patients in the first month after therapy terminated and in 1 patient in the third month. (36). Itraconazole is more active and less toxic than ketoconazole (37). It can be administered in lower doses than ketoconazole (19 g versus 47 g total dose) with a shorter duration of therapy (6 months versus 8 months), showing no interference with liver function or with bone marrow integrity (37).

In vitro studies (38) indicate that the Y phase of *P. brasiliensis* is more sensitive than the M phase to azoles in the following sequence: saperconazole > itraconazole > ketoconazole, with minimal inhibitory concentrations (MIC) and minimal fungicidal concentrations (MFC) fluctuating from 10^{-10} to 10^{-8}M. The M phase was more resistant than the Y phase to all drugs tested, MIC and MFC values indicating the same sequence of susceptibility, with inhibitory ranges from 10^{-10}M with saperconazole to 10^{-7}M with ketoconazole. This in vitro susceptibility of *P. brasiliensis* toward azoles is 10^2 to 10^3 times higher than the corresponding susceptibilities of *C. albicans* and *Aspergillus* spp. (39,40).

With regards to ultrastructure, azoles induce primary changes in most fungal species, *P. brasiliensis* among them, at the level of the cell wall and intracellular vacuoles. The Y phase of *P. brasiliensis*, in contact with azoles (Fig. 3B–H) at concentrations ranging from 10^{-10} to 10^{-8}M, produces vesicles in the periplasmic space that are particularly detached when saperconazole is used (Fig. 3B–D). As a general feature, the cell wall looks thicker in azole-treated Y cells (38).

Azole-treated mycelia at concentrations of 10^{-9} to 10^{-7}M are seen as deformed hyphae with vesicles in the periplasmic space. Contrary to the observations in the Y phase, ketoconazole instead of saperconazole induces a detachment of vesicles in the periplasmic space of the hyphae and the retraction of the cytoplasm (38).

As for their mode of action, the *N*-substituted azoles interfere with the cytochrome P450–dependent 14α-demethylation of lanosterol, a key step in the biosynthesis of ergosterol, the main sterol in most yeasts and fungi, which is an irreplaceable requisite for cell proliferation and an indispensable component of cellular membranes. Therefore, the azole-induced ergosterol depletion and the concomitant accumulation of membrane-disturbing 14α-methylsterols may be at the origin of their antifungal properties (41).

3. *Disturbance in Phospholipid Composition of the Membrane (Ajoene)*

Garlic (*Allium sativum*) extracts and allicin (one of its components) have been used as inhibitors of fungal growth, particularly of *C. albicans*, where it acts either by affecting lipid metabolism, inhibiting acetyl-CoA synthase, or inactivating essential thiols (42–44). Ajoene [(E,Z)-4,5,9-trithiadodeca-1,6,11-triene 9-oxide], a chemical derivative of allicin, has been introduced as an inhibitor of platelet aggregation, probably through an effect on the

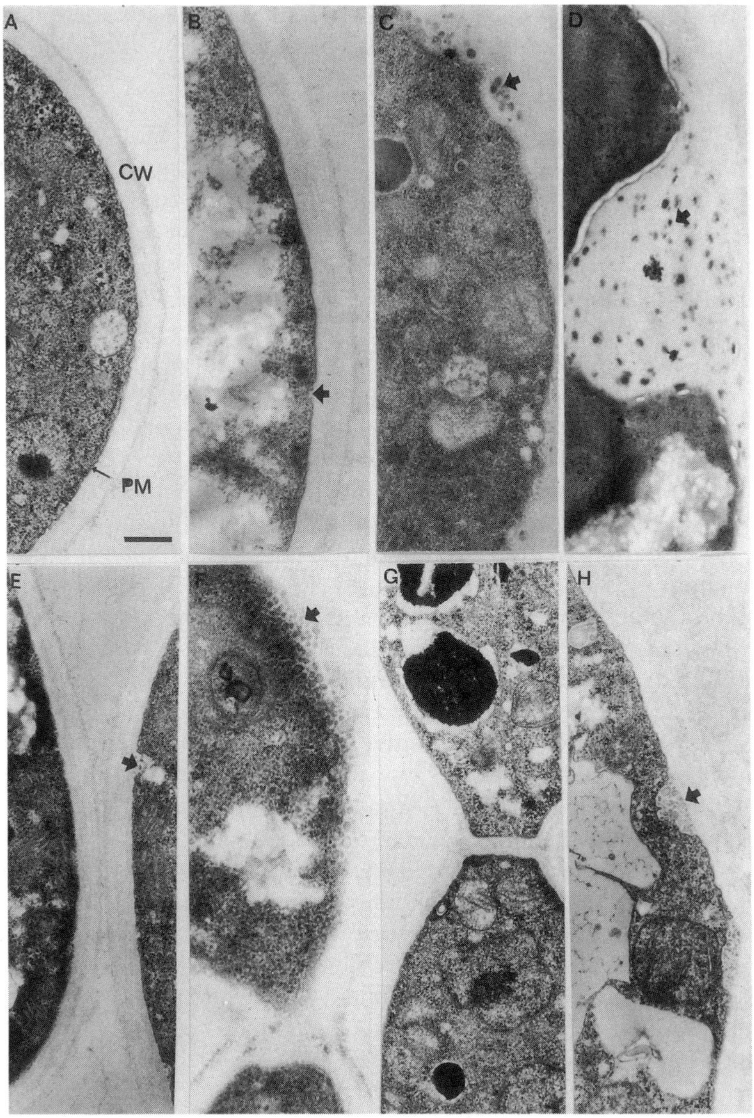

Figure 3 Effect of azoles on *P. brasiliensis* Y phase. Thin sections: (A) control; (B) saperconazole 10^{-10}M; (C) saperconazole 10^{-9}M; (D) saperconazole 10^{-8}M; (E) itraconazole 10^{-9}M; (F) itraconazole 10^{-8}M; (G) ketoconazole 10^{-9}M; (H) ketoconazole 10^{-8}M. Arrows indicate sites of perturbation. Abbreviations: CW = cell wall; PM = plasma membrane. Bar = 600 nm. (From Ref. 38.)

plasma membrane internal viscosity (45). Its action as a possible antifungal antibiotic was first reported in in vitro studies with *A. niger* and *C. albicans* by Yoshida et al. (46), who suggested that ajoene blocked some steps in cell wall synthesis. In vitro, the growth of *P. brasiliensis* was inhibited by ajoene, the Y phase being more sensitive than the M phase, with 90% inhibition of growth at ajoene concentrations of 50 and 100 μM for the Y and M phases, respectively. Electron microscopic evidence suggested a primary interference with the cytoplasmic membrane (47). Cysteine and dithiothreitol, protectors of free sulfhydryl groups, were able to cancel out the inhibitory effect produced by ajoene on the growth of the Y phase of *P. brasiliensis* but not on the M phase. With respect to the dimorphic process, ajoene blocked M-to-Y transformation indefinitely, but not the reverse (48). In recent experiments on the lipid composition of *P. brasiliensis* (Y and M phases) grown with or without ajoene (San-Blas et al., submitted for publication), no significant differences were observed in the phospholipid species present in both morphological phases. However, ajoene altered the lipid composition of this fungus. Phosphatidyl-choline was reduced from 35% to 18% in both phases, while phosphatidyl-ethanolamine increased from 17% to 36% (Y phase) or 46% (M phase), suggesting inhibition of phosphatidyl-choline synthesis. Ajoene also induced the transformation of squalene (40% in the Y phase and 70% in the M phase, reduced to 5–6% with ajoene) to ergosterol and ergosta-5,22 dien-3-β-ol (near 70% in the presence of ajoene). The damage caused by ajoene to the fungal membrane after long-term exposure to the drug and the concomitant change in the head-group composition of *P. brasiliensis* phospholipids is reflected in a very unstable lipid bilayer built with predominance of phosphatidyl-ethanolamine and acidic phospholipids, and to the destabilization of the cellular membrane, as verified by the ultrastructural results (47). The large reduction in the squalene content of treated Y and M cultures with a concomitant increase in the sterol content indicate an increase in the activity of the sterol biosynthetic pathway, probably as a consequence of the altered phospholipid composition. In conclusion, the antiproliferative effects of ajoene in *P. brasiliensis* are associated with a marked reduction in the content of phosphatidyl-choline, linked to an increase in the content of its precursor, phosphatidyl-ethanolamine, a fact that can lead to important alterations in the stability of the cell membranes and the activity of enzymes associated with it. This biochemical effect is remarkably similar to that reported previously for the protozoan *Trypanosoma cruzi* (47a), suggesting that it could be the common antiproliferative mechanism of ajoene, an antiplatelet compound, against lower eukaryotes.

C. Cell-Wall Inhibitors

Because the fungal cell wall is composed mainly of polysaccharides not present in higher eucariotes (i.e., glucan, chitin), inhibitors of the synthesis of these components may be considered as potential antifungal antibiotics of high selectivity.

In *P. brasiliensis*, whose cell wall contains glucan (in the α-configuration in the Y phase and β-configuration in the M phase) (48,49), the effects of papulacandin B (51) and cilofungin (52), both inhibitors of β-glucan synthesis, were tested in vitro. The former did not affect Y morphology or growth but inhibited M growth and Y-to-M transformation, while the latter was not as efficient in inhibiting the growth of *P. brasiliensis* as it was with some *Candida* species. In both cases, it might be assumed that the presence of α-glucan in the Y cell wall of *P. brasiliensis* instead of β-glucan is the reason for the resistance of this fungus to the action of both antibiotics.

IV. FINAL REMARKS

Knowledge about *P. brasiliensis* and PCM is growing steadily. The isolation of highly specific antigens provides better diagnostic tools and follow-up treatment, while the incorporation of more effective drugs in clinical practice and the exploration of alternative inhibitory pathways in research laboratories will bring new hope for the treatment of a mycotic disease that is difficult to eradicate.

REFERENCES

1. Franco M. Host-parasite relationships in paracoccidioidomycosis. J Med Vet Mycol 1987;25:5–18.
2. Restrepo A. The ecology of Paracoccidioides brasiliensis: A puzzle still unsolved. Sabouraudia 1985;23:323–334.
3. Restrepo A. Immune responses to Paracoccidioides brasiliensis in human and animal hosts. In: McGinnis M, ed. Current Topics in Medical Mycology. Vol 2. New York: Springer-Verlag, 1988:239–277.
4. Goldani LZ, Coehlo IC, Machado AA, Martinez R. Paracoccidioidomycosis and AIDS (letter). Scand J Infect Dis 1991;23:393.
5. San-Blas G, San-Blas F. Antigenic structure of Paracoccidioides brasiliensis. In: Kurstak E, ed. Immunology of Fungal Diseases. New York: Marcel Dekker, 1989:171–192.
6. Azuma I, Kanetsuna F, Tanaka Y, et al. Chemical and immunological properties of galactomannans obtained from Histoplasma duboisii, Histoplasma

capsulatum, Paracoccidioides brasiliensis, and Blastomyces dermatitidis. Mycopathol Mycol Appl 1974;54:111–125.
7. Camargo ZP, Unterkircher C, Travassos LR. Identification of antigenic polypeptides of Paracoccidioides brasiliensis by immunoblotting. J Med Vet Mycol 1989;27:407–412.
8. Puccia R, Takaoka DT, Travassos LR. Purification of the 43 kDa glycoprotein from exocellular components excreted by Paracoccidioides brasiliensis in liquid culture (TOM medium). J Med Vet Mycol 1991;29:57–60.
9. Mendes-Giannini MJ, Moraes RA, Ricci TA. Proteolytic activity of the 43,000 molecular weight antigen secreted by Paracoccidioides brasiliensis. Rev Inst Med Trop Sao Paulo 1990;32:384–385.
10. Puccia R, Travassos LR. The 43 kDa glycoprotein from the human pathogen Paracoccidioides brasiliensis and its deglycosylated form: Excretion and susceptibility to proteolysis. Arch Biochem Biophys 1991;289:298–302.
11. Taba MRM, Da Silveira JF, Travassos LR, Schenkman S. Expression in Escherichia coli of a gene coding for epitopes of a diagnostic antigen of Paracoccidioides brasiliensis. Exp Mycol 1989;13:223–230.
12. Puccia R, Travassos LR. 43-kilodalton glycoprotein from Paracoccidioides brasiliensis: Immunological reactions with sera from patients with paracoccidioidomycosis, histoplasmosis, and Jorge Lobo's disease. J Clin Microbiol 1991;29:1610–1615.
12a. Taborda CP, Camargo ZP. Diagnosis of paracoccidioidomycosis by dot immunoblotting assay for antibody detection using the purified and specific antigen gp43. J Clin Microbiol 1994;32:554–556.
12b. Camargo ZP, Gesztesi JL, Saraiva EC, et al. Monoclonal antibody capture enzyme immunoassay for detection of Paracoccidioides brasiliensis antibodies in paracoccidioidomycosis. J Clin Microbiol 1994;32:2377–2381.
13. Figueroa JI, Hamilton AJ, Bartholomew MA, et al. Preparation of species-specific murine monoclonal antibodies against the yeast phase of Paracoccidioides brasiliensis. J Clin Microbiol 1990;28:1766–1769.
14. Casotto M. Characterization of the cellular antigens of Paracoccidioides brasiliensis, yeast form. J Clin Microbiol 1990;28:1188–1193.
15. Casotto M, Paris S, Camargo ZP. Antigens of diagnostic value in three isolates of Paracoccidioides brasiliensis. J Med Vet Mycol 1991;29:243–253.
16. Arango M, Yarzábal L. T-cell dysfunction and hyperimmunoglobulinemia E in paracoccidioidomycosis. Mycopathologia 1982;79:115–123.
17. Singer-Vermes LM, Burger E, Franco MF, et al. Evaluation of the pathogenicity and immunogenicity of seven Paracoccidioides brasiliensis isolates in susceptible inbred mice. J Med Vet Mycol 1989;27:71–82.
18. de Oliveira SL, da Silva MF, Soares AM, Silva CL. Cell wall fractions from Paracoccidioides brasiliensis induce hypergammaglobulinemia. Mycopathologia 1993;121:1–5.
19. Ferreira-da-Cruz MF, Francesconi-do-Vale AC, et al. Study of antibodies in paracoccidioidomycosis: Follow-up of patients during and after treatment. J Med Vet Mycol 1990;28:151–157.

19a. Taborda CP, Camargo ZP. Diagnosis of paracoccidioidomycosis by passive haemagglutination assay of antibody using a purified and specific antigen-gp43. J Med Vet Mycol 1993;31:99–113.
20. Giannini MJ, Bueno JP, Shikanai-Yasuda MA, et al. Antibody response to the 43 kDa glycoprotein of Paracoccidioides brasiliensis as a marker for the evaluation of patients under treatment. Am J Trop Med Hyg 1990;43: 200–206.
21. Bhotta MH, Camargo ZP. Immunological response to cell-free antigens of Paracoccidioides brasiliensis: Relationships with clinical forms of paracoccidioidomycosis. J Clin Microbiol 1993;31:671–676.
21a. Singer-Vermes LM, Caldeira CB, Burger E, Calich LG. Experimental murine paracoccidioidomycosis: Relationship among the dissemination of the infection, humoral and cellular immune responses. Clin Exp Immunol 1993; 94:75–79.
22. Brummer E, Hanson LH, Stevens DA. Gamma-interferon activation of macrophages for killing of Paracoccidioides brasiliensis and evidence for nonoxidative mechanisms. Int J Immunopharmacol 1988;10:945–952.
23. Brummer E, Hanson LH, Stevens DA. Kinetics and requirements for activation of macrophages for fungicidal activity: Effect of protein synthesis inhibitors and immunosuppressants on activation and fungicidal mechanisms. Cell Immunol 1991;132:236–245.
24. Goihman-Yahr M, Rothenberg A, Bretaña A, et al. Digestion of killed Paracoccidioides brasiliensis by neutrophils. Mycopathologia 1989;106:53–58.
24a. Crott LS, Valim YM, Silva CL, Barbosa JE. The role of the complement system in the neutrophil functions stimulated in vitro by an alkali-insoluble cell wall fraction of Paracoccidioides brasiliensis. J Med Vet Mycol 1993; 31:17–27.
24b. Bretaña A, Goihman-Yahr M, Tapia FJ, et al. Comparative ultrastructure and immunolabeling of MHC-II antigens of alveolar macrophages obtained from patients with paracoccidioidomycosis and other lung diseases. J Leuk Biol 1993;57:101–109.
24c. Munk ME, Kaufman SH. Human cord blood T-cell receptor alpha beta cell responses to protein antigens of Paracoccidioides brasiliensis yeast forms. Immunology 1995;84:98–104.
24d. Munk ME, Fazioli RA, Calich VL, Kaufman SH. Paracoccidioides brasiliensis–stimulated human gamma/delta T cells support antibody production by B cells. Infect Immun 63:1608–1610.
25. Mota NGS, Peracoli MTS, Mendes RP, et al. Mononuclear cell subsets in patients with different clinical forms of paracoccidioidomycosis. J Med Vet Mycol 1988;26:105–111.
26. Bava AJ, Mistchenko AS, Palacios MF, et al. Lymphocyte subpopulations and cytokine production in paracoccidioidomycosis patients. Microbiol Immunol 1991;35:167–174.
27. Moscardi-Bacchi M, Soares A, Mendes R, et al. In situ localization of T lymphocyte subsets in human paracoccidioidomycosis. J Med Vet Mycol 1989;27:149–158.

27a. Marques M, Moscardi-Bacchi M, Marques S, Franco M. Immunohistochemical characterization of mononuclear cells in delayed hypersensitivity reactions to Paracoccidioides brasiliensis (paracoccidioidin test). Mycopathologia 1993;124:7–11.
28. Peracoli MTS, Soares AMVC, Mendes RP, et al. Studies of natural killer cells in patients with paracoccidioidomycosis. J Med Vet Mycol 1991;29: 373–380.
29. Peracoli MT, Montenegro MR, Soares AM, Mota NG. Transfer of cell-mediated immunity to Paracoccidioides brasiliensis in hamsters with dialysable leukocyte extracts. J Med Vet Mycol 1990;28:35–46.
30. Peracoli MT, Rezkallah-Iwasso MT, Mota NG, Montenegro MR. Dialysable leukocyte extracts modify the course of experimental paracoccidioidomycosis in the Syrian hamster. Mycopathologia 1993;121:149–156.
31. Del Negro G. Tratamento, controle de cura, profilaxia. In: Del Negro G, Lacaz CS, Fiorillo AM, eds. Paracoccidioidomicose, Blastomicose Sul-Americana. Sao Paulo: Sarvier, 1982:271–283.
32. Restrepo A, Arango MD. In vitro susceptibility testing of Paracoccidioides brasiliensis sulfonamides. Antimicrob Ag Chemother 1980;18:190–194.
33. Barraviera B, Pereira PCM, Mendes RP, et al. Evaluation of acetylator phenotype, renal function and serum sulfadiazine levels in patients with paracoccidioidomycosis treated with cotrimazine (a combination of sulfadiazine and trimethoprim). Mycopathologia 1989;108:107–112.
34. Restrepo A, Bedoutand C, Tabares AM. In vitro susceptibility of Paracoccidioides brasiliensis yeast form to antifungal agents. Rev Inst Med Trop Sao Paulo 1984;26:322–328.
35. Köller W. Antifungal agents with target sites in sterol functions and biosynthesis. In: Koller W, ed. Target Sites of Fungicide Action. Boca Raton, FL: CRC Press, 1992:119–206.
36. Heel RC. Paracoccidioidomycosis. In: Levine HB, ed. Ketoconazole in the Management of Fungal Disease. New York: ADIS Press, 1982:119–125.
37. Van Cutsem J, Van Gerven F, Janssen PAJ. The in vitro and in vivo antifungal activity of itraconazole. In: Fromtling RA, ed. Recent Trends in the Discovery, Development and Evaluation of Antifungal Agents. Barcelona: Prous Science, 1987:5–20.
38. San-Blas G, Calcagno AM, San-Blas F. A preliminary study of in vitro antibiotic activity of saperconazole and other azoles on Paracoccidioides brasiliensis. J Med Vet Mycol 1993;31:169–174.
39. Odds, FC. Antifungal activity of saperconazole (R66 905) in vitro. J Antimicrob Chemother 1989;24:533–537.
40. Denning DW, Hanson LH, Stevens DA. In vitro activity of saperconazole (R66 905) compared with amphotericin B and itraconazole against Aspergillus species. Eur J Clin Microbiol Infect Dis 1990;9:693–697.
41. Vanden Bossche H. Mode of action of pyridine, purimidine and azole antifungals. In Berg D, Plempel M, eds. Sterol Biosynthesis Inhibitors. Chichester, England: Horwood, 1988:79–119.

42. Adetumbi M, Javor GT, Lau BHS. Allium sativum (garlic) inhibits lipid synthesis by Candida albicans. Antimicrob Ag Chemother 1986;30:499–501.
43. Barone FE, Tansey MR. Isolation, purification, identification, synthesis, and kinetics of activity of the anticandidal component of Allium sativum and a hypothesis for its mode of action. Mycologia 1977;69:793–825.
44. Ghannoum MA. Studies on the anticandidal mode of action of Allium sativum (garlic). J Gen Microbiol 1988;134:2917–2924.
45. Rendu F, Daveloose D, Debouzy JC, et al. Ajoene, the antiplatelet compound derived from garlic, specifically inhibits platelet release reaction by affecting the plasma membrane internal microviscosity. Biochem Pharmacol 1989;38:1321–1328.
46. Yoshida S, Kasuga S, Hayashi N, et al. Antifungal activity of ajoene derived from garlic. Appl Environm Microbiol 1987;53:615–617.
47. San-Blas G, San-Blas F, Gil F, et al. Inhibition of growth of the dimorphic fungus Paracoccidioides brasiliensis by ajoene. Antimicrob Ag Chemother 1989;33:1641–1644.
47a. Urbina JA, Marchan E, Lazardi K, et al. Inhibition of phosphatidylcholine biosynthesis and cell proliferation in Trypanosoma cruzi by ajoene, an antiplatelet compound isolated from garlic. Biochem Pharmacol 1993;45:2381–2387.
48. San-Blas G, Mariño L, San-Blas F, Apitz-Castro R. Effect of ajoene on dimorphism of Paracoccidioides brasiliensis. J Med Vet Mycol 1993;31:133–141.
49. Kanetsuna F, Carbonell LM, Azuma I, Yamamura Y. Biochemical studies on the thermal dimorphism of Paracoccidioides brasiliensis. J Bacteriol 1972;110:208–218.
50. San-Blas F, San-Blas G. Paracoccidioides brasiliensis. In Szaniszlo P, ed. Fungal Dimorphism. New York: Plenum Press, 1985:93–120.
51. Dávila T, San-Blas G, San-Blas F. Effect of papulacandin B on glucan synthesis in Paracoccidioides brasiliensis. J Med Vet Mycol 1986;24:193–202.
52. Hanson LH, Stevens DA. Evaluation of cilofungin, a lipopeptide antifungal agent, in vitro against fungi isolated from clinical specimens. Antimicrob Ag Chemother 1989;33:1391–1392.

13

Histoplasmosis Susceptibility in Humans

L. JOSEPH WHEAT
Indiana University
Indianapolis, Indiana

I. INTRODUCTION

Histoplasmosis is the most common systemic mycosis and a major cause of morbidity in patients who live in endemic areas. Diagnosis requires recognition of its clinical syndromes, a high index of suspicion, and knowledge of the accuracy and limitations of tests used for the diagnosis of fungal infections. Antifungal treatment is indicated in patients with disseminated or chronic pulmonary histoplasmosis and is highly effective. Itraconazole offers an effective alternative to amphotericin B for mild cases.

II. EPIDEMIOLOGY

Histoplasmosis is worldwide in distribution but more prevalent in certain parts of North and Latin America (Fig. 1) (1). *Histoplasma capsulatum* var. *capsulatum* is found in "microfoci," such as bird roosts, caves, chicken coops, and environmental sites enriched with bird and bat droppings (Table 1). While most outbreaks have been caused by disturbance of blackbird roosts, sites contaminated with seagull and bat guano also have been sources for exposure to *H. capsulatum*.

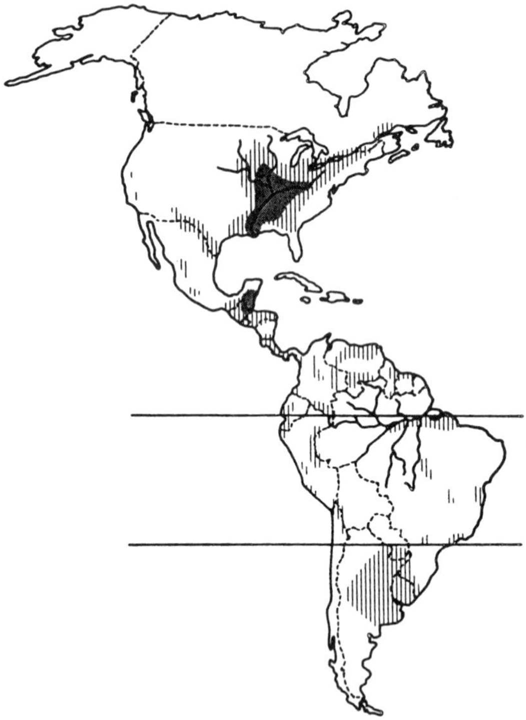

Figure 1 Endemic distribution of histoplasmosis in the Americas. The highest incidence is in the finely stippled areas of North and Central America. (From Ref. 1.)

Table 1 Microfoci and Activities That Result in Exposure to *Histoplasma capsulatum*

Sources	Activities
Old buildings	Construction/excavation
Farms	Wood gathering/cutting
Bird roosts	Camping
Wood piles	Spelunking
Caves	Gardening
Bat-inhabited structures	

III. PATHOGENESIS

Spores or mycelial fragments are inhaled and cause a primary infection in the lungs. Some 10 to 14 days later, cellular immunity develops in the lungs and mediastinal lymph nodes, followed by systemic immunity throughout the reticuloendothelial system. Immune thymus-derived lymphocytes activate macrophages to assume fungicidal properties (2,3). These defense mechanisms control the infection in immunocompetent individuals, explaining the subclinical or self-limited course characteristic of acute histoplasmosis. Progressive illnesses highlighted by hematogenous dissemination occur in persons with impaired cellular immunity (4).

IV. CLINICAL MANIFESTATIONS

A. Self-Limited Syndromes

The severity of infection depends on the level of exposure and underlying immunity of the host. Fewer than 5% of exposed individuals develop symptomatic self-limited disease after low-level exposure (Fig. 2) (5). Dissemination is characteristic in immunocompromised individuals (4,6). Most symptomatic cases (about 80%) present with a variety of self-limited manifestations. Following more intense exposure, patients often suffer

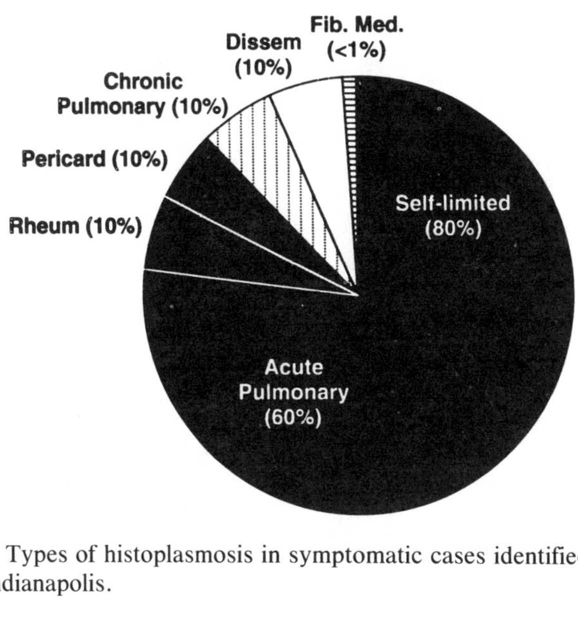

Figure 2 Types of histoplasmosis in symptomatic cases identified during outbreaks in Indianapolis.

respiratory insufficiency caused by diffuse reticulonodular or miliary pulmonary infiltrates (7,8).

About 10% of patients present with arthritis and erythema nodosum (9–11) or pericarditis (12,13). Neither is caused by infection of the involved tissues but by an immunological reaction to histoplasmosis.

B. Chronic Pulmonary Histoplasmosis

Patients with underlying lung disease often develop chronic pulmonary infection following exposure to *H. capsulatum* (14,15). Chest radiograms

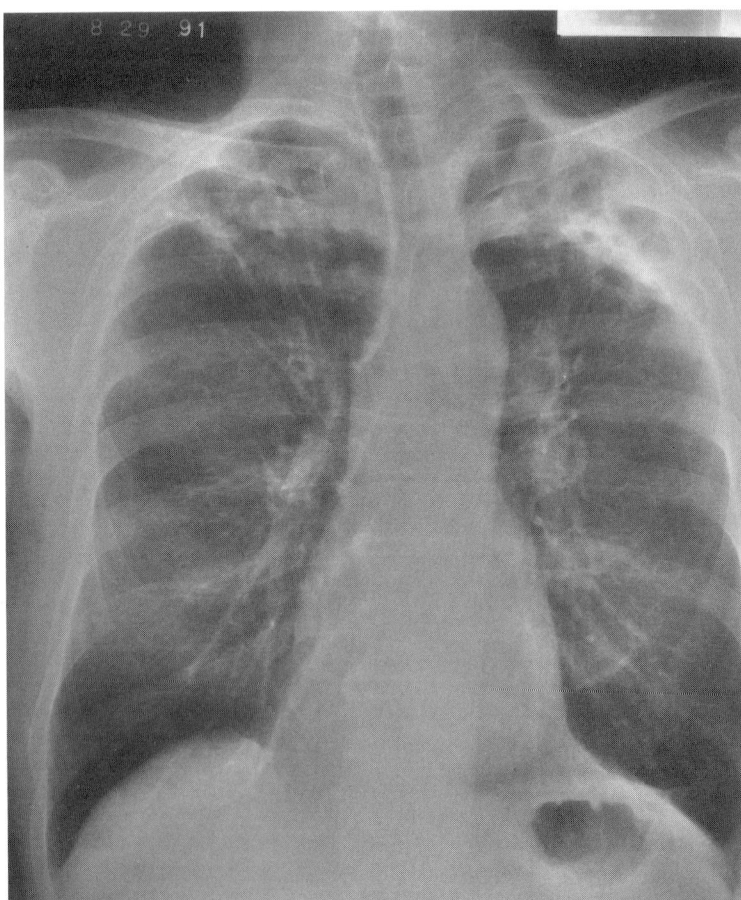

Figure 3 Chest radiograph showing fibrotic upper lobe infiltrates with pleural thickening and cavitation in a patient with chronic pulmonary histoplasmosis.

show fibrotic apical infiltrates, usually with cavitation (Fig. 3). Chronic pulmonary histoplasmosis is progressive in most patients (8,14,15).

C. Disseminated Histoplasmosis

Disseminated histoplasmosis is illustrated by systemic and progressive illness with clinical or laboratory evidence for extrapulmonary involvement (6,16,17). Severity varies with the degree of immune deficiency and extent of exposure. An acute, rapidly fatal course with diffuse reticuloendothelial involvement characterizes the infection in infants and others who are severely immunosuppressed, while a chronic course with focal organ distribution is more typical in nonimmunocompromised individuals (16).

Clinical findings of disseminated histoplasmosis are nonspecific (16,17), and the diagnosis is often unsuspected during life (17). Patients present with fever, fatigue, and weight loss, (Table 2) (8,16,17). Examination may reveal hepatomegaly, splenomegaly, or lymphadenopathy in one-third to two-thirds of cases and, less frequently, adrenal, central nervous system, skin or mucosal lesions, or chronic meningitis (10–20%). Chest radiographs, abnormal in 70% of cases, usually show diffuse interstitial or reticulonodular infiltrates (about 40%) (Fig. 4).

D. Mediastinal Fibrosis

Exuberant extranodal mediastinal fibrosis that invades adjacent structures is characteristic of this disorder (18,19). Obstructive complications are more common in fibrosing mediastinitis (about 80%) than in granulomatous mediastinitis (about 25%) (20).

Table 2 Clinical Findings in Disseminated Histoplasmosis

Common	Uncommon
Fever (95%)	Meningitis (15%)
Weight loss (95%)	Adrenal (12%)
Diffuse pneumonitis (50%)	Septicemia (10%)
Hepatosplenomegaly (25%)	Gastrointestinal (10%)
Lymphadenitis (20%)	Cerebritis (5%)
	Skin (5%)

Rare (<5%): Eye, pericardium, prostate, pancreas, omentum, pleura

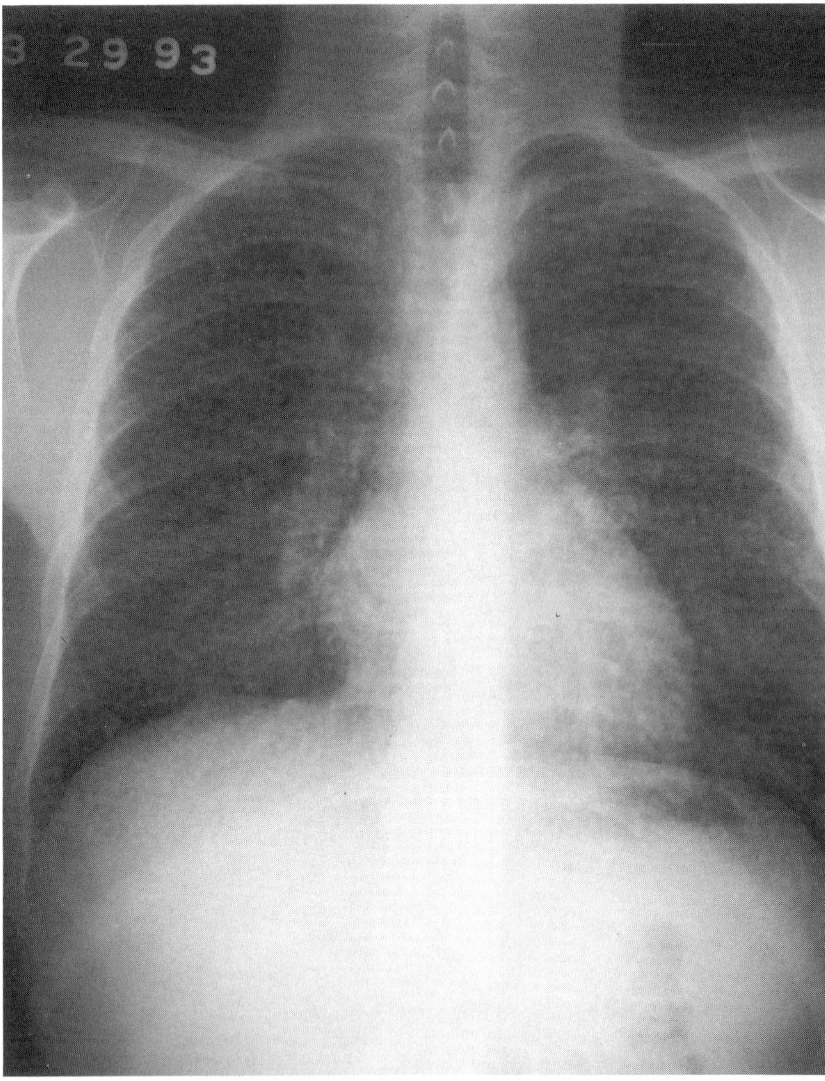

Figure 4 Chest radiograph showing the miliary reticulonodular pattern characteristic of heavy-inoculum acute pulmonary histoplasmosis or disseminated histoplasmosis in patients without heavy exposure.

V. DIAGNOSIS

A. Sensitivity of Tests for Fungal Diagnosis

Cultures, fungal stains, antigen detection, and serological tests for antibodies are useful for diagnosis of histoplasmosis (21,22). All are reasonably specific and can serve as the basis for diagnosis when combined with good clinical judgment. The sensitivities of these different tests vary with the type of histoplasmosis, providing a basis for their selection (Table 3).

B. Antigen Detection

Detection of a glycoprotein antigen in the blood or urine of infected patients offers a rapid approach to the diagnosis of more severe cases (22). With a sensitivity of over 90% in disseminated infection and at least 50% in extensive pulmonary histoplasmosis (Wheat, unpublished observation), this test is useful for diagnosing clinical forms of histoplasmosis, which require prompt recognition and treatment. Tests for antigen should be performed on urine and serum specimens in all patients with suspected disseminated histoplasmosis. Specimens should be sent to the Histoplasmosis Reference Laboratory (1-800-HISTO DG) in Indianapolis, Indiana; results are available within 1 or 2 days.

C. Description of Diagnostic Approach

A diagnostic approach can be formulated based on the relative sensitivity of the different tests in histoplasmosis.

1. Self-Limited Syndromes

In patients with suspected self-limited histoplasmosis, serological tests for antibodies should be performed in all cases. Tests for antigen and

Table 3 Sensitivity of Diagnostic Tests in Different Clinical Types of Histoplasmosis

Test	Disseminated	Chronic pulmonary	Self-limited
	←	Sensitivity %	→
Antigen	92	21	39
Culture	85	85	15
Stain	43	17	9
Serology	71	100	98

Source: From Ref.

bronchoalveolar lavage for fungal stain, culture, and antigen detection should be considered in patients with diffuse pulmonary infiltrates who are dyspneic or hypoxic, as antifungal therapy may be indicated. Tests for antigen may also be useful in patients who present within the first month of suspected exposure, when tests for antibodies may be negative.

2. *Chronic Pulmonary Histoplasmosis*

In chronic pulmonary histoplasmosis, serological tests for antibodies and fungal cultures of sputum should be performed in all cases. Bronchoalveolar lavage should be considered if sputum cannot be obtained or if sputum cultures are negative. If other causes for the pulmonary infiltrate—such as tuberculosis, other infectious or inflammatory processes, or cancer—are thought to be unlikely, positive serological tests for anti-*H. capsulatum* var. *capsulatum* antibodies would provide an acceptable basis for diagnosis and initiation of antifungal therapy.

3. *Disseminated Histoplasmosis*

In patients with suspected disseminated disease and in those with AIDS or who are otherwise immunocompromised, tests for antigen and fungal stains of lesions should be performed, as they allow for a rapid diagnosis. Serological tests for antibodies may provide a basis for performance of additional biopsies and assist in interpretation of positive tests for antigen in patients with negative cultures.

VI. TREATMENT

A. Self-Limited

Antifungal therapy is unnecessary in most patients with acute pulmonary histoplasmosis (Table 4). Patients typically recover spontaneously in a few weeks following mild exposure (23) but may remain symptomatic for months following heavier exposure (8). Therapy is reasonable in patients

Table 4 Summary of Treatment Indications in Histoplasmosis

Treatment indicated	Treatment not indicated
Disseminated	Rheumatologic
Chronic pulmonary	Pericarditis
Acute pulmonary with hypoxia	Fibrosing mediastinitis
Acute pulmonary > 1 month	Presumed ocular
	Histoplasmema

with moderately severe symptoms who have not improved after 2 or 3 weeks of observation.

Patients with extensive acute pulmonary histoplasmosis following intense exposure who are dyspneic and hypoxic respond to a 1- or 2-week course of amphotericin B and corticosteroids (7,24). Treatment might be changed to ketoconazole or itraconazole following clinical response to amphotericin B, for a total course of treatment of 6 to 12 weeks.

B. Chronic Pulmonary Histoplasmosis

Treatment is indicated in all patients with chronic pulmonary histoplasmosis. Although some patients may recover spontaneously (14,15), the illness is progressive, with further loss of pulmonary function in most patients, and death ensues in up to half (8,14,25–27). Treatment halts progression of the illness and halves mortality (27). Treatment with amphotericin B is effective in 59–100% of cases (25–28) (Table 5). Ketoconazole and itraconazole also are effective treatments for chronic pulmonary histoplasmosis, inducing responses in about 75–85% of cases (29,30).

Relapse occurs in at least 10% of patients treated with amphotericin B (25–27,31), itraconazole (30), or ketoconazole (Wheat, unpublished), supporting prolonged oral therapy (1 to 2 years) and careful follow-up. Therapy should be continued for 3 to 6 months after stabilization of radiographic findings and normalization of elevated erythrocyte sedimentation rate.

Table 5 Outcome of Treatment for Chronic Pulmonary Histoplasmosis

Treatment	No.	Response % (No)	Deaths % (No)	Relapse % (No)	Reference
Amphotericin B	89	59 (52)	16 (14)	10 (14)[a]	(27)
	32	100 (32)	0		(28)
	16	81 (13)	6 (1)	12.5 (2)	(26)
	56	96 (2)	0	9 (5)	(31)
	238	99 (236)		14.7 (35)	(25)
Itraconazole	20	80 (16)	5 (1)	15 (3)	(30)
Ketoconazole	23	74 (17)	0 (0)	4 (1)	(29)
	7	86 (6)			(34)

[a] Relapses were more common in patients treated with less than 25 mg/kg, 8/55 (14.5%) than in those receiving larger doses, 6/89 (6.7%).

C. Disseminated Histoplasmosis

Treatment is indicated in all patients with disseminated histoplasmosis. The mortality of untreated disseminated histoplasmosis is 80% (8), but it can be reduced to less than 25% with antifungal therapy (17,27,32,33). Several treatment regimens have proven to be effective for patients with disseminated histoplasmosis, inducing a response in at least two-thirds of cases (17,27,29,30,32–35) (Table 4) Itraconazole is effective treatment for patients with mild clinical manifestations of disseminated histoplasmosis. Amphotericin B induces a more rapid response than does itraconazole (35), supporting its selection for more severe cases. Fluconazole's role in histoplasmosis should be established soon.

Relapse occurs in 10–20% of patients treated with amphotericin B, particularly in those who received less than 35 mg/kg total doses (Table 5) (15–17,27,33). Presence of underlying immunosuppression also may increase the likelihood of relapse (Wheat, unpublished observations). Consistent with this hypothesis is the high relapse rate (near 80%) observed in patients with AIDS who have completed prolonged courses of amphotericin B (6).

D. Fibrosing Mediastinitis

Neither antifungal nor anti-inflammatory treatment ameliorates the outcome of this complication of histoplasmosis (18,19). Contrasted to the active inflammatory reaction characteristic of acute granulomatous mediastinitis, inflammation is not a feature of fibrosing mediastinitis. While organisms may be seen by fungal stain in fibrotic mediastinal tissues, rarely are they viable (18). Improvement has been reported following resection of the scar tissue, but operative mortality is high (about 25%) (36). The role of surgery for this complication has not been established (19).

VII. SPECIFIC TREATMENT RECOMMENDATIONS

A. Severe or Moderately Severe Disease

Amphotericin B, based on its fungicidal mode of action and rapid effect, is the treatment of choice for patients with moderately severe or severe clinical manifestations of disseminated histoplasmosis (Table 5). Amphotericin B is also preferred treatment for patients with severe acute pulmonary histoplasmosis. Adjunctive corticosteroid therapy is helpful in these patients. Severe manifestations rarely complicate chronic pulmonary histoplasmosis; thus amphotericin B therapy usually can be avoided.

Amphotericin B also would be a better choice for initial treatment in patients with malabsorption or who were receiving medications that impair absorption or accelerate metabolism of itraconazole or ketoconazole. These include H_2-receptor antagonists, rifampin and rifabutin, phenytoin, carbamazepine, and barbiturates.

Amphotericin B should be administered 50 mg daily or at a dose of 1 mg/kg in patients weighing less than 50 kg. Treatment may be changed to itraconazole or ketoconazole within 5 to 14 days, since improvement is rapid in most patients.

B. Mild Disseminated, Chronic Pulmonary, Acute Pulmonary, and Granulomatous Mediastinitis

Ketoconazole or itraconazole would be appropriate in patients with chronic pulmonary histoplasmosis or mild disseminated disease and in those with acute pulmonary histoplasmosis requiring therapy (Table 6). Ketoconazole, however, should not be used in patients who are immunosuppressed. Itraconazole is preferred in patients who are immunosuppressed, intolerant to ketoconazole, or who are receiving H_2-receptor antagonists or antacids.

Although treatment with oral antifungal agents is moderately expensive, ranging from $150 for ketoconazole to over $600 for itraconazole per month for doses of 400 mg daily, amphotericin B administered every other day at home under appropriate supervision costs up to $3000 monthly and is toxic and inconvenient.

Table 6 Outcome of Treatment for Disseminated Histoplasmosis

Treatment	No	Response % (No)	Deaths % (No)	Relapse % (No)	Reference
Amphotericin B	22	68(15)	23(5)	9(2)	27
	43	74(32)	16(7)	7(3)	17
	17	76(13)	23(4)		32
	24	91(22)	8(2)	20(5)	33
Itraconazole	10	100(10)	0(0)		30
Ketoconazole	31	56(17)[a]		10(3)	29
	10	70(7)	40(4)		34

[a] Only 6 from progression/relapse.

Itraconazole and ketoconazole are eliminated exclusively by hepatic metabolism, and their blood concentrations are markedly reduced by hepatic enzyme inducers. Rifampin and phenytoin reduce ketoconazole levels by up to 90% (37). Itraconazole may also be tried in patients who have failed therapy with ketoconazole, fluconazole, or amphotericin B, as cross-resistance has not been observed.

Ketoconazole and itraconazole dosage should be 200 mg three times daily for 3 days as a loading dose and then twice daily as a treatment dose. They should be given with food or an acidic beverage such as a cola. Considering the variable absorption, blood levels should be measured during the second week of therapy, 2 to 4 hr after a dose. Concentrations of at least 2 μg/ml should be regarded as therapeutic. Dosage may be reduced in patients with levels above 10 μg/ml.

Fluconazole can be used in patients with mild illnesses who cannot take or do not absorb itraconazole or ketoconazole, require treatment with interacting medications such as rifampin, or develop infection with other fungi that are resistant to itraconazole. However, more complete understanding of fluconazole's role in the treatment of histoplasmosis awaits final analysis of completed trials. Fluconazole dosage for disseminated histoplasmosis in patients with AIDS should be 800 mg daily, while lower doses may be adequate in other cases. Absorption does not require gastric acidity and is highly predictable, and drug interactions reducing fluconazole concentrations are rare. Thus, routine measurement of blood concentrations is unnecessary.

C. Duration of Ketoconazole, Itraconazole, or Fluconazole Therapy

The duration of therapy is unknown but probably should be at least 12 months for disseminated and probably longer for chronic pulmonary histoplasmosis. Shorter courses should be adequate in patients with acute pulmonary histoplasmosis or granulomatous mediastinitis. Treatment should be continued until all clinical and laboratory findings of histoplasmosis have resolved.

Erythrocyte sedimentation rate and *H. capsulatum* antigen levels should be normal before stopping therapy (Table 7).

D. Chronic Suppressive Maintenance Therapy

Suppressive treatment to prevent relapse is indicated in all patients with AIDS and in others who have relapsed after adequate courses of amphotericin B (about 35 mg/kg). Weekly or biweekly amphotericin B (50 to 100

Table 7 Recommendations for Treatment of Histoplasmosis

	Drug	Dose	Duration
Induction			
Mild	Itraconazole[a]	400 mg/d	3 months
Moderate or Severe	Amphotericin then	50 mg/d	3 days to 2 weeks
	Itraconazole	400 mg/d	10 weeks
Maintenance			
	Itraconazole[a]	200 mg/d[b] or	Life
		400 mg/d	Life

[a] Ketoconazole 400 mg daily is an alternative in nonimmunocompromised patients. Fluconazole is an alternative if the patient cannot take itraconazole or ketoconazole. Fluconazole dosage should be 800 mg daily for induction and 400 mg daily for maintenance. Amphotericin B 50 to 100 mg weekly or biweekly is also effective maintenance therapy for patients who cannot take or fail treatment with ketoconazole, itraconazole, or fluconazole.
[b] If itraconazole concentration in serum or plasma is at least 4 μg/dl by bioassay on 400 mg/day, induction dose may be reduced to 200 mg/day.

mg) and itraconazole (200 to 400 mg daily) are effective (>90%) maintenance therapies (6,38) and appear to be better than ketoconazole, being near 50% effective.

ACKNOWLEDGMENTS

This work was supported in part by the AIDS Program of the National Institutes of Allergy and Infectious Diseases and the Department of Veterans' Affairs.

REFERENCES

1. Wheat LJ. Histoplasmosis. Infect Dis Clin North Am 1988;2:841–859.
2. Deepe GS Jr, Bullock WE. Histoplasmosis: A granulomatous inflammatory response. In: Gallin JI, Goldstein IM, Snyderman R, eds. New York: Raven Press, 1992:943–958.
3. Wu-Hsieh B, Howard DH. Histoplasmosis. In: Murphy JW, ed. Fungal Infections and Immune Responses. New York: Plenum Press, 1993:213–250.
4. Wheat LJ, Slama TG, Norton JA. Risk factors for disseminated or fatal histoplasmosis. Ann Intern Med 1982;96:159–163.
5. Wheat LJ. Diagnosis and management of histoplasmosis. Eur J Clin Microbiol Infect Dis 1989;8:480–490.

6. Wheat LJ, Connolly-Springfield PA, Baker RL. Disseminated histoplasmosis in the acquired immune deficiency syndrome: Clinical findings, diagnosis and treatment, and review of the literature. Medicine 1990;69:361–374.
7. Kataria YP, Campbell PB, Burlingham BT. Acute pulmonary histoplasmosis presenting as adult respiratory distress syndrome: Effect of therapy on clinical and laboratory features. South Med J 1981;74:534–537.
8. Rubin H, Furcolow ML, Yates JL, Brasher CA. The course and prognosis of histoplasmosis. Am J Med 1959;27:278–288.
9. Leznoff A, Frank H, Telner P, et al. Histoplasmosis in Montreal during the fall of 1963, with observations on erythema multiforme. Can Med Assoc J 1964;91:1154–1160.
10. Sellers TF Jr, Price WN Jr, Newberry WM Jr. An epidemic of erythema multiforme and erythema nodosum caused by histoplasmosis. Ann Intern Med 1965;62:1244–1262.
11. Rosenthal J, Brandt KD, Wheat LJ, Slama TG. Rheumatologic manifestations of histoplasmosis in the recent Indianapolis epidemic. Arthr Rheum 1983;26:1065–1070.
12. Picardi JL, Kauffman CA, Schwarz J, et al. Pericarditis caused by Histoplasma capsulatum. Am J Cardiol 1976;37:82–88.
13. Wheat LJ, Stein L, Corya BC. Pericarditis as a manifestation of histoplasmosis during two large urban outbreaks. Medicine 1983;62:110–119.
14. Goodwin RA Jr, Owens FT, Snell JD. Chronic pulmonary histoplasmosis. Medicine 1976;55:413–452.
15. Wheat LJ, Wass J, Norton J, et al. Cavitary histoplasmosis occurring during two large urban outbreaks: Analysis of clinical, epidemiologic, roentgenographic, and laboratory features. Medicine 1984;63:201–209.
16. Goodwin RA Jr, Shapiro JL, Thurman GH, et al. Disseminated histoplasmosis: Clinical and pathologic correlations. Medicine 1980;59:1–33.
17. Sathapatayavongs B, Batteiger BE, Wheat LJ, et al. Clinical and laboratory features of disseminated histoplasmosis during two large urban outbreaks. Medicine 1983;62:263–270.
18. Goodwin RA, Nickell JA, des Prez RM. Mediastinal fibrosis complicating healed primary histoplasmosis and tuberculosis. Medicine 1972;51:227–246.
19. Loyd JE, Tillman BF, Atkinson JB, des Prez RM. Mediastinal fibrosis complicating histoplasmosis. Medicine 1988;67:295–310.
20. Schowengerdt CG, Suyemoto R, Beachley F. Granulomatous and fibrous mediastinitis. J Thorac Cardiovasc Surg 1969;57:365–379.
21. Wheat LJ, French MLV, Kohler RB. The diagnostic laboratory tests for histoplasmosis: Analysis of experience in a large urban outbreak. Ann Intern Med 1982;97:680–685.
22. Wheat LJ, Kohler RB, Tewari RP. Diagnosis of disseminated histoplasmosis by detection of Histoplasma capsulatum antigen in serum and urine specimens. N Engl J Med 1986;314:83–88.
23. Brodsky AL, Gregg MB, Kaufman L, Mallison GF. Outbreak of histoplasmosis associated with the 1970 Earth Day activities. Am J Med 1973;54:333–342.

24. Wynne JW, Olsen GN. Acute histoplasmosis presenting as the adult respiratory distress syndrome. Chest 1974;66:158–161.
25. Parker JD, Sarosi GA, Doto IL, et al. Treatment of chronic pulmonary histoplasmosis. N Engl J Med 1970;283:225–229.
26. Sutliff WD, Andrews CE, Jones E, Terry RT. Histoplasmosis cooperative study: Veterans Administration-Armed Forces Cooperative Study on histoplasmosis. Am Rev Respir Dis 1964;89:641–650.
27. Furcolow ML. Comparison of treated and untreated severe histoplasmosis. JAMA 1963;183:121–127.
28. Putnam LR, Sutliff WD, Larkin JE. Histoplasmosis cooperative study: Chronic pulmonary histoplasmosis treated with amphotericin B alone and with amphotericin B and triple sulfonamide. Am Rev Respir Dis 1968;97: 96–102.
29. Dismukes WE, Cloud G, Bowles C. Treatment of blastomycosis and histoplasmosis with ketoconazole: Results of a prospective randomized clinical trial. Ann Intern Med 1985;103:861–872.
30. Dismukes WE, Bradsher RW Jr, Cloud GC. Itraconazole therapy for blastomycosis and histoplasmosis. Am J Med 1992;93:489–497.
31. Baum GL, Larkin JC, Sutliff WD. Follow-up of patients with chronic pulmonary histoplasmosis treated with amphotericin B. Chest 1970;58:562–565.
32. Reddy P, Gorelick DF, Brasher CA, Larsh H. Progressive disseminated histoplasmosis as seen in adults. Am J Med 1970;48:629–636.
33. Sarosi GA, Voth DW, Dahl BA, et al. Disseminated histoplasmosis: Results of long-term follow-up. Ann Intern Med 1971;75:511–516.
34. Slama TG. Treatment of disseminated and progressive cavitary histoplasmosis with ketoconazole. Am J Med 1983;70:70–73.
35. Wheat LJ, Hafner RE, Ritchie M, Schneider D. Itraconazole is effective treatment for histoplasmosis in AIDS: Prospective multicenter non-comparative trial (abstr). Prog Abstr 32nd Intersci Conf. Antimicrob Agents Chemother 1992;1206.
36. Mathisen DJ, Grillo HC. Clinical manifestation of mediastinal fibrosis and histoplasmosis. Soc Thorac Surg 1992;54:1053–1058.
37. Tucker RM, Denning DW, Hanson LH. Interaction of azoles with rifampin, phenytoin, and carbamazepine: In vitro and clinical observations. Clin Infect Dis 1992;14:165–174.
38. McKinsey DS, Gupta MR, Driks M, et al. Histoplasmosis in patients with AIDS: Efficacy of maintenance amphotericin B therapy. Am J Med 1992; 92:225–227.

14

Relationship of *Cryptococcus neoformans* to Human Neutrophils

MALCOLM D. RICHARDSON
University of Glasgow and Western Infirmary
Glasgow, Scotland

I. INTRODUCTION

Cryptococcus neoformans is an encapsulated basidiomycetous yeast capable of causing life-threatening human disease. Two varieties of the organism have been described, *C. neoformans* var. *neoformans* and *C. neoformans* var. *gattii*, which differ in their geographical distribution, antigencity, and epidemiology. Exposure to *C. neoformans* occurs via inhalation of the yeast from the environment, but in the majority of cases this is not associated with symptomatic disease. Clinical infection can occur in apparently healthy individuals, but most cases are associated with conditions of impaired cell-mediated immunity and, in particular, defects in macrophage and T-cell function. *Cryptococcus neoformans* is a significant opportunistic pathogen in hematological malignancies, such as Hodgkin's lymphoma or in renal transplant recipients. However, most significantly, with the global emergence of acquired immunodeficiency syndrome (AIDS), the incidence of cryptococcosis is increasing and *C. neoformans* represents the major life-threatening fungal infection in these patients. The incidence of infection with *C. neoformans* in AIDS patients varies from approximately 3–15%, although it has been said to approach 30% in some regions of Africa. The reader is referred to Hay (1) for a recent overview of cryptococcosis.

II. HOST DEFENSE IN CRYPTOCOCCOSIS

Clinical and experimental evidence indicates that the initial pulmonary defenses against cryptococcosis involve the responses to T cells and the activities of alveolar macrophages. Recent murine studies suggest that natural killer (NK) cells may contribute to natural immunity against *C. neoformans* (2), and human NK cells appear to be equally effective against the yeast (3). Neutrophils and monocytes also effectively counteract the proliferation of *Cryptococcus*.

III. THE CAPSULE AND HOST DEFENSE

Cryptococcus is unique among the pathogenic fungi in expressing an extensive polysaccharide capsule, which is the primary determinant of virulence in vivo. The capsular polysaccharides possess important immunomodulatory properties, including a potent antiphagocytic action and the capacity to induce immunological suppression. Thus, defining the interaction between encapsulated yeasts and the immune system is essential in understanding the mechanisms of host resistance.

A number of biological properties have been attributed to the capsule of *C. neoformans*. It is likely that one or more of these functions is associated with virulence. Perhaps the most important property of the capsule is inhibition of phagocytosis. Encapsulated isolates of the yeast are less readily phagocytosed than acapsulate variants. However, acapsulate yeasts become more resistant to phagocytosis when isolated cryptococcal polysaccharide is added to media containing capsule-free mutants (4,5). In addition, acapsular mutants reverting to the encapsulated state become resistant to ingestion by phagocytes (6). Moreover, *C. neoformans* is a potent activator of the complement cascade, and opsonization of the encapsulated yeast via the alternative pathway is essential for phagocytosis (see below). Crucial to our understanding of the steps that take place in the sequence of events resulting in phagocytosis is an appreciation of the biochemical and physical nature of the capsular material surrounding the yeast cell of *C. neoformans*.

A capsule is a discrete slimy layer external to the yeast cell wall. The capsule of *C. neoformans* is composed of long, thin (0.3–0.4 nm in diameter) microfibrils proceeding radially from the outer surface of the cell wall. Capsular fibrils usually interwine and coil, often forming a fibrillar network of thicker fibrils along the capsule's periphery. Radial orientation of capsular polysaccharides, in contrast to the tangential orientation of cell-wall polysaccharides, is also demonstrable by polarizing microscopy. The mean thickness and size of capsules change during growth of cultures.

The mean thickness of capsules is minimal during the exponential phase of growth—i.e., the period of active budding. It then increases rapidly and achieves maximum thickness at the beginning of the stationary phase of growth. Measurements of capsules using India-ink mounts have shown that growing buds have very think capsules and that capsules are often not seen in the part of the bud projecting from the capsule of the mother cell. Only on completion of budding do newly formed buds and young daughter cells actively form their own capsules. The subsequent decrease in capsule size is caused by the release and dissolution of capsular material into the medium.

It is evident that the growth environment influences capsule formation. *Cryptococcus neoformans* usually develops large capsules in vivo, but their size is smaller when cells are grown in laboratory media. These observations suggest that in infected tissues, the yeast finds specific conditions that stimulate capsule production. A comparison of available data makes it possible to define a number of culture conditions that promote capsule synthesis. The best carbon source for capsule production in *C. neoformans* is D-mannose. Nitrogen-containing inorganic compounds promote formation. Increased concentrations of sugars, salts, and a low pH value suppress it. In the laboratory, 4% malt agar stimulates capsule production.

The polysaccharide capsule is predominantly composed of glucuronoxylomannan, which consists of a linear α (1–3) mannose backbone substituted with D-xylose and D-glucuronic acid. The capsular polysaccharide is shed from viable yeasts during in vitro culture and is present in the serum and cerebrospinal fluid of infected individuals. Circulating levels of cryptococcal antigen can be exceedingly high, with titers up to 10^6 being reported in cases of cryptococcal meningitis associated with AIDS. The detection of cryptococcal antigens at these sites allows a specific diagnosis of cryptococcal meningitis in over 90% of cases. The pathways of synthesis and extracellular organization of the cryptococcal polysaccharide are still being defined. Glucuronyltransferase and xylosyltransferase activities have recently been described in *C. neoformans*, but the mechanism of secretion of the capsular components to the cell surface is still unknown. Important information has been obtained by studying the interaction of purified capsular polysaccharides with acapsular yeasts in vitro. Binding of polysaccharide occurs in a rapid and specific manner, suggesting the presence of a receptor for the capsule polysaccharide on the fungal cell wall. It is possible that the initial saturable binding of polysaccharides to the cell wall is followed by self-association between polysaccharides, resulting in an extensive capsule structure.

IV. OPSONIZATION OF THE YEAST CELL

Phagocytosis by neutrophils of encapsulated cryptococci is depending upon opsonization of the yeast cell by opsonic ligands of the complement cascade (7). The inactive decay product of the C3 component of complement binds to the perimeter of the *Cryptococcus* capsule and is necessary for attachment of neutrophils prior to their phagocytosis (8). Cryptococci that are phagocytosed by human neutrophils are killed by mechanisms dependent on the generation of H_2O_2 and by nonoxidative mechanisms.

The process of phagocytosis of *C. neoformans* by neutrophils is very much dependent upon opsonization. Opsonization of encapsulated cryptococci involves cooperation between opsonic fragments of the complement system and antibody of the IgG class. The interrelationship of complement and antibody in opsonization appears to differ for encapsulated and acapsular varieties of the yeast. Wilson and Kozel (9) demonstrated that encapsulated and acapsular strains differ in their activation of the complement system. Incubation of acapsular cryptococci in normal human serum initiated both the classic and alternate pathways. This activation was characterized by an immediate, synchronous activation and binding of C3 to the yeast cells. Conversely, encapsulated cryptococci were found to activate only the alternative pathway. Here complement activation was characterized by a delayed (4 to 5 min), asynchronous activation and binding of C3. Furthermore, antibodies in normal human serum appeared to mediate immediate, synchronous binding of C3 to acapsular cells. The capsule size seems to be the major determinant of the amount of C3 deposited, as demonstrated recently when more C3 fragments were found on encapsulated than acapsular cryptococci when incubated with normal human serum, although this relationship was not linear (10). Thus, inhibition of encapsulate cryptococci requires a functional complement system to opsonize the yeasts so that they can bind to phagocytes and trigger engulfment.

V. BINDING AND THE NEUTROPHIL CYTOSKELETON—COMPARISONS BETWEEN ENCAPSULATED AND ACAPSULAR ISOLATES

Although there are sufficient data implicating the role of the capsule as a virulence factor in vitro, many of these in vitro data were obtained with *C. neoformans* long maintained in the laboratory, and there are still remarkably few studies comparing freshly isolated clinical isolates of varying capsule width. One in vivo study, however, found no correlation in the degree of in vitro encapsulation with virulence in vivo (11). This is probably because the "poorly encapsulated" isolates used were constructs on restrictive laboratory media and quickly reverted to the encapsulated state in vivo.

In order to overcome the limitations of using laboratory-maintained isolates of *C. neoformans*, we have conducted a series of studies using fresh encapsulated and acapsular clinical isolates from AIDS patients to look at various aspects of yeast-cell binding to neutrophil membranes. It is evident that the host cell receptors, which bind *Cryptococcus*, and the consequences of that binding will be important in determining whether or not *Cryptococcus* can establish itself as a pathogen. The role of the cytoskeleton in neutrophil fluidity and receptor clustering may be important in this reaction. The precise contribution of the cytoskeleton can be probed by exposing neutrophils to cytochalasins, which bind to the barbed ends of actin filaments and prevent both their polymerization and depolymerization and consequently inhibit neutrophil membrane ruffling (12). Of the cytochalasins, cytochalasin D is the most appropriate to study neutrophil mobility, since it is specific for actin and can be used in low concentrations to minimize nonspecific interactions. Our approach to this question has been to examine whether phagocytosis of encapsulated cryptococci by neutrophils is sterically inhibited, and if so, to examine at which stage phagocytosis is inhibited by the capsule (i.e., binding or internalization by neutrophils). Comparison was made with the binding characteristic of acapsular yeast cells isolated as wild types from AIDS patients. Complement receptors appeared to be involved in binding of both types of yeasts to neutrophils, but that the two isolates are bound by markedly different mechanisms. Acapsular yeasts bound in an independent manner, which did not require actin filaments and led, in some cases, to interalization, whereas encapsulated cryptococci competed for binding; binding required actin and did not appear to lead to phagocytosis of the yeast. These results are consistent with those from studies involving macrophages where acapsular but not encapsulated yeast-cell binding led to internalization (13).

In further experimentation, the finding that complement-depleted serum completely prevented binding of both isolates implicated complement receptors as essential for binding. Opsonization of both isolates with C3 fragments via activation of the alternative complement pathway (14) and binding to neutrophils through complement receptors seem likely to be central to both binding mechanisms. Studies with cultured macrophages, using anticomplement receptor monoclonal antibodies, showed complement receptors 3 and 4 mainly involved in binding, but a small amount of binding occurred in the absence of complement (13). Macrophages can produce some complement components (15); therefore it is possible that they could opsonize the cryptococci themselves. Neutrophils are unable to produce complement components, thus no opsonins would be present.

In neutrophil monolayer assays, competition between encapsulated yeasts for binding to neutrophils was shown by the observation that the binding index for a given number of neutrophils with one or more yeasts was lower in all experiments than expected for independent binding (16). The capsule has been shown to bind very large amounts of iC3b (13); therefore it is possible that the yeasts competed for complement. Although this seems an unlikely explanation, it cannot be dismissed until studies with varying amounts of complement have been performed. Competition between encapsulated cells for neutrophil binding sites seems a more plausible explanation. The differential effect of cytochalasin D on the percentage binding of the two isolates (i.e., increasing the concentration of cryptococci could overcome the effect of cytochalasin D for acapsular but not for encapsulated yeasts) suggests that actin filament inhibition abrogated binding of encapsulated yeasts in a way other than by inhibiting neutrophil mobility. Studies with macrophages have also shown that encapsulated yeast-cell binding is energy- and actin-dependent and acapsular yeast binding to be energy-dependent (13).

Our findings suggest a number of hypotheses. For encapsulated cryptococci, active receptor clustering on the neutrophil surface by rearrangement of actin filaments may be necessary. Localization of complement receptors to the area of cryptococcal binding has been seen with macrophages (13). Clustering would have been prevented by cytochalasin D, thus explaining its inhibitory effect. It could also explain the competition for binding and the maximum of four encapsulated cells bound per neutrophil. Only a limited number of clusters could form per neutrophil (possibly four); thus competition would be necessary. Clustering may have been necessary to reach the critical strength needed to hold cryptococci to neutrophils. The dynamic nature of the capsule may have prevented iC3b from clustering. Ligand clustering has previously been shown to increase the efficacy of binding (17).

For acapsular cryptococci, it is possible that binding to unclustered complement receptors was sufficient for attachment to neutrophils, since no capsule was present. It is possible that other receptors were involved in the binding of acapsular cells to neutrophils. This may explain the independence of acapsular yeast binding and the observation that up to 12 cells could bind to a single neutrophil, since the number of binding sites would not have been limited.

VI. PHAGOCYTOSIS OF THE ORGANISM

Phagocytes, primarily neutrophils and alveolar macrophages, are thought to play a major role in host defense against *C. neoformans* (13,18,19). Incubation of the yeast in normal human serum (NHS) leads to deposition of large amounts of the C3 degradation product, iC3b, in and on the surface of the capsule via activation of the alternative complement pathway (14). However, despite the presence of these potential opsonic ligands, phagocytosis of encapsulated cryptococci by neutrophils and macrophages is very limited, but acapsulate cryptococci can be ingested quite readily (19).

Thus, a key factor in resistance to cryptococcosis is the ability of phagocytes to overcome the antiphagocytic properties of the cryptococcal capsule. A recent study with human cultured macrophages implicated multiple complement receptors in binding of cryptococci and showed that binding of encapsulated but not acapsular yeast was an energy-dependent process which did not lead to phagocytosis.

Unlike mannose and Fc receptors, which are constitutively active at promoting ingestion of bound particles, complement receptors 1 and 3 (the major complement receptors on neutrophils that bind C3b and C3bi, respectively) exist in both active and inactive states with respect to promoting ingestion. The signals necessary to activate complement receptors are not known; however, it has been suggested that ligation of other receptors may provide signals to activate them. It is also possible that collaboration between receptors may occur, rather than interaction of signals. Complement receptors 1 and 3 have both been shown to associate with phagocyte cytoskeletons and to cluster. Complement receptor 3 clustering can occur in a ligand-independent fashion. Therefore, to alter properties of the receptors, it is possible that a second signal is required.

In our studies comparing the phagocytosis of encapsulated and acapsular strains of *C. neoformans* in neutrophil monolayer assays, no internalization of encapsulated cryptococci was observed. Complement receptors exist in active and inactive states with respect to promoting internalization of bound particles (20). Other studies have shown that neutrophils stimulated with supernatants from mixed leukocyte culture or phytohemagglutinatinin (PHA)–stimulated leukocyte cultures showed enhanced phagocytosis of *C. neoformans* (18), and PHA-stimulated ligand-independent clustering has been shown to lead to phagocytosis (21). Thus, a second signal may be required to enhance clustering and/or to activate complement receptors to stimulate ingestion of the yeast. There were no factors present in this system to act as a second signal, which may explain why no internalization of encapsulated cryptococci was observed.

We and others have shown that acapsulate cells of *C. neoformans* are internalized by neutrophils and macrophages (13). Acapsular cryptococci have exposed mannans, β-glucans, and other ligands in their cell walls. Receptors for these may have synergized with complement-coated zymosan (22) and *Leishmania* (15). We have also shown that acapsulate but not encapsulated cryptococci have exposed mannans, since FITC-labeled conconavalin A bound only to acapsular cells. These receptors may have provided a signal to activate the complement receptors or have collaborated with them (i.e., complement receptors providing strength of binding and mannose-receptors promoting internalization). The capsule of encapsulated cryptococci would mask these proposed ligands, thus preventing interaction with their receptors. That the capsule must be present on the yeast to inhibit phagocytosis has been shown previously (7); this is consistent with our own data, where we have shown that soluble capsular material was not inhibitory or binding (16). The capsule appeared to inhibit phagocytosis both at the level of binding, since only a limited number of sites were available, and possible ingestion, as complement receptors do not initiate ingestion unless activated.

VII. ENHANCEMENT OF PHAGOCYTOSIS

The nature of the interaction between phagocytes and *Cryptococcus* may be profoundly influenced by the culture surface, and presumably the cell type in vivo, upon which this interaction occurs. Levitz et al. (23) demonstrated that the phagocytic function of human peripheral blood monocytes, neutrophils, and monocyte-derived macrophages was enhanced by immobilized (solid-phase) mannose-binding protein and the complement subcomponent C1q. Interestingly, soluble mannose-binding protein had no effect on cryptococcal binding by phagocytes.

VIII. DIFFERENCES BETWEEN STRAINS IN BINDING AND PHAGOCYTOSIS

Little is known of the variation between strains (isolates) of *C. neoformans* in ingestion. An early study showed that isolates varied markedly in their sensitivity to phagocytosis (24). Kozel et al. (8) found variation between eight strains in phagocytosis but not in the degree of opsonization by complement. In a more recent study, which extends the number of isolates examined, Allendoerfer et al. (25) examined 20 clinical isolates of *C. neoformans*, 17 of which were from AIDS patients, in a murine model of cryptococcal meningitis. Based on LD_{50} analysis, these isolates were divided into two groups, namely high-virulence (HV) and low-virulence (LV) isolates. Capsule size, in vitro growth rate, phagocytosis, melanin formation, and minimum inhibitory concentration to the antifungal agent fluconazole were correlated with virulence in mice. Low-virulence isolates had similar growth rates as HV isolates. The range of capsule size was broad in both LV and HV isolates. No differences in phagocytosis were seen between LV and HV isolates. None of these characteristics correlated with virulence in mice. The study identified a broad range of virulence of *C. neoformans* from patients with AIDS. The inability of LV isolates to kill mice did not appear to depend critically on capsule size or binding to neutrophils. In a previous study, it was found that LV isolates were resistant to fluconazole (26). It was considered that larger capsules might impede access of fluconazole to the cell membrane, which might explain relative fluconazole resistance. However, in the study by Allendoerfer et al. (25), no such relationship was demonstrated between capsule size and fluconazole resistance.

IX. GROWTH INHIBITION BY PHAGOCYTES

Studies designed to assess the anticryptococcal activities of phagocytic cells have produced highly variable results. Disprepancies between results may be due to differences in (a) cell type, (b) manner of opsonization, (c) experimental model, (d) level of activation of the phagocytes, and (e) the species used as a source of phagocytic cells. Antibody-dependent anticryptococcal activity has been reported for mouse resident peritoneal macrophages, human nonadherent mononuclear cells, and human neutrophils. In contrast, opsonization of encapsulated cryptococci by anticapsular antibody does not facilitate the anticryptococcal activity of cultured human monocytes; indeed, the presence of anticapsular antibody significantly enhances fungal growth. Gamma interferon increases the in vitro anticryptococcal activity of cultured human monocytes.

Ingestion is not essential for the anticryptococcal action of phagocytes. Host defenses, including murine bone marrow–derived and peritoneal macrophages, may have found a way to overcome the phagocyte-inhibiting action of capsular polysaccharide. However, little evidence has accumulated to suggest that neutrophils can function in this way.

Several mechanisms have been proposed to account for the anticryptococcal activity of phagocytes. These include the myeloperoxidase-mediated fungicidal system, lysosomal granules, and an as yet unidentified product of the L-arginine–dependent nitrate-generating pathway.

X. VARIATION IN KILLING BETWEEN STRAINS

Different strains of *C. neoformans* exhibit considerable variation in the extent to which they are killed by neutrophils or monocytes (27). However, this variation was not consistently related to the size of the yeast cell and capsule. Furthermore, strains from AIDS patients were comparable in susceptibility as well as in cell and capsule dimensions to other strains. This study did not determine the basis for strain variation in killing.

XI. CONCLUSIONS

The role of phagocytosis in the killing of *C. neoformans* remains an intriguing area of research and speculation. Clearly, macrophages and natural killer cells play a major role in counteracting the proliferation of the yeast, but it is suggested from in vitro data that neutrophils equally play an important part in protection against *Cryptococcus*.

REFERENCES

1. Hay RJ. Clinical manifestations and management of cryptococcosis in the compromised patient. In: Warnock DW, Richardson MD, eds. Fungal Infection in the Compromised Patient, 2d ed. Chichester, England: Wiley, 1991: 85–115.
2. Hidmore MR, Nabavi N, Sonleitner F, Murphy JW. Murine natural killer cells are fungicidal to Cryptococcus neoformans. Infect Immun 1991;59: 1747–1754.
3. Murphy JW, Hidmore MR, Wong SC. Direct interactions of human lymphocytes with the yeast-like organism, Cryptococcus neoformans. J Clin Invest 1993;91:1553–1566.
4. Diamond RD, Root RK, Bennett JE. Factors influencing killing of Cryptococcus neoformans by human leukocytes in vitro. J Infect Dis 1972;125: 367–372.
5. Kozel TR. Non-encapsulated variant of Cryptococcus neoformans: II. Surface receptors for cryptococcal polysaccharide and their role in inhibition of phagocytosis by polysaccharide. Infect Immun 1977;16:99–105.
6. Bulmer GS, Sans MD. Cryptococcus neoformans: II. Phagocytosis by human leukocytes. J Bacteriol 1967;94:1480–1480.
7. Kozel TR, Gotschlich EC. The capsule of Cryptococcus neoformans passively inhibits phagocytosis of the yeast by macrophages. J Immunol 1982; 129:1657–1680.
8. Kozel TR, Pfrommer GST, Guerlain AS, et al. Strain variation in phagocytosis of Cryptococcus neoformans: Dissociation of susceptibility to phagocytosis from activation and binding of opsonic fragments of C3. Infect Immun 1988;56:2794–2800.

9. Wilson MA, Kozel TR. Contribution of antibody in normal human serum to early deposition of C3 onto encapsulated and nonencapsulated Cryptococcus neoformans. Infect Immun 1992;60:754–761.
10. Young BJ, Kozel TR. Effects of strain variation, serotype, and structural modification on kinetics for activation and binding of C3 to Cryptococcus neoformans. Infect Immun 1993;61:2966–2972.
11. Dykstra MA, Friedman L, Murphy JW. Capsule size of Cryptococcus neoformans: control and relationship to virulence. Infect Immun 1977;16:129–135.
12. Cooper JA. Effects of cytochalasin and phalloidin on actin. J Cell Biol 1987;105:1473–1478.
13. Levitz SM, Tabuni A. Binding of Cryptococcus neoformans by human cultured macrophages: Requirement for multiple complement receptors and actin. J Clin Invest 1991;87:528–535.
14. Kozel TR, Wilson MA, Murphy JW. Early events in the initiation of alternative complement pathway activation by the capsule of Cryptococcus neoformans. Infect Immun 1991;59:3101–3110.
15. Blackwell JM, Ezekowitz RAB, Roberts MB, et al. Macrophage complement and lectin-like receptors bind Leishmania in the absence of serum. J Exper Med 1985;162:324–331.
16. Richardson MD, White LJ, McKay IC, Shankland GS. Differential binding of acapsulate and encapsulated strains of Cryptococcus neoformans to human neutrophils. J Med Vet Mycol 1993;31:189–199.
17. Hermanowski-Vosatka A, Detmers PA, et al. Clustering of ligand on the surface of a particle enhances adhesion to receptor-bearing cells. J Biol Chem 1988;263:17822–17827.
18. Kozel TR, Pfrommer GST, Redelman D. Activated neutrophils exhibit enhanced phagocytosis of Cryptococcus neoformans opsonized with normal human serum. Clin Exp Immunol 1987;70:238–246.
19. Muller J. Immunological aspects of cryptococcosis in AIDS patients. In: Vanden Bossche H, Mackenzie DWR, Cauwenbergh G, et al, eds. Mycoses in AIDS Patients. New York: Plenum Press, 1990:123–132.
20. Silverstein SC, Greenberg S, Di Virgilio F, Steinberg TH. Phagocytosis. In: Paul WE, ed: Fundamental Immunology, 2d ed. New York: Raven Press, 1989:703–720.
21. Detmers PA, Wright SD, Olsen E, et al. Aggregation of complement receptors on human neutrophils in the absence of ligand. J Cell Biol 1987;105:1137–1145.
22. Ezekowitz RAB, Sim RM, Macpherson GG, Gordon S. Interaction of human monocytes, macrophages, and polymorphonuclear leukocytes with zymosan in vitro. J Clin Invest 1985;76:2368–2376.
23. Levitz SM, Tabuni A, Treseler C. Effect of mannose-binding protein on binding of Cryptococcus neoformans. Infect Immun 1993;61:4891–4893.
24. Mitchell TG, Friedman L. In vitro phagocytosis and intracellular fate of variously encapsulated strains of Cryptococcus neoformans. Infect Immun 1972;5:491–498.

25. Allendoerfer R, Richardson MD, Velez JD, et al. Broad range of virulence of Cryptococcus neoformans islates from patients with AIDS. J Infect Dis 1996. In press.
26. Velez JD, Allendoerfer R, Luther M, et al. Correlation of in vitro azole susceptibility with in vivo response in a murine model of cryptococcal meningitis. J Infect Dis 1993;168:508–510.
27. Miller MF, Mitchell TG. Killing of Cryptococcus neoformans strains by human neutrophils and monocytes. Infect Immun 1991;59:24–28.

15

Nocardia—Host Defenses and Immune Diagnosis

PATRICK BOIRON
Institut Pasteur
Paris, France

I. INTRODUCTION

Nocardiosis is a bacterial disease mainly caused by species of the *Nocardia asteroides* complex (including *Nocardia asteroides* new sense, *Nocardia farcinica*, and *Nocardia nova*), *Nocardia brasiliensis*, and *Nocardia otitidiscaviarum*. The spectrum of illness varies from asymptomatic colonization to localized or widely disseminated disease (1). This infectious disease is no longer rare, emerging as an important opportunistic as well as, in some instances, a primary pathogen both in human and animals. Regardless of their designation, *Nocardia* spp. are facultative intracellular pathogens that can infect both immunocompromised and normal individuals; their pathogenesis is incompletely understood. As with any infectious disease, the pathogenesis of nocardiosis is dependent upon the nature and extent of host defense and the virulence of the infecting microorganism. The virulence associated with nocardiae appears to reside primarily in their ability to evade or modulate host responses.

II. HOST DEFENSES

The mechanisms of host resistance to nocardial infections appear to be complex. Phagocytic cells of the reticuloendothelial system can eliminate

Nocardia cells from host tissues by nonselective phagocytosis of the invading organisms. Moreover, specific phagocytosis under the control of humoral and cell-mediated immunity can reinforce the host response against nocardial infection.

A. Innate Host Resistance

1. The Mechanical Barrier and the Superficial Microenvironment

a. The Skin, Mucosa, and Surface Secretions Nonspecific immune mechanisms represents the first line of defense against invasion by *Nocardia* cells. The skin and mucosal membranes form an effective superficial mechanical barrier to *Nocardia*. Nocardiae seems unable to colonize healthy skin for extended periods of time. Failure of the skin barrier, such as superficial trauma that breaches its surface integrity, may be necessary for cutaneous or subcutaneous infection to become established (2,3).

The mucosa secreted along the inner surfaces of the body is known to be a less effective mechanical barrier. However, it seems that the mucosal barrier provides some protection against nocardial adherence, trapping microbial particles that can then be removed by mechanisms such as ciliary movement of epithelial cells, coughing, or sneezing. Other fluids that bathe epithelial surfaces—such as saliva, tears, nasal secretions, and urine—and contain a variety of microbicidal substances (e.g., lysozyme) have a similar action. Disturbance of the integrity of the mucosal barrier, which may be caused by steroid or antitumor agents, may lead infection to become established here.

b. The Endogenous Flora Endogenous microflora, which is found in many parts of the body, can prevent overgrowth by opportunistic organisms. They compete for nutrients, block adherence sites, and may also produce inhibitory compounds such as colicins and acids. Indeed, after either intranasal or intravenous inoculation by nocardiae, germ-free mice are significantly more susceptible to the acute phase of infection than are the conventionally grown animals that possess a normal resident microflora. The brains, lungs, kidneys, and adrenals of the former are affected more dramatically than the latter, but no significant differences are observed on the clearance of nocardial cells from the liver, spleen, and blood. As was established by experiments of pretreatment with lipopolysaccharide that enhances macrophage activity and renders germ-free mice significantly more resistant than the conventionally grown mice, the normal flora could serve to increase the level of nonspecific activation of phagocytic cells in the host (4).

2. *The Inflammatory Response*

Once nocardiae penetrate below the epithelium into the deeper layers of the skin or mucosa or into deep organs (which are normally a sterile environment), they stimulate the inflammatory response, which is the most important of the nonspecific host defense mechanisms. The first element of the inflammatory response is the production of a variety of soluble chemical compounds that are toxic to invading organisms. These include lysozyme, cytokines, complement, and acute-phase proteins. The second element of the inflammatory response consists of polymorphonuclear neutrophils and the mononuclear phagocyte system.

Nocardia cells are readily phagocytized in vitro by cultured macrophages (5), even in the absence of antibody and complement. However, the intracellular fate of the nocardiae depends on several factors, including the degree of virulence and the growth phase of the strain and the metabolic state of the phagocyte (6–8).

Relatively avirulent *Nocardia* strains are destroyed following phagocytosis. Some nocardial cells of relatively more virulent strains are slowly degraded by macrophages, while a few of the intracellular organisms are capable of surviving for long periods of time in an altered, wall-less cellular state (L forms). Ultimately, the surviving intracellular bacteria grow out of the macrophage. Following phagocytosis, virulent strains of *Nocardia* are not killed; the cells grow rapidly and filaments cross the phagocytic cell membrane as they grow out of the macrophage. Therefore, virulent strains of *Nocardia* are facultative intracellular pathogens. Furthermore, cells of virulent strains of *Nocardia* that grow within macrophages appear to be cytotoxic for phagocytic cells. The virulent strains inhibit phagosome-lysosome fusion (6–8), block or neutralize phagosomal acidification (9), and modulate lysosomal enzyme content, probably by utilizing some of these enzymes, such as acid phosphatase, as growth substrate (10).

Moreover, virulent strains of *N. asteroides* are able to block the microbicidal oxygen-dependent mechanisms used by polymorphonuclear neutrophils to kill microorganisms. The survival and growth of virulent *N. asteroides* involve the synthesis of a surface associated and secreted superoxide dismutase and of intracytoplasmic catalase, whereas avirulent strains of *Nocardia* do not secrete superoxide dismutase. It was shown that both of these enzymes were important in protecting nocardiae from oxidative microbicidal activities in vitro (11,12). In addition, phagocytic cells contain myeloperoxidase, which catalyzes a reaction resulting in potent microbicidal substance for phagocytes.

The stage of growth of *Nocardia* cells is also an important factor that influences their intraphagocytic-cell fate. Log-phase cells of virulent *No-*

cardia strains are more toxic to the macrophage monolayer, their growth is not inhibited by macrophages from immunized animals, and they increase in number more rapidly than do stationary-phase cells (5).

B. Immune Response to *Nocardia*

Both humoral and cell-mediated responses are demonstrated during nocardial infection (13). The immune response of the "normal" host against *Nocardia* must be effective, since clinically apparent disease does not seem very frequent, in spite of probable contact with these relatively common environmental organisms occurring with most individuals. Comprehensive reviews in this field were recently published by Beaman (13,14).

1. The Humoral Response

Immunoglobulins of IgM, IgG, and IgA isotypes have been detected following experimental infection in animals and humans with progressive nocardial infections. Treatment of mice prior to infection with cyclophosphamide, a polyfunctional cytotoxic agent that can affect B-lymphocyte function, increased host susceptibility to nocardial infection. However, passive immunization studies utilizing sera from immunized animals injected into nonimmunized recipients have failed to show either significant protection in vivo when challenged with virulent nocardial cells or significant opsonic activity, microbicidal activity in either the presence or absence of complement, or enhancement of the microbicidal activities of macrophages (13).

On the contrary, some arguments suggest that antibodies, involved in immune complexes, that are produced in large amounts in chronic lesions exacerbate the severity and chronicity of the lesions and play a role in causing extensive tissue damage. Furthermore, following intravenous injection of nocardial cells, it was demonstrated that congenitally B-cell-deficient CBN mice were more resistant to infection than the "normal" mice, which had a good humoral response. Passive transfer of immunologically normal or T-cell-deficient mice with nocardia-specific antibody not only did not protect the mice from developing mycetomas following footpad injection of *N. brasiliensis* but furthermore enhanced the severity of the symptoms (15). Therefore, the requirement for functioning B cells appeared not to be important in enhanced host resistance to *N. asteroides* and *N. brasiliensis* (14).

However, high titers of purified antibodies specific for defined cell-surface antigens, such as polyclonal rabbit IgG or murine monoclonal IgM antibody, which neutralized nocardial superoxide dismutase activity, may enhance host resistance in exacerbating the polymorphonuclear neutrophils killing of *N. asteroides* cells (11).

2. Cell-Mediated Immunity

The observation that humans who are deficient in cell mediated immunity are more susceptible to developing progressive nocardiosis than are those who have an intact cell-mediated response, and research using a variety of animal models suggests that cell-mediated and not humoral immunity are most important in host defense against invasive nocardial infection (13,16).

T cells appear to be involved in at least two distinct mechanisms of host resistance to nocardial infection. The first is their well-established role in immunologically specific activation of subpopulations of other T cells and macrophages and stimulation of a cellular immune response. Nude mice (T-cell-deficient) were found to be more susceptible to nocardial infection induced with virulent *N. asteroides* strains than were their heterozygotous (Nu/+) littermates (16). Adoptive transfers of primed splenic T cells from immunized animals into T-cell-deficient recipients demonstrated that T cells significantly enhanced host clearance of virulent strains of *N. asteroides* from the liver, spleen, and brain.

Using in vitro maintained alveolar macrophages from normal and immunized rabbits, it was shown that the most effective macrophage activity occurred when macrophages from immunized rabbits were incubated with physically present primed T cells from lymph nodes of the same animal in the presence of immune serum and alveolar lining material, inducing a complete intact cell-mediated response.

A second role for T lymphocytes in host resistance to *Nocardia* depends upon the specific binding and direct killing capacity of the lymphocyte in vitro toward the nocardial cell (17). The killing capacity of lymphocytes from immunized animals was antibody independent and was enhanced by in vitro priming of the lymphocytes with nocardial cell-wall fragments before challenge. The surface membrane of the T lymphocyte tightly adheres to and damages the nocardial cell wall, resulting in bacterial lysis (17). The specific direct T-lymphocyte killing of *N. asteroides* could be important in host defense, but its exact role in human resistance to nocardial infections is not known.

3. Regulation of Immune Response

Several studies have suggested that the glycolipid cord factor may induce tumor necrosis factor (TNF), a cell-wall subunit structure may stimulate B cells directly (B-cell mitogen), and additional cell-wall components may affect the regulation and enhancement of the T-cell activity. However, contrary to other facultative intracellular pathogens such as *Coccidioides immitis*, *Listeria monocytogenes*, and *Toxoplasma gondii*, activation of macrophages by γ-interferon and TNF seem able to stimulate the growth of phagocytized *Nocardia* cells (13).

On the contrary, a role for TNF in resistance to *N. brasiliensis* infection was suggered by studies of treatment with anti-TNF antibody of mice infected with *N. brasiliensis* showing that the number of colony-forming units (CFU) recovered from spleens and livers was increased (18).

III. IMMUNE DIAGNOSIS

Nocardiosis is difficult to recognize on the basis of clinical, radiological, or histological findings. A definitive diagnosis depends on obtaining appropriate clinical samples, which may require the use of invasive procedures, and on the isolation and identification of a *Nocardia* spp., a procedure that can take 2 to 3 weeks (1). A high level of suspicion on the part of the physician, who should always alert the laboratory when nocardiae are suspected, and experience on the part of the laboratory personnel, are essential for early detection. Immunodiagnosis of patients with nocardial infection should permit an earlier and more rapid recognition of nocardia-induced disease. It should provide a basis for earlier chemotherapy, which could improve the prognosis.

Therefore, tests for the demonstration of delayed cutaneous hypersensitivity and for humoral antibodies for the diagnosis of nocardiosis have been investigated as alternatives to classical microbiological procedures.

It is now well known that members of the genera *Nocardia* and *Mycobacterium* have many properties in common, as attested by similarities of morphological, cultural, chemotaxonomic, and particularly serological characteristics. Nocardiae possess several polysaccharidic antigens, principally arabinomannan and arabinogalactan, which are shared mainly with mycobacteria, corynebacteria, and rhodococci (19–21). Nocardial ribosomal antigen also cross-react with ribosomal antigens of mycobacteria and corynebacteria (22). Consequently, cross reactivity was observed between *Nocardia* and *Mycobacterium* using immunodiffusion tests (23–26) or agglutination tests (27). However, specificity not apparent on direct test was demonstrated, either by hemagglutination assay using erythrocyte-sensitizing somatic antigen (28) or by combining hemagglutination (erythrocyte-sensitizing culture filtrate antigen) and the hemolytic inhibition test (29).

With an extracellular glycoprotein culture filtrate antigen and an immunodiffusion precipitin test, four major immunotypes were recognized within *N. asteroides* and *N. brasiliensis* (30,31). Factors I, II, and III are mutually exclusive, since a strain of *N. asteroides* produces only one or the other of these antigens. Factors II or III can be produced simultaneously with the factor IV, the latter being produced by *N. brasiliensis*. Eventual cross-reactions with *Mycobacterium* antigens have not been tested, and the biochemical nature of these antigens is unknown. Of interest, the ability of the four immunotypes to identify *N. asteroides* to the subspecies level has been reported to be useful as part of an epidemiological evaluation of an outbreak of nocardiosis in a renal transplant unit (32). Three other antigenic factors were further detected (16,33,34) that permitted the characterization of seven distinct immunotypes, each with its own antigenic determinants.

A. Delayed Cutaneous Hypersensitivity

The first antigens used in delayed cutaneous hypersensitivity that were prepared from culture filtrates from *N. asteroides* and *N. brasiliensis* showed contradictory results. Animals that were experimentally infected or patients with nocardiosis or mycetoma revealed positive or negative skin reactions following subcutaneous inoculation of these antigens (35). However, cross-reactions with tuberculin were systematically observed.

Several studies reported partial purification of antigenic fractions. In one study, an antigen of *Nocardia*, prepared following a method similar to that used to isolate purified protein derivatives from mycobacteria, made it possible to obtain positive cutaneous reactions on guinea pigs immunized with the *N. asteroides* strains used for antigenic preparation (36). The same kind of antigen prepared from *N. brasiliensis* was successfully used in skin tests on patients with mycetoma due to *N. brasiliensis* (37). Using ion-exchange chromatography, an antigen (F fraction) was isolated from the cell wall–less culture filtrate of *N. asteroides*. The F fraction was able to produce delayed cutaneous hypersensitivity on cattle experimentally infected with *N. asteroides* but not on those infected with *Mycobacterium* sp. (19,38–40). Precipitating antigens and those involved in complement fixation remained in this F fraction. Unfortunately, this F fraction was never tested on humans.

Concerning *N. brasiliensis*, a polysaccharidic antigen isolated by Gonzalez-Ochoa was able to produce delayed cutaneous hypersensitivity on patients with mycetoma due to *N. brasiliensis* but not on patients with pulmonary tuberculosis or actinomycosis (41). A ribosomal fractionless cellular extract was shown to be able to distinguish between *N. asteroides*–sensitized animals from *N. brasiliensis*–sensitized ones (42). These results were confirmed in vitro by the inhibition of migration of phagocytes sensitized with homologous antigen. This antigen did not induce any skin reaction on patients with tuberculosis or leprosy (43).

Better results were obtained by using partially purified antigens. Nocardin active polypeptide (NAP-A) was isolated from *N. asteroides* following a method similar to that used to isolate active peptides from mycobacteria (44). The NAP-A, of about 20,000 molecular weight, contained 15% of proteins and undetectable lipids or carbohydrates. Delayed skin reactions on sensitized guinea pigs (44,45) and in vitro lymphocyte transformation (46) with NAP-A showed a relative species specificity (no cross-reactions with *Mycobacterium* and *Streptomyces*; cross-reaction with *N. brasiliensis* and *N. otitidiscaviarum* using high antigenic concentration), and perhaps a strain specificity.

Polysaccharides were extracted from *N. asteroides* and *N. brasiliensis* (47). Two fractions were separated using differential solubility. The soluble fraction, Poly I (Poly I Na and Poly I Nb), was not precisely characterized, but could be arabinogalactan. The insoluble fraction, Poly II (Poly II Na and Poly II Nb), is made up of arabinose, galactose, and mannose and contained less than 1% proteins. Highly purified polysaccharides (containing less than 0.04% proteins) were produced from Poly I and II (48).

Poly I Na and Poly I Nb were apparently the same, showing cross-reactions in agar diffusion tests with rabbit antisera prepared against either *N. asteroides* or *N. brasiliensis* and total absorbtion of serum antibodies against either polysaccharide. Moreover, cross-reactions were observed with serum from patients with tuberculosis or leprosy.

Poly II Na and Poly II Nb were different, exhibiting different molecular ratios of constituent sugars and reacting only with homologous antisera. Using Poly Nb, precipitating antibodies were detected in sera of patients with mycetoma caused by *N. brasiliensis* (49). No cross-reactions were observed with sera from patients with other diseases, including tuberculosis, leprosy, actinomycosis, and mycetoma due to *Actinomadura madurae*.

B. Serological Diagnosis

Whole-cell and filtrate antigens were used in immunodiffusion tests (50,51). These tests were 45–47% sensitive. The use of reactions of identity, with serum from a human nocardiosis case as reference, was more specific and more predictive than the presence of any band, but less sensitive. Culture filtrate antigens were also used to develop a complement-fixation test with rabbit reference antiserum (21). An overall sensitivity of 81% was found. However, cross-reactivity with sera from patients with leprosy (three of three patients) and tuberculosis (two of five patients) was still evident. These data supported the suggestion that infected individuals can be identified but that a high degree of cross-reactivity seriously hinders the specificity of these tests. Moreover, because of the relatively poor sensitivity of each individual assay, they were unable to detect antibody response in immunosuppressed patients. In addition to the methods used for detection, considerable variation in the antigenic composition of *N. asteroides* could be attributed to the variable cultural conditions in these studies. On the contrary, using a panel of tests for recognition of nocardial infections, reactions occur frequently within a normal healthy population. In a study of the incidence of infection by nocardiae, 25% of healthy volunteers (71 of 284) had a subclinical exposure to *Nocardia* spp. based on seropositivity as compared with patients with culture-proven infection (14). Moreover, using immunofluorescent staining, antibodies to *Nocardia* were detected in the serum of patients with Parkinson's disease (52). These results suggest that individuals are routinely exposed to and naturally infected with *Nocardia*-related microorganisms.

In the search of an easy and reliable test for serodiagnosis of nocardiosis, an enzyme immunoassay was developed with whole *N. asteroides* cells adsorbed on microtitration plates (53). This simple assay appeared as an easy method of diagnosing nocardiosis in nonimmunosuppressed patients but lacked of sensitivity and specificity.

More recently, Sugar et al. have documented the presence of a major 55-kDa protein in culture filtrate of *N. asteroides* (54). This protein has been shown to be a highly specific marker for identifying patients infected with *N. asteroides*, *N. brasiliensis* and *N. otitidiscaviarum* (55). Ninety-one percent of the patients with nocardiosis, including immunocompromised and cutaneously infected patients, had positive antibody titers to this antigen (56). Pier and colleagues, in earlier studies, found a similar extracellular antigen that was useful for diagnostic purposes in monitoring infected dairy cattle. In Beaman's laboratory, Pier's diagnostic extracellular antigen appears to be the same as Sugar's 55-kDa extracellular diagnostic antigen (13).

Boiron and Provost reported the partial purification of a specific immunodominant 54-kDa antigen by immunoaffinity chromatography from a culture filtrate of *N. asteroides* (57,58). In all probability, this 54-kDa antigen is the same as the 55-kDa antigen used by Sugar et al. The Western blot technique, combined with immunodetection performed according to the biotin-avidin system, was applied to detecting the immunologic response to nocardiae. Each of 16 serum samples from immunosuppressed or immunocompetent patients infected with *N. asteroides* reacted with the 54-kDa band. There was only one reaction with serum samples obtained from patients with tuberculosis, and none with sera from patients with leprosy and from healthy controls.

Although the 54/55-kDa protein is the most promising diagnostic antigen that may be successfully used in the routine serodiagnosis of nocardiosis, Kjelstrom and Beaman (59) reported that not all clinical isolates of *Nocardia* spp. induced an antibody response to the 54/55-kDa antigen in experimental animals. Furthermore, these authors found that several humans with nocardiosis confirmed by culture did not have a demonstrable response against the 54/55-kDa antigen in an immunoblot assay (14).

Based upon several independent studies (54,57), it appears that several extracellular proteins secreted by *Nocardia* species (i.e., 31-, 43-, 54/55-, and 62-kDa proteins) could be useful antigenic markers, since individuals may have antibody to these antigens (in particular, 31- and 62-kDa). In order to avoid false-negative recognition of nocardiosis when using a single diagnostic antigen, Kjelstrom and Beaman developed a panel of serodiagnosis tests based on reactivity to a variety of antigens by using enzyme-linked immunosorbent assay of cytoplasmic, culture filtrate, and cord factor antigens; immunofluorescence assay against whole cells of *N. asteroides*; and Western blot analysis of secreted protein antigens of *N. asteroides* GUH-2 (59). When this diagnostic panel was applied to human sera, there was excellent sensitivity and specificity for culture-proven cases of clinical disease caused by nocardiae (14). This diagnostic panel was used in a study of the incidence of infection by nocardiae. It was estimated that at least one-third of all seropositive individuals (108 of 345 people tested were seropositive) evaluated in this study had either a clinical or subclinical infection with an organism closely related antigenically to *N. asteroides* GUH-2 (14).

The search for monoclonal antibodies (Mabs) was reported by several authors in view of the development of a sensitive and specific diagnostic test for nocardiosis. The immunosuppressed status of some patients may limit a diagnostic procedure that relies on the detection of antibodies. The use of an antibody probe specific to a *Nocardia*-specific antigen could result in the development of a specific and sensitive serodiagnostic test for systemic nocardiosis based on detection of such an antigen.

Antigenic factors displaying specificity for *N. asteroides* were characterized by El-Zaatari et al. (60) by the enzyme-linked immunoelectrotransfer blot technique adapted to isofocused polyacrylamide gels. The Mabs were produced against antigenic factors 1, 6, and 8. Mab against factor 8 cross-reacted with antigens of *Mycobacterium intracellulare* and *Mycobacterium fortuitum*. The Mabs against factors 1 and 6 did not cross-react with cytoplasmic antigens of *Mycobacterium chelonae*, *M. intracellulare* serotype 4B and 8A, *M. fortuitum*, *Mycobacterium gordonae*, and *Mycobacterium kansasii*.

The Mabs produced by Jiménez et al. (61) showed cross-reactivity with *M. tuberculosis*, *M. intracellulare*, *Mycobacterium scrofulaceum*, *M. kansasii*, and *M. fortuitum*; this may be viewed as undesirable for diagnostic purpose. The Mabs that reacted strongly with *Nocardia* were those that showed the highest degree of cross-reactivity with *Mycobacterium*.

Two Mabs reacting with the *Nocardia*-specific 54-kDa antigen were generated by Boiron et al. (62). These Mabs did not react with whole *Nocardia* cells, as evidenced from indirect immunofluorescence experiments indicating that the 54-kDa antigen is apparently not exposed to microbial surface. No or weak cross-reactivity was observed with mycobacterial antigens (culture-filtrate antigen and tuberculin), suggesting that at least one of these Mabs may be used as a specific reagent and could be a candidate for use in the development of a sensitive and specific diagnostic test for nocardiosis.

IV. CONCLUSION

The mechanisms of pathogenesis and host resistance to nocardiae have been shown to be multiple and complex. Although host-parasite relationships/mechanisms and the relative importance of cellular and humoral immunity begin to be more clearly understood, mainly owing to Beaman and Beaman's works, it is clear that much more research is necessary, in particular to investigate the long-term consequences of subclinical infection of humans by *Nocardia*.

Although the role of the humoral response to infection with *Nocardia* has not be claimed to play an important role in the mechanisms of host resistance, it appears to be useful for serological diagnosis. However, more studies are needed to develop a reliable and useful scheme for the recognition of nocardial infections.

REFERENCES

1. McNeil MM, Brown JM. The medically important aerobic actinomycetes: Epidemiology and microbiology. Clin Microbiol Rev 1994;7:357–417.
2. Hay RJ. Nocardial infection of the skin. J Hyg Camb 1983;91:385–391.
3. Rippon JW. Mycetoma. In: Rippon JW, ed. Medical Mycology: The Pathogenic Fungi and the Pathogenic Actinomycetes, 3d ed. Philadelphia: Saunders, 1988:81–118.
4. Beaman BL, Gershwin ME, Scates SM, Ohsugi Y. Immunobiology of germ-free mice infected with *Nocardia asteroides*. Infect Immun 1980;29:733–743.
5. Filice GA, Beaman BL, Remington JS. Effects of activated macrophages on *Nocardia asteroides*. Infect Immun 1980;27:643–649.

6. Davis-Scibienski C, Beaman BL. Interaction of *Nocardia asteroides* with rabbit alveolar macrophages: Association of virulence, viability, ultrastructural damage, and phagosome-lysosome fusion. Infect Immun 1980;28: 610–619.
7. Davis-Scibienski C, Beaman BL. Interaction of *Nocardia asteroides* with rabbit alveolar macrophages: Effect of growth phase and viability on phagosome-lysosome fusion. Infect Immun 1980;29:24–29.
8. Davis-Scibienski C, Beaman BL. Interaction of alveolar macrophages with *Nocardia asteroides*: Immunological enhancement of phagocytosis, phagosome-lysosome fusion, and microbicidal activity. Infect Immun 1980;30: 578–587.
9. Black CM, Palieschskey B, Beaman BL, et al. Acidification of phagosomes in murine macrophages: Blockage by *Nocardia asteroides*. J Infect Dis 1986; 154:952–958.
10. Beaman L, Paliescheskey M, Beaman BL. Acid phosphatase stimulation of growth of *Nocardia asteroides* and its possible relationship to the modulation of lysosomal enzymes in macrophages. Infect Immun 1988;56:1652–1654.
11. Beaman L, Beaman BL. Monoclonal antibodies demonstrate that superoxide dismutase contributes to protection of *Nocardia asteroides* within the intact host. Infect Immun 1990;58:3122–3128.
12. Filice GA, Beaman BL, Krick JA, Remington JS. Effects of human neutrophils and monocytes on *Nocardia asteroides*: Failure of killing despite occurrence of the oxidative metabolic burst. J Infect Dis 1980;142:432–438.
13. Beaman BL. Nocardial infections. In: Murphy JW, Friedman H, Bendinelli M, eds. Fungal infections and immune responses. New York: Plenum Press, 1993:533–554.
14. Beaman BL, Beaman L. *Nocardia* species: host-parasite relationships. Clin Microbiol Rev 1994;7:213–264.
15. Rico G, Ochoa R, Oliva A, et al. Enhanced resistance to *Nocardia brasiliensis* infection in mice depleted of antigen-specific B-cells. J Immunol 1982;129:1688–1693.
16. Krick JA, Remington JS. Resistance to infection with *Nocardia asteroides*. J Infect Dis 1975;131:665–672.
17. Deem RL, Doughty FA, Beaman BL. Immunologically specific direct T-lymphocyte-mediated killing of *Nocardia asteroides*. J Immunol 1983;130: 2401–2406.
18. Silva CL, Faccioli LH. Tumor necrosis factor and macrophage activation are important in clearance of *Nocardia brasiliensis* from the livers and spleens of mice. Infect Immun 1992;60:3566–3570.
19. Pier AC, Keeler RF. Extracellular antigens of *Nocardia asteroides*: I. Production and immunologic characterization. Am Rev Respir Dis 1965;91: 391–399.
20. Ridell M. Immunodiffusion studies of some *Nocardia* using mycobacterial precipitation reference systems. J Bacteriol 1973;113:1–7.
21. Shainhouse JZ, Pier AC, Stevens DA. Complement fixation antibody test for human nocardiosis. J Clin Microbiol 1978;8:516–519.

22. Laub R, Delville J, Cocito C. Immunological relatedness of ribosomes from mycobacteria, nocardiae and corynebacteria, and microorganisms in leprosy lesions. Infect Immun 1978;22:540–547.
23. Kwapinski JB, Kwapinski EH, Dowler J, Hosman G. The phyloantigenic position of nocardiae revealed by examination of cytoplasmic antigens. Can J Microbiol 1973;19:955–964.
24. Rajki K, Brehmer W, Hammer HJ, et al. Analysis of the soluble cytoplasmic components of mycobacteria and nocardia by crossed immunoelectrofocusing. Zbl Bakt Hyg I Abt Orig A 1982;251:389–398.
25. Ridell M. Crossreactivity between *Mycobacterium leprae* and various actinomycetes and related organisms. Int J Lepr 1983;51:185–190.
26. Ridell M. Immunodiffusion studies of some *Nocardia* strains. J Gen Microbiol 1981;123:69–74.
27. Schneidau JD, Jr, Shaffer MF. Studies on *Nocardia* and other actinomycetales: II. Antigenic relationships shown by slide agglutination tests. Am Rev Respir Dis 1959;82:64–76.
28. Savard EV, Snyder IS, Hawkins JE. Hemagglutinating antibodies to *Nocardia asteroides*. J Infect Dis 1966;116:439–446.
29. Thurston JR, Phillips M, Pier AC. Extracellular antigens of *Nocardia asteroides*: III. Immunologic relationships demonstrated by erythrocyte-sensitizing antigens. Am Rev Respir Dis 1968;97:240–247.
30. Pier AC, Fichtner RE. Serologic typing of *Nocardia asteroides* by immunodiffusion. Am Rev Respir Dis 1971;103:698–707.
31. Pier AC, Fichtner RE. Distribution of serotypes of *Nocardia asteroides* from animals, human, and environmental sources. J Clin Microbiol 1981;13:548–553.
32. Stevens DA, Pier AC, Beaman BL, et al. Laboratory evaluation of an outbreak of nocardiosis in immunocompromised hosts. Am J Med 1981;71:928–934.
33. Kurup VP, Scribner GH. Antigenic relationship among *Nocardia asteroides* immunotypes. Microbios 1981;31:25–30.
34. Kurup VP, Piechura JE, Ting EY, Orlowski JA. Immunochemical characterization of *Nocardia asteroides* antigen: Support for a single species concept. Can J Microbiol 1983;29:425–432.
35. Drake CH, Henrici AT. *Nocardia asteroides*: Its pathogenicity and allergic properties. Am Rev Tuberc Pulm Dis 1943;48:184–198.
36. Magnusson M, Mariat F. Delineation of *Nocardia asteroides* by delayed type skin reaction on guinea pigs. J Gen Microbiol 1968;51:151–158.
37. Bojalil LF, Magnusson M. Specificity of skin reactions of humans to *Nocardia* sensitins. Am Rev Respir Dis 1963;88:409–411.
38. Keeler RF, Pier AC. Extracellular antigens of *Nocardia asteroides*: II. Fractionation and chemical characterization. Am Rev Respir Dis 1965;91:400–408.
39. Pier AC, Enright JB. *Nocardia asteroides* as a primary pathogen of cattle: II. Immunologic reactions of infected animals. Am J Vet Res 1962;23:284–292.
40. Pier AC, Thurston JR, Larsen AB. A diagnostic antigen for nocardiosis:

Comparative tests in cattle with nocardiosis and mycobacteriosis. Am J Vet Res 1968;29:397–403.

41. Gonzalez-Ochoa A, Vasquez-Hoyos. Relaciones serologicas de los principales actinomycetes patogenos. Revta Inst Salubr Enferm Trop Mexico 1953; 33:177–187.
42. Ortiz-Ortiz L, Contreras MF. Cytoplasmic antigens from *Nocardia* eliciting a specific delayed hypersensitivity. Infect Immun 1972;5:879–882.
43. Ortiz-Ortiz L, Bojalil LF. Delayed skin reactions to cytoplasmic extracts of *Nocardia* organisms as a means of diagnosis and epidemiological study of *Nocardia* infection. Clin Exp Immun 1972;12:225–229.
44. Kingsbury EW, Slack JM. A polypeptide skin test antigen from *Nocardia asteroides*: I. Production, chemical and biological characterization. Am Rev Respir Dis 1967;95:827–832.
45. Kingsbury EW, Slack JM. A polypeptide skin test antigen from *Nocardia asteroides*: II. Further studies on the specificity of a nocardin active polypeptide. Sabouraudia 1972;7:85–89.
46. Hiramine CK, Hojo K, Yano I. Development of cell-mediated hypersensitivity in guinea pigs following infection with *Nocardia asteroides*. Int Arch Allergy Appl Immunol 1981;65:220–234.
47. Zamora A, Bojalil LF, Bastarrachea F. Immunologically active polysaccharides from *Nocardia asteroides* and *Nocardia brasiliensis*. J Bacteriol 1963; 85:549–555.
48. Ortiz-Ortiz L, Bojalil LF, Contreras MF. Delayed hypersensitivity to polysaccharides from *Nocardia*. J Immunol 1972;108:1409–1413.
49. Bojalil LF, Zamora A. Precipitin and skin tests in the diagnosis of mycetoma due to *Nocardia brasiliensis*. Proc Soc Exp Biol Med 1963;113:40–43.
50. Blumer SO, Kaufman L. Microimmunodiffusion test for nocardiosis. J Clin Microbiol 1979;10:308–312.
51. Humphreys DW, Crowder JG, White A. Serological reactions to *Nocardia* antigens. Am J Med Sci 1975;269:323–326.
52. Kohbata S, Shimokawa K. Circulating antibody to *Nocardia* in the serum of patients with Parkinson's disease. In: Narabayashi H, Nagatsu T, Yanagisawa N, Mizuno Y, eds. Advances in Neurology. New York: Raven Press, 1993:355–357.
53. Boiron P, Provost F. Enzyme immunoassay on whole *Nocardia asteroides* cells for human nocardiosis. Serodiagn Immunother Infect Dis 1988;2: 445–452.
54. Sugar AM, Schoolnik GK, Stevens DA. Antibody response in human nocardiosis identification of two immunodominant culture-filtrate antigens derived from *Nocardia asteroides*. J Infect Dis 1985;151:895–901.
55. Angeles AM, Sugar AM. Identification of a common immunodominant protein in culture filtrates of three *Nocardia* species and use in etiologic diagnosis of mycetoma. J Clin Microbiol 1987;25:2278–2280.
56. Angeles AM, Sugar AM. Rapid diagnosis of nocardiosis with an enzyme immunoassay. J Infect Dis 1987;155:292–296.

57. Boiron P, Provost F. Use of partially purified 54-kilodalton antigen for diagnosis of nocardiosis by Western blot (immunoblot) assay. J Clin Microbiol 1990;28:328–331.
58. Boiron P, Stynen D. Immunodiagnosis of nocardiosis. Gene 1992;115: 219–222.
59. Kjelstrom JA, Beaman BL. Development of a serologic panel for the recognition of nocardial infections in a murine model. Diagn Microbiol Infect Dis 1993;16:291–301.
60. El-Zaatari FA, Reiss E, Yakrus MA, et al. Monoclonal antibodies against isoelectrically focused *Nocardia asteroides* proteins characterized by the enzyme-linked immunoelectro-transfer blot method. Diagn Immunol 1986; 4:97–106.
61. Jimenez T, Diaz AM, Zlotnik H. Monoclonal antibodies to *Nocardia asteroides* and *Nocardia brasiliensis* antigens. J Clin Microbiol 1990;28:87–91.
62. Boiron P, Stynen D, Belkacem G, et al. Monoclonal antibodies to a specific 54-kilodalton antigen of *Nocardia* spp. J Clin Microbiol 1992;30:1033–1035.

16

On the Biology of Mucorales: The Etiological Agents of Mucormycoses

JOSE RUIZ-HERRERA
Centro de Investigación y de Estudios Avanzados del IPN
Irapuato, México

I. INTRODUCTION

Mucormycoses are diseases of a wide geographical distribution whose etiological agents are fungi, members of the order Mucorales. Most of the clinical cases are due to invasion by representatives of the family Mucoraceae, but members of other families of the order have also been described (Table 1) (see Ref. 1 for review). All these zygomycetous fungi (as well as the nonpathogenic species) are characterized by their coenocytic mycelium and the formation of zygospores during their sexual reproduction. They all have a saprophytic mode of life, but they behave as opportunistic pathogens, invading subjects who suffer from an underlying disease, trauma, or the abuse of certain drugs. Among the predisposing factors the most important is diabetes mellitus.

Mucormycoses are not restricted to any specific organ or tissue. They may appear in the form of skin lesions or invasion of wounds or burns; pneumonia, gastrointestinal lesions, kidney infections, brain lesions resulting from dispersion through blood vessels, sinusitis developing into rhinocerebral and craniofacial invasions, and others. In invaded tissues, Mucoraceous fungi appear mostly in the form of broad, nonpigmented, coenocytic hyphae, which characteristically invade blood vessels; but yeast forms (2) and conidiophores (3) have also been observed.

Table 1 Identified Pathogenic Species of Mucorales Responsible for Mucormycosis in Humans

Family	Genus
Mucoraceae	*Absidia*
	Apophysomyces
	Mucor
	Rhizomucor
	Rhizopus
Cunninghamellaceae	*Cunninghamella*
Thamnidiaceae	*Cokeromyces*
Saksenaceae	*Saksenaea*
Syncephalastraceae	*Syncephalastrum*

Unfortunately, there are no systematic studies on the factors involved in the pathogenesis of Mucorales. It may be tentatively suggested that host invasion is related to their high rate of growth, their capacity to secrete proteases, the low antigenicity of their cell walls, their high rates of sugar metabolism, and their ability to grow at the host's temperature. The image of a tissue infected with a mucoraceous fungus produces the impression that it is utilizing the living cells merely as an inert substrate.

II. GROWTH AND DEVELOPMENT

A. Spore Germination

The asexual life of Mucorales involves three different stages: spore, vegetative mycelium, and aerial mycelium. Spores of Mucorales are usually uninucleate, but some species, such as *Phycomyces blakesleeanus*, produce multinucleate spores. Measuring the DNA per spore, it was concluded that the only haploid *Mucor* species was *M. bacilliformis* (4). These data, however, appear to depend on the fact that, at least in *M. rouxii*, sporangiospores are in the G2 phase of the cell cycle (5). When spores are placed in a culture medium, nuclear division occurs in the absence of net DNA synthesis. Germination of sporangiospores normally occurs when they are placed into an appropriate medium, but in some cases, such as that of *P. blakesleeanus*, they require a previous activation step by a heat shock, or the addition of a chemical such as acetic acid. Spore germination of *Mucor* species requires the presence of a hexose when an inorganic nitrogen source is used. It appears that spore activation involves a rapid increase in the pool of cAMP (6). Regulation of cAMP concentration is mainly due to adenylate cyclase activity (7). Elevation in the pool levels of cAMP affect the activity of protein kinases (8,9), responsible, among other things, for trehalase activation (10,11). This enzyme transforms the accumulated disaccharide trehalose into glucose, which is used as the energy source during early phases of spore germination.

Spore germination of Mucorales has been divided into three stages (5,12). Stage Ia involves rounding of the normally ellipsoidal spore without a net increase in its larger diameter. During stage Ib, the spore increases in diameter to reach a maximal value about twice that of the initial spore's larger diameter. This stage involves net synthesis of macromolecules and organelles and not merely a swelling process. Stage II follows with the formation of germ tubes. Synthesis of specific proteins and mRNA occurs at each stage (5). In dimorphic Mucorales, spore germination may occur either in the form of germ tubes (mycelium), or buds (yeast), depending on the environmental conditions (see Fig. 1) (13). Of all the physiological effectors, the most important appear to be the presence or absence of oxygen in the atmosphere, the tension of CO_2 under anaerobic conditions, and the nature and concentration of the carbon source (7,14–16). The reported morphogenetic effect of some inhibitors or metabolites appears to be due to a derailment of the normal germination process or to interference with the action of the indicated effectors.

B. Dimorphism

It is an important observation that a large number of fungi pathogenic to humans are dimorphic, normally displaying different morphologies when invading the host or in their saprophytic living. Dimorphism thus appears an important factor in pathogenicity (17,18). Mucorales normally appear mycelial in invaded tissues, but whether yeast forms play a role during invasion, is a possibility to be analyzed. Yeast cells possess a thicker cell wall, which may help the fungus to escape from the defense mechanisms of the host. According to their growth pattern, we have recognized four groups in Mucorales (14): (a) species that grow only aerobically, in the form of mycelium; (b) species that grow mycelial under either aerobic or anaerobic conditions; (c) species that grow aerobically and anaerobically as hyphae but yeastlike if a high tension of CO_2 is supplied in anaerobiosis; and (d) species that grow mycelial in aerobiosis and yeastlike in anaerobiosis. Some species grow yeastlike when they are incubated aerobically in the presence of inhibitors of the respiratory chain (19–21); and most yeast monomorphic mutants are affected in their cytochrome content (22,23). On the other hand, as described above, anaerobiosis by itself does not

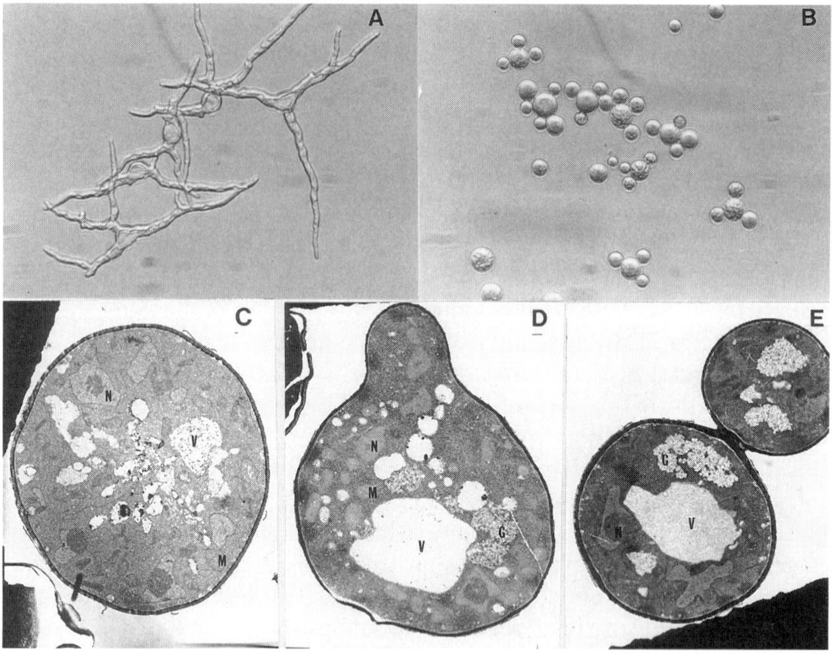

Figure 1 Dimorphic behavior of *Mucor rouxii*. A and B. Light microscopy (Nomarski); C, D, and E. Transmission electron microscopy. A and D. Germlings grown in aerobiosis. E. Yeast form grown under N_2/CO_2 (70%/30%, by vol). C. Swollen spore in stage lb. Key: N = nuclei; V = vacuoles; M = mitochondria, G = glycogen granules.

induce yeastlike growth in Mucorales belonging to group c, and at least one mutant of *M. racemosus* has been isolated that grows yeastlike in aerobiosis in the presence of glucose but whose respiratory pathway is not affected (24). These apparently contradictory data suggest that respiration by itself is not the physiological function responsible for the morphogenetic decision. We have recently made a reappraisal of the subject, and demonstrated that neither inhibitors or mutations that blocked the respiratory pathway nor ATPase inhibitors induced yeast development in *M. rouxii* (25). We have proposed that redox potential, plus catabolite repression (brought about by high concentrations of hexoses), or intracellular pH alterations (induced by CO_2), acted over a redox sensor triggering the morphogenetic response. The possibility that the sensor may have evolved from the system originally responsible for the respiratory-fermentative switch was entertained.

C. Signal Transduction in Development

Scant information exists on the mechanisms that link environmental effectors and the final morphogenetic effects. Apparently levels of cAMP constitute an important member of the transducing pathway. In dimorphic species of *Mucor* (6,9,26,27), addition of exogenous cAMP or dibutiryl cAMP inhibits germ tube emergence; instead spores continue growing isodiametrically, reaching large volumes. Spores of the monomorphic species *Mucor mucedo* (6) and *Mucor hiemalis* (28) incubated in the presence of exogenous cAMP gave rise to round and septate structures. It has also been demonstrated that addition of cAMP inhibits the yeast-to-mycelium transition and induces yeastlike growth of *M. racemosus* (29) and *M. rouxii* (30) in aerobiosis.

Evidence has accumulated suggesting that polyamine levels are involved in the cell differentiation of Mucorales. Initial observations have demonstrated that during the yeast-to-hyphae transition of *M. racemosus* (15), *M. rouxii*, and *M. bacilliformis* (31), there occurred significant elevations in the levels of ornithine decarboxylase (ODC), which is the first and most regulated enzyme of the pathway for the biosynthesis of the polyamines putrescine and spermidine [Mucorales do not contain spermine, (31,32)]. A further piece of evidence was the observation that a group of yeastlike monomorphic mutants of *M. bacilliformis* (23) all contained very low levels of ODC. Later on it was observed that the increase in enzyme and products occurred not only during the dimorphic transition but also during spore germination and sporangiophore formation (phorogenesis) of *M. rouxii* and *P. blakesleeanus* (33,34). Moreover, inhibition of ODC by the competitive inhibitor 1,4, diaminobutanone (DAB) blocked all these differentiative steps without a significant decrement in growth (33–35). Evidence has been obtained that ODC is located in at least two cellular compartments in *M. rouxii*. One of these compartments is accessible to DAB (36). Accordingly, ODC present in this compartment would be responsible for the morphogenetic phenomena. The mode of action of polyamines appears to be related to DNA methylation (37,38). It is known that methylation of DNA regulates the transcription of specific genes in many eucaryotic systems.

Protein methylation also appears to play an important role in development. Cycloleucine, an inhibitor of S-adenosylmethionine (SAM) synthetase, prevented the yeast-to-mycelium conversion in *M. racemosus* (39). This SAM is the methylating agent in biological systems. It was also demonstrated that levels of SAM correlated with morphogenesis in the same fungus (40). Analysis of methylated proteins demonstrated that their concentrations were higher in mycelial cells. The most prominent one was identified as elongation factor 1a (EF-1a) (41); it was shown that its activity in protein synthesis was directly proportional to its degree of methylation.

D. Phorogenesis

Despite the fact that the giant sporangiophore of *P. blakesleeanus* has been extensively analyzed as a model for behavior because the variety of its tropic responses (42), our knowledge on the mechanism of sporulation or phorogenesis in Mucorales is very limited. In other systems, such as *Aspergillus nidulans*, it is known that a complex mechanism involving sequential expression of regulatory and structural genes operates during sporulation (43). The data described above indicate that previous to the onset of phorogenesis in Mucorales, there occur elevations in the levels of ODC and polyamines. Addition of the ODC inhibitor DAB prevents elevation in the pool of putrescine and inhibits phorogenesis but not vegetative growth. The period of sensitivity to DAB corresponds to formation of sporangiophore primordia. Once this step has occurred, DAB has no further effect on phorogenesis. The fact that 5-methylcytosine, an inhibitor of DNA methylation, counteracts the effect of DAB was considered to be evidence that genes involved in the onset of phorogenesis are regulated by methylation (34). Blue light stimulates phorogenesis of different species. In *P. blakesleeanus*, it not only stimulates phorogenesis, but also separates two different pathways in the process. The fungus produces two kinds of aerial structures: the most typical giant sporangiophores (macrophores), and dwarf sporangiophores (microphores), roughly the size of sporangiophores of *Mucor* species. Blue light represses microphore production and stimulates macrophorogenesis. The response of the fungus revealed the existence of two photoreactions, each responding to different levels of light intensity (44,45).

III. CELL-WALL STRUCTURE AND BIOSYNTHESIS

A. General Features

One of the most salient features of Mucorales is the chemical composition and structure of the cell wall. Bartnicki-Garcia (46) proposed a division of the fungal kingdom into eight groups according to the chemical composition of their cell walls. This division agrees with other taxonomic indicators, and it is clearly in agreement with the polyphyletic origin of fungi. Cell walls of Zygomycetes are characterized by their large amounts of chitosan. Chitosan is the partially deacetylated product of chitin and contains variable proportions of glucosamine (GlcN) and *N*-acetyglucosamine (GlcNAc) moieties, joined through β 1,4 linkages. Chitosan reacts with iodine solution, producing a characteristic purple color. The possibility of utilizing this cytochemical reaction to identify hyphae from Mucorales in invaded tissues is an attractive one. In *Mucor*, *Phycomyces*, and probably other members of the group, a characteristic chemical differentiation of the cell wall occurs during spore germination. Cell wall from the spore contains large amounts of glucans. Upon germination, a new cell wall is synthesized beneath the one from the spore. This wall, which gives rise to the one from the germ tube, lacks glucans (46), but it contains small amounts of galactose and fucose (46,47). Comparison of the chemical composition of the cell wall from hyphae and yeasts of *M. rouxii* demonstrated that the latter contained larger amounts of mannans and proteins (46). Other polysaccharides present in significant amounts in the cell walls of Mucorales are polyuronides. Two polyuronides have been described in *M. rouxii*: mucoric acid, made only of glucuronic acid, and mucoran, which contains also mannose, galactose, fucose, and glucose (48). In *M. mucedo*, it was described that both, homo- and hetero-polyuronides constituted a single macromolecule (49).

B. Chitin

Rigidity of the cell wall, as occurs in most fungi, is due to the presence of the microfibrillar polysaccharide chitin. According to current models of cell-wall organization, it is considered that chitin is embedded into the amorphous components, the former being responsible for the tensile strength of the wall and the latter compounds for the resistance to pressure (see Ref. 50).

The synthesis of chitin has been amply studied in several fungi (reviewed in Refs. 50–52). The final step in the reaction, polymerization of GlcNAc units, is catalyzed by an ill-defined enzyme called chitin synthetase. It has been demonstrated that all chitin synthetases utilize uridine-diphosphate-GlcNAc (UDPGlcNAc) as the sugar donor for the polymerization reaction. Decisive evidence that the polymerization reaction does not involve a lipid intermediate was provided in *M. rouxii* (52). A group of chitin synthetases are activated in vitro by exogenous proteases, indicating that they are either zymogenic or bound to a protease-sensitive inhibitor. In *M. rouxii* (53) and *P. blakesleeanus* (54,55), the exogenous protease activates not chitin synthetase itself but an endogenous activating factor. Mycelial cells of *M. rouxii* contain a soluble acid protease that rapidly inactivates chitin synthetase (56). More recently, a second group of chitin synthetases that are not activated by exogenous proteases has been described (57).

Synthesis of chitin microfibrils in vitro was achieved for the first time using "solubilized" enzyme from the yeast form of *M. rouxii* (58). The physical nature of the enzyme was studied by electron microscopy. It appeared in the form of microvesicles that we called chitosomes (59). Chitosomes were later identified in representatives of all chitinous fungi, including other Mucorales (60). They appear to be the natural conveyors of chitin synthetase in fungi from its site of synthesis (endoplasmic reticulum?) to the cell surface, where chitin synthesis occurs (61).

Chitin synthetase is stimulated by GlcNAC that plays the role of an allosteric stimulator substituting for the real effector which is UDPGlcNAc. The catalytic reaction is cooperative and requires a divalent metal (50–52). All chitin synthetases are sensitive to two families of antibiotics of nucleoside-peptide nature. These are the polyoxins (62) and the nikkomycins (63), which behave as analogues of the substrate, UDPGlcNAc. Active concentrations in vitro are in the μmolar range, but much higher concentrations are required in vivo. Inefficacy of these compounds in most fungal systems is due to their instability and to permeability problems. Considering the absence of chitin in higher animals (and plants), inhibition of its synthesis appears as the most attractive target for therapeutic strategies. It seems reasonable to expect that chemical modifications of these antibiotics will, in the near future yield effective products for the treatment of mycoses.

Chitin synthetase from *M. rouxii* has been thoroughly purified after solubilization with digitonin. It appears in the form of a multiprotein aggregate of about 500 kDa, containing at least four polypeptides of 21, 23, 33, and 39 kDa (64). Genes coding for chitin synthetase have been cloned from several fungi. It has been demonstrated that most fungi contain more than one gene coding for the enzyme. In general, two families of genes designated respectively as *CHS* and *CSD* (or *CAL*) have been described (65). Using oligonucleotides designed for the most conserved regions of *CHS* genes and polymerase chain reaction (PCR), homologous genes have been detected in *M. rouxii* (S. Bartnicki-Garcia, personal communication) and *P. blakesleeanus* (E. Cerdá-Olmedo, personal communication). In the latter organism, genetic and biochemical studies of nikkomycin-resistant mutants defined the existence of a gene (*CHSA*) coding for the catalytic polypeptide of chitin synthetase (66).

C. Chitosan

Chitosan, the deacetylated analog of chitin, is an important component of the cell wall of Mucorales, constituting its most characteristic feature.

We have presented evidence that chitin and chitosan synthesized in vitro by membrane fractions of *M. rouxii* represent two separate polymers, having roughly the same degree of polymerization (67). Chitosan is synthesized through deacetylation of chitin by a specific deacetylase. The crystalline polymer is extremely resistant to deacetylation. The process apparently occurs simultaneously to its synthesis, or at least before crystallization of chitin takes place (67,68).

D. Polyuronides

Synthesis of polyuronides has been studied mostly in *M. rouxii*. Synthesis of the sugar donor UDP-glucuronic acid (UDPGlr) occurs by oxidation of UDP-glucose (UDPGlc) by a specific dehydrogenase that utilizes NAD and has been partially purified from both mycelial and yeast forms of the fungus. The enzymes differed in size and kinetic properties. Membrane-bound glucuronosyl transferases catalyzing the addition of glucuronosyl (Glr) residues from UDPGlr to large Mr acceptors, showed also different properties according their source, yeast or mycelial cells (69). Published evidence suggests that synthesis of the large Mr products involves the previous formation of small soluble oligodextrins which latter on are transferred to protein-bound larger polymers (70).

E. Mannoproteins

Three kind of mannoproteins have been detected in the cell walls of *M. rouxii*: high Mr acidic mannoproteins and high and low Mr neutral glycoproteins (71). Mannosyl transferases involved in their synthesis have been identified in *M. rouxii*. Activity of the enzymes was noticeably elevated during spore germination and yeast-to-hyphae transition (72). It is most likely that mannoprotein biosynthesis follows the same pathway described for *Saccharomyces* and higher eucaryotic cells (reviewed in Ref. 50). In these systems, nascent polypeptides are recognized by a ribonucleoprotein complex (signal recognition particle, or SRP), which stops their further elongation and binds to specific sites (docking proteins) located on the cytoplasmic surface of the endoplasmic reticulum (ER). Peptide elongation is resumed, and they are internalized into the ER lumen, where they become glycosylated at serine or threonine residues (O-glycosylation), and/or at asparagine residues (N-glycosylation). Whereas O-glycosylation involves the sequential transfer of mannosyl residues to make short oligomers constituted by 1 to 4 mannosyl residues, N-glycosylation involves a series of complex reactions. Acetylglucosaminyl, mannosyl, and glucosyl residues are transferred to a lipid intermediate (a dolichol). When the oligosaccharide with the composition $(GlcNAc)_2(Mann)_9(Glc)_3$ has been completed, it is transferred to the protein. At this stage the chain is processed ("trimmed") by removal of the three glucose units and one mannose unit to constitute the "oligosaccharide core." Further on, sequential addition of mannosyl units occurs, giving rise to the high-Mr mannoproteins. This growth of the "outer chain" takes place during the transfer of the proteins through the ER and the Golgi apparatus or its physiological equivalent, since Zygomycetes do not possess recognizable dictyosomes. Finally glycoproteins reach the surface of the cell by means of secretory vesicles and become associated to the wall or secreted to the surrounding medium.

IV. CELL-WALL ASSEMBLY AND MORPHOGENESIS

The final mechanism of morphogenesis in Mucorales (and the rest of fungi), must be searched out in the cell wall, which is, in turn, responsible for the shape of the fungal cells. As originally demonstrated in *M. rouxii*, wall shape is not due to gross chemical differences but mostly to its growth pattern (73). In spherical yeast cells, wall deposition occurs isodiametrically, whereas in mycelial cells it occurs at the apex—i.e., it is polarized. Using the the giant sporangiophore of *P. blakesleeanus*, it was demonstrated that this pattern of growth was due to the accumulation of chitin synthetase in the apical region (74). From theoretical considerations and experimental data (74,75), it was concluded that cell-wall polarization was the result of the short half-life of chitin synthetase. It has been concluded that cell and wall growth are dependent on the operation of the vesicular apparatus, which continuously transfers to the cell surface components and precursors of the plasmalemma and the cell wall. Vesicles accumulate at the hyphal apex and close to developing septa.

A two-dimensional model of fungal cell expansion, which represents the projection of the three-dimensional cell, has been developed by means of computer simulation (76). According to this model, cell shape is the result of the operation and spatial location in the cell of a hypothetical organelle named "vesicle delivery center" (VSC), responsible for the discharge of vesicles to the cell surface. Location of VSC in its center gives rise to an expanding spherical "cell." Its transfer toward the surface originates departure from spherical growth. When permanently located close to the advancing "hyphal" apex, it generates a cylindrical shape equivalent to mycelial growth. The mathematical derivation of the model revealed that cell shape was dependent on two parameters, the coordinates of VSC location and the rate of "vesicle" discharge. The cytological correlate was found to be the "Spitzenkörper," a complex array of vesicles and microvesicles (chitosomes) with some cytoskeletal and other ill-defined elements which exist at the apex of fungal hyphae. Association of Spitzenkörper with hyphal growth has been deduced from structural and time-lapse microphotographic studies (77,78).

It has been suggested that cytoskeletal elements constitute the mechanism involved in driving either (or both), Spitzenkörper or vesicles (reviewed in Ref. 50), although no firm evidence for this proposal has been obtained. Electrical, ionic, or pH gradients detected in all fungal hyphae studied thus far have also been proposed as likely guiding mechanisms (reviewed in Ref. 50), although several authors have proposed that electrical currents accompany but are not responsible for hyphal growth (79). We have demonstrated that dissipation of the calcium gradient in *P. blakesleeanus* by means of the addition of the calcium ionophore A23187 stops chitin synthesis, hyphal elongation and glycoprotein secretion almost immediately (75). Through electron microscopy studies, it was demonstrated that the effect of the ionophore was due to inhibition of the formation of vesicles and chitosomes.

REFERENCES

1. Kwon-Chung KJ, Bennet JE. Medical Mycology. Philadelphia: Lea & Febiger, 1992.
2. Cooper BH. A case of pseudoparacoccidioidomycosis: Detection of the yeast phase of *Mucor circinelloides* in a clinical specimen. Mycopathologia 1987; 97:189–193.
3. La Touche CJ, Sutherland, TW, Telling M. Histopathological and mycological features of a case of rhinocerebral mucormycosis (phycomycosis) in Britain. Sabouraudia 1964;3:148–150.
4. Stork R, Morrill RC. Nuclei, nucleic acids and protein in sporangiospores of *Mucor bacilliformis* and other *Mucor* species. Mycologia 1977;69:1031–1041.
5. Cano C, Ruiz-Herrera J. Developmental stages during the germination of *Mucor* sporangiospores. Exp Mycol 1988;12:47–59.
6. Orlowski M. Cyclic adenosine 3′, 5′-monophosphate and germination of sporangiospores from the fungus *Mucor*. Arch Microbiol 1980;129:133–140.
7. Orlowski M. *Mucor* dimorphism. Microbiol Rev 1991;55:234–258.
8. Moreno S, Passeron S. Further studies on cyclic adenosine 3′, 5′-monophosphate protein kinase from dimorphic fungus *Mucor rouxii*. Arch Biochem Biophys 1980;199:321–330.
9. Orlowski M. Changing pattern of cyclic AMP-binding proteins during hyphal germ tube emergence from sporangiospores of *Mucor*. Biochem J 1979;182: 547–554.
10. Van Laere AJ, Hendrix P. Cyclic AMP-dependent in vitro activation of trehalase from dormant *Phycomyces blakesleeanus* spore. J Gen Microbiol 1983; 129:3287–3290.
11. Dewerchin MA, Van Laere AJ. Trehalase activity and cyclic AMP content

during early development of *Mucor rouxii* spores. J Bacteriol 1984;158: 575–579.
12. Bartnicki-Garcia S, Nelson N, Cota-Robles E. Electron microscopy of spore germination and cell wall formation in *Mucor rouxii*. Arch Microbiol 1968; 63:242–255.
13. Bartnicki-Garcia S. Mold-yeast dimorphism of *Mucor*. Bacteriol Rev 1963; 27:297–304.
14. Ruiz-Herrera J. Dimorphism in *Mucor* species with emphasis on *M. rouxii* and *M. bacilliformis*. In: Szaniszlo JP, ed. Fungal Dimorphism. New York: Plenum Press, 1985:361–384.
15. Inderlied CB, Petres J, Cihlar RL. *Mucor racemosus*. In: Szaniszlo JP, ed. Fungal Dimorphism. New York: Plenum Press, 1985:337–359.
16. Ruiz-Herrera J. Dimorphism in *Mucor* species. In: Vanden Bossche H, Odds FC, Kerridge D, eds. Dimorphic Fungi in Biology and Medicine. New York: Plenum Press, 1993:257–265.
17. Szaniszlo JP, ed. Fungal Dimorphism. New York: Plenum Press, 1985.
18. Vanden Bossche H, Odds FC, Kerridge D, ed. Dimorphic Fungi in Biology and Medicine. New York: Plenum Press, 1993.
19. Friedenthal M, Epstein A, Passeron S. Effect of potassium cyanide, glucose and anaerobiosis on morphogenesis of *Mucor rouxii*. J Gen Microbiol 1974; 82:15–24.
20. Schulz BE, Kraepelin G, Hinkelman W. Factors affecting dimorphism in *Mycotypha* (Mucorales): A correlation with fermentation-respiration equilibrium. J Gen Microbiol 1974;81:1–13.
21. Zorzopulos J, Jobbagy AJ, Terenzi HF. Effects of ethylenediamine tetraacetate and chloramphenicol in *Mucor rouxii*. J Bacteriol 1973;115:1198–1204.
22. Storck R, Morrill R. Respiratory-deficient yeastlike mutant of *Mucor bacilliformis*. Biochem Genet 1971;5:467–479.
23. Ruiz-Herrera J, Ruiz A, Lopez-Romero E. Isolation and biochemical analysis of *Mucor bacilliformis* monomorphic mutants. J Bacteriol 1983;156: 264–272.
24. Borgia PT, Gokul NK, Phillips GJ. Respiratory-competent conditional developmental mutant of *Mucor racemosus*. J Bacteriol 1985;164:1049–1056.
25. Salcedo-Hernandez R, Ruiz-Herrera J. Isolation and characterization of a mycelial cytochrome aa_3-deficient mutant and the role of mitochondria in dimorphism of *Mucor rouxii*. Exp Mycol 1993;17:142–154.
26. Pereyra E, Zaremberg V, Moreno S. Effect of dibutyryl cAMP on growth and morphology of germinating *Mucor rouxii* sporangiospores. Exp Mycol 1992;16:93–102.
27. Wertman KF, Paznokas JL. Effects of cyclic nucleotides upon germination of *Mucor racemosus* sporangiospores. Exp Mycol 1981;5:314–322.
28. Jones BE, Bullock JD. The effect of N^6, O^2-dibutyryl adenosine 3′, 5′-monophosphate on morphogenesis in Mucorales. J Gen Microbiol 1977;103:29–36.
29. Larsen AD, Sypherd PS. Cyclic adenosine 3′, 5′-monophosphate and morphogenesis in *Mucor racemosus*. J Bacteriol 1974;117:432–438.

30. Paveto C, Epstein A, Passeron S. Studies on cyclic adenosine 3′, 5′-monophosphate levels, adenylate cyclase and phosphodiesterase activities in the dimorphic fungus *Mucor rouxii*. Arch Biochem Biophys 1975;169:449–457.
31. Calvo-Mendez C, Martinez-Pacheco M, Ruiz-Herrera J. Regulation of ornithine decarboxylase in *Mucor bacilliformis* and *Mucor rouxii*. Exp Mycol 1987;11:270–277.
32. Marshall M, Russo G, Van Etten J, Nickerson K. Polyamines in dimorphic fungi. Curr Microbiol 1979;2:187–190.
33. Martinez-Pacheco M, Rodriguez G, Reyna G, et al. Inhibition of the yeast-mycelial transition and the phorogenesis of Mucorales by diamino butanone. Arch Microbiol 1989;151:10–14.
34. Reyna-Lopez G, Ruiz-Herrera J. Polyamines and the phorogenesis of Mucorales. Exp Mycol 1993;17:79–89.
35. Ruiz-Herrera J, Calvo-Mendez C. Effect of ornithine decarboxylase inhibitors on the germination of sporangiospores of Mucorales. Exp Mycol 1987; 11:287–296.
36. Martinez-Pacheco M, Ruiz-Herrera J. Differential compartmentation of ornithine decarboxylase in cells of *Mucor rouxii*. J Gen Microbiol 1993;139: 1387–1394.
37. Cano C, Herrera-Estrella L, Ruiz-Herrera J. DNA methylation and polyamines in regulation of development of the fungus *Mucor rouxii*. J Bacteriol 1988;170:5946–5948.
38. Cano-Canchola C, Sosa L, Fonzi W, et al. Developmental regulation of CUP gene expression through DNA methylation in *Mucor* spp. J Bacteriol 1992; 174:362–366.
39. Garcia JR, Sypherd PS. S-adenosylmethionine and morphogenesis in *Mucor racemosus*. Curr Microbiol 1984;10:111–116.
40. Garcia JR, Hiatt WR, Peters J, Sypherd PS. S-adenosylmethionine levels and protein methylation during morphogenesis of *Mucor racemosus*. J Bacteriol 1980;142:196–201.
41. Hiatt WR, Garcia R, Merrick WC, Sypherd PC. Methylation of elongation factor 1a from the fungus *Mucor*. Proc Natl Acad Sci USA 1982;79: 3433–3437.
42. Cerdá-Olmedo E. Behavioral genetics of *Phycomyces*. Annu Rev Microbiol 1977;31:535–547.
43. Timberlake WE. Molecular genetics of *Aspergillus* development. Annu Rev Genet 1990;24:5–36.
44. Corrochano L, Cerdá-Olmedo E. Photomorphogenesis in *Phycomyces*: Dependence on environmental conditions. Planta 1988;174:309–314.
45. Corrochano L, Galland P, Lipson ED, Cerdá-Olmedo E. Photomorphogenesis in *Phycomyces*: Fluence-response curves and spectra. Planta 1988;174: 315–320.
46. Bartnicki-Garcia S. Cell wall chemistry, morphogenesis, and taxonomy of fungi. Annu Rev Microbiol 1968;22:87–108.
47. Obregon A, Monzalvo S, Calvo-Mendez C, Ruiz-Herrera J. Ultrastructural

and chemical alterations in germinating spores of *Mucor rouxii* (Zygomycetes) induced by two compounds which inhibit their developmental pattern. Crypt Bot 1990;1:323–332.

48. Bartnicki-Garcia S, Reyes E. Polyuronides in the cell walls of *Mucor rouxii*. Biochim Biophys Acta 1968:54–62.
49. Datema R, Van Den Ende H, Wessels JGH. The hyphal wall of *Mucor mucedo*. 1. Polyanionic polymers. Eur J Biochem 1977;80:611–619.
50. Ruiz-Herrera J. Fungal Cell Wall. Structure, Synthesis and Assembly. Boca Raton, FL: CRC Press.
51. Ruiz-Herrera J, Martinez JP, Sentandreu R. Chitin biosynthesis in fungi. In: Arora DK, Elander RP, Mukerji KG, ed. Handbook of Applied Mycology. Vol. 4. New York: Marcel Dekker, 1992:281–312.
52. Ruiz-Herrera J. Synthesis of chitin microfibrils in vitro. In: Brown RM, ed. Cellulose and other Natural Polymer Systems. New York: Plenum Press, 1982:207–223.
53. Ruiz-Herrera J, Bartnicki-Garcia S. Regulation of chitin synthetase in Mucorales. In: Muzzarelli RAA, ed. Chitin Enzymology. Ancona, Italy, European Chitin Society, 1993:35–45.
54. Reyna G, Ruiz-Herrera J. Fotoactivacion in vitro de la quitina sintetasa de los esporangioforos de *Phycomyces blakesleeanus*. Rev Mex Micol 1987;3: 249–263.
55. Martinez-Cadena G, Ruiz-Herrera J. Activation of chitin synthetase from *Phycomyces blakesleeanus* by calcium and calmodulin. Arch Microbiol 1987; 148:280–285.
56. Diaz S, Ruiz-Herrera J. Purification of an acid protease from *Mucor rouxii* that inactivates chitin synthetase. Antonie van Leeuwenhoeck 1987;53: 279–291.
57. Orlean P. Two chitin synthetases in *Saccharomyces cerevisiae*. J Biol Chem 1987;262:5732–5739.
58. Ruiz-Herrera J, Bartnicki S. Synthesis of cell wall microfibrils in vitro by a "soluble" chitin synthetase from *Mucor rouxii*. Science 1974;186:357–359.
59. Bracker CE, Ruiz-Herrera J, Bartnicki-Garcia S. Structure and transformation of chitin synthetase particles (chitosomes) during microfibril synthesis in vitro. Proc Natl Acad Sci USA 1976;73:4570–4574.
60. Bartnicki-Garcia S, Bracker CE, Reyes E, Ruiz-Herrera J. Isolation of chitosomes from taxonomically diverse fungi and synthesis of chitin microfibrils in vitro. Exp Mycol 1978;2:173–192.
61. Ruiz-Herrera J. The role of chitosomes in the apical growth of fungi. In: Nombela C, ed. Microbial Cell Wall Synthesis and Autolysis. Amsterdam: Elsevier, 1984:113–120.
62. Endo A, Kakiki K, Misato T. Mechanism of action of the antifungal agent polyoxin D. J Bacteriol 1970;104:189–196.
63. Dahn U, Hagenmeier H, Hohne H, et al: Stoffwechselsprodukte von Mikroorganismen, 154 Mitteilung. Nikkomycin, ein neuer Hemmstoff der Chitinsynthese bei Pilzen. Arch Microbiol 1976;107:143–160.

64. Lending CR, Leal-Morales CA, Flores-Martinez A, et al: Purification and characterization of 16S chitin synthetase particles from cell walls of *Mucor rouxii*. Exp Mycol 1991;15:11–25.
65. Bulawa CE. Genetics and molecular biology of chitin synthesis in fungi. Annu Rev Microbiol 1993;147:505–534.
66. Cubero B, Ruiz-Herrera J, Cerdá-Olmedo E. Chitin synthetase mutants of *Phycomyces blakesleeanus*. Mol Gen Genet 1993;40:9–16.
67. Calvo-Mendez C, Ruiz-Herrera J. Biosynthesis of chitosan in membrane fractions from *Mucor rouxii* by the concerted action of chitin synthetase and a particulate deacetylase. Exp Mycol 1987;11:128–140.
68. Davis LL, Bartnicki-Garcia S. The coordination of chitosan and chitin synthesis in *Mucor rouxii*. J Gen Microbiol 1984;130:2095–2102.
69. Dow JM, Olona PM, Villa VD. Glucuronosyl transferase from the dimorphic fungus *Mucor rouxii*. Exp Mycol 1982;6:329–334.
70. Dow JM, Carreon RR, Villa VD. Role of membranes of mycelial *Mucor rouxii* in synthesis and secretion of cell wall matrix polymers. J Bacteriol 1981;145:1088–1093.
71. Dow JM, Rubbery PH. Chemical fractionation of the cell walls of mycelial and yeast-like forms of *Mucor rouxii*: A comparative study of the polysaccharides and glycoprotein components. J Gen Microbiol 1977;99:29–41.
72. Gutierrez F, Ruiz-Herrera J. Mannosyl transferase from yeast and hyphal forms of *Mucor rouxii*. Exp Mycol 1979;3:351–362.
73. Bartnicki-Garcia S, Lippman E. Fungal morphogenesis: Cell wall construction in *Mucor rouxii*. Science 1969;165:302–304.
74. Herrera-Estrella L, Ruiz-Herrera J. Light response in *Phycomyces*: Evidence for roles of chitin biosynthesis and breakdown. Exp Mycol 1983;7: 362–369.
75. Ruiz-Herrera J, Valenzuela C, Martinez-Cadena G, Obregon A. Alterations in the vesicular pattern and wall growth of *Phycomyces* induced by the calcium ionophore A23187. Protoplasma 1989;148:15–25.
76. Bartnicki-Garcia S, Hergert F, Gierz G. Computer simulation of fungal morphogenesis and the mathematical basis for hyphal (tip) growth. Protoplasma 1989;153:46–57.
77. Girbardt M. Die Ultrastruktur der Apikalregion von Pilzhyphen. Protoplasma 1969:413–441.
78. Grove SN. Bracker CE. Protoplasmic organization of hyphal tips among fungi: Vesicles and Spitzenkörper. J Bacteriol 1970;104:989–1009.
79. Harold FM, Caldwell JH. Tips and currents: Electrobiology of apical growth. In: Heath IB, ed. Tip Growth in Plant and Fungal Cells. New York: Academic Press, 1990:59–90.

17

Antifungal Vaccinology

LUCIANO POLONELLI, STEFANIA CONTI, MARA GERLONI, PAOLA FISICARO, CRISTINA CANTELLI, and WALTER MAGLIANI
University of Parma
Parma, Italy

I. INTRODUCTION

The science of vaccinology introduced by Jenner and developed by Pasteur has represented a crucial factor in the control and, in some cases, the eradication of numerous infectious diseases with a bacterial or viral etiology. More limited success has been attained in the control of mycotic and parasitic diseases. The opportunistic nature of the fungi, the predisposition of patients with congenital and acquired deficiencies to fungal infections, and the evident natural immunity to reinfection have spurred the search for efficacious and safe antifungal vaccines. Aside from the prevention of the dermatophytoses, of interest primarily to veterinarians, in that large-scale immunization of animals has drastically reduced the number of dermatophytic infections among the involved laborers, especially in the countries of Eastern Europe (1,2), research in medical mycology was turned toward the development of effective vaccines against the etiological agents of the systemic mycoses, such as aspergillosis, blastomycosis, candidiasis, coccidioidomycosis, cryptococcosis, histoplasmosis capsulati, and zygomycosis, which can lead to fatalities in immunocompromised hosts. Efforts have been made to induce protective immunity to the superficial infections caused by dermatophytes, *Candida*, and *Malassezia*. The results of the investigations indicate that a vaccine for prophylaxis of the corresponding diseases is not forthcoming (3). The majority of the studies for preventing deep-seated mycoses were carried out on laboratory animals and only a few of the experimental efforts led to results that encouraged clinical trials on humans.

II. VACCINES AGAINST ASPERGILLOSIS

Aspergillosis is a cosmopolitan disease, primarily pulmonary in nature, which results from the inhalation of the airborne conidia of several species of the genus *Aspergillus* (*A. fumigatus*, *A. flavus*, *A. niger*, and *A. terreus* in particular), which are environmentally ubiquitous. In its varied clinical manifestations—allergic bronchopulmonary aspergillosis, aspergilloma, invasive aspergillosis—this mycosis primarily affects individuals predisposed to infection who are afflicted with neoplasms or cystic fibrosis, who have serious forms of neutropenia or who have been subjected to long-term therapy with immunosuppressive medications or antibiotics. In view of the fact that disseminated aspergillosis can lead to a poor prognosis and even to a high rate of fatalities, studies directed to the prevention of this important opportunistic disease have been relatively few in number. Experimental attempts to induce immunoprotection have been carried out in mice (*Mus musculus*) treated with cortisones and utilizing live conidia of *A. fumigatus* (4). The vaccinated animals demonstrated, in the course of the experimental infections, a significant extension of survival, presumably referable to the clearance of most of the fungal propagules from their lungs. In more recent studies, turkeys (*Meleagris gallopavo*) were immunized with two different vaccines and three different adjuvants. Acquired immunity was verified by exposing the birds to sublethal conidial aerosols of *A. fumigatus*. It was observed that the germling (germinated conidia) vaccines of this *Aspergillus* species gave greater protection according to their growth on different media and especially when associated with the lipopolysaccharide of *Pasteurella multocida*, which was used as an adjuvant. The immunoprotection of the vaccinated turkeys was verified in comparison to that of nonimmunized animals on the basis of the number of pulmonary lesions and on the semiquantitative culture data per gram of pulmonary tissue (5). In respect to allergic bronchopulmonary aspergillosis, however, the concept of vaccination should be directed more specifically to the possibility of desensitization.

III. VACCINES AGAINST BLASTOMYCOSIS

Blastomycosis is an unevenly distributed mycosis that is endemic in certain regions of North America (Canada, the United States), Europe (Poland), Africa, the Middle East (Israel, Saudi Arabia), and Asia (India). This systemic disease is caused by the dimorphic fungus *Blastomyces dermatitidis*, whose conidia, produced by its mycelial form, are inhaled from the natural environment, being naturally present in suitable ecological niches. The disease is basically pulmonary, even though, in immunocompromised hosts, it can disseminate to various organs, including the skin, by way of the venous and lymphatic systems. Resistance to infection is essentially represented by cellular immunity as revealed by the classic reaction of delayed hypersensitivity. Attempts to induce immunity to blastomycosis were carried out utilizing subcellular fractions of the etiologic agent's yeast forms (6), the living organism (7,8), or substances capable of nonspecifically stimulating immunity with muramyl dipeptide and its dismethyl analogue (9). Utilizing the insoluble fraction of the yeast form of *B. dermatitidis*, obtained by sonication, as a vaccine, it was possible to obtain a significant increase of survival in the mice infected intraperitoneally and intravenously with the conidia from the mycelial form. In contrast, no protection resulted with the use of the yeast form cells. Increments of survival were observed in mice inoculated subcutaneously with viable propagules and infected intraperitoneally after 2 weeks. The resistance was clearly related to cell-mediated immunity. This was demonstrable through a retarded hypersensitivity reaction and the possibility of transferring immunity through T lymphocytes but not with serum.

IV. VACCINES AGAINST CANDIDIASIS

The majority of the completed studies in relation to vaccines have been directed toward *Candida albicans* on the basis of the multiplicity and importance of its clinical manifestations. Its endogenicity in humans has also been an important stimulus. These characteristics make this polymorphic yeast the most prevalent opportunistic pathogen among immunocompromised hosts. Early immunization studies in respect to candidiasis have been pursued in animals, especially in mice and rabbits (*Lepus cuniculus*). Heat-killed cells of *C. albicans*, when inoculated intravenously into rabbits (10), as well as viable cells (11) were not capable of conferring active immunity when challenged with experimental infections. This failure occurred notwithstanding a demonstrable elevated agglutination titer in the immune serum, which was incapable of conferring passive immunity to nonimmunized animals. On the other hand, contrasting results were obtained with the same experimental model using those vaccines of *C. albicans* made up of yeast cells that had been killed, attenuated by heat, or with ethanol or irradiated with γ-rays. These vaccines gave evidence that cellular immunity played a protective role in the vaccinated animals, which could be inferred histologically from the reactivity state of the lymph nodes (12–14). Comparative experimental studies, utilizing either living cells of *C. albicans* or cells killed with merthiolate or sonication when inoculated subcutaneously in mice, demonstrated, following intravenous infection with yeast cells, a significantly reduced mortality rate in comparison to unvaccinated controls, which suffered a complete mortality (15). It is interesting to note how the serum from the animals vaccinated with the most efficaceous immunogen, the yeast cells of *C. albicans* killed by sonication, was capable of conferring passive immunity to unvaccinated animals (16,17). Mechanically disintegrated cells have been shown, through experiments based on their capacity to protect against muscle damage, to possess an elevated immunological protective capacity for mice (18). On the other hand, contradictory experiments have led to postulations that immunity against candidiasis can be exclusively acquired through vaccination with living cells of *C. albicans* (19).

Comparative studies, carried out as a function of survival times, have made it possible to single out in the cell walls of *C. albicans*, inoculated either subcutaneously or intraperitoneally, the cellular component with the greatest immunogenic potential in mice experimentally infected intravenously (20). Repeated subcutaneous inoculations have demonstrated, on the other hand, the capacity to confer efficaceous immunoprotection to a significant number of the vaccinated mice. The protective effect was correlated subsequently to the immunostimulatory potential of the cell walls and cytoplasmic extracts of *C. albicans* (21), which could also be increased by nonspecific immunostimulators such as the P40 fraction of *Corynebacterium granulosum*. The enhancement by *Bordetella pertussis* vaccine given alone or as an adjuvant when administered with a sublethal dose of *C. albicans* cells on acquired resistance to murine candidiasis has been also reported (22). A mouse model has been also used for the study of resistance to reinfection following the cure of cutaneous candidiasis (23).

In regard to the endogenous saprophytism of *C. albicans*, studies have been carried out among gnotobiotic animals in order to establish the role played by natural immunity against candidiasis (24). It was revealed that axenic rats (*Rattus norvegicus*) were significantly more susceptible to intravenous infection with cells of *C. albicans* than animals already colonized. This resistance, however, could be induced by vaccination with formalin-killed yeast cells associated with complete Freund's adjuvant. Immunoprotection was definite in respect of the histological aspects and to kidney colonization on the basis of microscopic findings and semiquantitative cultural data.

Later studies downplayed the importance of cell-mediated immunity in comparison to that of humoral immunity against candidiasis (25). Mice immunized intraperitoneally with live cells of *C. albicans* and which demonstrated delayed-type hypersensitivity in antigenic confrontations, were rendered, in respect to survival time, more protected against systemic infection challenge than unvaccinated mice. On the contrary, absence of correlation between delayed-type hypersensitivity and immunoprotection against systemic candidiasis has been reported also in mice (26). In addition, it was revealed that the transfer of specific antibodies to mice that gave positive delayed hypersensitivity reactions could increase resistance to candidiasis, while no effect was observable in the control animals. This allows one to presume a role, although a secondary one, in humoral immunity united to the predominant cellular immunity in the control of infections.

A study involving a patient with chronic mucocutaneous candidiasis demonstrated, following vaccination with heat-killed cells of *C. albicans*, a transient abrogation of immunosuppression, suggesting how different immune responses can independently provide protection against superficial and systemic candidiasis and how an eventual failure of the response to superficial infections does not necessarily imply the absence of protection against dissemination (27). Clinical observations and experimental studies attest that although T lymphocytes are important in preventing mucocutaneous candidiasis, an antibody response to the immunodominant 47-kDa antigen of *C. albicans*, which is associated with the recovering, could play an important role against the dissemination of the infection (28). The occurrence of these antibodies could account for the rarity of systemic candidiasis in patients with chronic mucocutaneous candidiasis and AIDS. The 47-kDa antigen characterized as the heat-shock protein enolase could represent a potential vaccine for immunization against disseminated candidal infections.

On the basis of the information acquired on the efficacy of antimicrobial ribosomal vaccines (29), numerous studies have been undertaken to evaluate their effectiveness in the field of medical mycology. The experimental results have revealed that ribosomal vaccines can be equally protective to animals that were immunocompetent, immunocompromised, or afflicted with neoplasmas when confronted with systemic candidiasis (30,31). This immunoprotection became evident by a significant increase in survival time as well as by a reduction in parasitized tissue in the kidney, the target organ in disseminated candidiasis (32). Vaccines made up of *C. albicans* ribosomes were protective even against infections caused by other species of *Candida* (33) and were capable of providing a specific humoral or cell-mediated response (34). In addition, candidacidal cells appeared in the spleen of mice vaccinated with *C. albicans*.

A clinical study was carried out on women who experienced frequent episodes of recurring vulvovaginal candidiasis utilizing an oral vaccine made up of ribosomes extracted from cultures of the A and B serotypes of *C. albicans* and utilizing, as an adjuvant, the proteoglycan from the membrane of an acapsulated isolate of *Klebsiella pneumoniae* with clear signs of a reduction in recurrent infections (41).

An alternative experimental approach against systemic and mucosal candidiasis was carried out in a model of idiotypic vaccination in mice and oophorectomized, estradiol-treated rats. The animals were concurrently immunized along with Freund's adjuvant with a monoclonal antibody that neutralized a killer toxin of *Pichia anomala* that is active against an isolate of *C. albicans* which is used for intravenous or vaginal infections. The significant immunoprotection, as measured in regard to prolongation of survival time or a decrease in the time of colonization of the vaccinated animals in respect to the unvaccinated ones or those treated with an irrelevant isotype-matched monoclonal antibody and similarily inoculated, was referable to the elevated titer in circulation or in vaginal fluid of yeast killer toxin–like antiidiotypic antibodies. These antibodies, when purified against the complementary monoclonal antibody, had shown that they expressed in vitro the same antimycotic action as the internal imaged killer toxin. The recognition of passive immunoprotection by transfer of yeast killer toxin–like antibodies permitted one to presume an in vivo antibiotic activity (42,43).

V. VACCINES AGAINST COCCIDIOIDOMYCOSIS

Coccidioidomycosis is a mycosis caused by the dimorphic fungus *Coccidioides immitis*, exclusively endemic in certain regions of the United States, Mexico, and Central and South America. The disease is contracted through the inhalation of the arthroconidia of the saprophytic form of the fungus, which lives in the soil of desertlike areas of the New World. In parasitized tissues, the mold develops in the form of spherules which, when mature, are filled with endospores that can also be induced in vitro when the fungus is grown on special media. Even though coccidioidomycosis may remain asymptomatic or manifest itself in a self-limited mild respiratory infection, it may, in some immunocompromised patients, disseminate and often prove fatal. On the basis of epidemiological observations of acquired immunity following exposure to the fungus in the endemic areas, numerous studies have been carried out with the objective of obtaining an effective vaccine against the disease. The initial experiments had utilized such immunogens as heat-killed spherules developed in the amniotic sac of chicken embryos (44) or heat-killed arthroconidia (45). Both methods conferred some immunity in dogs that had been exposed to an infectious aerosol or intraperitoneally inoculated with the arthroconidia of *C. immitis*. The degree of protection was measured on the basis of survival time and histological study of the number of foci of pulmonary infection or in the lymph nodes of the vaccinated animals in comparison to the controls (46).

The best results on the prevention of coccidioidomycosis were obtained in the studies that utilized vaccines made from the cell walls of spherules grown in vitro (47,48). These preparations were developed to the stage where they were used in human experiments (49–51). Those studies revealed that the intramuscular route of immunization was the most effective (52,53), especially if it was repeated with several doses (54). This vaccine was especially effective, even in primates, against infections experimentally produced with living arthroconidia from the fungal isolate used as an immunogen as well as heterologous isolates that were administered intranasally, the route most similar to the natural one (55,56). The intramuscular route of immunization was especially efficient, moreover, in establishing cell-mediated immunity, the most effective type against infections. Immunoprotection was manifested in the reduction of proliferation of the fungus in host tissue and reduced dissemination from the initial site of the infection, generally the lungs, which significantly augmented survival time. The vaccine, however, did not hinder the development of infections (57) with the formation of granulomas which, nevertheless, prevented the risk of dissemination.

The human experiments, even though they gave equivocal results (58), permitted verification that the vaccine was relatively safe. It only rarely produced side effects in the immunized individuals, who developed specific responses that were either humoral or cell-mediated (59,60).

A clone encoding for a β-galactosidase fusion protein stimulating a murine T cell line responding to a soluble conidial cell wall fraction of *C. immitis* has been isolated from a λgt11 library. The predicted amino acid sequence has shown partial identity with the corresponding regions of F antigens, a model protein for the study of immunoreactivity and self-tolerance in mice. Amino acid homology of murine F antigens with human 4-hydroxyphenylpyruvate led to speculate that the T-cell-stimulating protein is likely to be the *C. immitis* form of the same enzyme, which might represent a good candidate for vaccination studies (61).

VI. VACCINES AGAINST CRYPTOCOCCOSIS

Cryptococcosis is a disease caused by the basidiomycetes yeast *Cryptococcus neoformans* var. *neoformans* (serotypes A or D) or var. *gattii* (serotypes B and C). The *neoformans* variety of *C. neoformans* is primarily found in soil contaminated with the feces of domestic pigeons (*Colum-*

bus livia). The disease is generally contracted through inhalation of this yeast's blastoconidia from the environment. Infections by the *gattii* variety are rare outside of Australia. There, this variety has been found to be associated with *Eucalyptus camaldulensis* (river red gum tree) and *Eucalyptus tereticornis* (forest red gum tree) (62,63). The infection initially involves the lungs but, in patients compromised in their cell-mediated immunity and in particular afflicted with AIDS, it can rapidly disseminate to the central nervous system due to the clearcut neurotropism of this yeast.

The first experimental studies on conferring active or passive immunity against disseminated infection—which, if not treated early, may end fatally—have not given satisfactory results. Such failure underlines how a certain amount of immunoprotection can be induced exclusively by utilizing living cell vaccines even though an enhancing effect of a *Bordetella pertussis* vaccine with a nonviable *C. neoformans* yeast cell vaccine had been reported on resistance to murine cryptococcosis (64–68). Later studies were based on the use of vaccines made from acapsular isolates of *C. neoformans* var. *neoformans* rendered avirulent by exposure to γ-rays (69). The results obtained were satisfactory in relation to the level of survival following infection after immunization either by subcutaneous or intraperitoneal routes. Encouraging results were also obtained with a variant of *C. neoformans* that produced pseudohyphae and was rendered avirulent by being grown with a soil amoeba (70). More recent studies have been carried out for the induction of cell-mediated immunity to cryptococcosis through a localized skin infection (71,72). This procedure, although conferring some protection against experimental systemic infection, was precluded from the necessity of utilizing live yeasts. Complementary experiments have shown, among other things, the possibility of immunizing against lethal infections by employing formalin-killed blastocells of *C. neoformans* var. *neoformans* for intranasal vaccination, the most natural infectious route, in presumable relation to the phagocytic activity of the alveolar macrophages (71). Vaccines, potentially utilizable against the rising tide of cryptococcosis, have been sought by taking advantage of the immunogenic characteristics of the various antigenic fractions of *C. neoformans* var. *neoformans* to stimulate cell-mediated immunity. The antibody response of mice to serotype A *C. neoformans* capsular polysaccharide compared after experimental cryptococcal infection and immunization with a serotype A glucuronoxylomannan–tetanus toxoid conjugate vaccine has shown that some antibodies elicited by infection or by immunization bind to the same antigenic determinant (O-acetyl groups) in the glucuronoxylomannan (73). The *C. neoformans* serotype

A glucuronoxylomannan protein conjugate has been synthesized, characterized, and retested for antigenicity, appearing suitable for clinical evaluation as a vaccine (74). Encouraging results have been also obtained by utilizing a noncapsular carbohydrate (75). Experiments on humans have centered almost exclusively on testing the effectiveness of a cryptococcal vaccine made up of alcohol-killed blastoconidia combined with nystatin for the treatment of pulmonary cryptococcosis. The results were apparently satisfying (76).

VII. VACCINES AGAINST HISTOPLASMOSIS CAPSULATI

Histoplasmosis capsulati is a disease caused by the *capsulatum* variety of *Histoplasma capsulatum*, which commonly is recovered, throughout the world, in its saprophytic form from soil enriched with the feces of birds or bats. When its microconidia are inhaled, the fungus can multiply in tissues in the form of yeast cells, especially in the cells of the reticuloendothelial system. The infection, which may develop asymptomatically, can evolve into a disease initially confined to the lungs, and, in immunocompromised hosts, becoming invasive and disseminating to other internal organs, i.e., the central nervous system. The epidemiological observation that asymptomatic individuals become positive for a delayed hypersensitivity reaction with histoplasmin attests that the infection may induce an acquired state of immunity even through vaccination. This would constitute a means of prevention which could be of value to the great number of individuals who are potentially subject to infection in the endemic areas.

Initial studies have indicated the possibility of conferring partial immunity for a limited period of time to mice vaccinated with the yeast form cells of *H. capsulatum* var. *capsulatum* that were either killed with formalin or dried in acetone and infected with living cells intracerebrally (77,78).

Similarly, it has been ascertained that a sublethal infection by the var. *capsulatum* is capable of inducing partial immunoprotection to a successive lethal dose in mice or guinea pigs. In this instance, it was determined that the immunoprotective antigen resided in a cell wall fraction of the yeast form (79) or in its autolysate from a broth culture (80). Immunoprotection by acellular antigens against high infectious dosages, although less than that provided by whole killed yeast cells of the *capsulatum* variety of *H. capsulatum*, which are more immunogenic by various inoculation routes, was verified even when a polysaccharidic preparation of this fungus was used (81). Experimental evidence supporting the possibility of vaccination against histoplamosis capsulati spurred more research featuring different approaches for administrating the antigens, in preparing the reagents, and in the use of experimental animals. Some animal models were studied to prevent dissemination from the primary site of infection, the lung, utilizing as antigen a cell-wall polysaccharide of *H. capsulatum* var. *capsulatum*. It was administered intramuscularly to guinea pigs successively infected intratracheally and monitored for immunoprotection through culturing the spleens of the animals spontaneously dead or sacrificed during the experiment (82). Comparative studies carried out on other animal models, including primates, and with a variety of antigens and inoculation routes, revealed how the living yeast form cells of the *capsulatum* variety of *H. capsulatum* were the most immunogenic and most capable of inducing the highest titer of complement fixing antibodies as well as a reaction of cell-mediated immunity correlated to a certain level of immunoprotection (82). Studies directed toward the determination of the immune mechanism implied in the resistance to histoplasmosis capsulati were carried out utilizing, in a comparative way, antigens derived from the cell walls of this fungus or from living cells (83,84). Both of these antigens induced a measurable cell-mediated response in vivo utilizing histoplasmin and in vitro with assays of lymphocytic transformation involving cell-wall glycoproteins or soluble cytoplasmic extracts. The greatest immunoprotection, however, was manifest in the animals that had been actually infected. The use of athymic mice, moreover, made it possible to demonstrate the vital importance of T lymphocytes in the immunological process against infections caused by the *capsulatum* variety of *H. capsulatum* (85). Ribosomal fractions, composed essentially of proteins, were successively investigated for their immunogenicity, demonstrating how, under optimal conditions, such vaccines would confer a high degree of specific protection against histoplasmosis capsulati caused by the same or heterologous ones (86), stimulating a specific response that was either humoral or cell-mediated (87,88) and played a predominant role in the immunological process.

An alternative approach to immunity against histoplasmosis capsulati has been proposed employing *p*-chloromercuriphenylsulphonic acid (PCMS) a sulfhydryl inhibitor with the capability to specifically prevent the conversion of the mycelial form of *H. capsulatum* var. *capsulatum* to its yeast form (89). The impossibility of the mycelial form of this fungus to convert to its yeast form when treated with this compound was permanent and irreversible. Mycelium treated in this manner was incapable of infecting laboratory animals. The mycelium could immunologically stimulate resistance against infection by isolates of *H. capsulatum* var. *capsulatum* that had not been treated with PCMS.

VIII. VACCINES AGAINST ZYGOMYCOSIS

Zygomyçosis (cutaneous, subcutaneous, and systemic) is an opportunistic mycosis that especially involves immunocompromised individuals. It is caused most frequently by species of *Absidia*, *Rhizomucor*, and *Rhizopus*. Zygomycosis has a global distribution and the systemic form, the most serious one, results from the inhalation of the sporangiospores of the pathogenic species that are diffused into the environment. Some of the zygomycetes tend, in hosts with a predisposition to acidotic diabetes and uremia, to develop in rhinocerebral sites an almost inevitably fatal infection. Although such patients would need an effective vaccine, such pertinent studies have been rare. Experimental immunizations have been carried out on mice utilizing various immunogens extracted from *A. ramosa* (90). These represented formalin-killed spores, hyphal cell walls, and extracts from mechanically disrupted mycelium used either singly or collectively with Freund's incomplete adjuvant. These studies revealed, under some conditions, a certain level of immunity inferable from clinical, histological, and cultural observations, as given by an evident humoral and cell-mediated response. This immunity, however, was not comparable to that obtained by using as immunogen a sublethal concentration of live sporangiospores. A passive immunization was achieved against zygomycosis in an animal model with mice vaccinated intraperitoneally with a soluble antigen prepared from *Rhizomucor pusillus*. Ascitic fluid taken from the vaccinated animals and transferred to mice that were unvaccinated but had been rendered immunopredisposed with cortisone and injected intranasally with spores of *R. pusillus* demonstrated a certain level of immunoprotection and limitations in the process of dissemination (91).

IX. CONCLUSIONS

In regard to other diseases caused by bacterial and viral infections, additional studies are needed with the objective of obtaining antifungal vaccines that can be satisfactorily used clinically on humans, especially for such mycoses as aspergillosis, blastomycosis, and zygomycosis. Up to now, one of the major obstacles in antifungal vaccinology is represented by the endosaprophytic nature of some etiological agents and by the necessity to use vaccines made up of living microorganisms in order to obtain effective immunoprotection. Such a situation is completely unacceptable for preventing mycotic diseases. Conceivably, the administration modalities in fungal vaccination should be more properly considered in order to simulate the natural route of the infection. However, the development of new subcellular or acellular immunogens and new vaccination modalities, sought especially with rccombinant DNA technologies, and eventually combined with cytokines therapy, are promising for use in an immunological strategy even against the most epidemiologically relevant mycoses.

REFERENCES

1. Sarkisov AK, Koromyslov G. The prevention and control of animal dermatophytoses. Clin Insight 1988;3:313–316.
2. Sarkisov AK, Kolesnikov AY. Towards eradication of dermatomycoses. Veterinariya (Moskva) 1989;12:36–38.
3. Segal E. Vaccines for the management of dermatophyte and superficial yeast infections. Curr Top Med Mycol 1989;3:36–49.
4. Kisch AL, Echols RM, Maydew RP. Protective efficacy of antifungal immunization in opportunistic murine pulmonary aspergillosis. Clin Res 1979;27: 2685–2689.
5. Richard JL, Peden WM, Sacks JM. Effects of adjuvant augmented germlings vaccines in turkey poults challenged with *Aspergillus fumigatus*. Avian Dis 1991;35:93–99.
6. Landay ME, Hotchi M, Soares N. Effect of prior vaccination on experimental blastomycosis. Mycopathol Mycol Appl 1972;46:61–64.
7. Brummer E, Morozumi PA, Stevens DA. Protection against pulmonary blastomycosis: Adoptive transfer with T-lymphocytes, but not serum, from resistant mice. Cell Immunol 1982;73:349–359.
8. Spencer WD, Cozad GC. Role of delayed hypersensitivity in blastomycosis of mice. Infect Immun 1973;7:329–334.
9. Morozumi PA, Brummer E, Stevens DA. Immunostimulation with muramyl dipeptide and its desmethyl analogue: studies of non-specific resistance to pulmonary blastomycosis in inbred mouse strains. Mycopathologia 1983;81: 35–39.
10. Hurd RC, Drake CH. *Candida albicans* infections in actively and passively immunized animals. Mycopathol Mycol Appl 1953;6:290–297.
11. Winner HI. Immunity in experimental moniliasis. J Path Bacteriol 1956;71: 234–237.
12. Balogh E, Kakuk G, Halmy K, Szabolcsi M. Experimental investigation of immunoreactivity against *Candida albicans*: I. Reaction of rabbits immunized with *Candida albicans* and challenged with living *Candida albicans*. Mykosen 1971;14:385–392.
13. Kuttin ES, Muller J, Douchet C, Vogt A. Immunological and pathological observations with *Candida albicans* infected animals. Sabouraudia 1983;21: 185–194.
14. Mikami Y, Tabeta H, Arai T. Role of active immunization in the resistance to *Candida albicans* infection in mice. Jpn J Med Mycol 1983;24:165–171.
15. Mourad S, Friedman L. Active immunization of mice against *Candida albicans*. Proc Soc Exp Biol Med 1961;106:570–572.

16. Mourad S, Friedman L. Passive immunization of mice against *Candida albicans*. Sabouraudia 1968;6:103–105.
17. Pearsall NN, Adams BL, Bunni R. Immunologic responses to *Candida albicans*: III. Effects of passive transfer of lymphoid cells or serum on murine candidiasis. J Immunol 1978;120:1176–1180.
18. Oblack DL, Holder IA. Active immunization of mice against muscle damage mediated by *Candida albicans*. J Med Microbiol 1979;12:503–506.
19. Hasenclever HF, Mitchel WO. Acquired immunity to candidiasis in mice. J Bacteriol 1963;86:401–406.
20. Dobias B. Specific and nonspecific immunity in *Candida* infections: Experimental studies on the role of *Candida* cells constituents and review of the literature. Acta Med Scand 1964;176:1–79.
21. Drouhet E, Dupont B. Immunisation par *Candida albicans* et immunostimulation non specifique par *Corynebacterium granulosum* et BCG dans la candidose experimentale. CR Acad Sci Paris 1976;283:1385–1388.
22. Hasenclever HF, Corley EJ. Enhancement of acquired resistance in murine candidiasis by *Bordetella pertussis* vaccine. Sabouraudia 1968;6:289–295.
23. Giger DK, Domer JE, McQuitty JT Jr. Experimental murine candidiasis: Pathological and immune responses to cutaneous inoculation with *Candida albicans*. Infect Immun 1978;19:496–509.
24. Rogers TJ, Balish E. Immunity to experimental renal candidiasis in rats. Infect Immun 1978;19:737–740.
25. Kagaya K, Shinoda T, Fukazawa Y. Murine defense mechanism against *Candida albicans* infection: I. Collaboration of cell-mediated and humoral immunities in protection against systemic *C. albicans* infection. Microbiol Immunol 1981;25:647–654.
26. Hurtrel B, Lagrarge PH, Michel JC. Absence of correlations between delayed-type hypersensitivity and protection in experimental systemic candidiasis in immunized mice. Infect Immun 1981;31:95–101.
27. Burford-Mason AP, Matthews RC, Williams JR. Transient abrogation of immunosuppression in a patient with chronic mucocutaneous candidiasis following vaccination with *Candida albicans*. J Infect 1987;14:47–57.
28. Matthews R, Burnie J, Smith D, et al. *Candida* and AIDS. Evidence for protective antibody. Lancet 1988;2:263–265.
29. Youmans AS, Youmans GP. Immunogenic activity of a ribosomal fraction obtained from *Mycobacterium tuberculosis*. J Bacteriol 1965;89:1291–1298.
30. Levy R, Segal E, Eylan E. Protective immunity against murine candidiasis elicited by *Candida albicans* ribosomal fractions. Infect Immun 1981;31: 874–878.
31. Segal E, Sandovsky-Losica H. Experimental vaccination with *Candida albicans* ribosomes in cyclophosphamide treated animals. Sabouraudia 1981;19: 267–273.
32. Levy R, Segal E, Barr-Nea L. Systemic candidiasis in mice immunized with *Candida albicans* ribosomes. Mycopathologia 1985;91:17–22.
33. Segal E, Nussbaum S, Barr-Nea L. Protection against systemic infections

with various *Candida* species elicited by vaccination with *Candida albicans* ribosomes. Sabouraudia J Med Vet Mycol 1985;23:275–285.
34. Levy R, Segal E, Eylan E. Detection of antibodies against *Candida albicans* ribosomes by the enzyme linked immunosorbent assay. Mycopathologia 1984;87:167–170.
35. Levy R, Segal E. Induction of a candicidal activity in mice by immunization with *Candida albicans* ribosomes. FEMS Microbiol Lett 1986;36:213–217.
36. Hiatt JS Jr, Martin DS. Recovery from pulmonary moniliasis following serum therapy. JAMA 1946;130:205–206.
37. Al-Doory Y. An immune factor in baboon anti-*Candida* serum. Sabouraudia 1970;8:41–47.
38. Waldman RH, Cruz JM, Rowe DS. Intravaginal immunization of humans with *Candida albicans*. J Immunol 1972;109:662–664.
39. Gravina-Sanvitale G, Gravina E, De Negri M. Vaccine therapy of a case of onychomycosis caused by *Candida albicans*. Arch Sci Med 1977;134:95–98.
40. Schalla WO, Johnson W. Immunogenicity of ribosomal vaccines isolated from group A, type M *Streptococcus pyogenes*. Infect Immun 1975;11: 1195–1202.
41. Levy DA, Bohbot JM, Catalan F, et al. Phase II study of D.651, an oral vaccine designed to prevent recurrences of vulvovaginal candidiasis. Vaccine 1989;7:337–340.
42. Polonelli L, Lorenzini R, De Bernardis F, et al. Idiotypic vaccination: Immunoprotection mediated by anti-idiotypic antibodies with antibiotic activity. Scand J Immunol 1993;37:105–110.
43. Polonelli L, De Bernardis F, Conti S, et al. Idiotypic intravaginal vaccination to protect against candidal vaginitis by secretory, yeast killer toxin-like anti-idiotypic antibodies. J Immun 1994;152:3175–3182.
44. Vogel RA, Fether BF, Conant NF, Lowe EP. Preliminary studies on artificial active immunization of guinea pigs against respiratory challenge with *Coccidioides immitis*. Am Rev Tuberc 1954;70:498–503.
45. Friedman L, Smith CE. Vaccination of mice against *Coccidioides immitis*. Am Rev Tuberc 1956;74:245–248.
46. Levine HB, Cobb JM, Smith CE. Immunity to coccidioidomycosis induced in mice by purified spherule, arthrospore and mycelial vaccine. Trans NY Acad Sci 1960;22:436–449.
47. Kong J, Levine HB, Smith CE. Immunogenic properties of nondisrupted and disrupted spherules of *Coccidioides immitis* in mice. Sabouraudia 1963; 2:131–142.
48. Pappagianis D, Hector R, Levine HB, Collins MS. Immunization of mice against coccidioidomycosis with a subcellular vaccine. Infect Immun 1979; 25:440–445.
49. Levine HB, Smith CE. The reaction of eight volunteers injected with *Coccidioides immitis* spherule vaccine: First human trials. In: Ajello L, ed. Proc. 2d Symp. Coccidioidomycosis. Phoenix: University of Arizona Press, 1967: 197–200.

50. Levine HB, Pappagianis D, Cobb JM. Development of vaccines for coccidioidomycosis. Mycopathol Mycol Appl 1970;41:177–185.
51. Pappagianis D, Levine HB, Smith CE. Further studies on vaccination of human volunteers with killed *Coccidioides immitis*. In: Ajello L, ed. Proc 2d Symp Coccidioidomycosis. Phoenix: University of Arizona Press, 1967: 201–220.
52. Levine HB, Kong YCM. Immunologic impairment in mice treated intravenously with killed *Coccidioides immitis* spherules: Suppressed response to intramuscular doses. J Immunol 1966;96:297–305.
53. Scalarone GM, Levine HB. Attributes of deficient immunity in mice receiving *Coccidioides immitis* spherule vaccine by the intravenous route. Sabouraudia 1969;7:169–177.
54. Kong YCM, Savage DC, Levine HB. Enhancement of immune responses in mice by a booster injection of *Coccidioides* spherules. J Immunol 1965; 95:1048–1056.
55. Huppert M, Levine HB, Sun SH, Peterson ET. Resistance of vaccinated mice to typical and atypical strains of *Coccidioides immitis*. J Bacteriol 1967; 94:924–927.
56. Levine HB, Miller R, Smith CE. Influence of vaccination on respiratory coccidioidal disease in cynomolgus monkeys. J Immunol 1962;89:242–251.
57. Kong YCM, Levine HB, Machin SH, Smith CE. Fungal multiplication and histopathologic damages in vaccinated mice infected with *Coccidioides immitis*. J Immunol 1964;92:779–790.
58. Gunby P. Coccidioidomycosis vaccine trial planned with 3000 volunteers. JAMA 1981;245:1711–1715.
59. Kong YCM, Savage DC, Kong LNL. Delayed dermal hypersensitivity in mice to spherule and mycelial extracts of *Coccidioides immitis*. J Bacteriol 1966;91:876–883.
60. Levine HB, Cobb JM, Scalarone GM. Spherule coccidioidin in delayed dermal sensitivity reactions of experimental animals. Sabouraudia 1969;7:20–32.
61. Cole GT, Kirkland TN. Identification of antigens of *Coccidioides immitis* which stimulate immune T lymphocytes. Arch Med Res 1993;24:281–291.
62. Ellis DH, Pfeiffer TJ. Natural habitat of *Cryptococcus neoformans* var. *gattii*. J Clin Microbiol 1990;28:1642–1644.
63. Pfeiffer TJ, Ellis DH. Environmental isolation of *Cryptococcus neoformans* var *gattii* from *Eucaliptus tereticornis*. J Med Vet Mycol 1992;30:407–408.
64. Abrahams I, Gillerman TG. Studies on actively acquired resistance to experimental cryptococcosis in mice. J Immunol 1960;85:629–635.
65. Abrahams I. Further studies on acquired resistance to murine cryptococcosis: Enhancing effect of *Bordetella pertussis*. J Immunol 1966;96:525–529.
66. Louria DB. Specific and non-specific immunity in experimental cryptococcosis in mice. J Exp Med 1960;111:643–665.
67. Louria DB, Kaminski T, Finkel G. Further studies on immunity in experimental cryptococcosis. J Exp Med 1963;117:509–520.

68. Louria DB, Kaminski T. Passively acquired immunity in experimental cryptococcosis. Sabouraudia 1965;4:80–84.
69. Reiss F, Alture-Weber E. Immunization of mice with a mutant of *Cryptococcus neoformans*: Characterization of the mutant, actively acquired resistance to experimental cryptococcosis in mice. Dermatologica 1976;152:16–22.
70. Fromtling RA, Blackstock R, Hall NK, Bulmer GS. Immunization of mice with an avirulent pseudohyphal form of *Cryptococcus neoformans*. Mycopathologia 1979;68:179–181.
71. Anderson DM, Dykstra MA. Resistance to challenge and macrophage activity in mice previously vaccinated with formalin-killed *Cryptococcus neoformans*. Mycopathologia 1984;86:169–177.
72. Dykstra MA, Friedman L. Pathogenesis, lethality, and immunizing effect of experimental cutaneous cryptococcosis. Infect Immun 1978;20:446–455.
73. Casadevall A, Mukherjee J, Devi SJ, et al. Antibodies elicited by a *Cryptococcus neoformans*-tetanus toxoid conjugate vaccine have the same specificity as those elicited in infection. J Infect Dis 1992;165:1086–1093.
74. Devi SJ, Schneerson R, Egan W, et al. *Cryptococcus neoformans* serotype A glucuronoxylomannan conjugate vaccines: Synthesis, characterization and immunogenicity. Infect Immun 1991;59:3700–3707.
75. Graybill JR, Straus DC, Nealou TJ, et al. Immunogenic fractions of *Cryptococcus neoformans*. Mycopathologia 1982;78:31–39.
76. Beemer AM, Davidson W, Kuttin ES, et al. Vaccine and mycostatin in treatment of cryptococcosis of the respiratory tract. Sabouraudia 1976;14: 171–179.
77. Kong YCM, Levine HB. Experimentally induced immunity to the mycoses. Bacteriol Rev 1967;31:35–53.
78. Salvin SB. Immunization of mice against *Histoplasma capsulatum*. J Immunol 1953;70:267–270.
79. Salvin SB, Ribi E Antigens from yeast phase of *Histoplasma capsulatum*: II. Immunologic properties of protoplasm vs. cell walls. Proc Soc Exp Biol Med 1955;90:287–294.
80. Salvin SB, Smith RF. Antigens from the yeast phase of *Histoplasma capsulatum*: III. Isolation, properties, and activity of a protein carbohydrate complex. J Infect Dis 1959;105:45–53.
81. Hill GA, Marcus S. Resistance induced against *Histoplasma capsulatum*: quantitative aspects. J Infect Dis 1959;105:26–30.
82. Bauman DS, Chick EW. Immunoprotection against extra-pulmonary histoplasmosis in hamsters. Am Rev Respir Dis 1969;100:82–85.
83. Domer JE. In vivo and in vitro cellular responses to cytoplasmic and cell wall antigens of *Histoplasma capsulatum* in artificially immunized or infected guinea pigs. Infect Immun 1976;13:790–799.
84. Domer JE, Ichinose H. Cellular immune responses in guinea pigs immunized with cell walls of *Histoplasma capsulatum* prepared by several different procedures. Infect Immun 1977;16:293–301.
85. Williams DM, Graybill JR, Drutz DJ. Adoptive transfer of immunity to *Histoplasma capsulatum* in athymic nude mice. Sabouraudia 1981;19:39–48.

86. Feit C, Tewari RP. Immunogenicity of ribosomal preparations from yeast cells of *Histoplasma capsulatum*. Infect Immun 1974;10:1091–1097.
87. Tewari RP, Sharma D, Solotorovsky M, et al. Adoptive transfer of immunity from mice immunized with ribosomes or live yeast cells of *Histoplasma capsulatum*. Infect Immun 1977;15:789–795.
88. Tewari RP, Khardori N, Connachie MC, et al. Blastogenic responses of lymphocytes from mice immunized by sublethal infection with yeast cells of *Histoplasma capsulatum*. Infect Immun 1982;36:1013–1018.
89. Medoff G, Sacco M, Maresca B, et al. Irreversible block of the mycelial-to-yeast phase transition of *Histoplasma capsulatum*. Science 1986;231: 476–479.
90. Corbel MJ, Eades SM. Experimental phycomycosis in mice; examination of the role of acquired immunity in resistance to *Absidia ramosa*. J Hyg 1976; 77:221–223.
91. Waldorf AR, Halde C, Vedros NA. Passive immunization in murine mucormycosis. Mycopathologia 1983;83:149–155.

18

Dermatophyte Vaccines

ALLAN C. PIER
University of Wyoming
Laramie, Wyoming

Dermatophytosis is a frequent disease of companion animals and livestock, where it usually occurs as classic ''ringworm,'' with circular lesions of hair loss over areas of thickened, scaly skin. Ringworm of animals produces clinical lesions that persist for 8 to 16 weeks. Infected animals shed large numbers of arthrospores in skin scales and hairs from active lesions; these spores can remain viable and infectious in the animal's bed, stall, or environment for several years, creating a continuity of infection. Because of the highly contagious nature of the infection, animals with clinically apparent lesions are barred from performance, show, and sale arenas. Other economic losses are incurred by damage to affected hides (1–5).

The major ringworm agents of animals are zoonotic and frequently cause infections of the head, face, hands, arms, and bodies of human companions and attendants. When humans are infected by zoophilic dermatophytes, they often develop lesions with an exaggerated inflammatory response called kerion formation, and scarring is a frequent sequela (2,3,6). Zoophilic dermatophytes constitute an important public health problem in many social and geographic areas of the world. *Trichophyton verrucosum*, the major agent of ringworm in cattle, is also the major agent of severe clinical dermatophyte infections in human attendants of infected cattle. *Trichophyton mentagrophytes* var. *mentagrophytes* is a major agent of dermatophytosis in laboratory animals, wild rodents, and furbearing animals as well as being a frequent agent of infection in dogs, cats, horses, and other domestic animals. Human infection with this variety of *T. mentagrophytes* often involves the face, hands, arms, and bodies of people who work around infected animals and grain storage bins contaminated with hairs and scales from infected wild rodents. *Microsporum canis*, the major agent of ringworm in dogs and cats, is the chief agent of tinea capitis in young persons in many major cities of the United States and Europe (2,3). The source of this infection is often infected stray cats, which abound in such metropolises. *Microsporum canis* is also a major problem in catteries and kennels, where infection, once established, is extremely difficult to eradicate. Several other zoophilic dermatophytes also cause occasional zoonotic infections in humans, chiefly *T. equinum* and *M. equinum* (2).

Ringworm in companion animals and livestock usually involves young animals. The animal generally is infected by only a single species of dermatophyte and, once the infection has cleared, subsequent reinfection with the same or different dermatophyte is rare. These facts argue strongly for the establishment of an effective broad-based immunity against recurrent ringworm in animals. (This represents a much different situation than that of persistent, recurring, recrudescing, or new infection of humans with tinea pedis or tinea unguium.) There have been a great many studies of the immunological events that accompany or follow dermatophytosis (4,5,7–9). The delivery system for an effective immune response remains in question. Dermatophytes parasitize dead, keratinized, avascular tissue; they virtually never reach living cells with their associated humoral and cellular defense mechanisms. Rippon (3) correctly noted that "there is no single clearcut mechanism that will explain all aspects of susceptibility and immunity to dermatophyte infection." Current information suggests that both cell-mediated and humoral immune mechanisms are involved with resistance to and clearance of dermatophyte infections in animals (7,9). The fact that animals are rarely reinfected with different dermatophytes suggests that the immunity acquired from infection is broad and may protect across species as well as generic lines (3,5,10).

Immunization of livestock and companion animals against prevalent dermatophytes has been proposed to alleviate economic losses among affected animals as well as to reduce the reservoir of zoonotic infections of humans (2,6,10). Active immunization of calves against ringworm caused by *Trychophyton verrucosum* was accomplished by Florian et al. (14). Some years later, Sarkisov et al. (11) utilized a suspension of viable *T. verrucosum* from a strain of reduced virulence for cattle (TF 130) and immunized a large number of cattle in Russia. This latter vaccine has proven to be highly effective in reducing the incidence of new infection in vaccinated herds. A lyophilized version of the live *T. verrucosum* vaccine (LTF 130) has been applied to cattle in extensive field trials in Norway (12) and other European countries with generally effective results. The vaccine is applied intramuscularly in two doses at a 10- to 14-day interval. Protection from infection of over 90% in fully vaccinated animals has been claimed from these trials.

The safety of the viable *T. verrucosum* vaccine relies on its reduced virulence for cattle and its intramuscular application. A small inflammatory focus with a scab often appears at the cutaneous injection site, particularly after the second dose. The scab contains viable *T. verrucosum* organisms, but they are of reduced virulence for cattle, and spread from the injection site or to other cattle is rare. Limited experimental data have shown that the viable vaccine may infect the skin of laboratory animals and the scarified skin of humans when directly applied experimentally. However extensive field use has not been hampered by problems with adventitious infection, and a high degree of effectiveness has resulted from use of the LTF 130 product. This vaccine is currently being produced commercially for use in countries where it has been approved. Two other viable vaccines of Russian origin have also been used in animals; one was prepared from *T. equinum* for use in horses, the other from *T. mentagrophytes* for use in fur-bearing animals. Neither has gained the degree of acceptance of the *T. verrucosum* vaccine.

It is not clear why viable vaccines should be necessary to induce a reliable dermatophyte immunity. Live fungal elements do not persist in the tissues below the skin for more than 7 days following intramuscular injection (5). The dermatophyte is incapable of colonizing or reproducing in those tissues. Its persistence in the subcutaneous tissues is of approximately the same duration as one would expect from nonviable particulate or precipitated antigens. And even when strains of reduced virulence are used, a potential for adventitious infection in closely grouped animal populations causes some anxiety with their use.

In recent studies in the United States, killed dermatophyte vaccines have been used in horses against *T. equinum* infection (13) and in laboratory animals, cats and dogs against *M. canis* infection (5,10). Both of the latter preparations employed adjuvanted suspensions of conidia and aerial mycelium. Two intramuscular doses were used at a 10- to 20-day interval and a 4-month booster dose was recommended when infection pressure in the animal's environment was excessive. Protection from infection approximated or exceeded 90% in vaccinated animals in controlled exposure studies and effectively reduced new infection in field studies (5,10,13). The killed dermatophyte vaccines offer the advantages of safety, in that they cannot cause infection in the vaccinated animal or in the human administering the vaccine. They can also utilize a number of adjuvants to enhance the immune response. The killed adjuvanted dermatophyte vaccines have yet to be made available commercially.

Both live and killed dermatophyte vaccines cause detectable induration at the vaccine site, but only the live products produce a localized scab. The immunity resulting from dermatophyte vaccination is not absolute. However vaccination does produce an enhanced resistance to infection in young animals. If the challenge of infection is excessive, lesions may result in some vaccinated animals, but they are generally smaller and fewer than those that occur in unvaccinated animals. Thus the vaccine reduces the production and dissemination of infectious particles that colonize other animals, their environment, and their human attendants.

The control of epizootics of dermatophytosis among populations of companion animals and livestock, and thereby the reduction of the resultant dermatophytic zoonoses of humans, rests on one of two approaches: (a) Limiting access of susceptible animals to the dermatophyte through extensive sanitation of corral boards, tack, brushes, bedding etc., and isolation or culling of infected animals or (b) Limiting access of the dermatophyte to susceptible animals through removing the animals' susceptibility by means of immunization. It is the latter approach that has been recommended by WHO/ISHAM Liaison Committee consultation on prevention and control of dermatophytosis (6). Dermatophyte vaccines are clearly a means whose time has come to help control these highly contagious diseases of veterinary and public health importance.

REFERENCES

1. Jungerman RF, Schwartzman RM. Veterinary Medical Mycology. Philadelphia: Lea & Febiger, 1972.
2. Pier AC. Superficial mycoses (dermatophytoses). In: Beran G, ed. Handbook Series in Zoonoses, 2d ed. Boca Raton, FL: CRC Press, 1994.
3. Rippon JW. Medical Mycology, 3d ed. Philadelphia: Saunders, 1988.
4. Scott DW. Large Animal Dermatology. Philadelphia: Saunders, 1988.
5. Smith JMB, Aho R, Mattsson R, Pier AC. Progress in Veterinary Mycology. J Med Vet Mycol 1992;30(suppl 1):307–316.
6. World Health Org./ISHAM Liaison Committee. Proceedings of the ISHAM consultation on prevention and control of dermatophytosis with special reference to immunity and immunization. Oslo, Norway: National Veterinary Institute, 1987:1–40.
7. Calderone RA. Immunological aspects of dermatophyte infection. Proc X Congress Int Soc Hum and Animal Mycol 1988:29–35.

8. Grappel SF, Bishop CT, Blank F. Immunology of Dermatophytes and Dermatophytosis. Bacteriol Rev 1974;38:222–250.
9. Pier AC, Ellis JA, Mills KA. Development of immune response to experimental bovine *Trichophyton verrucosum* infection. Vet Dermatol 1993;3: 131–138.
10. Pier AC, Hodges AB, Lauze JM, Raisbeck M. Experimental immunity to *M. canis* and cross reactions with other dermatophytes of veterinary importance. J Med Vet Mycol 1995;33:93–97.
11. Sarkisov AK, Pctrovich SV, Nikiforose LL. Immunization of cattle against Trichophytosis. Veterinary 1971;48:54–56.
12. Gudding R, Naess B. Vaccination of cattle against ringworm caused by *Trichophyton verrucosum*. Am J Vet Res 1986;47:2415–2417.
13. Pier AC, Zancanella PJ. Immunization of horses against dermatophytosis caused by *Trichophton equinum*. Equine Pract 1993;15:23–27.
14. Florian E, Nemeseri L, Louas G. Active immunization of calves against ringworm. Magy Allatorv Lap 1964;19:529–530.

19

Basis for *Candida albicans* Adhesion and Penetration

ESTHER SEGAL and HANA SANDOVSKY-LOSICA
Sackler School of Medicine
Tel-Aviv University
Tel-Aviv, Israel

I. INTRODUCTION

Candida albicans is a versatile organism living as a commensal of the gastrointestinal tract and having the ability to invade host tissues and to initiate serious diseases under the appropriate environmental conditions (1,2). In the normal host, the fungus has evolved to become a successful commensal. It expresses variable traits critical for existence on mucosal surfaces, where constant but dynamic interplay occurs between innate and acquired host-defense mechanisms. In the abnormal host, these same traits may become virulence characteristics, accounting for invasive abilities as the delicate balance of *C. albicans* with host shifts in favor of the fungus.

Current understanding of candidal virulence derives largely from studies in which potential virulence attributes are assessed one at a time in vitro or in attenuated *C. albicans* variants. But it must be taken into account that a wholesome picture of the fungus's virulence requires a combination of traits that can be expressed individually, mutually, or in succession (3,4).

The most extensively investigated putative virulence factors of *Candida* include the ability of the fungus to attach to host tissues (5–11) followed, apparently, by penetration. The basis for each of these steps involves specific components, such as the adhesins or hydrolytic enzymes—molecules facilitating the penetration (4,12,13), and hypha formation—a morphogenetic transformation also associated with penetration (4,14,15). Moreover, as indicated above, it is reasonable to hypothesize that no single *C. albicans* factor accounts for virulence, and not all expressed virulence attributes are necessary for a particular stage or site of infection.

In this chapter we focus on the virulence factors associated with adherence of *C. albicans* to host tissues and its penetration into the tissues.

II. ADHERENCE

Adherence is regarded (16,17) as a first step of the infectious process, thus enabling the organism to survive on host tissue. Information relating the adherence of *C. albicans* to virulence and studies of mechanisms of adherence involve in vitro and in vivo investigations. A number of specific and review articles have focused on this subject in recent years (5,11–18). Thus, for the sake of avoiding redundancy, we aim in this chapter only to summarize briefly the major issues of this topic, concentrating on adherence studies from the point of view of association with virulence and disease, putative molecules involved in the binding process, as deduced primarily from the personal experience of the authors.

In vitro adherence systems involve on one side the fungus *Candida*, especially *C. albicans*, mostly in its yeast form, and the counterpart target, which can be various cells, tissues, or inert plastic surfaces. In vitro adherence was shown to a variety of surfaces: various human exfoliated epithelial cells—buccal (Fig. 1), vaginal, urogenital, or corneocytes (7,19–25); various cell lines such as HeLa, CCL-6; or endothelial cells (26–29); tissue segments such as murine gastrointestinal tissue disks (30–32); or specific systems, such as fibrin clots (33) or spleen, and lymph node tissues (34). All of these experimental systems may be of relevance, as they represent analogous sites of candidal infections, superficial or systemic forms. Thus these in vitro models of *Candida* interactions with host tissues may reflect the in vivo interactions within the host.

Simple in vitro adherence tests are usually performed by incubating the epithelial cells with the yeast form of *C. albicans*, followed by microscopic examination for evaluation. Evaluation of adherence using this method is based on microscopic counting of epithelial cells with adherent yeasts and/or counts of adhering yeasts. This method suffers from subjectivity and lack of standardized criteria. Other methods for evaluating adherence involves use of radiolabeled fungi, enzyme-linked immunosorbent assay (ELISA), or flow cytometry (35).

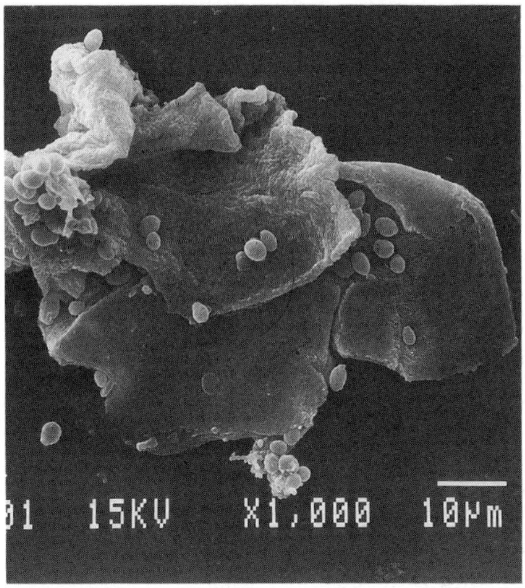

Figure 1 Scanning electron microscopy of in vitro adherence of *Candida albicans* to human buccal epithelial cells. (Original magnification, ×1000.) (From a collaborative study with Dr. I. Berdicevsky.)

Using in vitro assays to measure the attachment of various *Candida* species to exfoliated epithelial cells, it was found that in vitro adherence could be correlated with relative pathogenicity of *Candida* species. It was found that *C. albicans* adhered most avidly, while less pathogenic species such as *C. krusei* or *C. guillermondii* adhered minimally (9). It was also found by Segal et al. that *C. albicans* was more adherent to methacrylate than less pathogenic species (36).

Furthermore, more cells from susceptible populations, known for their high susceptibility to candidal infections, adhered to fungi than did cells from nonsusceptible populations. This was confirmed by Segal et al. using human vaginal cells (23) and corneocytes (25) as well as animal cells—murine vaginal cells collected from mice with continuous estrus (37) and murine gastrointestinal tissue disks from mice treated with cytotoxic anticancer drugs (31,32). Thus, these data support the hypothesis that increased binding capacity of host cells may be a contributing factor in the development of candidal infection.

It is believed that in vitro experiments, in addition to reflecting the reaction in vivo between the fungi and the host tissues, may also make it possible to study the basis or mechanisms of adherence and the molecules involved. Adherence is based on the interaction between the fungal surface molecules called adhesins (ligands) and host components. The *C. albicans* cell surface possesses several ligands, which bind to host components such as C3d, iC3b, fibrinogen, laminin, fibronectin, fucose and *N*-acetylglucosamine (NAG) (5–8,38–40). Most surface ligands apparently help fungal cells to adhere to host surfaces. However, the complement binding factors and the fibrinogen binding factor (18,40) may play an additional role in pathogenesis. The surface adhesins of *C. albicans* can be categorized into several types. According to Calderone (18), five adhesin systems have been described. Four of these adhesin systems involve mannoprotein or mannan, while the fifth relates to chitin.

In several experimental systems involving various epithelial cells (24,41), tissue disks (30,32) or acrylics (42), it was shown by Segal and coworkers that the in vitro adherence of *C. albicans* to these various targets could be blocked by chitin, NAG, or a chitin derivative (chitin-soluble extract—CSE). A summary of these experiments is shown in Table 1. Inhibition of adherence was 50–70% when vaginal epithelial cells were pretreated with NAG, CSE, chitin, or chitin hydrolysate. The ability of these chitinous sustances, and CSE in particular, to block the adhesion of *C. albicans* in vitro was also noted when human buccal epithelial cells, human corneocytes, or murine gastrointestinal tissue disks were substituted for vaginal epithelial cells in the adhesion assay.

Similarly, other investigators showed that a blocking effect of adherence of *C. albicans* could be achieved by the other putative adhesins of *C. albicans* (4–6,18,29,38). Mannan, mannoprotein complexes, or the proteinous component of *C. albicans* are considered natural candidates for molecules with adhesive activity, constituting a major component of the *Candida* cell wall. Evidence pointing to the role of mannan or mannoprotein was obtained in a number of studies using a variety of experimental systems. These systems included the blocking of the adhesion of *C. albicans* to epithelial cells in vitro by mannose (43), pretreatment of the yeasts with mannose specific lectin (44), or exposing the yeasts to tunicamycin (45), which inhibits mannoprotein synthesis. Evidence that the protein alone may serve as an adhesin or that the protein portion of the mannoprotein complex is more important than the carbohydrate moiety is evident from other studies showing decreased adherence after pretreatment of *C. albicans* with proteolytic enzymes (38).

The host-cell ligand (4,5) is either a carbohydrate or a protein, namely, fucosyl, glucosamine, fibronectin or argenine-glycine-asparagine (RGD), respectively (7,18,40,46), depending upon the type of host cell, epithelial or endothelial.

Table 1 Effect of a Chitin Extract (CSE) on in vitro Adherence of C. albicans to Various Targets

Fungus	Type of cell	Effect of CSE, % inhibition[a]	Reference
CBS-562[b]	Buccal (H)[c]	63.4[d]	73
Various isolates[e]	Buccal (H)[c]	43–88[f]	73
CBS-562	Vaginal (H)[c]	68[d]	20,41,47
4918	Vaginal (H)[c]	72.4[d]	47
CBS-562	Corneocytes (H)[c]	56[d]	24
CBS-562	GI tissue disks (M)[g]		
	Naive	73[d]	31,32
	Irradiated	79[d]	
	MTX	56[d]	
	5-FU	64[d]	
CBS-562	Acrylic[h]	82[d]	42

[a] Inhibition (%), calculated by dividing the adhesion value in presence of CSE by the value of the control devoid of CSE.
[b] CBS-562: Type strain from Centraalbureau voor Schimmelcultures, Delft, Netherlands.
[c] H = human exfoliated epithelial cells.
[d] Mean value.
[e] *C. albicans* isolates from various sources and sites.
[f] Range.
[g] M = murine gastrointestinal tissue disks from naive, 600R irradiated, methotrexate (MTX) or 5-fluorouracil (5-FU)–treated animals.
[h] Methacrylate = denture resin.

There are several additional lines of evidence indicating that adhesins are important to the virulence of the organism. First, mutants of *C. albicans* that adhere less readily than parental cells are less virulent in animal models of candidiasis (26,47). Second, treatment of animals with soluble ligand prior to infection prevented or decreased infection (37,41,48–51).

Blocking the attachment and thereby preventing infection strengthens the notion of the importance of in vivo adherence as the first step of the infection. Segal et al., in several experimental systems (described in Table 2), found that a chitin-soluble extract applied to test animals prior to their inoculation with the fungus could prevent development of candidiasis, thus decreasing infection rate and mortality.

Interestingly, such findings were also noted by Ghannoum et al. (49) using the chitin-soluble extract or chitin itself in gastrointestinal candidiasis induced in an infant mouse model. In another model, Suzuki et al. (52)

Table 2 Effect of CSE in vivo in Experimental Murine Candidiasis

Type of infection	Application	Effect	Reference
Vaginal			
Naive	Intravaginal	80% prevention[a]	41
Constant estrus[b]	Intravaginal	45.4% prevention[a]	37
Diabetic[c]	Intravaginal	30% prevention[a]	48
		Clearance[d] day 21–28, (35)	
Gastrointestinal			
Naive—Colonization	Oral	49% prevention[e]	50
Systemic			
MTX[f]—Infection[g]	Oral	60% prevention	50
Mortality		60% decrease	

[a] Prevention of development of infection versus untreated controls.
[b] Constant estrus induced in mice by subcutaneous inoculations of estradiol benzoate.
[c] Diabetic mice, rendered diabetic by intraperitoneal inoculation of streptozotocin.
[d] Day of clearance of infection in treated mice versus day of control in parentheses.
[e] Prevention of GI colonization as compared to controls.
[f] Methotrexate-treated animals.
[g] Development of systemic infection determined by fungal colonization of viscera.

showed that chitin administered intraperitoneally to mice prolonged the survival of those challenged intravenously with *C. albicans* as compared to mice that received only the fungus. Klotz et al. (3,53) blocked attachment of *C. albicans* to vascular endothelium in vivo by administering an RGD-containing peptide, which represents the competitive use of the host cell receptor.

In this context, it should be added that discrepancies and controversial results obtained in the various studies by different investigators regarding the nature of the adhesin could be explained by the possible existence of more than a single adhesive molecule, a situation typical of various microorganisms (17). Expression of different adhesins may be a function of the specific fungal isolate or the specific environmental and growth conditions (11,53a,54).

In addition to adhesion based on interaction(s) between specific binding molecules, it is believed that nonspecific mechanisms also play a role. Relative hydrophobicity of a microorganism influences how well it adheres nonspecifically to surfaces (55). *Candida albicans* can adhere to various biomaterials (9,56–58) such as contact lenses, urinary catheters, or prosthetic devices. Invasion of the human host can occur by vascular dissemination of yeasts attached to intravenous catheters; thus, this mechanisms may have implications of clinical relevance. Electrostatic forces and hydrophobicity have been reported to be responsible for such interactions (56–58).

Interest in the cell-surface hydrophobicity of *Candida*, particularly *C. albicans*, has developed. These studies have shown that hydrophobic interactions contribute to fungal attachment to plastic, but fungal growth conditions, the type of plastic and assay conditions, can influence the degree to which the hydrophobic interactions participate (58). Hazen et al. (58) showed that hydrophobic *C. albicans* cells cultured at 25°C are more virulent than their more hydrophilic counterparts cultured at 37°C. The degree of surface hydrophobicity of *C. albicans* cells contributes to epithelial adherence and also to the speed of hyphal germ tube formation. Germ tubes and strongly hydrophobic *Candida* cells adhere better to epithelia than do yeast forms and hydrophilic cells, but hydrophobicity also influences germ tube formation. As an overall conclusion, Hazen claims that the clinical significance of fungal cell surface hydrophobicity in candidiasis is unknown, as *C. albicans*, the most frequent agent of nearly all forms of candidiasis, has been variously ranked as one of the most hydrophobic species to one of the least.

In summary, discrepancies and controversial results obtained in various studies by different investigators regarding the adherence phenomena could be explained by the fact that current understanding of the virulence of *Candida* derives from studies performed under various conditions involving different strains of *C. albicans*, thereby reducing uniformity. Thus, although the phenomenon of candidal adhesion to host tissues is apparently of importance in the pathogenesis of candidiasis, a comprehensive overview of its mechanistic basis is still not available and leaves the field open for further research.

III. PENETRATION

The factors necessary for a *Candida* yeast cell to attach to and colonize host surfaces are not necessarily the same as those required for penetration.

Penetration of *C. albicans* into the host is assumed to be associated with the formation of hyphae and hydrolytic enzymes, thus pointing to their role as virulence factors of *Candida* (4).

Hyphae formation by *C. albicans* is regarded as a virulence factor relating to invasiveness (13), whereas yeast forms are thought to be responsible for colonizing epithelia. This, although there is no direct proof that *C. albicans* in the commensal state exists uniquely in the yeast form. Histopathological observations show that both yeasts and hyphae are found in infected tissues (59).

Among the potential virulence factors of *Candida* associated with hydrolytic enzymes, extracellular proteolysis exhibited by *C. albicans* has attracted much attention. The extracellular proteolytic activity of *Candida* is due to aspartyl proteinase enzymes (12,60,61).

The enzyme has been purified from the culture media of various strains of *C. albicans*; it is characterized as an acid carboxyl proteinase with broad substrate specificity including keratin, dermal collagen, albumin, hemoglobin, immunoglobulin heavy chains, and extracellular matrix proteins and has activity in the range of pH 2.0–7.0.

Candida acid proteinase is expressed by *C. albicans* after attachment of yeast cells to host epithelium in vitro. Only the pathogenic *Candida* species produce proteinases (12). Moreover, proteinase-deficient mutants are less virulent than parental strains in mice following intravenous challenge (62,63).

The secreted acid proteinase of *C. albicans* is thought to play a role in the virulence of this organism for several reasons. It facilitates adherence to eukaryotic tissue, enhances resistance against phagocytosis, provides nitrogen sources during the infection, activates inflammatory mediators, and possibly facilitates tissue invasion by degrading keratin and collagen.

The availability of spontaneous mutants of *C. albicans* that are unable to invade mucosal tissue, mutagenized strains which have lost their ability to secrete the aspartyl proteinase of the parental strain, and other species of *Candida* showing lower levels of candidal acid proteinase production versus decreased pathogenicity provide the experimental basis pointing to candidal acid proteinase as a virulence factor.

A possible role of candidal acid proteinase in the pathogenesis of *Candida* can also be deduced from other evidence. A specific inhibitor of aspartyl proteinase, pepstatin-A, interfered with the adherence of *C. albicans* to, and its invasion of, human oral epithelium (12).

The most recent developments in the research of aspartyl proteinase involve molecular biology techniques (64,65). Sequencing of the enzyme and cloning of the gene(s) encoding for the enzyme have been described. This line of research may provide additional, more basic information as to the role of these enzymes in fungal tissue penetration and the pathogenesis of disease.

EXPERIMENTAL ANIMAL MODELS

Experimental animal models (66,67) of candidiasis serve as means to investigate interactions of *Candida* with host tissues in vivo. Numerous studies have been published describing different types of *Candida* infections, ranging from the superficial mucocutaneous entities to deep-seated disseminated disease. The studies varied in the animal species, the *Candida* isolate used, the mode of induction of infection, and the specific goals of the experimental models. In this chapter the authors will refer only to specific animal models of relevance to adhesion and penetration.

Various murine models of vaginal candidiasis were studied by Segal et al. (37,41,48). In these models, naive, estrogen-treated or diabetic mice were infected intravaginally with *C. albicans*. The vaginal infections developed in these different types of animals aim to represent the differences in susceptibility to vaginal candidiasis of various human populations. As mentioned before, studies assessing the ability of human vaginal cells collected from groups with different susceptibility (23) to adhere Candida in vitro were carried out. Such studies revealed that cells from pregnant women, women using contraceptives, or diabetics were highly adhesive for *C. albicans* as compared with cells from a control population. Thus, the animal studies could corroborate experimentally, under controlled conditions, the epidemiological observations made in human studies. Microscopy from vaginal lavages or histopathology of tissues from experimental vaginal infections demonstrated that, 2 hr postinfection, blastospores adhering to vaginal mucosa were seen, followed by formation of hyphae that penetrated into the mucosa (41).

These findings were also noted in ultrastructural studies (19). In the case of deep-seated and systemic candidiasis, a model of gastrointestinal candidiasis developing into systemic infection in debilitated mice was studied (59,68). An immunosuppressed state renders the animals susceptible to infection (69,70). Immunosuppression induced by certain anticancer treatments or otherwise is known also for its damage of the gastrointestinal mucosa, thus enabling passage of the fungi across the mucosa into the viscera. As indicated above, in vitro studies in our laboratory with gastrointestinal tissue disks from anti-cancer-treated mice tested for their adherence with *C. albicans* were carried out (31,32). These revealed increased in vitro adherence levels to gastrointestinal tissue disks taken from the immunosuppressed mice. Thus, these findings point to adherence as a first step in the infectious process and its increased level in susceptible populations as an important factor in the infection. Gross examination of the gastrointestinal tract of the compromised mice postchallenge revealed macroscopic changes (68) in the mucosa of the stomach, especially in the cardial atrium line. Direct examination of calcofluor-stained tissue homogenates from the stomach tissue of compromised mice revealed fungal elements, including hyphae and budding yeasts. Tangential sections of stomach tissue showed hyphal elements associated with the squamous epithelium in the region of the cardial atrium line. These observations together with observations made by others (11,13,14,71,72) show that penetration involves primarily hyphae, but the first association with the outermost layers of the mucosa involves the association of yeasts with the intestinal contents, the mucus gel, and the epithelium proper. Penetration of stomach mucosa by germ tubes plays an important role in the systemic spread of the fungus from the gastrointestinal tract.

Special emphasis should be given to the use of CSE in the experimental model of systemic candidiasis originating from the gastrointestinal tract of mice compromised by methotrexate (50). Addition of CSE to the drinking water significantly reduced candidal colonization, especially in the stomach, and the extent of subsequent development of systemic infection as well as the mortality rate. These in vivo findings corroborate the inhibitory effect of CSE noted previously (32) in vitro and point to inhibition of adherence as a means of preventing infection by blocking adherence as the first step in the infectious process.

The experimental models described in this section did not intend to cover all aspects of this topic but rather to illustrate by in vivo experiments the fungal virulence attributes associated with the initial infiltration of the pathogen within the host and the following invasion.

REFERENCES

1. Odds FC. Candida and Candidosis. 2d ed. London: Balliére Tindall, 1988: 68–72.
2. Bodey GP. Candidiasis, Pathogenesis, Diagnosis and Treatment. New York: Raven Press, 1993.
3. Cutler JE. Putative virulence factors of Candida albicans. Annu Rev Microbiol 1991;45:187–218.
4. Odds FC. Candida species and virulence. ASM News 1994;60:313–318.
5. Calderone RA, Braun P. Adherence and receptor relationships of Candida albicans. Microbiol Rev 1991;55:1–20.
6. Douglas J. Adhesion of Candida species to epithelial surfaces. CRC Crit Rev Microbiol 1987;15:27–43.
7. Hostetter MK. Adhesins and ligands involved in the interaction of Candida spp. with epithelial and endothelial surfaces. Clin Microbiol Rev 1994;7: 29–42.
8. Kennedy MJ, Calderone RA, Cutler JE, et al. Molecular basis of Candida albicans adhesion. J Med Vet Mycol 1992;30(suppl 1):95–122.
9. Rotrosen D, Calderone RA, Edwards JE. Adherence of Candida species to host tissues and plastic surfaces. Rev Infect Dis 1986;8:73–85.
10. Segal E. Pathogenesis of human mycoses: Role of adhesion to host surfaces. Microbiol Sci 1987;4:344–347.

11. Kennedy MJ. Adhesion and association mechanisms of Candida albicans. Curr Top Med Mycol 1988;2:73–169.
12. Ruchel R, De Bernardis F, Ray TL, et al. Candida acid proteinase. J Med Vet Mycol 1992;30(suppl 1):123–132.
13. Kennedy MJ. Candida blastospore adhesion, association, and invasion of the gastrointestinal tract of vertebrate. In: Cole GT, Hoch HC, eds. The Fungal Spore and Disease Initiation in Plants and Animals. New York: Plenum Press, 1991:157–180.
14. Kennedy MJ. Regulation of Candida albicans populations in the gastrointestinal tract: Mechanisms and significance in GI and systemic candidiasis. Curr Top Med Mycol 1989;3:315–402.
15. Cole GT, Seshan KR, Pope LM, Yancey RJ. Morphological aspects of gastrointestinal tract invasion by Candida albicans in the infant mouse. J Med Vet Mycol 1988;26:173–185.
16. Beachey EH, Eisenstein B, Ofek I. Bacterial adherence in infectious diseases. In: Current Concepts: A Scope Publication. Kalamazoo, MI: Upjohn Company, 1982:1–52.
17. Ofek I, Doyle RJ. Principles of bacterial adhesion. In: Ofek I, Doyle RJ, eds. Bacterial Adhesion to Cells and Tissues. New York: Chapman & Hall, 1994:1–15.
18. Calderone RJ. The recognition of host cells by the pathogenic yeast Candida albicans. Jpn J Med Mycol 1994;36:9–18.
19. Calderone RA, Lehrer N, Segal E. Adherence of Candida albicans to buccal and vaginal epithelial cells—Ultrastructural observations. Can J Microbiol 1984;30:1001–1007.
20. Lehrer N, Segal E, Lis H, Gov Y. Effect of Candida albicans cell wall components on the adhesion of the fungus to human and murine vaginal mucosa. Mycopathologia 1988;102:115–121.
21. Ray TL, Digre KB, Payne CD. Adherence of Candida species to human epidermal corneocytes and buccal mucosal cells: Correlation with cutaneous pathogenicity. Invest Dermatol 1984;83:37–41.
22. Segal E, Lehrer N, Ofek I. Adherence of Candida albicans in vitro to human vaginal epithelial cells: Inhibition by amino sugars. Exp Cell Biol 1982;50: 13–17.
23. Segal E, Soroka A, Schechter A. Correlative relationship between adherence of Candida albicans to human vaginal epithelial cells in vitro and Candida vaginitis. J Med Vet Mycol 1984;22:191–200.
24. Kahana M, Segal E, Schewach-Millet M, Gov Y. In vitro adherence of Candida albicans: Inhibition by chitin soluble extract. Acta Derm Venerol 1988; 68:98–101.
25. Srebrnik A, Segal E. Comparison of Candida albicans adherence to human corneocytes from various populations. Acta Derm Venerol 1990;70:459–462.
26. Calderone RA, Cihlar RL, Lee D, et al. Yeast adhesion in the pathogenesis of endocarditis due to Candida albicans: Studies with adherence-negative mutants. J Infect Dis 1985;152:710–715.

27. Mayer CL, Filler SG, Edwards JE. Candida adherence to endothelial cells. Microvasc Res 1992;43:218–226.
28. Kalo A, Segal E. Interaction of Candida albicans with genital mucosa: Effect of sex hormones on adherence of yeasts in vitro. Can J Microbiol 1988;34: 224–228.
29. Segal E. Virulence factors. In: Segal E, Baum GL, eds. Pathogenic Yeasts and Yeast infections. Boca Raton, FL: CRC Press, 1994:49–59.
30. Segal E, Savage DC. Adhesion of Candida albicans to mouse intestinal mucosa in vitro: Development of the assay and test of inhibitors. J Med Vet Mycol 1986;24:477–479.
31. Sandovsky-Losica H, Segal E. Interaction of Candida albicans with murine gastrointestinal mucosa: Effect of irradiation on adherence in vitro. J Med Vet Mycol 1989;27:345–352.
32. Sandovsky-Losica H, Segal E. Interaction of Candida albicans with murine gastrointestinal mucosa from methotrexate and 5-fluorouracil treated animals: In vitro adhesion and prevention. J Med Vet Mycol 1990;28:274–287.
33. Maisch PA, Calderone RA. Adherence of Candida albicans to a fibrin-platelet matrix formed in vitro. Infect Immun 1980;27:650–656.
34. Kanbe T, Han Y, Redgrave B, et al. Evidence that mannans of Candida albicans are responsible for adherence of yeast forms to spleen and lymph node tissue. Infect Immun 1993;61:2578–2584.
35. Segal E, Sandovsky-Losica H. Interaction of Candida with mammalian tissues in vitro and in vivo. In: Doyle RJ, Ofek I. eds, Adhesion of Microbial Pathogens, vol. 253 of Methods in Enzymology, Academic Press, 1995: 439–452.
36. Segal E, Lehrman O, Dayan D. Adherence in vitro of various Candida species to acrylic surfaces. Oral Surg Oral Med Oral Pathol 1988;66:670–673.
37. Segal E, Gottfried L, Lehrer N. Candidal vaginitis in hormone treated mice: Prevention by a chitin extract. Mycopathologia 1988;102:157–163.
38. McCurtie J, Douglas JL. Extracellular polymer of Candida albicans: Isolation, analysis and role in adhesion. J Gen Microbiol 1985;131:495–503.
39. Tosh FD, Douglas LJ. Characterization of a fucoside-binding adhesion of Candida albicans. Infect Immun 1992;60:4734–4739.
40. Tronchin G, Bouchara JB, Annaix V, et al. Fungal adhesion molecules in Candida albicans. Eur J Epidemiol 1991;7:23–33.
41. Lehrer N, Segal E, Barr-Nea L. In vitro and in vivo adherence of Candida albicans to mucosal surfaces. Ann Microbiol 1983;134:239–306.
42. Segal E, Kremer I, Dayan D. Inhibition of adherence of Candida albicans to acrylic by a chitin derivative. Eur J Epidemiol 1991;8:350–355.
43. Sandin RL, Rogers AL, Patterson RJ, Beneke AS. Evidence for mannose-mediated adherence of Candida albicans to human buccal cells in vitro. Infect Immun 1982;35:79–85.
44. Sandin RL. The attachment to human buccal epithelial cells by Candida albicans: an in vitro kinetic study using concanavalin A. Mycopathologia 1987;98:179–184.

45. Douglas LJ, McCourtie J. Effect of tunicamycin on the adherence of Candida albicans to human buccal epithelial cells. FEMS Microbiol Lett 1983;16: 199–202.
46. Critchley IA, Douglas LJ. Role of glycosides as epithelial cell receptors for Candida albicans. J Gen Microbiol 1987;133:637–643.
47. Lehrer N, Segal E, Cihlar R, Calderone RA. Pathogenesis of vaginal candidiasis: Studies with a mutant which has reduced ability to adhere in vitro. J Med Vet Mycol 1986;24:127–131.
48. Segal E, Josef-Lev A. Induction of candidal vaginitis in diabetic mice and attempts to prevent the infection. J Med Vet Mycol, 1995;33:1–8.
49. Ghannoum MA, Abu-Elteen K, Ibrahim A, Stretton R. Protection against Candida albicans gastrointestinal colonization and dissemination by saccharides in experimental animals. Microbios 1991;67:95–105.
50. Sandovsky-Losica H, Segal E. Effect of a chitin derivative on experimental candidiasis of gastrointestinal origin in compromised mice. Immunol Infect Dis 1993;3:155–159.
51. Schwarzpeter M. Experimental cutaneous candidiasis in animals: Attempts of prevention by a chitin soluble extract. Tel Aviv University Thesis. 1991.
52. Suzuki K, Okawa Y, Hashimoto K, et al. Protecting effect of chitin and chitosan on experimentally induced murine candidiasis. Microbiol Immunol 1984;28:903–912.
53. Klotz S, Smith R, Stuart B. Effect of an arginine-glicine-aspartic acid-containing peptide on hematogenous candidal infections in rabbits. Antimicrob Agents Chemother 1992;36:132–136.
53a. Kennedy MJ, Sandin RL. Influence of growth conditions on Candida albicans adhesion, hydrophobicity and cell wall structure. J Med Vet Mycol 1988;26:79–92.
54. McCurtie J, Douglas JL. Relationship between cell surface composition, adherence, and virulence of Candida albicans. Infect Immun 1984;45:6–12.
55. Hazen KC, Brawner DL, Riesselman MH, et al. Differential adherence of hydrophobic and hydrophilic Candida albicans yeast cells to mouse tissues. Infect Immun 1991;59:907–912.
56. Minagi S, Miyake Y, Inagaki K, et al. Hydrophobic interactions in Candida albicans and Candida tropicalis adherence to various denture base resin materials. Infect Immun 1985;47:11–14.
57. Miyake Y, Fujita Y, Minagi S, Suginaka H. Surface hydrophobicity and adherence of Candida to acrylic surfaces. Microbios 1986;46:7–14.
58. Hazen K. Cell surface hydrophobicity of medically important fungi, especially Candida species. In: Doyle RJ, Rosenberg M. eds. Microbial Cell Surface Hydrophobicity. Washington, DC: ASM, 1990:249–295.
59. Kwon-Chung KJ, Bennett JE. Candidiasis. In: Medical Mycology. Philadelphia: Lea & Febiger, 1992:280–336.
60. Ray TL, Payne CD, Morrow BJ. Candida albicans acid proteinase: Characterization and role in candidiasis. Adv Exp Med Biol 1991;306:173–183.
61. White TC, Miyasaki SH, Agabian N. Three distinct secreted aspartyl proteinases in Candida albicans. J Bacteriol 1993;175:6126–6133.

62. Kwon-Chung KJ, Lehman D, Good C, Magee PT. Genetic evidence for role of extracellular proteinase in virulence of Candida albicans. Infect Immun 1985;49:571–575.
63. Ross IK, De Bernardis F, Emerson GW, et al. The secreted aspartate proteinase of Candida albicans: Physiology of secretion and virulence of a proteinase-deficient mutant. J Gen Microbiol 1990;136:687–694.
64. Hube B, Turver CJ, Odds FC, et al. Sequence of the Candida albicans gene encoding the secretory aspartate proteinase. J Med Vet Mycol 1991;29: 129–132.
65. Lott TJ, Page LS, Boiron P, et al. Nucleotide sequence of the Candida albicans aspartyl proteinase gene. Nucleic Acids Res 1989;17:1779.
66. Guentzel MN, Cole GT, Pope LM. Animal models for candidiasis. Curr Top Med Mycol 1985;1:57–116.
67. Segal E. Experimental infection. In: Segal E, Baum GL, eds. Pathogenic Yeasts and Yeast Infections. Boca Raton, FL: CRC Press, 1994;61–77.
68. Sandovsky-Losica H, Barr-Nea L, Segal E. Fatal systemic candidiasis of gastrointestinal origin: An experimental model in mice compromised by anticancer treatment. J Med Vet Mycol 1992;30:219–231.
69. De-Repentigny L, Phaneuf M, Mathieu LG. Gastrointestinal colonization and systemic dissemination by Candida albicans and Candida tropicalis in intact and immunocompromised mice. Infect Immun 1992;60:4907–4914.
70. Narayanan R, Joyce WA, Greenfield RA. Gastrointestinal candidiasis in a murine model of severe combined immunodeficiency syndrome. Infect Immun 1991;59:2116–2119.
71. Cole GT, Lynn KT, Seshan KR. An animal model for oropharingeal, esophageal and gastric candidiasis. Mycoses 1990;33:7–19.
72. Pope LM, Cole GT. Comparative studies of gastrointestinal colonization and systemic spread by Candida albicans and non-lethal yeast in the infant mouse. Scanning Electron Microsc 1982;IV:1667–1676.
73. Trygerman O. Interaction of Candida with buccal epithelial cells. M.Sc. Thesis, Tel-Aviv University 1994.

20

Immunomodulation by *Candida albicans*

JUDITH E. DOMER
Tulane University
New Orleans, Louisiana

I. INTRODUCTION

Candida albicans is the consummate opportunist, an organism that is part of the normal microbial flora, usually of the gut, causing disease only in those individuals in whom some underlying abnormality allowing for fungal overgrowth exists. The conditions that predispose to the development of candidiasis are many and varied, as are the clinical syndromes produced. Reduced to the lowest common denominator, however, it is convenient to think of human candidiasis existing in one of four clinical entities based upon the primary site(s) of involvement, namely, cutaneous, mucocutaneous, disseminated, and "focal."

Cutaneous candidiasis is usually an occupational disease (e.g., those who wear rubber gloves frequently develop candidiasis on the skin of their hands) or related to such conditions as obesity, wherein candidal organisms thrive on the surface between folds of the skin. Mucocutaneous candidiasis may be limited to the vagina, mouth, or esophagus, but it may also be a more involved and chronic phenomenon encompassing mucous membranes and skin, in which case it is referred to as the syndrome of chronic mucocutaneous candidiasis (CMC). Mucocutaneous disease correlates most frequently with underlying conditions such as diabetes, pregnancy, T-lymphocyte defects, endocrine abnormalities, and antibiotic therapy. Disseminated candidiasis (DC), fortunately, is relatively rare but usually involves multiple organs, including the spleen and liver, and is often complicated by immunosuppressive therapy, granulocytopenia, and leukemia. Focal infections—for example, heart valve involvement or peritonitis—may follow fungemia associated with indwelling catheters or abdominal surgery, respectively.

Apart from the obvious pathology that results from infection and disease, CMC and DC have often been associated with reduced or absent cell-mediated immune (CMI) function, demonstrable in vivo by testing for delayed hypersensitivity (DH) and in vitro by testing isolated lymphocytes for various responses, such as uptake of tritiated thymidine (lymphocyte stimulation, or LS) and production of migration inhibition factor (MIF) when incubated with mitogens or candidal antigens. In many instances abnormalities have been linked to a circulating inhibitor of immune function; in a few instances the inhibitor was identified as a cell-wall component of *C. albicans*, either mannan or a mannan-containing compound. In addition to the immunosuppressive phenomena described in human disease, however, mannan or other components of the yeast-cell wall, derived from *C. albicans* as well as from other yeasts such as *Saccharomyces cerevisiae*, have been shown to be both immunostimulatory and immunosuppressive in experimental in vitro and in vivo systems in the laboratory. While there is a rather extensive literature detailing immunoregulatory events mediated by fungal polysaccharides from many sources, this review focuses on *C. albicans* and its components.

II. PREDOMINANTLY *CANDIDA*-SPECIFIC IMMUNOMODULATION

A. Observations of Immunosuppression in Vivo and in Vitro Associated with CMC or DC

Chilgren, et al. (1) in 1967 were among the first to report specific immunological abnormalities in CMC, observing three patients deficient in their ability to respond in vivo with DH to *Candida*-specific and noncandidal antigens, two of whom also had defects in *Candida*-specific IgA production. Subsequently a number of additional patients were studied, and in the early 1970s Kirkpatrick, et al. (2) suggested using CMC as a model for studying cellular immunity, and Lehner et al. (3) and Valdimarsson, et al. (4) both suggested stratifying CMC patients based on their in vivo and in vitro immune responses to *C. albicans*, unrelated antigens, and mitogens. However, CMC, the underlying conditions predisposing to its development, and the resultant immunological abnormalities observed have been so diverse (reviewed in Ref. 5) that classification schemes based on immunological abnormalities have not stood the test of time.

In general, patients with CMC are more likely to have *Candida*-specific defects than global suppression. Comprehensive data illustrating the nature of the immunological defects in CMC have been summarized by Odds (5), but the data on CMI responses of 43 patients collated from eight medical centers in the United States (6) illustrate well the general pattern of cell-mediated responses observed in CMC patients (Table 1). Only 18% of the CMC cohort had in vivo DH responses to *C. albicans* antigen, and lymphocytes from 86% of the same patients had diminished responses to *Candida* antigen in vitro. In contrast, *Candida*-specific DH in the population at large is generally considered to be quite high (7,8). In vitro reactivity to *Candida* antigens was shown to parallel closely in vivo sensitivity as well (7).

One of the most interesting observations made of CMC and DC patients was that a number of such patients had circulating inhibitors of immune function (reviewed in Ref. 9). The inhibitors from all patients were clearly not the same, as their physical properties were different. Moreover, while

Table 1 In Vitro and in Vivo Cell-Mediated Immune Responses of 43 Patients with Chronic Mucocutaneous Candidiasis Observed by Physicians Participating in a Pediatric Immunodeficiency Collaborative Study Group

	No positive/total	%
DH[a] responses in vivo to:		
Candida albicans antigen	7/39	18
Other antigens	10/21	48
	No decreased/total	**%**
LS[b] in vitro to:		
Phytohemagglutinin	3/31	10
Concanavalin A	4/31	13
Pokeweed mitogen	3/33	9
Candida antigen	25/29	86
Other antigens	7/10	70

[a] DH = delayed hypersensitivity.
[b] LS = lymphocyte stimulation.
Source: Ref. 6.

some suppressed LS when sera were added to lymphocyte cultures in vitro, others were shown to downregulate neutrophil or monocyte function. Many data were anecdotal, wherein observations involved one or two patients, but Fisher et al. (10) identified a population of 23 patients with CMC for study and provided solid evidence that at least one of the serum inhibitors in a significant portion of the patients was *Candida* mannan or a mannan-containing compound. The inhibitor disappeared after antifungal therapy; it was nontoxic, nondialyzable, and thermostable, could be absorbed with anti-*Candida* serum, and could not be precipitated with ammonium sulfate. Later, Fischer et al. (11) determined that mannan interfered with *Candida* antigen presentation by adherent cells to autologous T lymphocytes. At that time they also concluded that suppressor T lymphocytes were not involved in the downregulation. Data derived from more recent studies, however, some of which are summarized below, have emphasized the fact that the issue is much more complicated than previously thought.

B. Observations of Immunosuppression Using Peripheral Blood Lymphocytes from Patients with Recurrent Vaginal Candidiasis

Technically speaking, recurrent vaginal candidiasis (RVC) could be described as a form of CMC, albeit one that is localized to the vagina instead of the gastrointestinal tract. Although the number of women afflicted with this disorder is relatively small, the syndrome itself is of particular interest in the context of this review because of its apparent association with defects in CMI. Most of the immunological data come from one laboratory (12–16) in which human cells and serum have been investigated, although another laboratory has begun investigations in animal models to address the issue of the role of CMI in vaginal candidiasis (17,18). The original observations of abnormally low in vitro reactivity to *Candida* antigen were reported by Hobbs et al. (19).

Witkin (20) summarized much of the early data from his laboratory in an excellent review several years ago. In their initial studies Witkin et al. (12) showed that peripheral blood lymphocytes (PBL) from 6 patients with RVC were poorly responsive to *Candida* antigens, whereas PBL from 6 healthy individuals responded well. Next (13), data were provided supporting the conclusion that a macrophage defect occurred in some women with RVC, a conclusion supported by even more recent data from the same laboratory (14,16). Lymphocytes from RVC patients responded with values in the control range if they were incubated with monocytes from healthy individuals and inhibitors of prostaglandin E_2 (PGE_2) synthesis, such as ibuprofen and indomethacin, prevented patient macrophages from inhibiting the proliferative response (13). The mechanism in all patients would not appear to be the same, however, since PBL from only 50% of the RVC patients responded positively to the exogenous application of interleukin-2 (IL-2) to the culture system. On the basis of these and later studies (14), it has been proposed that PGE_2, produced by macrophages, blocks in vitro lymphoproliferative responses by activating suppressor cells and blocking IL-2 production.

Two additional factors have been suggested as contributors to chronic vaginal problems, namely, histamine release as a consequence of IgE-mediated immunity to multiple antigens (15), *Candida* and non-*Candida*, and fluctuating hormone levels during the menstrual cycle (14,16). Cell-mediated immunity specific for *Candida* antigens was reduced during the luteal phase of the menstrual cycle, particularly in women not on oral contraceptives, suggesting that the dramatic increase of progesterone during the third and fourth weeks of the cycle contributed to the immunosuppression and thus to increased susceptibility to episodes of RVC (14). As with PGE_2 production, the effect of progesterone on CMI may be related to monocyte activity. A significantly decreased proliferative response was noted when PBL from individuals in the luteal phase of the menstrual cycle were incubated with *Candida* antigens. Removal of monocytes from the PBL populations allowed for normal proliferative responses to occur (16). It is obvious from the above that multiple factors have the potential for being involved in the expression of RVC and in the concomitant immunosuppression observed.

C. *Candida albicans*–Specific Immunomodulation by *Candida albicans* or Components Thereof

1. In Vitro Studies of Antibody Production

Experimental studies of *C. albicans*-specific immunomodulation have been carried out primarily in two different systems: in vitro culture of human cells, designed to induce *Candida*-specific antibody production as well as detect CMI, and in vivo studies of CMI in animal models, predominantly the mouse. In order to study regulation of antibody responses in vitro, Durandy et al. (21) developed an in vitro system for the generation of *Candida*-specific antibodies and then coincubated various cell types derived from PBL of CMC patients with cells from healthy volunteers to attempt to identify the source of suppression (22). Complete cultures—i.e., cultures containing B and T lymphocytes and monocytes from CMC patients with active disease—produced no *Candida*-specific antibody under the same conditions in which cell cultures from normal volunteers did. Moreover, T lymphocytes from CMC patients with active candidiasis suppressed antibody formation by lymphocytes from healthy donors. The suppressor cells were irradiation-sensitive and the addition of indomethacin to the cultures had no effect on the suppressor activity, indicating that prostaglandins were not involved in the immunosuppression. The suppression was not limited to $CD8^+$ cells, in that $CD8^-$ cells were also effective. Addition of *C. albicans* mannan (MAN) to control monocytes and lymphocytes elicited the same effect, suggesting that the effect was mediated by MAN and was MAN-specific.

2. *In Vitro Studies of Lymphocyte Stimulation*

Mannan has also been shown to be immunoinhibitory in lymphocyte-stimulation (LS) assays in vitro when added to cultures of lymphoid cells derived from healthy individuals. In one of the first such studies (23), mannan derived from *Saccharomyces cerevisiae* by extraction with Fehlings solution (24), a procedure that involves precipitation of MAN as a copper complex and then removal of the copper with hydrochloric acid—inhibited the proliferation of lymphocytes to both mitogens and antigens. If residual copper was removed by passage of the preparation through an ion-exchange resin, the inhibitory effects were specific for *C. albicans* antigen. Moreover, if a MAN extraction procedure not involving copper was used,—namely, precipitation with cetryltrimethylammonium bromide (CTAB,25)—a *C. albicans* MAN was obtained, which was highly antigenic and not inhibitory in vitro (26). Disaccharides through hexasaccharides separated from bulk CTAB MAN by β-elimination, however, were highly inhibitory of *Candida*-specific lymphoproliferative responses, the latter of which were produced in response to the Hollistier-Stier *Candida* antigen. It should be remembered that the Hollistier-Stier antigen is a complex mixture of *C. albicans* antigens, one of which is MAN (27).

3. *In Vivo Studies of Cell-Mediated Immunity*

Candida-specific downregulation of CMI has been reported in response to the injection into mice of large numbers of viable *C. albicans* yeasts intraperitoneally (IP) (28), or of various *C. albicans* yeast cell–derived soluble cell-wall extracts intravenously (IV) (29,30). The cell-wall preparation in one instance was a glycoprotein consisting of both MAN and glucan (29,31); in the second instance it contained mannose as the only sugar moiety (30). Both extracts are associated with small amounts of protein as well. The most extensive investigations have been done with the MAN. Delayed hypersensitivity in mice given viable cells IP was determined by the injection of whole killed cells into the footpad, while that in the animals treated with cell-wall fractions was by the injection of the soluble cell-wall extracts.

The injection of particulate matter into the footpad to detect DH, as was done by Valdez et al. (28) using whole killed cells, is a cause for concern in the interpretation of the results, since the whole killed cells are more likely to elicit non-DH phenomena at the same time as DH. Nevertheless, T lymphocytes were shown to be involved in the regulatory activity associated with both viable *C. albicans* (28) and MAN (32), in that lymphoid suspensions from suppressed animals treated in vitro with antitheta and complement prior to transfer could not downregulate DH in immunized recipients. Further, Garner et al. (32), using anti-Lyt 2-specific antibody and complement prior to transferring cell suspensions to immunized recipients, identified the suppressor as an Lyt 2+ cell. Downregulation was MAN-specific in that only DH responses to MAN or a MAN-containing glycoprotein were inhibited (32). The presence of downregulatory cells specific for MAN has no negative influence on the development of protective immune responses, however (33). In fact, 8 of 12 groups of immunized animals treated with MAN under selected conditions and then challenged IV with viable *C. albicans* to detect the presence of protective immunity, had fewer *C. albicans* yeasts in their kidneys when cultured 4 weeks later than did their non-MAN-treated counterparts. These results emphasize the lack of correlation of DH with systemic protection in candidiasis and suggest that MAN may contain epitopes involved in the protective response.

III. IMMUNOMODULATION OF NON-*CANDIDA* IMMUNE RESPONSES BY *C. ALBICANS* OR COMPONENTS THEREOF AS DEMONSTRATED IN EXPERIMENTAL SYSTEMS

Most of the non-*Candida*-specific immunoregulatory phenomena reported have involved modulation of antibody responses either to sheep erythrocytes (SRBC) or pneumococcal polysaccharide type III (SSS-III). In one of the earliest studies, Vardinon and Segal (34) injected SRBC and 10^6 viable *C. albicans* intramuscularly and then assayed for SRBC-specific plaque-forming cells (PFC). Such cells were reduced about fivefold in *C. albicans*–treated mice. Since bacterial lipopolysaccharide (LPS) did not alter the number of SRBC-specific PFC, the authors felt that the effect of the *C. albicans* was on T cells. They did not however, do additional experiments to actually identify the cell.

Immunopotentiation of non-*Candida* antibody responses in vivo, rather than immunosuppression, was demonstrated by Cutler and Lloyd (35).

They used viable *C. albicans* also, but in addition tested heat-killed cells, cell walls, and a cell-wall polysaccharide extracted with phenol for their immunomodulatory capacity. All preparations were capable of potentiating the antibody response to SRBC and to chicken gamma globulin, especially if the latter was coated onto horse erythrocytes. No immunosuppressive phenomena were noted and no attempt was made to identify the cell(s) responsible for the immunopotentiation. Domer et al. (36) confirmed the immunopotentiating effects of cell-wall polysaccharides from *C. albicans*, one of which was extracted with ethylenediamine and the other with dilute alkali, using SRBC and SSS-III as immunogens. In contrast to the studies of Cutler and Lloyd (35), however, Domer, et al. (36) were able to achieve enhancement if the modulators were given by a different route than the immunogen and if given prior to immunization. Domer et al. (36) were not able to identify the cell(s) responsible for the modulation either, but the enhancement did not appear to be associated with mitogenicity or with the production of B-cell growth factors or IL-2.

It is important to note that the cell wall extracts used by Cutler and Lloyd (35) and Domer et al. (36) contained both glucan and MAN. As is emphasized in the discussion below, glucan has been identified only with immunopotentiation, and it is possible that it might override any suppressive influences that MAN might exert. *Candida albicans* MAN alone, in fact, depending upon the system employed to demonstrate its effect, was either suppressive or enhancing of SRBC or SSS-III responses (37). These opposing properties could be separated by chromatography on the basis of size and charge. Lower-molecular-weight substances were suppressive, as was one of the more highly charged fractions from a Sephadex A-50 column. As mentioned above, Podroski et al. (26) found that disaccharides through hexasaccharides, unlike the native MAN, separated from bulk CTAB MAN by β-elimination, were highly inhibitory of *Candida*-specific lymphoproliferative responses. Domer et al. (37) did not identify a specific mechanism responsible for the modulatory activities, but it was hypothesized that the MAN exerted its influence on a regulatory T cell, regulatory T cells being an important feature in both SSS-III and SRBC responses.

An in vitro SRBC-specific antibody production system using murine splenocytes has been used by Cuff et al. (38–40) to investigate immunosuppressive activity of formalin-killed *C. albicans* or a dithiothreitol extract of cells walls. B lymphocytes were proposed as the mediators of suppression induced by formalin-killed cells (38,40), but T cells, surprisingly L3T4^{+} and not Lyt 2^{+}, were responsible for the in vitro suppressor phenomena demonstrated in response to the cell-wall extract (39). The suppressor cells in both instances were generated by incubating normal splenocytes in vitro with either formalin-killed *C. albicans* or the cell-wall extract for 3 days prior to coculture with fresh splenocytes in an in vitro SRBC-specific antibody production culture. T cell–independent antibody responses were not influenced by the suppressor B cells. Interestingly, the suppressor B population also downregulated T-cell-specific but not B-cell-specific mitogen responses in vitro (38,40,41).

IV. ANTITUMOR ACTIVITY AND RELATED PHENOMENA INDUCED BY *C. ALBICANS* OR ITS COMPONENTS

About 30 years ago, Wooles and DiLuzio (42) demonstrated that glucan extracted from the *S. cerevisiae* cell wall activated macrophages of the reticuloendothelial system; since that time, a number of studies have attempted to develop fungal cell walls or extracts thereof as antitumor agents (reviewed in Refs. 43 and 44). Inactivated whole cells or cell wall components of *C. albicans* (45–48), as well as extracellular polysaccharide (49), were early targets of such studies, some of which are summarized in Table 2. Several studies were performed in mice using LSTRA, a Moloney-virus-induced lymphoma, Friend leukemia virus, or S-180 solid tumor, and efficacy of the fungus or its wall components given IP was measured in terms of mean survival time or tumor weight. Whole killed *C. albicans* and glucan ghosts derived from cell walls, when combined with antitumor chemotherapy, increased survival time after challenge with LSTRA (46–48). Soluble MAN and a glucomannan were ineffective in the same system, however. To the contrary, only whole killed cells stimulated antitumor activity against Friend leukemia virus (50), but chemotherapy was not required to stimulate the effect.

More recently, investigators have focused on the ability of *C. albicans* or its wall components, administered IP to mice (51–57) or added to in vitro cultures of human cells (58–60) to stimulate natural killer (NK), activated-macrophage, or lymphokine-activated killer (LAK) activity in vitro against selected tumor cell lines (e.g., YAC-1 and U937, NK-sensitive lines and P-815, an activated macrophage-sensitive line, which is NK-resistant). A number of these studies are summarized in Table 3. In early studies, conflicting data were reported, in that one group (56) detected no increases in activated macrophages or splenic NK activity in response to whole cells, whereas another did (57); later (51,52), however, significant NK activity was detected in peritoneal exudate cells (PEC) and a transient increase in NK activity was noted in the spleen.

In the most recent investigations (54,55), using single and multiple injections of inactivated *C. albicans* or cell-wall fractions thereof, evidence has been obtained for the induction of two types of cells in PEC. The

Table 2 Antitumor Activity of Whole Killed Yeast Cells or Cell-Wall Fractions in Animal Systems Following the Introduction of the Model Intraperitoneally

	K-CA	Mannan-rich alkali-soluble fraction	Glucan-protein alkali-soluble fraction	Glucan ghosts	Assay	Comments	Reference
Line-10 hepatoma[a]	Yes[b]	—[c]	—	—	Tumor size	PEC primed for tumoricidal activity in presence of LPS	45
LSTRA (with chemotherapy)	Yes	—	—	—	Survival		46
LSTRA (with chemotherapy)	Yes	No	No	Yes	Survival	Effect was radiation-sensitive	47
LSTRA (with chemotherapy)	Yes	—	—	—	Survival	1. Radiation-sensitive 2. No increase splenic NK 3. Athymic mice unprotected	56
Friend leukemia virus (no chemotherapy)	Yes	No	Partial	Yes	Tumor size	No direct effect on virus	50

[a] Guinea pig model; all other data are from mouse models.
[b] Effective (yes) or ineffective (no) as antitumor agent.
[c] No data available.
Abbreviations: K-CA = whole killed yeast cells; LSTRA = a Moloney virus-induced lymphoma; PEC = peritoneal exudate cells; LPS = lipopolysaccharide; NK = natural killer.

earliest response is that of the NK-type cell effective against YAC-1 cells. It is asialo-GM1+, Lyt 2−, partially sensitive to anti-Thy 1, and previously had been shown to be nonadherent and nonphagocytic (53). The second and later response was that of a LAK-like cell effective against NK-insensitive targets. Its identification as a LAK-like cell is based on (a) lack of characteristic features associated with macrophages, such as adherence, (b) sensitivity to antiasialo GM1 and anti-Thy but not anti-Lyt 2, (c) isolation by discontinuous Percoll gradient separation with the large granular lymphocyte population, and (d) in vivo the cells had to be cultured with IL-2 to sustain their antitumor cell activity. Moreover, multiple injections of *C. albicans* were required to induce LAK-like cells, and none of the cell-wall fractions induced them, although mannoprotein used as a booster dose in animals pretreated with whole cells could recall LAK-like activity.

In summary, it is clear that inactivated yeasts and to a lesser extent selected cell-wall components are capable of inducing the expansion and differentiation of cells that have antitumor cell properties, such as NK, activated macrophage, or LAK-like cells. The application of this information to therapy in human disease, however, is not likely to occur any time soon, as the applicability of *Candida* wall preparations to the regression of human tumors has not been demonstrated. In contrast to the minimal information available for *Candida* walls, there is an extensive body of literature available on glucans derived from *S. cerevisiae*, but that topic is beyond the scope of this review. In spite of the relatively meager experimental data available on *Candida* cell walls and their efficacy as immunomodulatory agents in humans, there is a commercial preparation of glucan derived from *C. albicans* that is available for testing (61). Nicoletti et al. (61) did not test its antitumor activity; however, they demonstrated its ability to increase resistance to infection with *C. albicans* and *Staphylococcus aureus* when administered orally.

V. POTENTIAL MECHANISMS, INCLUDING CYTOKINE INVOLVEMENT, IN *CANDIDA*-INITIATED IMMUNOMODULATION IN HUMANS

The proposed mechanisms responsible for immunosuppression observed in humans or when using human cells in vitro have been varied, ranging from suppressor T cells (62,63) to an impairment in the generation of helper T cells (64) to the production of a soluble "nonspecific" inhibitor produced by macrophages (65). The early studies were done, of course, without benefit of knowledge of the many cytokines and soluble products of lymphoid cells known today. More recent studies, therefore, have fo-

Table 3 Natural Killer–Activated-Macrophage and Lymphokine-Activated Killer–Like Activities in Peritoneal Exudates or Splenic Lymphoid Populations of Mice Treated Intraperitoneally with Whole Killed Yeast Cells or Cell Wall Fractions

Cell source	K-CA	MAN-rich alk-sol	Mannoprot (Peat)	Man-Prot (ethanol)	Glucan ghosts	Assay	Response	Reference
PEC	Yes[a]	—[b]	—	—	—	YAC-1	Cytotoxicity present	51
Spleen	No	—	—	—	—	YAC-1	No cytotoxicity detected	
Spleen	Yes	—	—	—	—	LS, mitogens	Suppressed response	
Spleen	Yes	—	—	—	—	YAC-1	Cytotoxicity present (transiently) Effector cell was: 1. Nonadherent 2. Nonphagocytic 3. Asialo GM1 + 4. Partially sensitive to anti-Thy	52
Spleen	Yes	—	—	—	—	YAC-1	Cytotoxicity present	57
PEC	Yes	No	No	Yes	Yes	YAC-1	Cytotoxicity present early (cell characteristics same as above)	58,53
						P-815	Cytotoxicity present later	

							1. Adherent 2. Phagocytic 3. Sensitive to anti-Thy	
PEC (single)[c]	Yes	Yes	—	Yes	Yes	YAC-1	NK-like cells detected:	54,55
(multiple)	Yes (best)	Yes		Yes	Yes		1. Asialo GM1+ 2. Lyt 2− 3. Partially sensitive to anti-Thy 4. Found in athymic mice	
(single)	No	No	—	No	No	P-815	LAK-like cells detected:	
(multiple)	Yes	No		No (Yes) (As booster)	No		1. Asialo GM1+ 2. Lyt 2− 3. Sensitive to anti-Thy 4. Found in athymic mice	

[a] Yes or no: positive or negative modulatory activity.
[b] Not tested.
[c] Number of injections of immunomodulator.
Abbreviations: NK = natural killer; LAK = lymphokine-activated killer; PEC = peritoneal exudate cells; MAN-rich alk-sol = mannan-rich alkali-soluble; mannoprot (Peat) = mannoprotein extracted by Peat method; Man-Prot = mannoprotein precipitated with ethanol; YAC-1 = NK-sensitive cell line; P-815 = NK-insensitive cell line; LS = lymphocyte stimulation assay.

cused on specific cytokine production in response to in vitro incubation with *C. albicans* or cell-wall components.

Interpretation of the data generated in vitro studies with human cells is complicated because most human cells are not naive with respect to *C. albicans*, as many humans are colonized with the organism and have CMI responses capable of being recalled with *Candida* antigens. Thus, it comes as no surprise that inactivated *C. albicans* stimulated the production of IL-2 by human cells which peaked 1 to 2 days after the initiation of culture, and gamma interferon (IFNγ), which peaks at 3 days (66). Both of these cytokines can be produced by Th1 lymphocytes in response to a recall antigen. Moreover, selected fractions of cell wall mannoprotein, designated F1 and F2, separated by chromatography on DEAE Sephadex A-50 stimulated the production of IL-2 and IFNγ just as well as did whole cells (67). Cytokine profiles in response to stimulation with the unseparated mannoprotein indicated that long-lasting mRNAs were induced early for not only IL-2 and IFNγ but also IL-1B, TNFα, IL-6, and GM-CSF (68), whereas they were not induced for IL-4, IL-5, and IL-10. Gamma interferon appears to be a critical cytokine for the generation of LAK-like cells in PBL in response to the F2 fraction (60). Using the U937 cell line, uninfected or persistently infected with the human immunodeficiency virus (HIV), Gomez, et al. (60) found that F2 stimulated LAK-like cells in normal PBL capable of killing infected or uninfected cells, but that F2, unlike recombinant-IL-2, was unable to stimulate the production of LAK-like cells in PBL from patients with advanced acquired immunodeficiency syndrome (AIDS). Using antibodies to various cytokines, including tumor necrosis factor α (TNFα) and IFNγ, anti-IFNγ antibodies destroyed the ability of normal PBL to produce LAK-like activity against U937. These and several other lines of data pointed to a pivotal role for IFNγ in the induction of the LAK-like activity.

Other investigators have concentrated on the production of cytokines more often associated with macrophages—namely, IL-1 and TNFα. Since TNFα has tumoricidal activity (69), it is of particular interest in situations where NK activity can be demonstrated. F2, a subfraction of MAN mentioned above, was capable of stimulating the production of TNFα (70), and another MAN-rich antigen designated MPPS induced the release of IL-1(71). Opposing data were obtained, however, when viable and heat-killed blastospores were compared for their cytokine-stimulating capacity, in that viable cells preferentially induced IL-1 production in cultures of unseparated PBL from healthy women of childbearing age, whereas heat-killed cells induced higher levels of TNFα (72). To the contrary, TNFα production varied little when live and heat-killed *C. albicans* were incubated with human mononuclear cells and large granular lymphocytes separated from PBL (73). Finally, Raponi, et al. (74) have demonstrated the release of IL-6, one of the cytokines for which Ausiello, et al. (68) detected mRNA, when human monocytes were incubated with culture filtrate antigens or heat-killed *C. albicans*.

It is difficult to synthesize a unified hypothesis based on the anecdotal information available. It is clear that cytokines associated with CMI and the recall of specific immune responses are expressed in the presence of viable and inactivated *C. albicans* as well as in the presence of cell walls and MAN or MAN-containing fractions thereof. Moreover, the stimulation of the production of TNFα would help to explain the antitumor effects observed in selected assays. The nonspecific inhibitor detected, but never identified, after 6 days of culture in the presence of a MAN-containing antigen in the early studies of Lombardi et al. (65,75) might be explained on the basis of prostaglandin E_2 (PGE_2) production in the in vitro cultures. As mentioned earlier, Witkin et al. (13), using PBL from women with recurrent vaginitis, noted that *Candida*-specific proliferative responses were greatly diminished when inhibitors of prostaglandin synthesis were added to the cultures, whereas proliferative responses to *Candida* antigens were normal if monocytes from healthy volunteers were substituted for those of the patients. Moreover, it is known that PGE_2 induces TNFα and IL-1 synthesis (76) and then feeds back to suppress subsequent TNFα but not IL-1 production (77). PGE_2 is also known to inhibit IL-2 synthesis and stimulate the production of down-regulatory T cells (reviewed in Ref. 78). What is clear from these and many other studies is that the effects shown by various cytokines are dose-dependent, that both synergistic and antagonistic effects can occur between the same two cytokines depending upon the experimental conditions, and that the net response detected depends upon the balance between various groups of cytokines (79).

VI. CONCLUSION

In summary, then, while in vitro studies are useful for attempting to identify the components involved in the response, there are so many redundancies in the immune system that a factor/cell identified as the key immunoregulatory agent in vitro may well have minimal importance in vivo. It will be necessary therefore, to wait for correlative data from in vivo systems before making firm commitments to any one mechanism being responsible for the immunomodulation observed. Moreover, it has been our observation in in vivo systems (29,30) that immunosuppression is often antigen-specific and can be induced by almost any antigen which is immunogenic if that antigen is presented to the immune system by the appropriate route and in the appropriate concentration. The site of initial contact with the antigen and its concentration when administered are critical. It is difficult, therefore, to determine whether the immunoregulatory events detected have a cause-and-effect relationship with *Candida* disease or whether they are simply concomitant events.

REFERENCES

1. Chilgren RA, Meuwissen HJ, Quie PG, Hong R. Chronic mucocutaneous candidiasis deficiency of delayed hypersensitivity and selective local antibody defect. Lancet 1967;2:688–693.
2. Kirkpatrick CH, Rich RR, Bennett JE. Chronic mucocutaneous candidiasis: Model-building in cellular immunity. Ann Intern Med 1971;74:955–978.
3. Lehner T, Wilton JMA, Ivanyi L. Immunodeficiencies in chronic mucocutaneous candidosis. Immunology 1971;22:775–786.
4. Valdimarsson H, Higgs JM, Wells RS, et al. Immune abnormalities associated with chronic mucocutaneous candidiasis. Cell Immunol 1973;6:348–361.
5. Odds FC. *Candida* and Candidosis: A Review and Bibliography, 2d ed. London: Bailliére Tindall, 1988:146–147.
6. Herrod HG. Chronic mucocutaneous candidiasis in childhood and complications of non-*Candida* infection: A report of the pediatric immunodeficiency collaborative study group. J Pediatr 1990;116:377–382.
7. Ferguson AC, Kershnar HE, Collin WK, Stiehm ER. Correlation of cutaneous hypersensitivity with lymphocyte response to *Candida albicans*. Am J Clin Pathol 1977;68:499–504.
8. Shannon DC, Johnson G, Rosen FS, Austen KF. Cellular reactivity to *Candida albicans* antigen. N Engl J Med 1966;275:690–693.
9. Domer JE. *Candida* cell wall mannan: A polysaccharide with diverse immunologic properties. CRC Crit Rev Microbiol 1989;17:33–51.
10. Fischer A, Ballet JJ, Griscelli C. Specific inhibition of in vitro *Candida*-induced lymphocyte proliferation by polysaccharidic antigens present in serum of patients with chronic mucocutaneous candidiasis. J Clin Invest 1978;62:1005–1013.
11. Fischer A, Pichat L, Audinot M, Griscelli C. Defective handling of mannan by monocytes in patients with chronic mucocutaneous candidiasis resulting in a specific cellular unresponsiveness. Clin Exp Immunol 1982;47:653–660.
12. Witkin SS, Yu R, Ledger WJ. Inhibition of *Candida albicans*-induced lymphocyte proliferation by lymphocytes and sera from women with recurrent vaginitis. Am J Obstet Gynecol 1983;147:809–811.
13. Witkin SS, Hirsch J, Ledger WJ. A macrophage defect in women with recurrent *Candida* vaginitis and its reversal in vitro by prostaglandin inhibitors. Am J Obstet Gynecol 1986;155:790–795.
14. Kalo-Klein A, Witkin SS. *Candida albicans*: Cellular immune system interactions during different stages of the menstrual cycle. Am J Obstet Gynecol 1989;161:1132–1136.

15. Witkin SS, Kalo-Klein A, Galland L, et al. Effect of *Candida albicans* plus histamine on prostaglandin E_2 production by peripheral blood mononuclear cells from healthy women and women with recurrent candidal vaginitis. J Infect Dis 1991;164:396–399.
16. Kalo-Klein A, Witkin SS. Regulation of the immune response to *Candida albicans* by monocytes and progesterone. Am J Obstet Gynecol 1991;164: 1351–1354.
17. Sobel JD, Muller G, McCormick JF. Experimental chronic vaginal candidosis in rats. Sabouraudia 1985;23:199–206.
18. Fidel PL, Lynch ME, Sobel JD. *Candida*-specific cell-mediated immunity is demonstrable in mice with experimental vaginal candidiasis. Infect Immun 1993;61:1990–1995.
19. Hobbs JR, Brigden D, Davidson F, et al. Immunological aspects of candidal vaginitis. Proc R Soc Lond (Med) 1977;70(suppl 4):11–13.
20. Witkin SS. Immunology of recurrent vaginitis. Am J Reprod Immunol Microbiol 1987;15:34–37.
21. Durandy A, Fischer A, Griscelli C. Specific in vitro antimannan-rich antigen of *Candida albicans* antibody production by sensitized human blood lymphocytes. J Clin Invest 1983;71:1602–1613.
22. Durandy A, Fischer A, le Deist F, et al. Mannan-specific and mannan-induced T-cell suppressive activity in patients with chronic mucocutaneous candidiasis. J Clin Immunol 1987;7:400–409.
23. Nelson RD, Herron MJ, McCormack, RT, Gehrz RC. Two mechanisms of inhibition of human lymphocyte proliferation by soluble yeast mannan polysaccharide. Infect Immun 1984;43:1041–1046.
24. Peat S, Whelan WJ, Edwards TE. Polysaccharide of baker's yeast: Part IV. Mannan. J Chem Soc (Lond) 1961;1:29–34.
25. Lloyd KO. Isolation, characterization and partial structure of peptido galactomannans from the yeast form of *Cladosporium werneckii*. Biochemistry 1970;9:3446–3453.
26. Podzorski RP, Gray GR, Nelson RD. Different effects of native *Candida albicans* mannan and mannan-derived oligosaccharides on antigen-stimulated lymphoproliferation in vitro. J Immunol 1990;144:707–716.
27. Syverson RE, Buckley HR. Cell wall antigens in soluble cytoplasmic extracts of *Candida albicans* as demonstrated by crossed immunoelectrophoresis with concanavalin A. J Immunol Methods 1977;18:149–156.
28. Valdez JC, Meson OE, Sirena A, de Alderete NG. Characteristics of DTH suppressor cells in mice infected with *Candida albicans*. Mycopathologia 1987;98:121–126.
29. Carrow EW, Domer JE. Immunoregulation in experimental murine candidiasis: Specific suppression induced by *Candida albicans* cell wall glycoprotein. Infect Immun 1985;49:172–181.
30. Domer JE, Garner RE, Befidi-Mengue RN. Mannan as an antigen in cell-mediated immunity (CMI) assays and as a modulator of mannan-specific CMI. Infect Immun 1989;57:693–700.

31. Lyon FL, Domer JE. Chemical and enzymatic variation in the cell walls of pathogenic *Candida* species. Can J Microbiol 1985;31:590–597.
32. Garner RE, Childress AM, Human LG, Domer JE. Characterization of *Candida albicans* mannan-induced, mannan-specific delayed hypersensitivity suppressor cells. Infect Immun 1990;58:2613–2620.
33. Garner RE, Domer JE. Lack of effect of *Candida albicans* mannan on the development of immune responses in experimental candidiasis. Infect Immunol 1994;62:738–741.
34. Vardinon N, Segal E. Suppressive action of *Candida albicans* on the immune response in mice. Exp Cell Biol 1979;47:275–280.
35. Cutler JE, Lloyd RK. Enhanced antibody responses induced by *Candida albicans* in mice. Infect Immun 1982;38:1102–1108.
36. Domer JE, Elkins KL, Ennist DL, et al. Enhancement of non-*Candida* antibody responses by *Candida albicans* cell wall glycoprotein. Infect Immun 1987;55:2619–2624.
37. Domer JE, Stashak PW, Elkins K, et al. Separation of immunomodulatory effects of mannan from *Candida albicans* into stimulatory and suppressive components. Cell Immunol 1986;101:403–414.
38. Cuff CF, Rogers CM, Lamb BJ, Rogers TJ. Induction of suppressor cells in vitro by *Candida albicans*. Cell Immunol 1986;100:47–56.
39. Cuff CF, Taub DD, Rogers TJ. The induction of T-suppressor cells with a soluble extract of *Candida albicans*. Cell Immunol 1989;122:71–82.
40. Cuff CF, Packer BJ, Rogers TJ. A further characterization of *Candida albicans*–induced suppressor B-cell activity. Immunology 1989;68:80–86.
41. Rivas V, Rogers TJ. Studies on the cellular nature of *Candida albicans*–induced suppression. J Immunol 1983;130:376–379.
42. Wooles WR, Di Luzio NR. The phagocytic and proliferative response of the reticuloendothelial system following glucan administration. J Reticuloendothel Soc 1964;1:160–169.
43. DiLuzio NR, McNamee RB, Williams DL, et al. Glucan induced inhibition of tumor growth and enhancement of survival in a variety of transplantable and spontaneous murine tumor models. In: Escobar MR, Friedman H, eds. Macrophages and lymphocytes. Part A. New York: Plenum Press, 1980: 269–290.
44. Domer JE, Garner RE. Fungal wall components and immunostimulation. In: Latge JP, Boucias, D, eds. Fungal cell wall and immune response. Cell Biol 1991;53:415–430.
45. Weinberg JB, Hibbs JB Jr. Enhanced macrophage tumoricidal activity and tumor suppression or regression caused by heat-killed *Candida albicans*. JNCI 1979;63:1273–1278.
46. Bistoni F, Marconi P, Pitzurra M, et al. Combined effects of BCG or *Candida albicans* (CA) with anti tumor agents against a virus-induced lymphoma in mice. Eur J Can 1979;15:1305–1314.
47. Cassone A, Marconi P, Biston F, et al. Immunoadjuvant effects of *Candida albicans* and its cell wall fractions in a mouse lymphoma model. Cancer Immunol Immunother 1981;10:181–189.

48. Cassone A, Bistoni F, Cenci E, et al. Immunopotentiation of anticancer chemotherapy by *Candida albicans*, other yeasts and insoluble glucan in an experimental lymphoma model. Sabouraudia 1982;20:115–125.
49. Saltarelli CG, Coppola CP. Inhibitory effects of *Candida albicans* extracellular polysaccharides on mouse sarcoma 180. J Surg Oncol 1980;15:99–106.
50. Cassone A, Scaringi L, Pesce CD, et al. Suppression of Friend leukemia cell-induced tumors by cellular preparations of *Candida albicans*. Microbiologica 1983;6:207–220.
51. Marconi P, Scaringi L, Cassone A, Tissi L. Effect of inactivated *C. albicans* on natural killer (NK) cell activity and blastogenesis in mice. In: Aaronson A, Frati L, Verna R, eds. Genetic and Phenotypic Markers of Tumors. London: Plenum Publishing, 1985:145–151.
52. Marconi P, Scaringi L, Tissi L, et al. Induction of natural killer cell activity by inactivated *Candida albicans* in mice. Infect Immun 1985;50:297–303.
53. Scaringi L, Marconi P, Boccanera M, et al. Cell wall components of *Candida albicans* as immunomodulators: Induction of natural killer and macrophage-mediated peritoneal cell cytotoxicity in mice by mannoprotein and glucan fractions. J Gen Microbiol 1988;134:1265–1274.
54. Scaringi L, Cornacchione P, Rosati E, et al. Induction of LAK-like cells in the peritoneal cavity of mice by inactivated *Candida albicans*. Cell Immunol 1990;129:271–287.
55. Scaringi L, Rosati E, Cornacchione P, et al. In vivo modulation of lymphokine-activated killer cell activity by cell wall components of *Candida albicans*. Cell Immunol 1992;139:438–454.
56. Marconi P, Cassone A, Tissi L, et al. Cellular mechanisms underlying the adjuvant activity of *Candida albicans* in a mouse lymphoma model. Int J Cancer 1982;29:403–408.
57. Wojdani A, Ghoneum M. In vivo augmentation of natural killer cell activity by *Candida albicans*. Int J Immunopharmacol 1987;9:827–832.
58. Cassone A, Marconi P, Bistoni F. Cell wall of *Candida albicans* and host response. CRC Crit Rev Microbiol 1987;15:87–95.
59. Ausiello CM, Palma C, Spagnoli GC, et al. Cytotoxic effectors in human peripheral blood mononuclear cells induced by a mannoprotein complex of *Candida albicans*. Cell Immunol 1989;121:349–359.
60. Gomez MJ, Torosantucci A, Quinti I, et al. Mannoprotein-induced anti-U937 cell cytotoxicity in peripheral blood mononuclear cells from uninfected or HIV-infected subjects: role of interferon-γ and tumor necrosis factor-α. Cell Immunol 1993;152:530–543.
61. Nicoletti A, Nicoletti G, Ferraro G, et al. Preliminary evaluation of immunoadjuvant activity of an orally administered glucan extracted from *Candida albicans*. Arzneimittel-Forschung 1992;42:1246–1250.
62. Piccolella E, Lombardi G, Morelli R. Generation of suppressor cells in the response of human lymphocytes to a polysaccharide from *Candida albicans*. J Immunol 1981;126:2151–2159.
63. Barnaba V, Zaccari E, Levroro M, Balsano F. Suppressor T cells role in

the unresponsiveness to *Candida albicans* in chronic mucocutaneous candidiasis. Boll Ist Sieroter Milan 1985;64:126–130.
64. Ruiz-Arguelles A, Jett JR, Ritts RE Jr. Impaired generation of helper T cells in a patient with chronic mucocutaneous candidiasis and malignant thymoma. J Clin Lab Immunol 1983;10:165–169.
65. Lombardi G, Piccolella E, Vismara D, et al. Monocyte subsets in the production of inhibitory factor by *Candida albicans*-activated human T cells. Immunology 1985;56:373–376.
66. Spagnoli G, Ausiello C, Caslinuova I, et al. *Candida albicans* and a phosphorylated glucomannan-protein fraction of its cell wall induce production of immune interferon by human peripheral blood mononuclear cells. IRCS Med Sci 1985;13:1190–1191.
67. Torosantucci A, Palma C, Boccanera M, et al. Lymphoproliferative and cytotoxic responses of human peripheral blood mononuclear cells to mannoprotein constituents of *Candida albicans*. J Gen Microbiol 1990;136: 2155–2163.
68. Ausiello CM, Urbani F, Gessani S, et al. Cytokine gene expression in human peripheral blood mononuclear cells stimulated by mannoprotein constituents from *Candida albicans*. Infect Immun 1993;61:4105–4111.
69. Feinman R, Henricksen-DeStefano D, Tsujimoto M, Vicek J. Tumor necrosis factor is an important mediator of tumor cell killing by human monocytes. J Immunol 1987;138:635–640.
70. Vecchiarelli A, Puleti M, Torosantucci A, et al. In vitro production of tumor necrosis factor by murine splenic macrophages stimulated with mannoprotein constituents of *Candida albicans* cell wall. Cell Immunol 1991;134:65–76.
71. Lombardi G, Piccolella E, Vismara D, et al. *Candida albicans* polysaccharide extract (MPPS) and PPD stimulate the production of interleukin-1 and lymphocyte proliferation. Clin Exp Immunol 1984;58:581–586.
72. Jeremias J, Kalo-Klein A, Witkin SS. Individual differences in tumour necrosis factor and interleukin-1 production induced by viable and heat-killed *Candida albicans*. J Med Vet Mycol 1991;29:157–163.
73. Djeu JY, Blanchard DK, Richards AL, Friedman H. Tumor necrosis factor induction by *Candida albicans* from human natural killer cells and monocytes. J Immunol 1988;141:4047–4052.
74. Raponi G, Ghezzi MC, Mancini C, Filadoro F. Culture filtrates and whole heat-killed *Candida albicans* stimulate human monocytes to release interleukin-6. Microbiologica 1993;16:267–274.
75. Lombardi G, Vismara D, Piccolella E, et al. A nonspecific inhibitor produced by *Candida albicans* activated T cells impairs cell proliferation by inhibiting interleukin-1 production. Clin Exp Immunol 1985;60:303–310.
76. Le J, Vilcek J. Biology of Disease. Tumor necrosis factor and interleukin 1: Cytokines with multiple overlapping biological activities. Lab Invest 1987; 56:234–247.
77. Scales WE, Chensue SW, Otterness I, Kunkel SL. Regulation of monokine gene expression: Prostaglandin E_2 suppresses tumor necrosis factor but not

interleukin-1α or β-mRNA and cell-associated bioactivity. J Leuk Biol 1989; 45:416–421.
78. Chouaib S, Bertoglio JH. Prostaglandins E as modulators of the immune response. Lymphokine 1988;7:237–245.
79. Modlin RL, Nutman TB. Type-2 cytokines and negative immune regulation in human infections. Curr Opin Immunol 1993;5:511–517.

21

Candida Strain Typing

FRANK C. ODDS
Janssen Research Foundation
Beerse, Belgium

I. INTRODUCTION

Members of the species *Homo sapiens* are able to differentiate individual organisms within the species on the basis of a diversity of recognizable characters. Definitions of strains, grouped by common characters, also exist within this species. The present state of microbial technology does not permit such differentiation of each individual organism within a population of cells of the pathogenic fungus *Candida albicans*, but a need exists at least for differentiation of populations with a similar genotype (strains) as a means of solving problems in the epidemiology of *Candida* infections. This article gives an overview of the methods available for typing strains beyond the species level in *C. albicans* and in other yeasts of clinical importance within the genus *Candida*. It will also summarize the findings of surveys designed to elucidate aspects of epidemiology and transmission of strains in the context of *Candida* colonization of human hosts and the pathogenesis and treatment of symptomatic *Candida* infections.

The topic of *Candida* strain typing has been reviewed elsewhere (1,2), and these reviews should be consulted for more detailed coverage of the subject.

II. A BRIEF HISTORY OF *CANDIDA* STRAIN TYPING

The single species *C. albicans* accounts for 50–90% of all diseases grouped under the general clinical heading of *Candida* infections, and the species can be found as part of the normal commensal flora in up to 50% of the healthy population (3). Investigations of sources, routes of transmission, and pathogenesis of such infections therefore require a facility for detecting strain-specific markers within *C. albicans*. This pressing need has been filled only very slowly.

A. Serotyping

Possibilities for typing *C. albicans* isolates by agglutination reactions with strain-specific antisera were studied independently in the United States and Japan during the late 1950s and early 1960s. The groups of Hasenclever and Mitchell (4) and of Tsuchiya et al. (5) both succeeded in dividing *C. albicans* strains into two serotypes, called A and B by Hasenclever and Mitchell. Despite many subsequent efforts, serological recognition of more than two variable epitopes in intact *C. albicans* cells has not become possible.

B. Morphotyping

In 1968, Brown-Thomsen (6) proposed a scheme for typing strains based on the morphology of *C. albicans* colonies formed from heavy inocula on a rich growth medium. This approach was later refined by others (7,8), but it lacks ideal reproducibility, since many strains change colony morphotypes between subcultures and many strains belong to a single, predominant colony phenotype and therefore cannot be distinguished by the method. (The latter limitation has beset many phenotypic discrimination approaches with *C. albicans*.)

C. Physiological Typing

Also in 1968, Blaschke-Helmessen in Germany (9) typed *C. albicans* strains on the basis of their susceptibilities to nystatin and pimaricin and the activity zones they produced on agar plates designed to detect proteinase and lipase production. She showed that in 95% of *C. albicans* isolations made soon after birth, the strains found in the mouths of 94 mother-baby pairs matched each other in terms of physiological phenotype. Blaschke-Helmessen's method was later used by others in epidemiological studies of *Candida* carriage and infection (10,11).

Differentiation of strain phenotypes by their patterns of resistance to inhibitory chemicals in an agar growth medium was an approach developed in the United Kingdom by Warnock and his colleagues (12,13). A hybrid physiological biotyping approach was devised by Odds and Abbott (14,15) in which assimilation properties, flucytosine and boric acid susceptibility, and proteinase activity of *C. albicans* strains were determined on a series of test media that allowed simultaneous testing of up to 60 isolates. These various "agar-plate typing" methods have been used to study several epidemiological problems (see below), but they suffer from difficulties of reproducibility, particularly interlaboratory reproducibility (16), and isolates must exhibit several test differences to demonstrate convincingly that they represent different strains.

D. "Yeast Killer Factor" Typing

An entirely novel approach to *C. albicans* typing was introduced in 1983 by Polonelli et al. in Italy (17,18). This involved the use of yeast strains with the power to kill *C. albicans* isolates differentially. The method is analogous to bacteriocin typing as practiced with bacteria.

E. DNA Typing

Typing of *C. albicans* strains at the DNA level was first described in 1987 and was achieved by analysis of DNA restriction fragment length polymorphisms (RFLPs) (19–21) and by electrophoretic karyotyping (22,23). The introduction soon after of repeat-sequence DNA probes (24,25) further enhanced the elegance of *Candida* DNA typing by improving both the reproducibility and the discriminatory power of the techniques. As the methods for *C. albicans* strain typing at the level of both genotype and phenotype continued to proliferate, Hunter (26) conducted a thorough statistical review of the published methods and showed that many lacked fine discriminatory power.

The latest developments in *Candida* strain typing include randomly amplified polymeric DNA typing (27) and typing by isoenzyme polymorphisms (28). Many different methods of typing based on genotype or phenotype analysis are now available. All of them are still used essentially as research tools rather than as routine tests. The methods have been used to study *Candida* epidemiology in a variety of clinical situations; the findings will be summarized later. For those interested in typing *Candida* strains, it is important to achieve a good basic understanding of the principles and pitfalls of different approaches. Many investigators underestimate the complexity both of the necessary technology and of the analysis of epidemiological data; therefore a brief review of these aspects is provided below.

III. GENERAL PRINCIPLES OF MICROBIAL STRAIN TYPING

A. Genotype and Phenotype as the Basis for Strain Delineation

Microorganisms are presently assigned Latin binomial (genus and species) names on the basis of their defined morphological, behavioral, and physiological properties. However, it is a common observation that different isolates within each microbial species show variability with respect to certain properties beyond the level of those that constitute the species definition. Among bacteria, characteristics such as serotype, phage type, and bacteriocin type have been used for many years as a means of discriminating between strains of the same species, and such properties are often used to determine sources, reservoirs, and routes of transmission of strains in epidemiological investigations. For some organisms, including many yeasts and molds, the species name is qualified by the addition of descriptors such as "var." and "subsp.," with a third Latin name to indicate that an isolate belongs to a definable race or strain at a level below that considered to define the species itself.

For many years, phenotypic characters have formed the basis of descriptive taxonomies of microorganisms and have afforded the essential means of species identification. With the advent of technology capable of distinguishing differences at the level of DNA in a microbial isolate, an evolutionary process is taking place in which phenotypic characteristics are being overtaken by more direct examination of microbial genotype as a basis for recognition of isolates at both the species and subspecies levels. The ultimate reference criterion for definition and description of an individual isolate would be a listing of its entire DNA base sequence, but both determination of the sequence for a new isolate and its comparison with sequences from large numbers of other isolates fall beyond current technical capabilities. However, the differentiation of strains at the DNA level *is* now possible at a level of stringency lower than that of the complete base sequence but perfectly adequate for most epidemiological studies. Cost and complexity of DNA approaches to typing are the usual reasons given for the persistence of more traditional phenotypic tests as a basis for strain differentiation.

However, it is possible to overstate the scientific importance of genotype determination, and investigators studying epidemiological problems should be aware that determination of phenotypic characters remains of value as evidence in many real-life situations. For example, two microbial isolates may have apparently identical strain types as determined by DNA analysis at the present level of typing technology, yet one isolate nevertheless consistently expresses resistance to a particular antimicrobial agent while the other is always sensitive when tested. The phenotypic difference in susceptibility behavior of such isolates is more likely to be of as much or more significance to the clinical epidemiologist than the knowledge that their genotypes appear to be identical.

A case can therefore be made (at least in the absence of simple methodology for determination and comparison of entire DNA base sequences) for a combined approach to strain typing in which both genotypic and phenotypic markers are measured. In this approach, each of the two components of the strain typing must be optimized in a different way. Genotypic markers should be chosen so as to offer the maximum possible sensitivity of discrimination between strains at the DNA level, while phenotypic markers should be chosen to offer the greatest relevance to the process of microbial transmission, colonization, or pathogenesis under study.

B. Interpretation of Strain-Typing Experiments: "Identical" and "Different" Strains

The greatest problem confronting the investigator of microbial strain types is not choice of methodology or choice of sources and isolates for study but that of interpreting the findings from procedures designed to differentiate strains. This point is very commonly overlooked. It is statistically simple to measure the certainty with which a particular method reveals strain *differences* between isolates, and this is true whether genotype or phenotype has been determined. However, no method (at least not in the absence of the complete DNA base sequence) can produce a result that unequivocally defines two isolates as *identical*. When two isolates are shown as giving identical DNA fingerprints by one of the methods useful for such fingerprinting, those isolates should be described in terms such as "indistinguishable by the method used," not as "identical," since the possibility has not been excluded that a more refined typing method might yet reveal differences between isolates. This criticism is particularly applicable in studies based on patterns of electrophoretically separated chromosomes from organisms such as *Candida*. Chromosomes of apparently identical size in an electrophoresis gel may have measurably dissimilar DNA base sequences, so that only differences, not similarities in chromosomal patterns, provide reasonable evidence for use in typing experiments.

Most investigators desire a typing scheme in which a name or code can be attached to each definable strain type. Such a scheme greatly facilitates analysis of typing data, since it reduces to a readily understood level the concept of strain similarity and difference. Unfortunately, not many methods of strain typing lend themselves to black-and-white definitions suitable for coded typing schemes. DNA typing methods, in particular, produce data for each strain tested that lie on a continuum of variability (of properties such as RFLP or chromosome band intensity and position) rather than the conveniently discrete packets of variability necessary for codifying strains. Because of this limitation, analyses of typing data are nowadays often statistically based, and the previously familiar type of conclusion that, for example, "strain type X was isolated from 95% of the infected patients" is less likely to be found in the modern literature.

IV. METHODS FOR *CANDIDA* STRAIN TYPING

Almost all of the available methods for microbial strain typing can be applied to *Candida* strain differentiation. Phage typing of *Candida* strains is not possible, since *Candida*-specific viruses have rarely been described and, where known, they do not cause the yeast cells to form lysis plaques that would allow easy detection of their invasion. Bacteriocins are not known among yeasts, but they have a parallel in the form of yeast "killer toxins," which can be used for strain typing in a manner similar to bacteriocin typing. The various methods of strain delineation belong to one of three general groups. The first comprises methods that permit direct or indirect analysis of the DNA base sequence of an isolate. DNA typing methods represent the ideal approach to strain differentiation independent of phenotypic expression. The second general class of typing method consists of tests that detect the presence or absence of a single gene product. Approaches such as serotyping, "killer factor" typing, and isoenzyme detection belong to this class, since the method involves detection of a specific macromolecular conformation (epitope, receptor, or enzyme) and thus a specific gene product. These methods are normally highly reproducible and must be contrasted with other phenotypic typing methods such as carbohydrate assimilation patterns, susceptibility testing, and suchlike, where the measurement depends on the activity or behavior of multiple gene products. The level to which a particular isolate assimilates a particular sugar, for example, depends on a pathway of uptake and metabolism of the sugar substrate, whose individual steps may be susceptible to small variations in test performance variables.

A. Methods for Delineating DNA Profiles

The present level of technology offers several different approaches to determination of strain differences at the level of DNA. A simple and popular approach is electrophoretic karyotyping. This involves lysis of *Candida* cells in situ in an agarose gel, followed by electrophoretic separation of the chromosomes with pulsed electrical fields. It has been established that electrophoretic karyotype patterns indeed vary between strains of *C. albicans*, *C. glabrata*, *C. guilliermondii*, *C. tropicalis*, and other yeast species (1,22). However, karyotyping should probably be regarded as the least attractive approach to DNA typing of *Candida* strains. It suffers from substantial run-to-run reproducibility problems that make analysis difficult; one *C. albicans* chromosome (chromosome R) has highly variable mobility that can lead to karyotype pattern changes in subcultures of a clonal isolate; the method is comparatively complex; it allows analysis of relatively few strains per experiment; and the electrophoresis takes a long time—from 2 to 5 days (29,30).

Determination of DNA RFLPs is a more refined means of detecting differences in DNA base sequences between strains. In this method, DNA is digested with a suitable restriction endonuclease enzyme, and the fragments that result are separated electrophoretically. Because distances between restriction sites specific for the chosen endonuclease vary between strains, so do the band patterns of separated DNA fragments (19,21). This approach suffers from difficulties of interpretation, since the band patterns in practice usually appear as continuous smears in electrophoretic gels, with positions that contain particularly high concentrations of material highlighted as rather vague bands.

The RFLP typing method becomes much more definitive when a well-chosen probe is used as a radiolabeled (or enzyme-labeled) marker specific to sequences that occur with moderate frequency in different parts of the genome under analysis. Two such probes—27A (21) and Ca3 (31,32)—contain moderately repetitive, dispersed base sequences specific to DNA from *C. albicans*. These probes have been widely used in *C. albicans* DNA fingerprinting studies. Alternatives to species-specific probes for RFLP delineation are synthetic oligonucleotides based on base dimer or trimer repeats. Sequences such as polyGT (33), $(GACA)_4$, $(GGAT)_4$, $(GTG)_5$, etc. (34), have been proposed as useful for RFLP strain delineation for various *Candida* species.

The polymerase chain reaction (PCR) is a method of iterative DNA copying that achieves exponential amplification of a chosen gene sequence from within a sample of DNA. The PCR oligonucleotide primers with specificity for variable-length repeat sequences in *Candida* DNAs could in theory be used to produce easily detectable DNA fragments whose size patterns differ between strains. This approach, based on selected species-specific primers, has not yet been applied to *Candida* strain typing.

"Randomly amplified polymorphic DNA" (RAPD) refers to the application of the PCR DNA sequence detection approach just described but in which arbitrary oligonucleotide primers, rather than specific primers, are used to generate the iterated fragments. The RAPD method has been applied to *Candida* strain typing, with considerable success according to the first report of its use (27). The method offers the potential for *Candida* species identification as well as strain differentiation. It is technically straightforward and highly reproducible and may well become the favored DNA typing method of the future.

B. Methods for Typing Based on Detection of Single Gene Products

Serotyping of microbial isolates is based on the detection of differential expression of macromolecular epitopes between strains (surface macromolecules are favored for ease of technical performance). It has proved difficult to extend the principle of serotyping into *Candida* strain typing. Polyclonal antisera can differentiate only two serotypes of *C. albicans* (4,5), and the advent of monoclonal antisera has led to no obvious improvement in the discriminatory power of serotyping for this species. For other *Candida* species, no serotyping scheme has ever been devised for strain differentiation.

An alternative technique for serological analysis consists of immunoblotting (Western blotting) of *C. albicans* homogenates whose antigens have been separated by polyacrylamide gel electrophoresis. Lee et al. (35) found that isolates could be subtyped by this method on the basis of patterns of 14 major immunoreactive bands: however, 92% of the isolates they tested belonged to one or other of just two types. Ibrahim-Granet et al. (36) found several bands on immunoblots specific to the A and B agglutination serotypes of *C. albicans*, but the possible use of such bands for fine strain-typing purposes has not been followed up.

One-dimensional polyacrylamide gel electrophoresis (1-D PAGE) of *Candida* soluble proteins yields too complex a pattern for reliable strain typing, and two-dimensional electrophoresis is far too complex for routine application to reasonable numbers of clinical isolates. However, the detection of individual proteins in a 1-D PAGE gel by means of immunoblotting (35) or isoenzyme detection (28,37,38) reveals polymorphisms capable of strain differentiation.

Typing of *Candida* strains by their differential susceptibility to "killer toxins" has been developed in Italy by Polonelli et al. (17,18). This approach measures patterns of susceptibility of *C. albicans* isolates to a panel of yeasts (from the genera *Hansenula* and *Pichia*) that secrete peptides differentially toxic for *Candida* strains. The method has undergone subsequent technical enhancements to improve reproducibility and ease performance difficulties (39), but its potential for discrimination of large numbers of strain types is limited, and most *C. albicans* isolates belong to a single predominant type.

C. Methods for Typing Based on Complex Phenotypic Properties

Several approaches have been developed for *Candida* strain differentiation based on gross morphological or physiological phenotypic characters. Some investigators have relied on such easily measured properties as different sugar assimilation or enzyme activity patterns from commercial test kits as a basis for strain discrimination. The technical simplicity of such approaches is attractive, but the methods have not been widely evaluated for their reproducibility or dependability and they suffer from an inherently low potential for strain discrimination, since such kits were designed for species identification, not for strain typing, and the pattern variations encountered within a given species represent a small minority of the tests actually carried out.

Morphotyping of *Candida* isolates involves analysis of the appearance of a streak colony of the yeast on a nutrient-rich culture medium (6–8). The most recent version of a morphotyping scheme for *C. albicans* involves determination of colony edge morphology and color (arising from a tetrazolium salt indicator) (40). Once again, most clinical isolates usually belong to a single strain type. Inclusion of the colony indicator color measurement in the typing scheme somewhat improves this limitation, but the considerable technical ease of the method remains balanced by its limited discriminatory potential and the subjective nature of the readings.

Subjective reading difficulties, intermediate levels of colony growth, and a high tendency to irreproducibility between runs have confounded the use of methods variously referred to as "resistotyping" and "biotyping," in which *C. albicans* isolates were differentiated by their ability to grow on agar plates containing differential growth inhibitors or substrates (12–15). Such methods appear to be capable of strain discrimination in experienced hands within a single laboratory, but they lack inter-laboratory reproducibility and cannot be considered suitable for routine, wide-scale use (16).

Strain delineation by antifungal susceptibility testing was previously restricted to tests with flucytosine, since only flucytosine-resistant isolates were found frequently in clinical material. Now that increasing numbers of *Candida* isolates exhibit resistance to other agents such as fluconazole (41,42), the potential for design and development of an "antifungigram" method for phenotype differentiation has grown. Such an approach allows measurement of strain properties with possible direct relevance to clinical problems of *Candida* infection. A "quantitative relative growth" phenotyping method has been described (43) that combines objective growth measurement and comparative technical simplicity; it may facilitate future studies in which antifungal susceptibilities are measured as phenotypic strain-type markers.

V. CLINICAL APPLICATION OF *CANDIDA* STRAIN TYPING

A detailed review of all published studies in which clinical isolates of *Candida* spp. have been studied by strain-typing methodology is beyond the scope of this article. Instead, a selection of findings will be summarized to indicate the nature of observations that have been made in studies of this type. Many publications report only the number of different strain types found among isolates of *Candida* spp. from patients in a particular clinical setting. Since there is as yet no universal agreement concerning definitions of precisely what evidence indicates a strain difference for any particular typing test, it is of little use to set out the proportions of "identical" and "different" types found in any particular study. Most investigations show a tendency toward a predominant single strain type in any given test population of *Candida* isolates. This tendency is less apparent when DNA-level typing is used than with phenotyping methods. Pfaller et al. (44) showed that combination of DNA fingerprinting and biotyping methods gave a higher level of *C. albicans* strain discrimination than either method on its own.

A. Cross-Sectional and Longitudinal Studies of *Candida* Strain Similarities in Immunologically Intact Individuals

Many surveys, involving many different typing methods, have examined whether multiple isolates of a *Candida* sp. obtained from different anatomical sites at one time in the same healthy volunteer or patient with superficial mucosal infections are of the same strain type. They have also examined whether the same type is carried over a period of time at the same site in a given individual. The earliest phenotyping surveys strongly suggested a consistency of *C. albicans* strain types from each person studied, both between sites and with time, in a majority of cases. This general principle of clonal identity in a patient's yeast flora has been reinforced by surveys based on DNA typing methods, but in some of these studies the conclusion has been refined. Some data show major and minor strain differences occurring in some individuals which may relate to adaptation of strains to survive in particular anatomical microniches or in the presence of antifungal agents.

Table 1 summarizes several studies that examine cross-sectional differences in *Candida* strains in colonized and mucosally infected individuals. The findings are fairly consistent regardless of the typing methodology used. When *C. albicans* isolates from the urethra and the adjacent vagina are compared, strain differences are almost never found. By contrast, a measurable proportion of isolates show strain differences between other sites of isolation. Longitudinal surveys in populations of healthy volunteers and women undergoing gynecological examination similarly show carriage of a single strain type at a single site in most individuals studied (Table 2).

However, it is insufficient to assume that carriage of *Candida* strains is clonal and consistent in all circumstances. A careful statistical analysis of *C. albicans* DNA types isolated from healthy females suggested that, in some women, similar but nonidentical strain types could be found in different sites, and these data indicated possible selection of strain variants

Table 1 Similarities of *C. albicans* Strains from Different Anatomical Sites in the Same Individual[a]

Sites of yeast isolation	Typing method	No. of pairs	No. (%) not distinguishable	Reference
Vagina and urethra	Biotyping	140	138(99)	47
	RFLPs with Ca3 probe	9	9(100)	48
Vagina and anus	Resistogram	30	28(93)	12
	Biotyping	48	35(73)	45
	Biotyping + serotyping	10	9(90)	46
	Biotyping	124	116(94)	47
	RFLPs with 27A probe	10	9(90)	46
	RFLPs with Ca3 probe	7	4(57)	48
Vagina and mouth	Resistogram	20	13(65)	12
	Biotyping	63	47(75)	47
	RFLPs with Ca3 probe	11	4(36)	48
Anus and mouth	Resistotyping	19	14(74)	12
	Biotyping	53	41(77)	47
	RFLPs with Ca3 probe	9	5(56)	48

[a] Healthy volunteers and women undergoing gynecologic examination. The proportion of indistinguishable strain types between the pairs studied is taken or calculated from the published data. Criteria for determining whether strains are not distinguishable are those used in the publication in nearly all instances. These criteria differ between studies.

Table 2 Similarities of *C. albicans* Strain Types in Longitudinal Surveys of Isolates from the Same Anatomical Site in the Same Individual[a]

Site of repeated yeast isolation	Typing method	No. of cases	No. (%) not distinguishable	Reference
Vagina	Resistogram	20	18(90)	12
	Biotyping + serotyping	25	20(80)	46
	Biotyping	32	25(78)	47
	Biotyping	64	36(56)	45
	RFLPs with 27A probe	25	22(88)	46
Anus	Resistogram	30	29(97)	12
	Biotyping	13	11(85)	47
Mouth	Resistotyping	22	21(95)	12
	Biotyping	18	13(72)	47

[a] Healthy volunteers or women undergoing gynecologic examination. The proportion of indistinguishable strain types is taken or calculated from the published data. Criteria for determining whether strains are not distinguishable are those used in the publication in nearly all instances. These criteria differ between studies.

better adapted to survival in individual anatomical locations such as the vagina (48).

B. *Candida* Strain Types in Immunocompromised Hosts at Risk of Deep-Seated Infection

Several surveys have been made of *Candida* species and strain types isolated from patients at high risk of deep-seated *Candida* infections. Such patients include those with chemotherapy-induced neutropenia and other seriously debilitated patients receiving intensive therapy. In such patients, the tendency to *Candida* strain variations between sites of colonization and infection and with sequential samples has been observed with somewhat higher frequency than in healthy hosts.

A survey of 674 yeasts isolated from patients undergoing chemotherapy for hematological malignancies was based on biotyping technology to delineate strain types. Of 12 patients studied longitudinally, four harbored the same *Candida* sp. or *C. albicans* biotype in all samples, three showed major variations in the species or type carried, and the remaining five showed small longitudinal variations in *C. albicans* biotype that suggested a consistent underlying type (49). A similar survey done with yeasts from five neonates receiving intensive care showed carriage of indistinguishable types in each baby for from 7 to 63 days (50).

Pfaller et al. (44) used a combined biotyping/DNA fingerprint approach to achieve fine discrimination of strain types in a series of patients at high risk of nosocomial *Candida* infection. In seven patients with persistent *Candida* colonization, a trend toward a constant strain type was seen, but with some measurable variations in a minority of isolates. In each of eight patients with deep-seated *Candida* infections, all consecutive isolates from deep sites and catheter tips were indistinguishable. The strain types from all 15 patients studied differed from each other, strongly suggesting endogenous sources of colonization and infection.

Pittet et al. (51) used electrophoretic karyotyping to study surveillance cultures from 29 patients, of whom 24 were colonized with *C. albicans* and the rest with other species. In all 29, the species and karyotype remained the same for from 5 to 140 days of observation. In 11 patients, a serious *Candida* infection arose (candidemia in 8 cases) and the karyotype isolated from the deep site was indistinguishable from the colonizing strains in the same patient.

Van Belkum et al. (52) studied *C. albicans* strain types by RAPD in 27 neutropenic patients treated with fluconazole. The yeast phenotype changed from fluconazole-susceptible to -resistant in just 1 of the 24 patients. Seven patients showed longitudinal variation in strain type and the rest, including the patient whose strain became resistant, remained constant.

C. *Candida* Strain Types in AIDS Patients

Several investigators have examined the *Candida* types isolated from the mouths of patients infected with human immunodeficiency virus (HIV). The majority of these subjects, like immunologically intact hosts, retain a single *Candida* strain type in the mouth over time: when change in strain type is seen, the change does not always coincide with definable events that might influence strain carriage, such as antifungal therapy. Schmid et al. (53) found a reduced genetic diversity of *C. albicans* strains among a group of oral isolates from British patients with acquired immunodeficiency syndrome (AIDS) as compared with control strains from other patients in the same location. Repeated isolates from the same patients did not show variations in DNA fingerprint in the course of time.

Pujol et al. (28) used enzyme polymorphisms to demonstrate that *C. albicans* reproduces clonally in individual HIV-infected patients: no evidence was obtained for segregation and recombination, which implies that major changes in strain types in AIDS are probably evidence for exogenous replacement rather than for sexual or quasisexual reproduction. It should be noted that clonal development within a host is not the same as clonal restriction of particular types to a particular host group: Powderly et al. (54) showed that the strains colonizing the mouths of HIV-infected patients were similar to those colonizing other individuals.

Some investigators have examined the *Candida* strain types involved in cases where HIV-infected patients have developed resistance to fluconazole treatment during the course of therapy. One study based on killer-system typing found that the *C. albicans* strain type changed in 17/26 patients during their second episode of oral infection and in 10/14 during a third episode (55). However, this level of change may represent phenotypic rather than genotypic variation. Bart-Delabesse et al. (56) studied RFLPs of sequential isolates from four patients where the isolates developed resistance to fluconazole during treatment. In three of the four cases, there was no change in DNA type associated with the change to phenotypic resistance, whereas a change was seen in one case.

D. Hospital Cross-Infections

One obvious field of application for *Candida* strain typing is in the study of apparent nosocomial outbreaks of infection. Since typing of surveillance cultures of *Candida* has shown a tendency for most (though not all) individual patients to remain contaminated with the same clonal strain of *Candida*, the observation of a single strain type affecting several individuals in a closed area such as a hospital ward or intensive therapy unit should indicate cross-transmission of that strain. One early study indicated an outbreak of disseminated *C. albicans* infection caused by a strain with a similar phenotype in 13 patients in the course of 9 months in an intensive care unit (57). Subsequent RFLP typing of this and four other apparent *C. albicans* outbreaks showed that the strain types involved differed between outbreaks but were consistent within each set of isolates from a single outbreak (58), although more discriminatory DNA typing of outbreak isolates suggested some differences between them (59). There was evidence of possible transmission of *Candida* infection from nursing staff to patients in the original outbreak study (57), and Moro *et al.* (60) provided definitive evidence for probable cross-transmission of *C. albicans* to patients from a nurse involved in the preparation of parenteral nutrition fluids.

VI. CONCLUSIONS

The technology of *Candida* strain typing has advanced enormously from phenotypic analyses to methods that delineate differences at the DNA level. Indeed, a considerable profusion of competing methods is now available, and an approach to selection and standardization of typing methodology seems to be a desirable next step. Application of typing methodology to clinical problems of *Candida* infection has not revealed any single strain genotype or phenotype that has a higher than usual predilection for causing infection. However, the increasing sophistication of epidemiological studies and of their statistical analysis indicates the steadily growing value of strain typing for such research.

REFERENCES

1. Merz WG. Candida albicans strain delineation. Clin Microbiol Rev 1990;3: 321–324.
2. Pfaller MA. Epidemiological typing methods for mycoses. Clin Infect Dis 1992;14(S1):S4–S10.
3. Odds FC. Candida and Candidosis. 2d ed. London: Baillière Tindall, 1988.
4. Hasenclever HF, Mitchell WO. Antigenic studies of Candida: I. Observation of two antigenic groups in Candida albicans. J Bacteriol 1961;82:570–573.
5. Tsuchiya T, Fukazawa Y, Kawakita A. Serological classification of the genus Candida. In: Studies on Candidiasis in Japan. Tokyo: Research Committee of Candidiasis 1961:34–46.
6. Brown-Thomsen J. Variability in Candida albicans (Robin) Berkhout: I. Studies on morphology and biochemical activity. Hereditas 1968;60:355–398.
7. Hunter PR, Fraser CAM, Mackenzie DWR. Morphotype markers of virulence in human candidal infections. J Med Microbiol 1989;28:85–91.
8. Phongpaichit S, Mackenzie DWR, Fraser C. Strain differentiation of Candida albicans by morphotyping. Epidemiol Infect 1987;99:421–428.
9. Blaschke-Hellmessen R. Epidemiologische Untersuchungen zum Vorkommen von Hefepilzen bei Kinderen und deren Müttern. Mykosen 1968;11: 611–616.
10. Bernhard H. Untersuchungen zur Hefepilzbesiedlung des Menschen. Zentbl Bakteriol Hyg I Abt Orig A 1973;223:244–254.
11. Schönborn C. Nachweis stammspezifischer Lipaseaktivität als Beitrag zur Epidemiologie von Candida tropicalis. Dermatol Monatsch 1980;166: 541–550.
12. Warnock DW, Speller DCE, Day JK, Farrell AJ. Resistogram method for differentiation of strains of Candida albicans. J Appl Bacteriol 1979;46: 571–578.
13. McCreight MC, Warnock DW. Enhanced differentiation of isolates of Candida albicans using a modified resistogram method. Mykosen 1982;25: 589–598.
14. Odds FC, Abbott AB. A simple system for the presumptive identification of Candida albicans and differentiation of strains within the species. Sabouraudia 1980;18:301–317.

15. Odds FC, Abbott AB. Modification and extension of tests for differentiation of Candida species and strains. Sabouraudia 1983;21:79–81.
16. Odds FC, Auger P, Krogh P, et al. Biotyping of Candida albicans: Results of an international collaborative survey. J Clin Microbiol 1989;27:1506–1509.
17. Polonelli L, Archibusacci C, Sestito M, Morace G. Killer system: A simple method for differentiating Candida albicans strains. J Clin Microbiol 1983; 17:774–780.
18. Morace G, Archibusacci C, Sestito M, Polonelli L. Strain differentiation of pathogenic yeasts by the killer system. Mycopathologia 1984;84:81–85.
19. Magee BB, D'Souza TM, Magee PT. Strain and species identification by restriction fragment length polymorphisms in the ribosomal DNA repeat of Candida species. J Bacteriol 1987;169:1639–1643.
20. Olivo PD, McManus EJ, Riggsby WS, Jones JM. Mitochondrial DNA polymorphisms in Candida albicans. J Infect Dis 1987;156:214–215.
21. Scherer S, Stevens DA. Application of DNA typing methods to epidemiology and taxonomy of Candida species. J Clin Microbiol 1987;25:675–679.
22. Magee BB, Magee PT. Electrophoretic karyotypes and chromosome numbers in Candida species. J Gen Microbiol 1987;133:425–430.
23. Snell RG, Hermans IF, Wilkins RJ, Corner BE. Chromosomal variations in Candida albicans. Nucl Acid Res 1987;15:3625.
24. Scherer S, Stevens DA. A Candida albicans dispersed, repeated gene family and its epidemiologic applications. Proc Natl Acad Sci USA 1988;85: 1452–1456.
25. Soll DR, Langtimm CJ, McDowell J, et al. High-frequency switching in Candida strains isolated from vaginitis patients. J Clin Microbiol 1987;25: 1611–1622.
26. Hunter PR. A critical review of typing methods for Candida albicans and their applications Crit Rev Microbiol 1991;17:417–434.
27. Lehmann PF, Lin D, Lasker BA. Genotypic identification and characterization of species and strains within the genus Candida by using random amplified polymorphic DNA. J Clin Microbiol 1992;30:3249–3254.
28. Pujol C, Reynes J, Renaud F, et al. The yeast Candida albicans has a clonal mode of reproduction in a population of infected human immunodeficiency virus–positive patients. Proc Natl Acad Sci USA 1993;90:9456–9459.
29. Magee PT, Bowdin L, Staudinger J. Comparison of molecular typing methods for Candida albicans. J Clin Microbiol 1992;30:2674–2679.
30. Odds FC, Brawner DL, Staudinger J, et al. Typing of Candida albicans strains. J Med Vet Mycol 1992;30(suppl 1):87–94.
31. Schmid J, Voss E, Soll DR. Computer-assisted methods for assessing strain relatedness in Candida albicans by fingerprinting with the moderately repetitive sequence Ca3. J Clin Microbiol 1990;28:1236–1243.
32. Anderson J, Srikantha T, Morrow B, et al. Characterization and partial nucleotide sequence of the DNA fingerprinting probe Ca3 of Candida albicans J Clin Microbiol 1993;31:1472–1480.
33. Wilkinson BM, Morris L, Adams DJ, et al. A new, sensitive polynucleotide probe for distinguishing Candida albicans strains and its use with a computer

assisted archiving and pattern comparison system. J Med Vet Mycol 1992;30:123–131.
34. Sullivan D, Bennett D, Henman M, et al. Oligonucleotide fingerprinting of isolates of Candida species other than C. albicans and of atypical Candida species from human immunodeficiency virus–positive and AIDS patients. J Clin Microbiol 1993;31:2124–2133.
35. Lee W, Burnie J, Matthews R. Fingerprinting Candida albicans. J Immunol Methods 1986;93:177–182.
36. Ibrahim-Granet O, Delga JM, Granet C, Drouhet E. A program in BASIC for the determination of molecular weights and linear graphic representation of an electrophoretic protein pattern: Application to serotypes A and B of Candida albicans studied by polyacrylamide gel electrophoresis and immunoblotting. Electrophoresis 1986;7:316–323.
37. Caugant DA, Sandven P. Epidemiological analysis of Candida albicans strains by multilocus enzyme electrophoresis. J Clin Microbiol 1993;31:215–220.
38. Lehmann PF, Wu LC, Mackenzie DWR. Isoenzyme changes in Candida albicans during domestication. J Clin Microbiol 1991;29:2623–2625.
39. Polonelli L, Castagnola M, Rosetti DV, Morace G. Use of killer toxins for computer-aided differentiation of Candida albicans strains. Mycopathologia 1985;91:175–179.
40. Quindós G, Fernández-Rodríguez M, Burgos A, et al. Colony morphotype on Sabouraud-triphenyltetrazolium agar: A simple and inexpensive method for Candida subspecies discrimination. J Clin Microbiol 1992;30:2748–2752.
41. Odds FC. Resistance of yeasts to azole-derivative antifungals. J Antimicrob Chemother 1993;31:463–471.
42. Warnock DW. Azole drug resistance in Candida species. J Med Microbiol 1992;37:225–226.
43. Odds FC. Quantitative microculture system with standardized inocula for strain typing, susceptibility testing, and other physiologic measurements with Candida albicans and other yeasts. J Clin Microbiol 1991;29:2735–2740.
44. Pfaller MA, Cabezudo I, Hollis R, et al. The use of biotyping and DNA fingerprinting in typing Candida albicans from hospitalized patients. Diagn Microbiol Infect Dis 1990;13:481–489.
45. O'Connor MI, Sobel JD. Epidemiology of recurrent vulvovaginal candidiasis: Identification and strain differentiation. J Infect Dis 1986;154:358–363.
46. Mercure S, Poirier S, Lemay G, et al. Application of biotyping and DNA typing of Candida albicans to the epidemiology of recurrent vulvovaginal candidiasis. J Infect Dis 1993;168:502–507.
47. Odds FC, Webster CE, Fisk PG, et al. Candida species and C. albicans biotypes in women attending clinics in genitourinary medicine. J Med Microbiol 1989;29:51–54.
48. Soll DR, Galask R, Schmid J, et al. Genetic dissimilarity of commensal strains of Candida spp. carried in different anatomical locations of the same healthy women. J Clin Microbiol 1991;29:1702–1710.
49. Odds FC, Kibbler CC, Walker E, et al. Carriage of Candida species and

C. albicans biotypes in patients undergoing chemotherapy or bone marrow transplantation for haematological disease. J Clin Pathol 1989;42:1259–1266.
50. Sharp AM, Odds FC, Evans EGV. Candida strains from neonates in a special care baby unit. Arch Dis Child 1992;67:48–52.
51. Pittet D, Monod M, Filthuth I, et al. Contour-clamped homogenous electric field gel electrophoresis as a powerful epidemiologic tool in yeast infections. Am J Med 1991;91(suppl 3B):256S–263S.
52. Van Belkum A, Melchers W, de Pauw BE, et al. Genotypic characterization of sequential Candida albicans isolates from fluconazole-treated neutropenic patients. J Infect Dis 1994. In press.
53. Schmid J, Odds FC, Wiselka MJ, et al. Genetic similarity and maintenance of Candida albicans strains from a group of AIDS patients, demonstrated by DNA fingerprinting. J Clin Microbiol 1992;30:935–941.
54. Powderly WG, Robinson K, Keath EJ. Molecular typing of Candida albicans isolated from oral lesions of HIV-infected individuals. AIDS 1992;6:81–84.
55. Bruatto M, Vidotto V, Marinuzzi G, et al. Candida albicans biotypes in human immunodeficiency virus type 1-infected patients with oral candidiasis before and after antifungal therapy. J Clin Microbiol 1991;29:726–730.
56. Bart-Delabasse E, Boiron P, Carlotti A, Dupont B. Candida albicans geontyping in studies with patients with AIDS developing resistance to fluconazole. J Clin Microbiol 1993;31:2933–2937.
57. Burnie JP, Odds FC, Lee W, et al. Outbreak of systemic Candida albicans in intensive care unit caused by cross infection. Br Med J 1985;290:746–748.
58. Matthews R, Burnie J. Assessment of DNA fingerprinting for rapid identification of outbreaks of systemic candidiasis Br Med J 1989;298:354–357.
59. Stevens DA, Odds FC, Scherer S. Application of DNA typing methods to Candida albicans epidemiology and correlations with phenotype. Rev Infect Dis 1990;12:258–266.
60. Moro ML, Maffei C, Manso E, et al. Nosocomial outbreak of systemic candidosis associated with parenteral nutrition. Infect Control Hosp Epidemiol 1990;11:27–35.

22

Proteinase Gene Identification in Aspergillosis

PAUL E. STEELE and JUDITH C. RHODES
University of Cincinnati
Cincinnati, Ohio

I. INTRODUCTION

The cloning and characterization of proteinase genes from *Aspergillus* species has accelerated in recent years, for three reasons. First, evidence has been published that suggests involvement of proteinases in the virulence of clinical isolates (1,2). Second, high-level heterologous protein expression in *Aspergillus* (e.g., for industrial purposes) may depend upon inhibition, disruption, or modulation of particular proteinase genes in order to protect the intactness of the biosynthesized protein (3). Third, some of these *Aspergillus* enzymes are important in the food industry, and it may be advantageous to obtain cloned sources of them (4). Southern blot and nucleotide sequence data from these *Aspergillus* proteinase clones reveal interesting information about relationships among fungi, and the availability of these clones permits gene disruption and structure-function experiments.

This chapter focuses primarily on proteinase genes from the common clinical isolates *A. fumigatus* and *A. flavus*, but it will touch upon commercially important species such as *A. oryzae* and *A. niger*, particularly to describe enzymes and their genes, which are not well characterized in the former two species. The chapter is divided into sections on each of the four major classes of proteinases as categorized by inhibitor studies (5).

II. SERINE PROTEINASES

These proteinases can be subdivided into those of the subtilisin type and those of the chymotrypsin (trypsin) type (Table 1). Most of the published work on serine proteinases has focused on the extracellular subtilisin-like proteinase known as alkaline proteinase (Alp), which degrades such proteins as elastin, collagen, fibrinogen, casein, hemoglobin, and albumin.

Alp is of interest for three reasons. First, it is the enzyme of *A. fumigatus* responsible for in vitro secreted elastinolytic activity (6); the property of elastinolysis has been correlated to virulence (1,2), and loss of this property through chemical mutagenesis has been linked to hypovirulence (7). Second, Alp can be the predominant enzyme secreted in vitro (8) under particular culture conditions. Recent data indicate that this enzyme is secreted in vivo, and thus it is a candidate virulence factor (6,7,9). Third, polymerase chain reaction (PCR) analysis of bronchoalveolar lavage fluid, using primers specifically designed to detect Alp, may be useful as a sensitive assay for the presence of the organism (10).

It is controversial whether this elastinolytic activity resides with the Alp of *A. flavus*. We have found that the predominant elastinolyic activity displayed by this species resides in a metalloproteinase (see below) and that *A. flavus* Alp does not display appreciable elastinolytic activity; conversely, Ramesh et al. have reported the presence of elastinolytic activity in the *A. flavus* Alp (11).

Table 1 Proteinases of Aspergilli

Proteinase	References
Serine proteinases	
Subtilisinlike	
Alkaline proteinase	1,2,4, 6–15, 18–24
pepC	20, 26
Trypsinlike (not clonded)	27
Metalloproteinases	
Elastinolytic enzyme (*A. flavus*)	28, 29
Elastinolytic enzyme (*A. fumigatus*)	32
Neutral proteinase I	31
Neutral proteinase II	30
Asparatic proteinase	
pepA, *pepO*	33–36
pepB	37, 38
pepE	3

This discrepancy may be explained in part by differences in the enzyme being studied: the nucleotide sequence of Alp that we have studied is virtually identical to that described in the closely related species *A. oryzae* (4,12), while the coding sequence described by Ramesh et al. differs from the *A. oryzae* sequence by 18%. The reason why different genes have been identified from two strains of *A. flavus* remains unclear, however. Peptide mapping, amino acid analysis, pH optima, and molecular weight comparison data from Alp of *A. flavus* and *A. oryzae* support the assumption that the genes encoding the enzyme should be nearly identical if not completely identical (13).

The nucleotide sequences of genomic and cDNA clones harboring the Alp gene of *A. fumigatus* have been published (14). The genomic clone was obtained by screening libraries with degenerate oligonucleotide probes designed to detect areas of high homology among subtilisinlike serine proteinases. The cDNA sequence was obtained from PCR amplification of cDNA, using 5′ primers corresponding to (1) the *N*-terminal amino acid sequence of the mature protein or (2) the leader sequence beginning at the initiator methionine. The 3′ primer used corresponded to sequence just proximal to the putative stop codon. These studies revealed the presence of three small introns of 57, 63, and 72 base pairs (bp). The cDNA PCR data suggested the presence of a 121–amino acid leader sequence. The RNA start site was not determined, but a putative TATA box was noted 103 bp upstream of the initiator methionine. Four *N*-linked glycosylation sequences corresponding to Asn-X-Ser were present in the deduced amino acid sequence, although PAS staining of SDS-PAGE gels indicated lack of glycosylation.

Comparison of the *A. fumigatus* and *A. oryzae* Alp sequence revealed 46 deduced amino acid differences, or 17% of the amino acids (14). Among these differences must exist the basis for differences in substrate specificity of these two enzymes. Notably, the *A. oryzae* Alp exhibits twofold less activity against elastin as compared to the *A. fumigatus* Alp (15). Part of the sequence difference between the two enzyme genes results in a Ser-Asn (*A. fumigatus*) change to Gly-Gln (*A. oryzae*) in the region corresponding to the P1 substrate-binding pocket, which might account for substrate specificity differences. An analogous comparison can be drawn between the subtilisin-like gene of *Bacillus* strain Ya-B (which encodes an alkaline elastase activity) and *Bacillus subtilis* subtilisin E; the former gene exhibits a four–amino acid deletion in the P1 pocket region relative to the latter (16). Site-directed mutagenesis of the subtilisin E gene to produce a deletion in this region results in higher activity against synthetic substrate analogues for elastase (17).

Genomic Southern blot data, with the use of *A. fumigatus* Alp or *A.*

flavus Alp probes, reveal that Alp appears to be a single-copy gene in both species, although low stringency hybridization results suggest the existence of related genes in both species (18,19).

A homologue of Alp in *A. niger*, *pepD*, exhibits 70.7% amino acid identity with *A. oryzae* Alp and also appears to represent a single-copy gene by genomic Southern blot (20).

Because of the high degree of interest in Alp as a virulence factor, two research groups have carried out a total of four independent gene disruptions of this sequence in *A. fumigatus*, using a hygromycin resistance gene (18,21,22). The virulence comparisons of these disruptants with their isogenic parent in murine models of invasive aspergillosis fail to show any significant difference. Although these strains lack Alp activity, evidence for the persistence of some proteinase activity has been found, either in vitro (22) or in vivo (21).

The interpretation of these negative gene disruption data is of paramount importance with respect to future directions in *Aspergillus* virulence research. It is generally agreed that the virulence of Alp-negative strains could be related to the expression of other unspecified proteinases which substitute for Alp. Indeed it seems likely, given that Alp is a major secreted protein of *A. fumigatus* and *A. flavus*, that some compensatory proteinase expression might result from the Alp gene disruption. If so, the disruptant and isogenic parent could have significant differences other than their level of Alp expression.

Perhaps a useful alternative to gene disruption would be specific pharmacologic inhibition of Alp to assess its role in virulence. Unfortunately, other than passive immunization by monoclonal or polyclonal antibodies (23,24), few avenues exist to specifically inhibit Alp. Detailed structure-function studies, including design of specific inhibitors, would be desirable, but their priority may be jeopardized by the negative gene disruption results. Doubts have been raised about whether elastinolysis actually occurs in vivo (25), although it is unquestionable that the pathology of invasive aspergillosis includes the penetration of elastin-containing structures such as bronchi and blood vessels. This type of invasiveness is uncommonly encountered in many other fungal infections, including those caused by the dimorphic pathogens.

A second type of subtilisinlike serine proteinase is the intracellular form, a putative example of which been cloned in *A. niger*. Named *pepC*, the gene was selected with the yeast homologue *PRB1* as a probe (26). This gene exhibits 40% amino acid homology to *A. fumigatus* Alp, with scattered areas of high homology, including active site residues. Genomic Southern blot data indicate that *pepD* and *pepC* are each single-copy sequences with no cross-hybridization (20).

The other type of serine proteinase, a chymotrypsin- or trypsinlike proteinase, has been identified in *A. niger* (27), although its gene has not been cloned. A strategy to amplify a trypsinlike proteinase from *A. niger*, using degenerate primers based upon conserved active-site residues, failed to amplify any bona fide proteinase sequences (20).

III. METALLOPROTEINASES

At least three or possibly four distinct metalloproteinase genes appear to be present in *A. fumigatus* and *A. flavus* (Table 1).

One of these genes, which we have found encodes the enzyme (28,29) responsible for elastinolytic activity of *A. flavus* (but not *A. fumigatus*, see above), exhibits strong homology but not identity with the previously described neutral proteinase II (NpII) of *A. oryzae* (30). Both NpII and the specific elastinolytic proteinase genes appear to be present in *A. flavus*. They both encode proteinases of approximately 20–23 kDa but exhibit a markedly different pI: the pI of NpII is 4.1 (30) while the other specific elastinolytic enzyme has a pI of 7.6 (28). The two genes share some sequence homology, but they are distinct. Each of the two genes appears to represent a single-copy sequence in *A. flavus* genomic DNA as judged by genomic Southern blots.

A partial NpII gene from *A. oryzae* was cDNA cloned from an expression library and used as a probe to identify a full-length cDNA clone from the same organism (30). Like Alp, comparison of the deduced amino acid sequence with the *N*-terminal amino acid sequence of the mature protein revealed an apparent preproenzyme configuration. The gene was successfully expressed in yeast. Although its function is unknown, the relatively high level of in vitro expression of this protein suggests that it may be of importance (30).

Amino acid sequence analysis of the specific elastinolytic proteinase of *A. flavus* permitted the use of degenerate PCR amplimers to obtain a partial clone of its gene. Nucleotide sequence analysis of this clone reveals that it is related to but distinct from the sequence of NpII (19).

Two similar-sized but apparently distinct neutral proteinases of 40–43 kDa have also been described in *A. fumigatus*. The 40-kDa proteinase (31) is suggested to represent a homologue of the neutral proteinase I (NpI) of *A. sojae* on the basis of molecular weight and the presence of glycosylation; the gene is being cloned but has not been published yet. The 43-kDa proteinase (32) is not glycosylated, and unlike the 40-kDa protein, exhibits elastinolytic activity, at a level nearly comparable to that of *A. fumigatus* Alp. Immunogold electron microscopy revealed that this 43-kDa protein is secreted in vivo in a mouse model of invasive aspergillosis (32); the authors speculate that this enzyme could be a source of elastinolytic activity in a strain in which the Alp gene has been disrupted.

Partial amino acid sequence has been obtained for the 43-kDa proteinase (32). The complete cDNA has now been sequenced (GenBank Accession L29566).

IV. ASPARTIC PROTEINASES

Both extracellular and intracellular aspartic proteinases are expressed in aspergilli (Table 1). Most of the studies, including gene cloning, have focused upon commercially important organisms.

The most abundant extracellular aspartic proteinase in *A. niger* is encoded by *pepA*, which belongs to the family known as aspergillopepsins (33). The *pepA* gene was cloned by hybridization screening of a genomic library from *A. niger* with an oligonucleotide probe corresponding to the *N*-terminal portion of the mature protein (33). The gene is 1.3 kb and includes three introns of 51, 52, and 59 bp. The mature protein is missing 69 amino acid residues encoded by the gene, indicating the likely presence of a signal peptide and leader sequence. This gene was successfully disrupted by homologous recombination with a fragment of the gene, which harbored an auxotrophic marker (33).

The analogous gene in *A. oryzae* is *pepO*, which was cloned from a genomic DNA library with the use of a synthetic oligonucleotide corresponding to a portion of the active-site domain (34). The intron/exon structure of *pepO* is similar to that of *pepA*. Genomic Southern blotting suggested that this gene is a single copy sequence, which is interesting in view of the fact that two forms of the enzyme exist, only one of which contains carbohydrate (35,36).

A second extracellular aspartic proteinase, acid proteinase A, consists of a structure with a light chain of 39 amino acids linked noncovalently to a heavy chain of 173 amino acids (37). The gene encoding this unusual structure, *pepB*, has been obtained from an *A. niger* genomic library by using a PCR-generated probe (38). The gene is believed to encode a preproenzyme, which is processed to the mature form containing two separate chains. Interestingly, typical active site residues expected for aspartic proteinases are not found, and indeed, this enzyme has a unique inhibitor profile (38).

An intracellular aspartic proteinase gene, *pepE*, was cloned from *A. niger* by cross-species hybridization to a vacuolar proteinase gene of *Neurospora crassa* (3). Southern blot analysis of *A. niger* genomic DNA suggested that this gene represents a single-copy sequence. This gene is principally of industrial interest for understanding its role in heterologous protein expression and secretion.

V. OTHER PROTEINASES

An alkaline proteinase (''Exalp'') with extremely alkaline activity (a pH optimum for caseinolysis at 10.8) was identified by Reichard et al. (6) in *A. fumigatus*. Evidence for a cysteine proteinase produced by a clinical isolate of *A. flavus* has been described (39). These proteinases have not been further characterized by gene cloning.

VI. CONCLUSION: CLINICAL SIGNIFICANCE

Since the classic review of aspergillosis published a quarter century ago by Young et al. (40), little has changed with respect to the serious prognosis of disseminated disease. Although decreases in the incidence of aspergillosis in transplant patients accompanied the introduction of cyclosporin A, with preliminary evidence suggesting that further decreases will occur with FK506 (41), disseminated aspergillosis remains a highly lethal and difficult to diagnose infection in this setting. Aspergillosis is an important cause of morbidity and mortality in other settings, such as bone marrow transplantation and aplastic anemia (42,43).

The continuing need to identify therapeutic agents with acceptably low host toxicity has focused attention on proteinases as potential virulence factors and thus potential drug targets. Although gene knockout experiments provide some information about the relative importance of particular proteinase genes in virulence, assessment of the clinical relevance of proteinases as virulence factors may have to await the development and testing of specific proteinase inhibitors in vivo.

ACKNOWLEDGMENT

This work was supported by grant AI28392 from the National Institutes of Health.

REFERENCES

1. Kothary MH, Chase T Jr, MacMillan JD. Correlation of elastase production by some strains of Aspergillus fumigatus with ability to cause pulmonary invasive aspergillosis in mice. Infect Immun 1984;43:320–325.
2. Rhodes JC, Bode RB, McCuan-Kirsch CM. Elastase production in clinical isolates of Aspergillus. Diagn Microbiol Infect Dis 1988;10:165–170.

3. Jarai G, van den Hombergh H, Buxton FP. Cloning and characterization of the pepE gene of Aspergillus niger encoding a new aspartic protease and regulation of pepE and pepC. Gene 1994;145:171–178.
4. Tatsumi H, Ogawa Y, Murakami S, et al. A full length cDNA clone for the alkaline protease from Aspergillus oryzae: Structural analysis and expression in Saccharomyces cerevisiae. Mol Gen Genet 1989;219:33–38.
5. Barrett AJ, Salvesen G, eds. Proteinase inhibitors. Amsterdam: Elsevier, 1986.
6. Reichard U, Buttner S, Eiffert H, et al. Purification and characterisation of an extracellular serine proteinase from Aspergillus fumigatus and its detection in tissue. J Med Microbiol 1990;33:243–251.
7. Kolattukudy PE, Lee JD, Rogers LM, et al. Evidence for possible involvement of an elastolytic serine protease in aspergillosis. Infect Immun 1993; 61:2357–2368.
8. Klapper BF, Jameson DM, Mayer RM. The purification and properties of an extracellular protease from Aspergillus oryzae NRRL 2160. Biochim Biophys Acta 1973;304:505–512.
9. Moutaouakil M, Monod M, Prevost MC, et al. Identification of the 33-kDa alkaline protease of Aspergillus fumigatus in vitro and in vivo. J Med Microbiol 1993;39:393–399.
10. Tang CM, Holden DW, Aufauvre-Brown A, Cohen J. The detection of Aspergillus spp. by the polymerase chain reaction and its evaluation in bronchoalveolar lavage fluid. Am Rev Respir Dis 1993;148:1313–1317.
11. Ramesh MV, Sirakova T, Kolattukudy PE. Isolation, characterization, and cloning of cDNA and the gene for an elastinolytic serine proteinase from Aspergillus flavus. Infect Immun 1994;62:79–85.
12. Cheevadhanarak S, Renno DV, Saunders G, Holt G. Cloning and selective overexpression of an alkaline protease-encoding gene from Aspergillus oryzae. Gene 1991;108:151–155.
13. Turkova J, Mikes O, Hayashi K, et al. Alkaline proteinases of the genus Aspergillus. Biochim Biophys Acta 1972;257:257–263.
14. Jaton-Ogay K, Suter M, Crameri R, et al. Nucleotide sequence of a genomic and a cDNA clone encoding an extracellular alkaline protease of Aspergillus fumigatus. FEMS Microbiol Lett 1992;92:163–168.
15. Monod M, Togni G, Rahalison L, Frenk E. Isolation and characterisation of an extracellular alkaline protease of Aspergillus fumigatus. J Med Microbiol 1991;35:23–28.
16. Kaneko R, Koyama N, Tsai Y-C, et al. Molecular cloning of the structural gene for alkaline elastase YaB, a new subtilisin produced by an alkalophilic Bacillus strain. J Bacteriol 1989;171:5232–5236.
17. Takagi H, Matsuzawa H, Ohta T, et al. Studies on the structure and function of subtilisin E by protein engineering. Ann NY Acad Sci 1992;672:52–59.
18. Tang CM, Cohen J, Holden DW. An Aspergillus fumigatus alkaline protease mutant constructed by gene disruption is deficient in extracellular elastase activity. Mol Microbiol 1992;6:1663–71.
19. Rhodes JC, unpublished.

20. Jarai G, Kirchherr D, Buxton FP. Cloning and characterization of the pepD gene of Aspergillus niger which codes for a subtilisin-like protease. Gene 1994;139:51–57.
21. Tang CM, Cohen J, Krausz T, et al. The alkaline protease of Aspergillus fumigatus is not a virulence determinant in two murine models of invasive pulmonary aspergillosis. Infect Immun 1993;61:1650–1656.
22. Monod M, Paris S, Sarfati J, et al. Virulence of alkaline protease-deficient mutants of Aspergillus fumigatus. FEMS Microbiol Lett 1993;106:39–46.
23. Frosco M, Chase T Jr, MacMillan JD. Purification and properties of the elastase from Aspergillus fumigatus. Infect Immun 1992;60:728–734.
24. Frosco M, Fahed C, Chase T Jr, MacMillan JD. Inhibition of Aspergillus fumigatus elastase with monoclonal antibodies produced by using denatured elastase as an immunogen. Infect Immun 1992;60:735–741.
25. Denning DW, Ward PN, Fenelon LE, Benbow EW. Lack of vessel wall elastolysis in human invasive pulmonary aspergillosis. Infect Immun 1992; 60:5153–5156.
26. Frederick GD, Rombouts P, Buxton FP. Cloning and characterisation of pepC, a gene encoding a serine protease from Aspergillus niger. Gene 1993; 125:57–64.
27. Barthomeuf C, Pourrat H, Pourrat A. Properties of a new alkaline proteinase from Aspergillus niger. Chem Pharm Bull 1989;37:1333–1336.
28. Rhodes JC, Amlung TW, Miller MS. Isolation and characterization of an elastinolytic proteinase from Aspergillus flavus. Infect Immun 1990;58: 2529–2534.
29. Rhodes JC, Amlung TW. The elastinolytic proteinase of Aspergillus flavus is not glycosylated. J Med Vet Mycol 1991;29:407–411.
30. Tatsumi H, Murakami S, Tsuji RF, et al. Cloning and expression in yeast of a cDNA clone encoding Aspergillus oryzae neutral protease II, a unique metalloprotease. Mol Gen Genet 1991;228:97–103.
31. Monod M, Paris S, Sanglard D, et al. Isolation and characterization of a secreted metalloprotease of Aspergillus fumigatus. Infect Immun 1993;61: 4099–4104.
32. Markaryan A, Morozova I, Yu H, Kolattukudy PE. Purification and characterization of an elastinolytic metalloprotease from Aspergillus fumigatus and immunoelectron microscopic evidence of secretion of this enzyme by the fungus invading the murine lung. Infect Immun 1994;62:2149–2157.
33. Berka RM, Ward M, Wilson LJ, et al. Molecular cloning and deletion of the gene encoding aspergillopepsin A from Aspergillus awamori. Gene 1990;86: 153–162.
34. Berka RM, Carmona CL, Hayenga KJ, et al. Isolation and characterization of the Aspergillus oryzae gene encoding aspergillopepsin O. Gene 1993;125: 195–198.
35. Tsujita Y, Endo A. Purification and characterization of the two molecular forms of Aspergillus oryzae acid protease. Biochim Biophys Acta 1976;445: 194–204.
36. Tsujita Y, Endo A. Purification and characterization of the two molecular

forms of membrane acid protease from Aspergillus oryzae. Eur J Biochem 1978;84:347–353.

37. Takahashi K, Inoue H, Sakai K, et al. The primary structure of Aspergillus niger acid proteinase A. J Biol Chem 1991;266:19480–19483.
38. Inoue H, Kimura T, Makabe O, Takahashi K. The gene and deduced protein sequences of the zymogen of Aspergillus niger acid proteinase A. J Biol Chem 1991;266:19484–19489.
39. Zhu W-S, Wojdyla K, Donlon K, et al. Extracellular proteases of Aspergillus flavus: Fungal keratitis, proteases, and pathogenesis. Diagn Microbiol Infect Dis 1990;13:491–497.
40. Young RC, Bennett JE, Vogel CL, et al. Aspergillosis. The spectrum of disease in 98 patients. Medicine 1970;49:147–173.
41. Torre-Cisneros J, Manez R, Kusne S, et al. The spectrum of aspergillosis in liver transplant patients: comparison of FK 506 and cyclosporine immunosuppression. Transplant Proc 1991;23:3040–3041.
42. Guiot HFL, Fibbe WE, van't Wout JW. Risk factors for fungal infection in patients with malignant hematologic disorders: Implications for empirical therapy and prophylaxis. Clin Infect Dis 1994;18:525–532.
43. Weinberger M, Elattar I, Marshall D, et al. Patterns of infection in patients with aplastic anemia and the emergence of Aspergillus as a major cause of death. Medicine 1992;71:24–43.

23

Pathogenesis of Aspergillosis

HEINZ SEELIGER
Institute of Hygiene
University of Würzburg
Würzburg, Germany

I. INTRODUCTION

Aspergillosis was described as a clinical entity in humans under the names of *Broncho-* or *pneumomycosis aspergillina* by Virchow in 1856. This report (1) was illustrated with pictures of remarkable quality (Fig. 1). It was clearly pointed out for the first time that a fungal infection should be called a mycosis. Since then, aspergillosis was usually observed and studied in sporadic cases. Only recently has it occurred in epidemic proportions, and other syndromes associated with this group of fungi have been delineated.

II. ETIOLOGY AND DIAGNOSIS

The facultatively pathogenic aspergilli belong to a group of fungi the majority of which produce no sexual forms in their life cycle and hence are called "imperfect." Practically all aspergilli isolated from human beings and cultivated under appropriate conditions belong to such imperfect species as *Aspergillus (A.) fumigatus*, *A. flavus*, *A. niger*, and others but also to the perfect species *Emericella nidulans* (formerly *Aspergillus*). They form only a fraction of the total number of *Aspergillus* species as monographed by Raper and Fennell (1965) (2). Only those whose growth re-

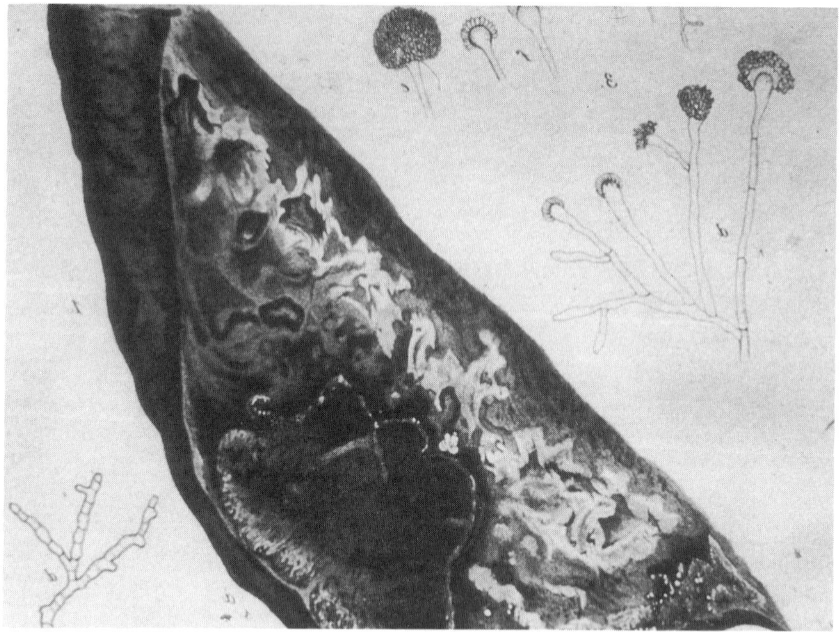

Figure 1 Illustration of human aspergillosis by Virchow (1856), with drawing of typical conidial and hyphal structures.

quirements comply with the conditions offered by the human (and animal) body are able to manifest themselves as opportunistic infectious pathogens.

Their identification is effected by a variety of measures that include the direct demonstration of hyaline, septate fungal elements in tissues and body fluids by all sorts of microscopy, including histopathology, and by their cultivation and identification on appropriate media in diagnostic laboratories. Laboratory work with aspergilli is carried out under normal conditions not requiring any special measures of protection, as is necessary with some other pathogenic fungi. Identification of the *Aspergillus* species is based on their growth requirements, macroscopic appearance of the cultivated colonies, and microscopic morphological characteristics (Fig. 2). In *A. fumigatus*, the colonies develop rapidly on fungal culture media between 25° and 45°C. The early growth of white mycelium is soon covered by a powdery layer of blue-green conidia developing on conidiphores in a typical arrangement (Fig. 3).

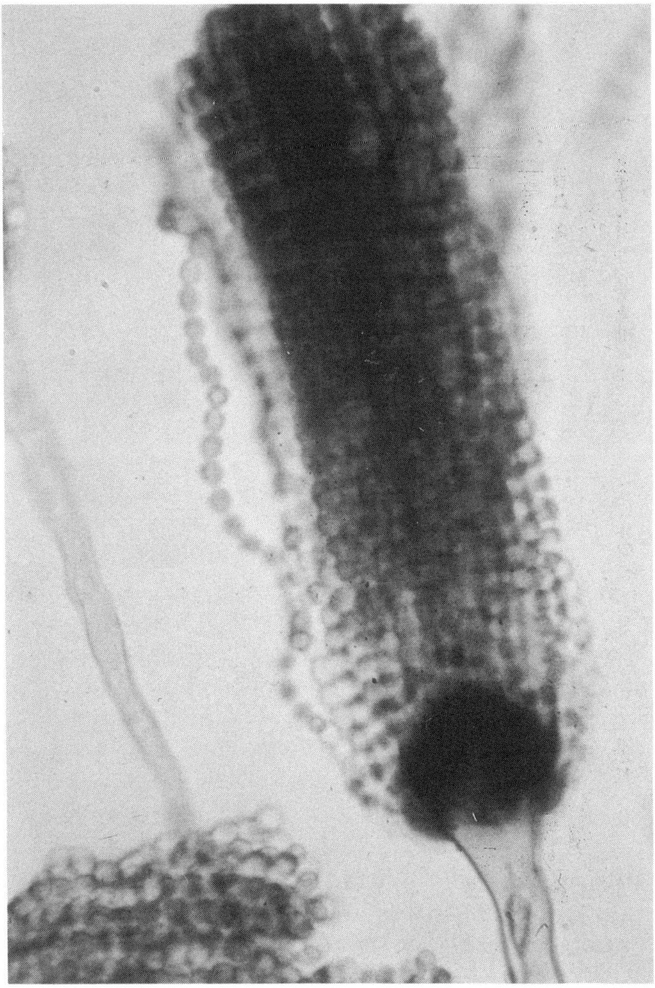

Figure 2 Microscopic appearance of typical conidial head of cultivated *A. fumigatus*.

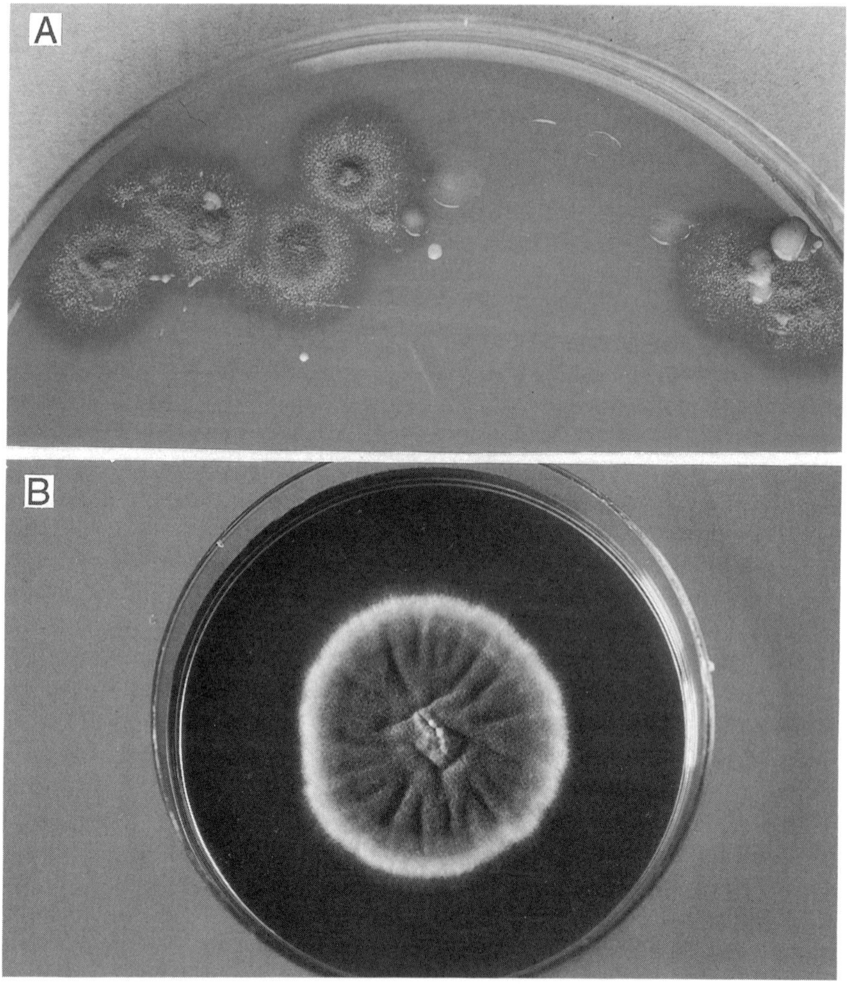

Figure 3 Macroscopic appearance of *A. fumigatus* colony grown on blood agar (A) and peptone agar (B).

III. SEROLOGY AS A DIAGNOSTIC AID

A great deal of work has been invested in the study of the serological response to aspergillosis. The classic methods of precipitation, complement fixation, and immune electrophoresis have been applied for diagnos-

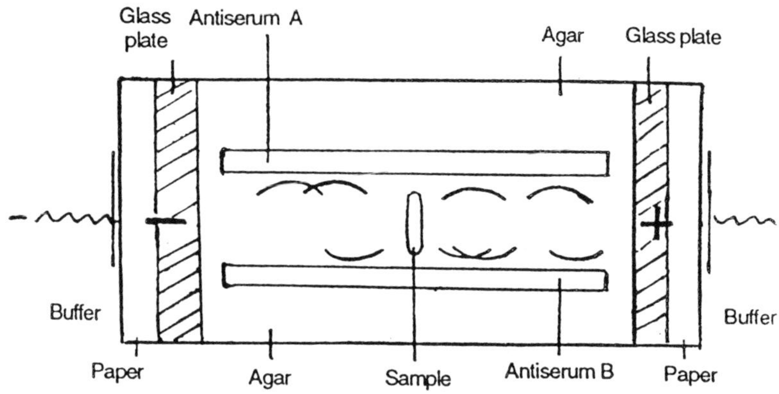

Figure 4 Positive results of immunoelectrophoresis performed with serum of patients with aspergilloma.

tic purposes (3). A typical picture of a positive outcome is presented in Fig. 4.

More recently, the *Aspergillus* galactomannan antigen has been found in patients' serum by the use of latex particles covered with antigalactomannan antibodies (4).

The successful application of this method depends on the availability of suitable commercial antigens, such as Pastorex *Aspergillus*.

Serology is useful in the diagnosis of many mycoses, and a minimum of precipitation lines is considered as diagnostic evidence.

Unfortunately the usually extremely rapid course of invasive aspergillosis leaves insufficient time for the development of guiding antibodies. Therefore the search for antigens may offer better help and has been found very useful (4–6) 0.5 and 1.0 ng of galactomannan could thus be detected in human urine and serum specimens.

The polymerase chain reaction—i.e., isolation of *Aspergillus* fractions from the serum and their subsequent multiplication and demonstration by serological methods—has already been attempted, but its clinical importance must still be proven.

IV. CLINICAL MANIFESTATIONS OF ASPERGILLOSIS IN THE HUMAN BEING

It should be noted that the manifestation of any form of aspergillosis requires abnormal reactions by the host, as in the development of hypersensitivity against fungal products in extrinsic asthma and extrinsic allergic bronchopulmonary forms as well as allergic alveolitis.

A. Allergic Manifestations of Aspergillosis

1. Hypersensitivity Due to Extrinsic Allergic Alveolitis

Bronchopulmonary allergies are frequently provoked by various kinds of organic dust particles. Hypersensitivity pneumonitis is found in nonatopic victims after repeated exposure to antigenic substances originating in their surroundings, such as thermophilic actinomycetes (cause of farmer's lung) and avian proteins, which induce bird fancier's lung. Such exposures, by inhalation of the conidia and mycelia of aspergilli originating from moldy grain, result 4–8 hr later in extrinsic allergic alveolitis. It is also the cause of so-called malt worker's lung (7), with cough, dyspnea, fever, and other clinical signs. Repeated attacks may eventually be followed by granulomatous lesions and pulmonary fibrosis. Bronchospasms, subsequent to inhalation of *Aspergillus* conidia and hyphae, are similar to those caused by allergies of other origin in atopic persons (8).

V. ALLERGIC BRONCHOPULMONARY ASPERGILLOSIS

First described in England (9), allergic pulmonary aspergillosis (ABPA) is almost invariably connected with inhalation of *Aspergillus* spp. conidia (mainly *A. fumigatus*) (10).

This condition, developing usually before the age of 35 years, is characterized by eight primary criteria (11): (a) episodic bronchial asthma; (b) peripheral blood eosinophilia—i.e., more 1000/mm^3; (c) type 1 skin reactions to *Aspergillus* antigen; (d) serum precipitins against *Aspergillus* antigens; (e) elevated IgE concentrations in serum; (f) elevated serum IgE and IgG antibodies reacting with *A. fumigatus*; (g) pulmonary infiltrates and (h) central saccular bronchiectasis'' (cited from Ref. 8).

Quite frequently the fungus can be cultured from sputum specimens. In chest x-ray films, atelectasis and cavitation is observed, as well as perihilar densities and dilated bronchi.

A. Superficial Infections

True infections may involve various sites of the body, such as the mucous membranes of the oral cavity, sinus tracts, the auditory meatus, or the cornea of the eye. Such superficial processes usually do not offer any diagnostic or therapeutic difficulties in view of the general susceptibility of the involved fungi to many kinds of superficially active antimycotic agents.

B. Pulmonary Aspergilloma

The predominant clinical entity up to a few years ago was pulmonary aspergilloma (8), caused in more than 95% of the recognized cases by *A. fumigatus*. This mycosis usually develops in various sorts of preformed cavities, such as pulmonary cysts or cystic scar tissue originating from previous lesions.

Aspergillomas may develop slowly and without signs of an infectious process until a sudden hemorrhage, bloody sputum, or both call for careful clinical examinations. X-rays will usually reveal a rather typical finding: within an area of shadowing, the fungal growth is recognized as a spherical structure—the so-called fungus ball—of various dimensions around 15–30 cm in diameter (see Fig. 5). Usually serum precipitins to *Aspergillus* spp. can be demonstrated.

Above this dense structure, a sickle-shaped halo indicates an area of the remaining cyst or cavity in which the fungal growth progresses slowly. The histopathology of a fungus ball shows that it consists of a mass of tangled hyphae. Pressure on pulmonary tissue and erosion of vessels eventually leads to bleeding and hemoptysis. Usually cultures from sputum or aspirated bronchial secretions will not reveal fungal elements or growth,

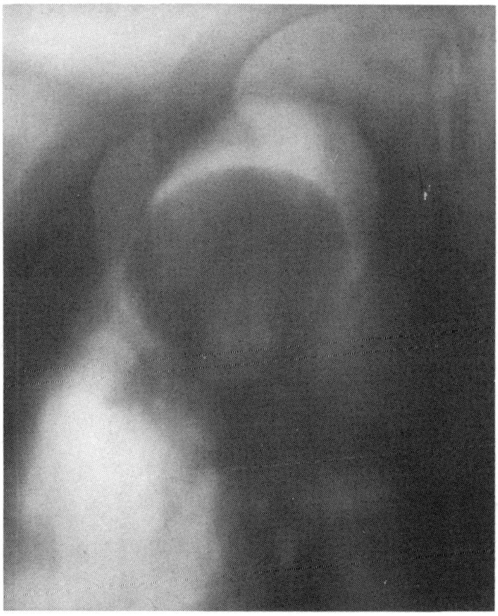

Figure 5 Fungus ball as seen on x-ray picture surrounded by halo.

because the structure of the compact fungus ball is such that conidia (asexual fungal "spores") are not produced (see Fig. 6).

It is obvious that this form of aspergillosis (a few other hyphomycetes may cause similar lesions) is only very exceptionally amenable to other than surgical treatment (8).

Systemic antifungal agents are useless, while intracavitary instillation of amphotericin B through a catheter, placed percutaneously, two to three times a week, may be advantageous to patients who cannot be subjected to surgery.

C. Bronchopneumonia

Although inhalation of the conidia of *A. fumigatus* usually does not lead to clinical infection—thus excluding allergic responses of various types (s.a.)—the use of antibiotic therapy in acute pneumonia of bacterial or viral origin may be followed by the development of fungal growth due to *A. fumigatus* in the previously damaged pulmonary tissue and may lead to a fatal outcome. Such cases were observed in the early sixties.

Histopathology in such autopsy material shows branched, septate my-

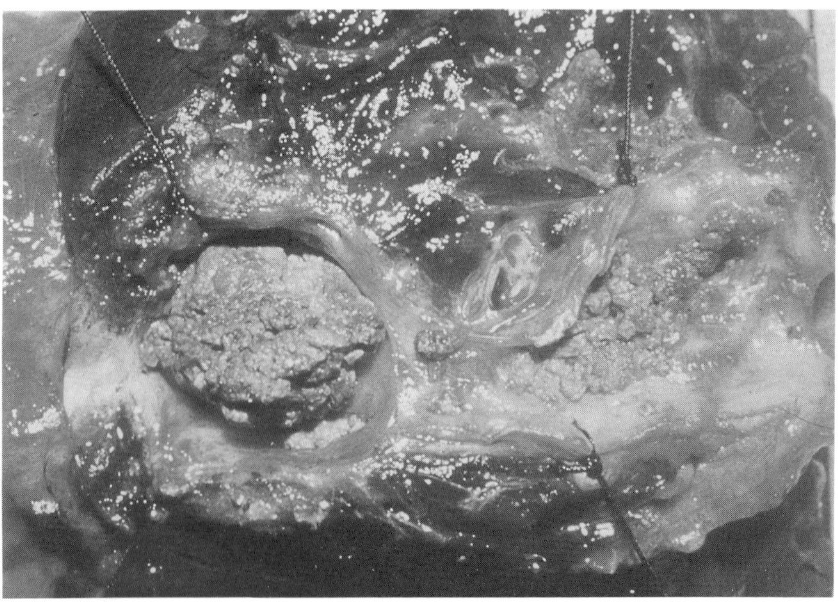

Figure 6 Fungus ball in surgically removed section of lung.

celium, usually with no sporulation, embedded in areas of leukocytic infiltration or microabcesses. This indicates very clearly a well-functioning defense system since the aspergilli provoke in tissues a normal cellular defense by granular leukocytes. These are, however, able to cope with the rapidly expanding growth only poorly or not at all unless antimycotic treatment is quickly applied. The developing mycelial structures can easily be identified with the use of a hematoxylin-eosin stain or by the Grocott stain, which reveal branched septate hyphae 3–4 μ in *width* (see Fig. 7).

D. Invasive Pulmonary Aspergillosis

This represents the most dangerous form of aspergillosis and is observed with increasing frequency throughout the world among susceptible patients (12). The common denominator is the lack of well-functioning leukocytes—i.e., leukopenia and agranulocytosis (12). This condition develops under various circumstances:

1. Treatment with corticosteroids in high dosages for extended periods of time.
2. Although not observed in the early stages of human immunodeficiency virus (HIV) infections, aspergillosis becomes a threat when the CD4 cells decrease to less than $100/mm^3$ and corticosteroids are administered for other concurrent infections.
3. Neutropenia in leukemic patients and others.
4. Leukemia and bone marrow transplantation.
5. Patients after liver and heart transplantation.
6. Agranulocytosis as a result of intolerance to medication.
7. Diabetic acidosis.
8. Granulomatous disease.

Invasive pulmonary aspergillosis is characterized by its rapid course, often ranging between 3 to 7 days. Inhaled *Aspergillus* spp. conidia may germinate in all sections of the respiratory tract without forming conidial structures (13,14). Secretory proteases and other metabolic products promote this invasion. The lack of conidial formation renders a quick diagnosis very difficult. Clumps of hyphae in sputum or aspirated material need special treatment (15) in order to become recognizable as such under the microscope. The procedure is as follows:

A droplet of the specimen is placed on a slide and exposed to an equal volume of 20% KOH for a few minutes in a moist chamber. Subsequently, a droplet of alkaline calcofluor white solution (Fungi-fluor-A, Polysciences Inc., Warrington, PA) is applied, the mount is covered with a

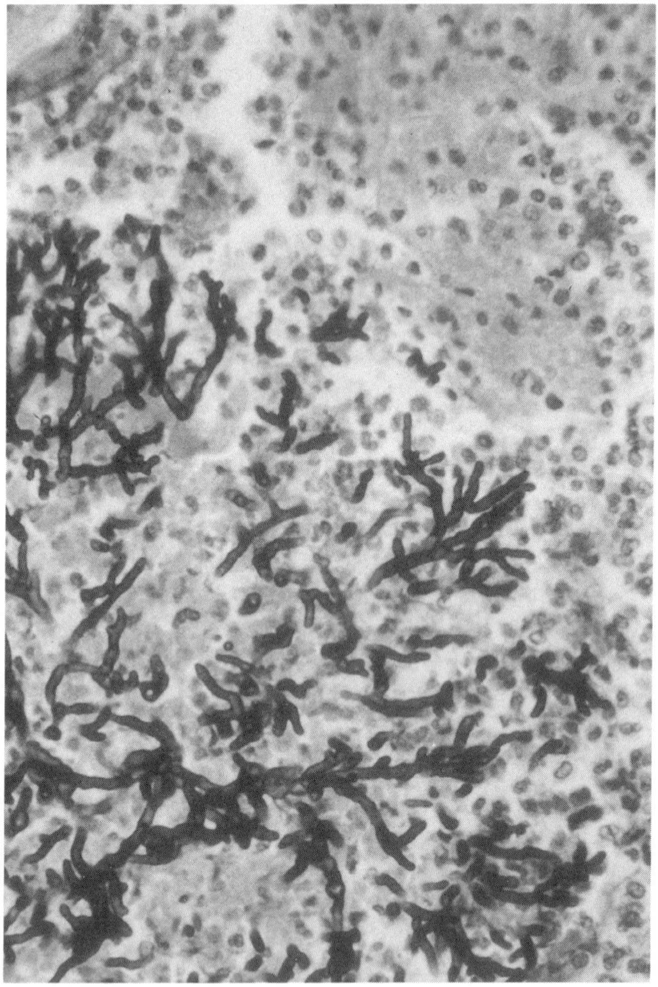

Figure 7 Mycelial structures of *A. fumigatus* in pulmonary infection. (Hematoxylin-eosin stain of section from autopsy.)

cover slip and examined with a fluorescence microscope (excitation 365–395 nm, barrier 420 nm).

The mycelium thus delineated is presented in Fig. 8.

The invasion of blood vessels usually occurs without symptoms other than fever and leads to thrombosis, embolism, and eventual infarction of distant organs.

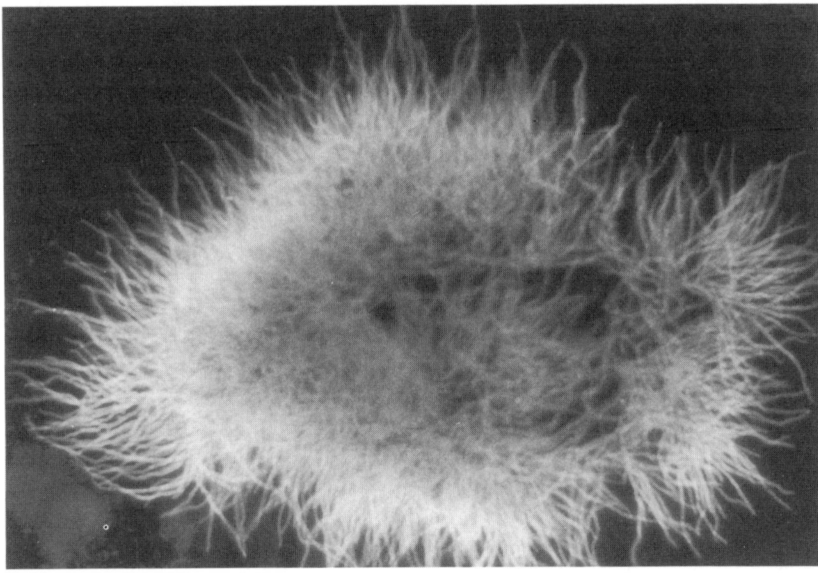

Figure 8 Mount of aspirated bronchial material as treated by the precipitation of Prof. Ruchel, Gottingen, Germany.

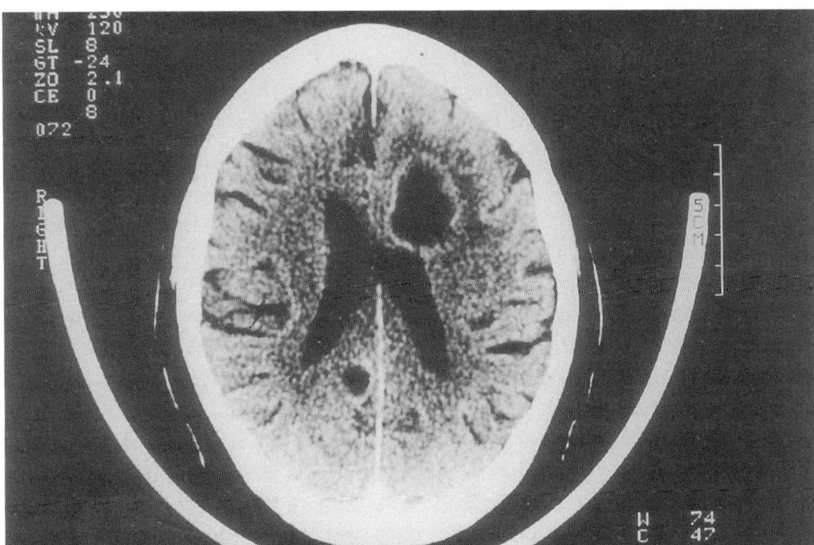

Figure 9 Multiple abscess formation in frontal area of brain as seen by computed tomography. (From Ref. 5.)

Fever resistant to antibacterial antibiotics is an early symptom and should immediately lead to suspicion of a visceral mycosis. Cerebral involvement may provoke central nervous system reactions (Fig. 9).

The reappearance of leukocytes, which are also essential in the defense under antimycotic therapy, stops the spread and introduces demarcation of the infection. As histological and microscopic examinations may give misleading results, daily attempts of cultivation are essential, this being eventually supported by serological demonstration of *Aspergillus* spp. galactomannan antigen (commercially available) in specimens of serum and urine twice weekly.

It should be noted that invasive aspergillosis is not restricted to the respiratory tract but, due to invasion of the bloodstream, may lead to life-threatening involvement of the brain and liver, with abscess formation.

The infectious dose, as expressed by numbers of fungal conidia, will depend on the actual susceptibility of the patient and perhaps on the site and circumstances of their inhalation or introduction.

VI. EPIDEMIOLOGY

Aspergilli are widely spread in nature and found in a great variety of habitats. Unfortunately the strains of the principal pathogen, *A. fumigatus*, are relatively uniform and differ only in a few characteristics that render intraspecies differentiation possible only with highly refined techniques (16) not available to the average hospital mycological laboratory. This situation makes the tracing of *Aspergillus* spp. infections to their eventual source extremely difficult if not impossible. Thus a multiplicity of contaminated sites has to be envisaged.

The habitat of aspergilli is strongly connected with vegetal materials: plants, compost, humus, soil—particularly in potted plants and flowers (17)—but also on various foods of plant origin such as nuts, black pepper, etc. Consequently a great deal of equipment and utensils may also become contaminated and carry infectious particles to susceptible patients in hospitals. This may even apply to the clothes of the medical personnel (14).

A great deal of attention has been devoted to polluted air conditioning systems and to all sorts of niches that harbor aspergilli (18,19). On walls and on or under wallpaper, they may be rather frequent and thus endanger susceptible individuals when such materials are removed during repair or demolition work. This is also of importance in all sorts of construction work done in hospitals and their vicinity, which generates dust that may carry fungal elements into the airstream and thus endanger patients.

This has been claimed in some instances (20) and has resulted in a demand to create in the respective hospital environment spore-free indoor conditions. The realization of such objectives is said to have considerably diminished the incidence of invasive infections due to aspergilli.

All this applies to all hospital patients and especially to those who are most endangered—that is, those who have received bone-marrow transplants, who must be confined to specially protected hospital areas.

There are, however, a growing number of susceptible persons who will continue to live as outpatients in their home environments or wait there until their time has come for therapeutic intervention in a hospital. They are also at risk.

It is obvious that the pharmacy area and food preparation rooms that serve high-risk patients should be free of *Aspergillus* conidia. In this connection, it must be noted that the containers set up to produce so-called "biowaste" and compost may become dangerous sources of fungal growth with the consequent production of infective particles (14).

VII. THERAPY

Except for the surgical removal of *Aspergillus*-infected tissue in aspergillomas and oral cavities, there were for a long time no drugs available against other than superficial *Aspergillus* infections.

Only with the introduction of amphotericin B and recently with its liposomal form and their intravenous application, could antimycotic drugs be administered in cases of systemic mycosis including aspergillosis (18–20).

The azole compounds improved this situation; particularly itraconazole has been reported to be the remedy of choice in cases of invasive aspergillosis. It should be administered in suspected cases as early as possible in order to cover the time until leukocytes reappear (22–26).

VIII. PROPHYLAXIS

A whole catalogue of preventive measures is recommended to possibly cope with the dangers of invasive aspergillosis (13,14).

1. Instructions to patients (and their caretakers) about their extreme susceptibility to the inhalation of airborne *Aspergillus* conidia (spores), particularly those who are leukopenic and under heavy immunosuppression.
2. Permanent (up to three times per week) mycological control by microscopy and culture techniques of specimens obtained from the respiratory tract and eventually from spinal fluid; furthermore,

search for *Aspergillus* galactomannan antigen in serum and urine (twice or more weekly) is strongly recommended.
3. No accommodation of immunocompromised patients in wards on the ground floor, surrounded by vegetation.
4. Complete avoidance of plants, etc., in the patient's hospital, including wards, floor, and departments for gymnastics, x-ray, radiation treatment, pharmacy, and others.
5. No unheated food (which is frequently contaminated by aspergilli), such as ground species (pepper), nuts, open packages of cereal, moist baked goods, and the like.
6. Elimination of the risk that *Aspergillus* spp. conidia are dispersed by carrier patients [“cough plate” (27)].
7. Routine mycological control (monitoring) of indoor air.
8. Air filtration facilities (28–30).
9. Eventual chemoprophylaxis.

ACKNOWLEDGMENT

The author wishes to express his gratitude to Dr. Libero Ajello, Emory University, Atlanta/Ga for his kindness in critically evaluating the manuscript.

REFERENCES

1. Virchow R. Beiträge zur Lehre von den beim Menschen vorkommenden pflanzlichen Parasiten. Arch Pathol Anat 1856;9:557–593.
2. Raper KB, Fennel DI. The genus Aspergillus. Baltimore: Williams & Wilkins, 1965.
3. Kappe, R., Seeliger, HPR. Serodiagnosis of deep seated fungal infections. Current Topics in Medical Mycology. Vol 5. New York: JR Prous, 1994. 247–280.
4. Dupont S, Improvisi L, Prevot F. Détection de galactomannane dans les aspergilloses invasives humaines avec un test au latex. Bull Soc Francaise Mycol Med 1990;19:35–41.
5. Tietz H-J, Tausch I, Engelmann, U, et al. Aspergillusinfektionen in der Intensivmedizin. Hautnah 1993;2:58–61.
6. Piens MA, Troncy Y, Nicolle MC, et al. Aspergilloses invasives chez des patients atteints d'hémopathies malignes: A propos de 29 obervations. J Mycol Med 1993;3:79–83.
7. Riddle HFV, Channel S, Blyth W. Allergic alveolitis in malt workers. Thorax 1968;23:271.
8. Levitz St M, Diamond RD. Changing patterns of aspergillosis infections. Adv Intern Med 1984;30:153–174.

9. Hinson KFW, Moon AS, Plummer NS. Bronchopulmonary aspergillosis. Thorax 1952;7:317.
10. Biguet J. Affections respiratoires secondaires à l'inhalation de spores fongiques et pneumopathies par hypersensibilité. Lille Médical, 3me Série 1971; 16:34–42.
11. Rosenberg M, Patterson R, Mintzer R. Clinical and immunological criteria for the diagnosis of allergic bronchopulmonary aspergillosis. Ann Intern Med 1977;86:407.
12. Rinaldi MG. Invasive aspergillosis. Rev Infect Dis 1983;5:1061–1072.
13. Gerson St L, Talbot GH, Hurwitz Sh, et al. Prolonged granulocytopenia: The major risk factor for invasive pulmonary aspergillosis in patients with acute leukemia. Ann Intern Med 1984;100:345–351.
14. Staib F. Problems associated with aspergilli and aspergillosis in the hospital. Eur J Hosp Pharm 1992;2:128–132.
15. Rüchel R. Diagnosis of invasive mycoses in severely immunosuppressed patients. Ann Hematol 1993;67:1–11.
16. Denning DO, Clemons KV, Hansen LH, Stevens DA. Restriction endonuclease analysis of total cellular DNA of Aspergillus fumigatus isolates of geographically and epidemiologically diverse origin. J Infect Dis 1990;162: 1151–1158.
17. Staib F, Tompak D, Thiel D, Abel Th. Aspergillus fumigatus in der Topferde von Zimmerpflanzen. Bundesgesundheitsblatt 1978;2:471–474.
18. Seeliger HPR. Extrinsic sources of nosocomial mycoses with particular reference to aspergillosis. In: Torres-Rodriguez, ed. Proceedings of the Xth Congress of ISHAM Barcelona: JR Prous, 1988:284–286.
19. Seeliger HPR, Tintelnot K. Epidemiology of aspergillosis. Second Symposium: Topics in Mycology. In: Bossche HV, Mackenzie R, Cauwenbergh G, eds. Aspergillus and Aspergillosis. New York: Plenum Press, 1988:23–33.
20. Medoff G, Kibayasshi GS. Strategies in the treatment of systemic fungal infections. N Engl J Med 1980;302:145.
21. Katz NM, Pierce PF, Anzeck RA. Liposomal amphotericine B for treatment of pulmonary aspergillosis in a heart transplant patient. J Heart Transplant 1990;9:14–17.
22. Ikemoto H. Bronchopulmonary aspergillosis: Diagnosis and therapeutic considerations. In: Borgers M, Hay R, Rinaldi MG, eds. Current Topics in Medical Mycology. Vol 4. New York: Springer-Verlag, 1992:64–87.
23. Denning DW, Tücker RM, Hanson LH, Stevens DA. Treatment of invasive aspergillosis with itraconazole. Am J Med 1989;86:791–800.
24. Kappe R, Osterziel KY, Rüchel R, Siehl S. Fluconazole in patients at risk from invasive aspergillosis. J Med Vet Mycol 1993;31:259–261.
25. Loeuille GA, Berthou C, Hilmarsdottir I, et al. Aspergilloses traitées par l'itraconazole: Analyse de 64 cas. J Mycol Med 1993;3:1–13.
26. De Beule K, De Doncker P, Cauwenbergh G, et al. The treatment of aspergillosis and aspergilloma with itraconazole: Results of an open international study (1982–1987). Mycoses 1988;31:476–485.

27. Staib F. Aspergillus fumigatus in der Ausatmungsluft eines Arztes: Hustean- und Sprechplatte zur Erfassung von A. fumigatus-Ausscheidern. Dtsch Med Wochenschr 1974;99:1804–1807.
28. Sherertz RJ, Belani A, Kramer BS, et al. Impact of air filtration on nosocomial Aspergillus infections. Am J Med 1987;83:709–718.
29. Warnock, DW.: Introduction to the management of fungal infection in the compromised patient. In: Warnock DS, Richardson MD, eds. Fungal Infection in the Compromised Patient, 2d ed. Chichester, England: John Wilegtsone 1991:23–33.
30. Cohen J. Clinical manifestation and management of aspergillosis in the compromised patient (see Ref. 29). 1991:117–152.

24

Iron Acquisition by *Aspergillus fumigatus*

ANGELA M. NILIUS
Abbott Laboratories
Abbott Park, Illinois

I. INTRODUCTION: INFECTION WITH *ASPERGILLUS*

Although the aspergilli are ubiquitous in nature and may be found as transient flora in the respiratory tract, they only infrequently cause disease in humans. A complex interplay of host and fungal factors is required for disease to occur, since the aspergilli have very low inherent virulence. Individuals who possess normal respiratory tracts, skin integrity, and immune systems are generally resistant to infection with *Aspergillus*. At most, transient colonization of the upper respiratory airways due to inhalation of fungal spores from environmental sources may occur; this colonization is unrelated to any infectious process (1,2). *Aspergillus fumigatus* is the species most frequently involved in human disease because of its prevalence in nature and its small conidia which facilitate respiratory infection. Also implicated in disease processes are *A. flavus*, *A. nidulans*, *A. niger*, *A. ochraceous*, *A. terrus*, and *A. clavatus* (1).

In particular, the immunocompromised patient is at risk of life-threatening, invasive disease caused by infection with *Aspergillus*. The primary risk factor for invasive aspergillosis is lowered phagocytic capacity caused by either a decrease in the number or effectiveness of the mononuclear phagocytes or polymorphonuclear leukocytes. Lowered phagocytic defenses may be a result of malignancies, granulocytopenia, infection with human immunodeficiency virus (HIV) or functional defects of the neutrophils. Phagocytic responses are also compromised by treatment with radiation or anntineoplastic, cytotoxic, and immunosuppressive drugs (2,3). Invasive disease of the lung is the most common form of aspergillosis in immunocompromised patients (2). The lack of intact phagocytic defenses allow inhaled spores of *Aspergillus* to germinate in the lung. The growing mycelia can then invade the lung parenchyma. In addition, spores inoculated through a skin break may germinate and invade local tissue unopposed by host defenses. The tissue invasion by mycelia causes an acute inflammatory response and tissue necrosis (2,3). Because the aspergilli are angioinvasive, thrombosis, hemorrhage, and secondary dissemination of the infection throughout the body by septic emboli of infectious mycelia may occur (3). Invasive and disseminated aspergillosis is often fatal because the early diagnosis of the infection is difficult, the patients are already debilitated by their initial disease, and antifungal therapy may be less effective in patients with defective immunological responses (2,3).

II. ROLE OF IRON IN INFECTION

Most invading microorganisms, like *A. fumigatus*, must proliferate at the site of infection in order to cause disease (4,5). Therefore, the site of infection must provide a suitable physical and nutritional environment to support microbial growth. One of the essential elements for both prokaryotic and eukaryotic cells is iron because of its role in nucleic acid synthesis, oxygen metabolism, energy generation, and cell differentiation. The minimum concentration of iron required by most cell types is 0.4 to 4 μM (6). However, iron is highly insoluble in aqueous solutions at neutral and alkaline pH so that the concentration of free ferric iron is limited to 10^{-11} μM (6). To circumvent the problem of insolubility of ferric iron, iron is usually bound to various chelators or is found as ferrous salts in acidic or anaerobic conditions (6). In humans, the bulk of the iron is intracellular and is inacessible to most microorganisms (7,8). The iron content of milk and plasma ranges from 10 to 65 μM, but it is bound to the iron transport proteins transferrin and lactoferrin. The level of saturation of transferrin and lactoferrin with iron is 30 and 15% respectively, creating a large reserve of unused iron binding capacity which can easily absorb changes in the circulating iron concentration (9). Therefore, the concentration of free iron in body fluids is calculated to be less than 10^{-15} μM (7,8), far lower than the amount required to support microbial growth during infection. Because iron is sequestered by the host so that it is not not readily available for microbial use, withholding iron may be an effective form of natural immunity. This type of immunity is described as nutritional immunity because the host environment does not meet the nutritional requirements for microbial growth (5,7–9).

Transferrin and lactoferrin have antimicrobial effects due to their ability to bind iron, preventing its use by microorganisms. Conversely, the antimicrobial effect of transferrin is lessened as its iron-binding capacity becomes more saturated through either decreased transferrin concentration or increased iron concentration (8,9). Both the antifungal effect of unsaturated transferrin and the loss of that effect by increasing the level of iron saturation can be demonstrated experimentally. For example, normal human sera inhibit the growth in vitro of *Candida albicans*, while thalassemic sera in which the iron-binding capacity of transferrin is fully saturated are not inhibitory (7). Similarly, the growth of *C. albicans* and *C. stellatoidia* is inhibited by adding unsaturated human transferrin to the growth medium, but the growth inhibition is reversed when the added transferrin has high levels of iron saturation (10). Last, the growth of yeast and hyphal forms of *Histoplasma capsulatum* is inhibited by sera containing transferrin at 10–80% iron saturation. The inhibition is reversed when the iron-binding capacity is fully saturated with exogenous iron (11).

III. FUNGAL IRON BINDING COMPOUNDS: THE SIDEROPHORES

Most aerobic and facultatively aerobic microorganisms synthesize ferric-specific ligands called siderophores. Siderophores are nonprotein, nonporphyrin ligands having molecular masses of 500 to 1000 Da. Most microbial siderophores are amino acid conjugates of either 2,3 dihydroxybenzoic acid (phenolate class) or are derivatives of secondary hydroxamic acids (hydroxamate class). Both classes bind Fe^{3+} via six coordinating electronegative atoms carried on one or more sets of bidentate functional units that form an octahedral configuration around the central Fe^{3+} ion. Hydroxamate siderophores usually contain D-*N*-hydroxyl-L ornithinine with various acyl substitutions. The groups used for iron chelation by the hydroxamate siderophores are arranged on a cyclic or linear peptide or a linear carbon chain. The association constants of siderophores for Fe^{3+} are at least 10^{30}; in contrast, they have little affinity for Fe^{2+} or other cations (5,12,13). It is the ability of the siderophores to specifically chelate Fe^{3+} that is responsible for their biological activities. The molecules function to solubilize inorganic Fe^{3+}, to transport it to the cells and across biological membranes, and to store it intracellularly. By virtue of their iron-binding properties, they act as germination factors, growth factors, virulence factors, and antibiotics (the ferrimycins) (5,12,14).

Aspergillus fumigatus synthesizes five extracellular, hydroxamate siderophores. *N,N′,N″*-triacetyl fusarinine C is the most prominent siderophore and ferricrocin is the second most prominent siderophore found in culture filtrates of *A. fumigatus* grown in low-iron medium (15,16). In our study (16), the extracellular siderophores produced by eight clinical and one environmental isolate of *A. fumigatus* were identified using thin-layer chromatography. All nine strains produced the same profile of five siderophores and in the same relative concentrations. *N,N′,N″*-triacetyl fusarinine C and ferricrocin were identified as the predominant siderophores, with three siderophores remaining unidentified. Similarly, the study of a single strain of *A. fumigatus* by Konetschny-Rapp et al. (15) identified the siderophores *N,N′,N″*-triacetyl fusarinine C and ferricrocin plus three unknown siderophores in culture filtrates using high-performance liquid chromatography. Other studies have also identified ferricrocin as a prominent siderophore in culture filtrates of *A. fumigatus*, along with other hydroxamate siderophores including triacetylfusigen, fusigen, ferrichrome, and sideramine B (17,18).

Hydroxamate-class siderophores are produced by other pathogenic fungi during growth in iron-limited media as well. These include the opportunistic pathogens *Rhizopus* sp., *Aspergillus* sp., and *Penicillium* (17,19,20,21) the dimorphic pathogens *Sporothrix schenckii*, *Histoplasma capsulatum*, and *Blastomyces dermatiditis* (21), the dermatophyte *Trichophyton mentagrophytes* (27), and the yeast *C. albicans* (22,27). As is described for *A. fumigatus*, more than one siderophore is produced by most fungi and different morphological forms of the same fungus such as spores and mycelia may contain different siderophores. These observations suggest that different siderophores may have specialized roles in fungal physiology and iron nutrition.

IV. ROLES OF SIDEROPHORES IN FUNGAL IRON METABOLISM

The locations and roles of different hydroxamate siderophores are best described for the fungus *Neurospora crassa*. Coprogen is excreted during mycelial growth, mycelia contain ferricrocin as the predominant siderophore as well as ferrichrome C, and spores contain the siderophores ferricrocin and ferrichrome C (14,23–25). In experiments using Mössbauer spectroscopic analysis to follow the transfer of iron (25), extracellular iron is bound by the iron-free coprogen excreted into the environment during mycelial growth. The iron-coprogen complex is taken up by the mycelium, using a specific iron-coprogen transport system. Once in the mycelium, the iron is transferred principally to the mycelial siderophore ferricrocin for storage. The remainder of the iron is incorporated into metabolically active molecules. At least some of the iron-free coprogen is then recycled back into the extracellular environment. Mycelial iron-ferricrocin is incorporated into the spore during sporulation to provide a readily available pool of iron for germination and early mycelia growth (14,25).

Fungal siderophores are taken up across the cytoplasmic membrane of mycelia by active transport of the iron-siderophore complex. The transport of iron-siderophores is an energy-dependent process that can be inhibited by metabolic poisons such as azide, cyanide, and *N*-methylmaleimide (26). In fungi, the transport system is operational immediately after the spores germinate (23). The transport of iron-siderophore complexes uses highly specific membrane-bound receptors. Iron must be bound to the siderophore to be recognized by the receptor. The reactions of the iron-siderophore complex with the corresponding receptor depends on the geometry of the metal center, the peripheral groups, the molecular backbone, molecular stereochemistry, and the molecule as an entity (12,13,26,27).

Assimilated iron is directly transferred into either storage forms or biosynthetic pathways (12). Because free iron is highly insoluble, mycelial iron stores are are likely to be in the form of iron-siderophore complexes, although iron-protein complexes may also be possible (25). The transfer of iron from a transport siderophore to a storage siderophore may occur by simple exchange of iron-binding ligands, since the association constants for most hydroxamate siderophores are similar. The exchange may be promoted by an excess of iron-free siderophore located in the mycelium (25). For example, transfer of extracellular iron via iron-coprogen to mycelial ferricrocin is demonstrated for *N. crassa* (25). Siderophores have been identified in the spores of many fungi including *Aspergillus* (20,24). Loss of siderophores from fungal spores blocks the ability of the spores to germinate (14,20). In spores, siderophores may act as either storage depots for immediately available iron when present as the iron chelates or as preformed, iron-free ligands for active iron acquisition during germination and early phases of mycelial growth (25).

For use in metabolically active molecules, two mechanisms have been proposed for the release of iron from the iron-siderophore complex. The first mechanism relies on the differences in affinity of siderophores for Fe^{3+} as compared with Fe^{2+}. In this mechanism, Fe^{3+} is reduced intracellularly to Fe^{2+} using a specific ferrisiderophore reductase. Since the affinity of siderophores for Fe^{2+} is low, the iron is released and the iron-free siderophore may be recycled (13,25). Iron-siderophore reductase activity is found in the cytoplasm of various fungi and bacteria and it can remove iron from trihydroxamate siderophores (13). Reductive release of iron from a siderophore may be coupled to insertion of Fe^{2+} into protoporphyrin through the use of a ferrichelatase, as is shown for *Ustilago sphaerogena* (26). Alternatively, iron-siderophore complexes may be hydrolyzed enzymatically to release the bound iron. This reaction is established for siderophores which contain ester bonds such as *N,N′,N″*-triacetyl fusarinine C produced by *Penicillium* sp. which also produces the corresponding esterase activity (12,26).

Low levels of extracellular, iron-free siderophores are synthesized by microorganisms in environments with adequate iron content and represent the amount needed to acquire iron for normal microbial growth and metabolism (5,16,20). For bacteria such as *Escherichia coli* grown in conditions of limited iron, the genes for molecules required to synthesize, transport, and utilize siderophores are derepressed and the concentration of the iron-free siderophores and their ancillary molecules is increased (8). Derepression of these genes when iron availability is limited enhances the ability of the bacteria to acquire this essential nutrient from environmental sources. Less is known about the regulation of iron acquisition in fungi. Siderophore synthesis has been shown to increase when fungi are grown in medium with low concentrations of iron (23). (A. Nilius unpublished observations). For example, the amount of extracellular, iron-free coprogen produced by *N. crassa* increases when the fungus is grown in medium with limited amounts of iron. And in conjunction with the increase in the amount of coprogen produced by the fungus, the rate of iron-siderophore transport is also increased. However, the relative concentrations of membrane proteins, including the siderophore transport proteins, remain unchanged. Increasing both the extracellular concentration of iron-free siderophores and the rate at which the iron chelates are taken up by the mycelium may provide sufficient iron for the survival and growth of *N. crassa* in environments where iron is limited (23).

V. POSSIBLE ROLE OF SIDEROPHORES IN FUNGAL INFECTIONS

Successful pathogens are known to adapt and evolve biochemical processes that allow them to compete with the host for iron. They may be able to accomplish this through the use of siderophores, which can chemically compete with the host for the available iron (7–9). In our study of clinical isolates, *A. fumigatus* did not produce distinctive extracellular siderophores that could be related to the ability of a particular strain to cause invasive and disseminated disease. Instead, all strains appear to produce the same profile of extracellular siderophores (15,16). In contrast, pathogenic strains of *E. coli* and *Yersinia enterocolitica* produce novel extracellular siderophores not found in nonpathogenic strains. The novel siderophores are associated with the virulence of the bacterial strains (28,29).

Unlike the antifungal activity demonstrated against *Candida* sp. (10), transferrin and lactoferrin at physiological levels of iron saturation (30 and 15% respectively) were unable to inhibit the germination and subsequent mycelial growth in vitro of three clinical isolates of *A. fumigatus* (A. Nilius, manuscript in preparation). Because all the iron in the medium was bound to the proteins, these results suggested that iron bound to transferrin or lactoferrin was available for use by *A. fumigatus*. Both *N,N′,N″*-triacetyl fusarinine C and ferricrocin were produced by *A. fumigatus* during growth in the medium containing transferrin, which may provide a mechanism for the fungus to acquire iron in the presence of a competing iron ligand like transferrin (A. Nilius, manuscript in preparation). Similarly, yeast-phase cells of *Paracoccidiodes braziliensis* can grow in brain-heart infusion agar containing 4% horse serum. Supplementing the medium with either a culture filtrate of *P. braziliensis* or the siderophores dimerumic acid and coprogen B enhances the recovery of yeast cells compared with the recovery of yeast cells on medium lacking the supplements. The siderophore supplements, either as pure compounds or culture filtrate constituents, may help the yeast cells overcome the iron-withholding properties of the transferrin found in the serum (the serum itself is likely to be required for improved yeast growth for reasons other than its iron content) (30). However, the possibility remains that iron-transferrin is utilized directly by opportunistic and pathogenic fungi for use as an iron source during growth, as is described for some bacterial pathogens like *Neisseria gonorrhoeae* (31).

No distinctive functions in fungal physiology other than providing a mechanism to assimilate iron have been assigned to any of the extracellular siderophores of *A. fumigatus*. However, the hydroxamate siderophores produced by *A. fumigatus* are ideally suited to participate in iron acquisition during infection. They are soluble in aqueous solutions, have a high affinity for iron, and retain bound iron at acid pH. They are nonantigenic and are not susceptible to proteolytic cleavage (9,13). In addition, equilibrium dialysis experiments have demonstrated that iron-free ferricrocin stimulated the release of more iron from iron-transferrin than is spontaneously released from the protein. The released iron was shown to be bound to ferricrocin. Stimulation of iron release by ferricrocin required that the concentration of ferricrocin exceed that of the transferrin by 100-fold and that the buffer pH be reduced to 5. In contrast, iron-free *N,N′,N″*-triacetyl fusarinine C could not stimulate the release of iron from transferrin under the same conditions, but it did bind the iron that was spontaneously released (A. Nilius, manuscript in preparation). It is known that the local pH of an abcess formed at the site of infection falls below 5 due to the release of components of phagocytic cells, local tissue destruction, and the formation of metabolic end products during microbial growth (32).

Since the affinity of transferrin for iron is reduced as the pH drops below 6.5 (9), if *A. fumigatus* siderophores are present at the site of infection, they may be able to compete for the iron released from transferrin and mediate its transport into the mycelium. Because the hydroxamate siderophores including ferricrocin and *N,N′,N″*-triacetyl fusarinine C retain bound iron in acidified environments, this would provide a mechanism for overcoming iron-withholding by the host at the site of infection.

Spores of *A. fumigatus* also contain siderophores. Two hydroxamate siderophores were isolated from spores of three pathogenic strains of *A. fumigatus* but could not be identified by thin-layer chromatography, although they were distinct from those secreted by the strains during mycelial growth (A. Nilius, unpublished observations). The spore siderophores of *A. fumigatus* may influence the germination of spores and the initiation of mycelial growth in vivo by providing a source of stored iron or a mechanism for quickly acquiring environmental iron without the need for molecular synthesis.

Clinical evidence indirectly supports a role for hydroxamate siderophores in iron acquisition by pathogenic fungi during infection. The use of the trihydroxamate siderophore deferoxamine (desferrioxamine B) to treat hemodialysis patients with chronic iron and aluminum overload is associated with invasive mucormycosis caused by the opportunistic fungal pathogen *Rhizopus* (33). This observation is corraborated by an experimental guinea pig model of mucormycosis using *R. rhizopodiformis* and *R. oryzae* as the infectious agents. Infected animals treated with desferoxamine have shortened survival times and more extensive dissemination of infection than untreated control animals. In addition, the in vitro growth of the two strains used in the animal model is improved when 0.001 to 1 mmol deferoxamine is added to iron-limited Sabouraud Dextrose agar (33). Although direct uptake of ferric complexes of deferoxamine by *Rhizopus* has not been shown, *Rhizopus* is known to synthesize hydroxamate siderophores and, therefore, should have the corresponding transport systems required for the assimilation of the iron-siderophore complexes (21). The fungus may be able to use that transport system for the uptake of iron-deferoxamine (8,33). In patients treated with deferoxamine, *Rhizopus* may be able to use the deferoxamine as a source of preformed, extracellular siderophores for iron acquisition to support and enhance fungal growth during infection.

VI. SUMMARY

Immunocompromised patients with invasive aspergillosis show histological evidence of mycelial growth in their infected tissues. Therefore, the tissues must provide a suitable nutritional environment for the growth and survival of *Aspergillus*. Although the host has mechanisms such as transferrin to withhold iron from the fungus as a nonspecific defense, *Aspergillus* may be able to effectively circumvent that defense. The hydroxamate siderophores of *A. fumigatus*, while not virulence factors, may act as growth factors in the microenvironment of the infectious process by chelating iron released from transferrin and mediating its transport into the fungus.

REFERENCES

1. Bardana EJ Jr. The clinical spectrum of aspergillosis: Part 1. Epidemiology, pathogenicity, infection in animals and immunology of Aspergillus. Crit Rev Clin Lab Sci 1980;21–83.
2. Saral R. Candida and Aspergillus infections in immunocompromised patients: overview. Rev Infect Dis 1991;13:487–492.
3. Bardana EJ Jr. The clinical spectrum of aspergillosis: Part II. Classification and description of saprophytic, allergic, and invasive variants of human disease. Crit Rev Clin Lab Sci 1980;13:85–159.
4. Garber ED. The host as a growth medium. Ann NY Acad Sci 1960;88: 1187–1194.
5. Weinberg E. Iron and susceptibility to infectious disease. Science 1974;184: 952–956.
6. Weinberg E. Cellular regulation of iron assimilation. Q Rev Biol 1989;64: 261–290.
7. Bullen JJ, Rogers HJ, Griffiths E. Role of iron in bacterial infection. Curr Top Microbiol Immunol 1978;80:1–33.
8. Finkelstein RA, Sciortino CV, McIntosh MA. Role of iron in microbe-host interactions. Rev Infect Dis 1983;5(suppl 4):S759–S777.
9. Weinberg ED. Iron withholding: A defense against infection and neoplasia. Physiol Rev 1984;64:65–102.
10. Shiraishi A, Tadashi A. Antifungal activity of transferrin. Sabouraudia 1979; 17:79–83.
11. Stucliffe M, Savage A, Alford R. Transferrin-dependent growth inhibition of yeast-phase Histoplasma capsulatum by human serum and lymph. J Infect Dis 1980;142:209–219.
12. Hider RC. Siderophore-mediated absorption of iron. Struct Bond 1984;58: 25–87.
13. Raymond KN, Muller G, Matzanke BF. Complexation of iron by siderophores: A review of their solution and structure chemistry and biological function. Top Curr Chem 1984;123:49–102.
14. Horowitz NH, Charlang G, Horn G, Williams NP. Isolation and identification of the conidial germination factor of Neurospora crassa. J Bacteriol 1976; 127:135–140.

15. Konetschny-Rapp S, Huschka H-G, Winkelmann G, Jung G. High performance liquid chromatography of siderophores from fungi. Biol Metals 1988; 1:9–17.
16. Nilius AM, Farmer SG. Identification of extracellular siderophores of pathogenic strains of Aspergillus fumigatus. J Med Vet Mycol 1990;28:395–403.
17. Diekmann H, Krezdorn E. Stoffwechselproducte von Mikroorganismen. 150 Mitteilun. Ferricrocin, Triacetylfusigen, und andere Sideramine aus Pilzen der Gattung Aspergillus, Gruppe fumigatus. Arch Mikrobiol 1975;106: 191–194.
18. Weibe C, Winkelmann G. Kinetic studies on the specificity of chelate-iron uptake in Aspergillus. J Bacteriol 1975;123:873–842.
19. Charlang G, Horowitz RM, Lowy PH, et al. Extracellular siderophores of rapidly growing Aspergillus nidulans and Penicillium chyrsogenum. J Bacteriol 1982;150:785–787.
20. Charlang G, Ng B, Horowitz NH, Horowitz RM. Cellular and extracellular siderophores of Aspergillus nidulans and Penicillin chyrsogenum. Mol Cell Biol 1981;1:94–100.
21. Holzberg M, Artis WM. Hydroxamate siderophore production by opportunistic fungal pathogens. Infect Immun 1983;40:1134–1139.
22. Ismail A, Bedell G, Lupan D. Siderophore production by the pathogenic yeast, Candida albicans. Biochem Biophys Res Comm 1985;130:885–891.
23. Huschka H-G, Winkelmann G. Iron limitation and its effect on membrane proteins and siderophore transport in Neurospora crassa. Biol Metals 1989; 2:108–113.
24. Matzanke BF, Bill E, Trautwein AX, Winkelmann G. Role of siderophores in iron storage in spores of Neurospora crassa and Aspergillus ochraceous. J Bacteriol 1987;169:5873–5876.
25. Matzanke BF, Bill E, Trautwein AX, Winkelmann G. Ferricrocin functions as the main intracellular iron-storage compound in mycelia of Neurospora crassa. Biol Metals 1988;1:18–25.
26. Emery T. The storage and transport of iron. In: Metal Ions in Biological Systems: Iron in Model and Natural Compounds. New York: Marcel Dekker, 1978;7:77–126.
27. Huschka H, Naegli HU, Leuenberger-Ryf H, et al. Evidence for a common siderophore transport system but different siderophore receptors in Neurospora crassa. J Bacteriol 1985;162:175–121.
28. Bullen JJ. The significance of iron in infection. Rev Infect Dis 1981;3: 1127–1138.
29. Haag H, Hantke K, Drechsel H, et al. Purification of yersiniabactin: A siderophore and possible virulence factor of Yersinia enterocolitica. J Gen Microbiol 1993;139:2159–2165.
30. Casteneda E, Brummer E, Perlman AM, et al. A culture medium for Paracoccidiodes braziliensis with high plating efficiency, and the effect of siderophores. J Med Vet Mycol 1988;26:351–358.
31. Blanton KJ, Biswas GD, Tsai J, et al. Genetic evidence that Neisseria gonorr-

hoeae produces specific receptors for transferrin and lactoferrin. J Bacteriol 1990;172:5225–5235.

32. Sriyosachti S, Cox CD. Siderophore-mediated iron acquisition from transferrin by Pseudomonas aeruginosa. Infect Immun 1986;52:885–891.
33. Van Cutsem J, Boelaert JR. Effects of deferoxamine, feroxamine, and iron on experimental mucormycosis (zygomycosis). Kidney Int 1989;36:1061–1068.

25

Is *Pityrosporum orbiculare* the Same Organism as *Pityrosporum ovale*?

JAN FAERGEMANN
Sahlgrens University Hospital
Gothenburg, Sweden

I. HISTORY

The genus *Pityrosporum* was first described by Rivolta in 1873 (1). The genus includes the lipophilic yeast *Pityrosporum ovale* and the nonlipophilic member *P. pachydermatis*. In 1873 Rivolta described the presence of round, double-contoured budding cells in a case of psoriasis (1). In 1874 Malassez described yeastlike cells in the stratum corneum of patients with various skin diseases and considered the organism responsible for scalp scaling (2). Baylon proposed the name *Malassezia furfur*. Numerous attempts have been made to culture the organism. In 1913, Castellani and Chalmers cultured the organism and characterized its growth properties. They introduced the name *Pityrosporum ovale*, and their description of the organism is based on the description of the fungus both in skin scales and in the laboratory (3). In 1951 Gordon isolated a round, double-contoured yeast that produces spherical to oval buds from both pityriasis versicolor scales and from normal skin (4). He named the round budding form of the organism *P. orbiculare* and the oval form which he found primarily in the scalp *P. ovale*. These characteristics are based primarily on the micromorphology.

A nonlipophilic member of the genus *Pityrosporum* was classified by Weidman in 1925 (5). There has been discussion concerning the genus name, and the International Commission on the Taxonomy of Fungi proposed that the genus name be changed to *Malassez*. Two species were accepted in the genus: *Malassezia furfur* for the lipophilic yeast and *M. pachydermatis* for the nonlipophilic species. It is still my opinion that the genus name *Pityrosporum* should be used. Malassez was certainly not the first to describe the organism or to culture it, and *Pityrosporum* has been used for many year both for *P. pachydermatis* and the oval form. Since Castellani and Chalmers were the first to both describe the yeast in skin scales and to culture the organism properly, I think that the name *P. ovale* has preference for the lipophilic yeast. Only this species will be discussed in the following sections.

II. MORPHOLOGY

As for many other yeasts, the size, color, and structure of the colonies depend on the culture medium. The following description of the colonies is based on the yeast being cultured on a glucose-neopeptone-yeast extract medium with the addition of olive oil, Tween 80, and glycerol monostearate (6). On this medium, colonies are slightly raised with irregular edges, white to cream in color, and 3–6 mm in diameter (7) (Fig. 1). When colo-

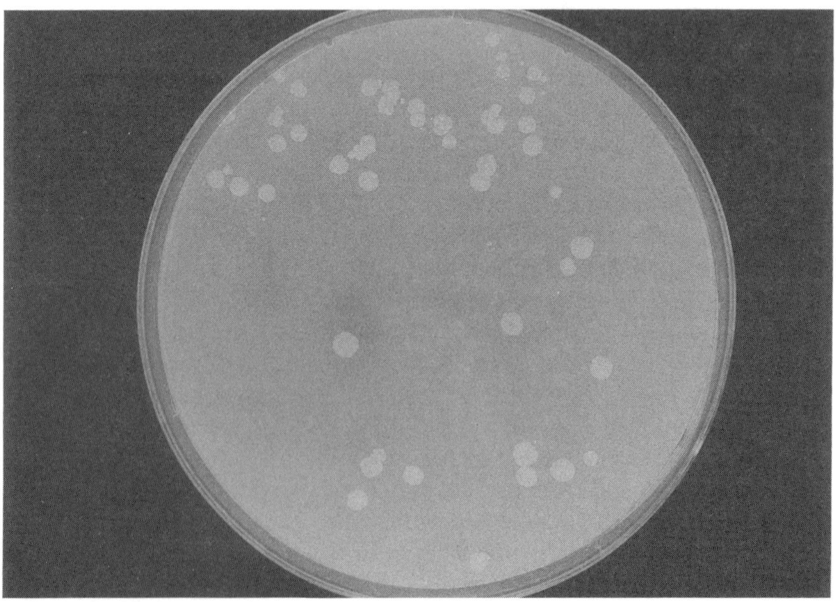

Figure 1 Colonies of *P. ovale*.

nies become older, they will turn yellow in color. On this medium, no differences in macromorphology are observed between the round and oval forms of the organism. However, the micromorphology between isolates may be different. The round-form (former *P. orbiculare*), cells are 3–6 μm in diameter, usually producing single spherical buds on a narrow base (Fig. 2). Sometimes two to four buds are produced in a row. In the oval form, the cells are oval to cylindrical, sometimes almost cigar-shaped; they are 2–3 μm wide and 4–5 μm long, producing single oval buds from a broad base (7) (Fig. 3). Electronmicroscopic studies have also shown a difference between the oval and round forms both in cell morphology and in the number and structure of mitochondria present (8).

Although the micromorphology is quite different in the oval and round forms of the organism, there have been reports about the changes of form in subcultures. Using a monospore technique, Randjandiche reported the change of the oval form in subcultures to a round form (9). The reverse was observed by Salkin and Gordon (10). The oval and round forms may represent different stages in a cell circle of the same organism. However, there have also been reports of stable oval or round forms in cultures. Midgley and coworkers have shown that, using their culture medium, *P. ovale* can be divided into a round form ("orbiculare") and an oval form ("ovale"). The latter can be subdivided into three variants (11). Using a culture medium developed by Leeming and Notman, Cunningham and coworkers have found that *P. ovale* (*M. furfur*) can be divided into three serotypes: A, B, and C (12–14). This description is based on serological differences in cell-surface antigens. The micromorphology and even the macromorphology of the organism clearly depend on the culture medium; more objective methods of classification, especially genome analyses, are necessary for a more exact classification of the genus.

By using certain culture media or changes in growth conditions, hyphae have been produced in vitro in both the oval and round forms of the organism. Dorn and Roehnert were able to produce hyphae in vitro in the round form of the organism but not in the oval form, using a culture medium containing glycine (15). Nazzaro-Porro et al. were able to produce identical hyphae in both forms of the organism using a mixture of cholesterol, cholesteryl stearate, and glyceryl monostearate added to Bacto-Yeast Morphology Agar containing oleic acid (16). We have been able to produce hyphae on sheets of human stratum corneum in vitro, with the longest hyphae being 50–60 μm in around 30–35% of the cells (17). We observed not only the production of hyphae from a large proportion of cells but also the conversion from one form to another (17). Finally, the changes in form of the organism have also been observed when experimental infections were produced (6).

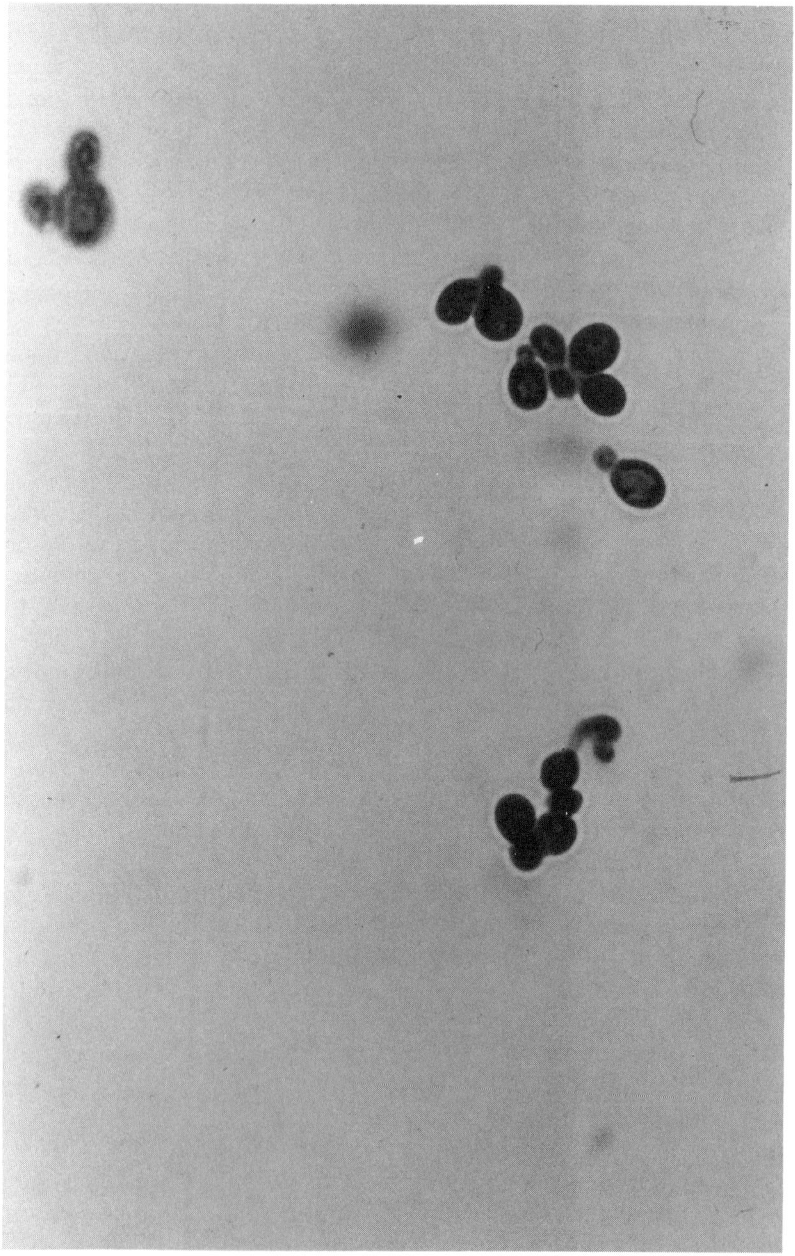

Figure 2 Microscopic view of the round form of *P. ovale* (former *P. orbiculare*).

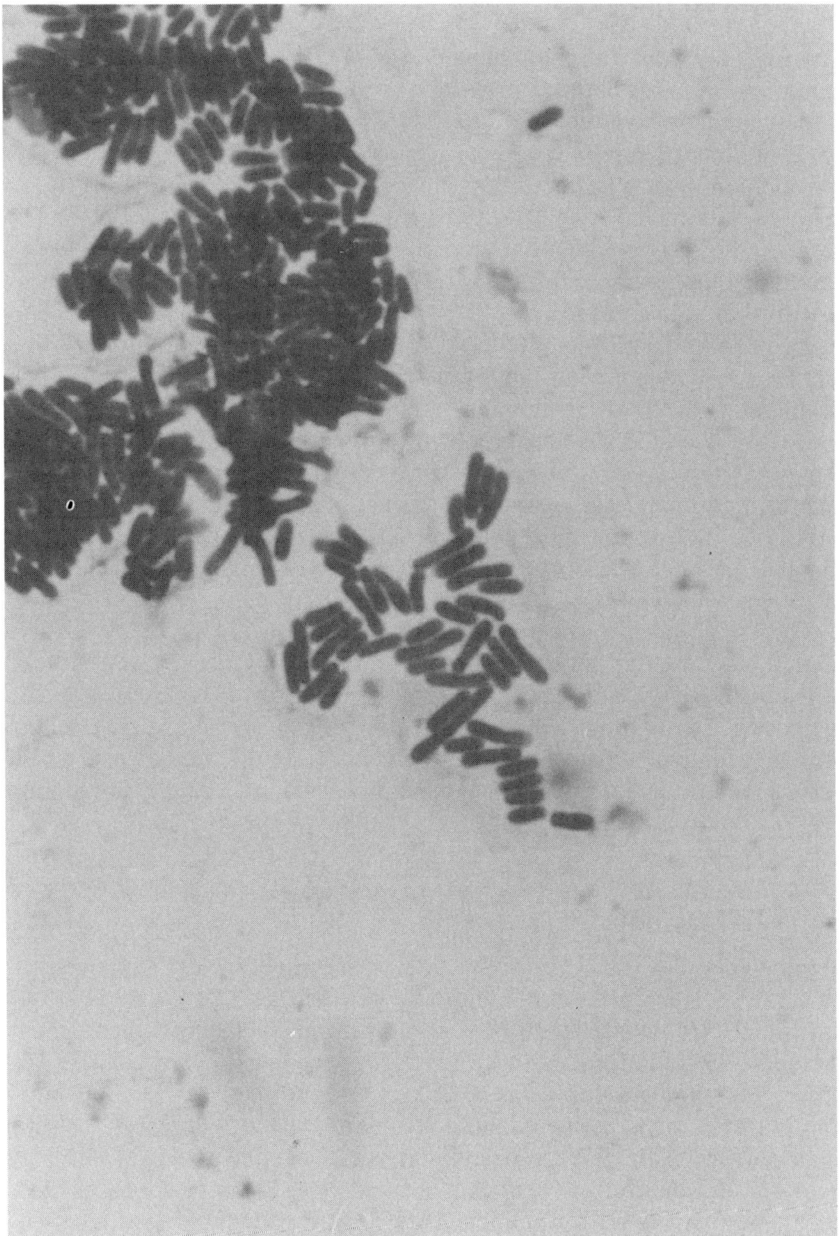

Figure 3 Microscopic view of the oval form of *P. ovale*.

III. GROWTH REQUIREMENTS

Pityrosporum ovale is lipophilic and requires the addition of lipids to the culture medium for optimal growth. It can be cultured on ordinary media if the surface is covered with olive oil. However, a medium into which lipids are incorporate is much easier to work with. The organism needs the addition of fatty acids of C_{12}–C_{14} or higher chain lengths for growth (18,19). They have lipase activity in vitro (20) and in vivo (21). With the addition of fatty acids of chain lengths C_{12} or more, the yeast is able to synthesize longer-chain fatty acids. The addition of glycose and asparagine further stimulates growth. One medium that I have used for several years contains glycose-neopeptone-yeast extract with the addition of olive oil, Tween 80, and glycerol monostearate (6). On this medium, growth is visible after 2 days of incubation and optimal growth is obtained after 3–4 days. The lipid substance is incorporated into the medium, and it is therefore easy to work with. Another medium that produces even better growth, especially for isolation of the organism, is the culture medium developed by Leeming and Notman (12). This medium contains, as lipid extracts, ox bile, glycerol, glycerol monostearate, Tween 60, and whole-fat cow's milk.

The organism is able to grow in the temperature range of 28–37°C. I have found that the optimal temperature is 37°C. The organism is very sensitive to drying and the humidity in the incubator should therefore be increased. The optimal pH for growth is between 5.5 and 6.5. Optimal growth is obtained not only under aerophilic conditions but also in an aerobic environment with 7% CO_2 and under microaerophilic conditions (22).

IV. IMMUNOLOGY

Serum antibodies (IgG) against *P. ovale* are present in sera from healthy adults (23). Titers are very low in children and also low in 80-year-old individuals as compared with 30-year-old subjects (24). Antibodies against the yeast are produced when an individual becomes colonized with the yeast. With immunofluorescense (direct and indirect) (25,26), Ouchterlony gel diffusion (26), and quantitative immunoelectrophoresis (27), antigenic similarities have been found between the round and oval forms of *P. ovale* and differences between *P. ovale* and *P. pachydermatis* have been noted. However, differences between the round and oval forms of the organism have also been described. Midgley used rocket immunoelectrophoresis and sodium dodecylsulfate (SDS) protein polyacrylamide gel electrophoresis (PAGE) pattern analysis (11). Using these techniques, she was able to find immunological differences between the four different forms of the organism that she saw using her culture medium. Subdivisions within *P. ovale* have also been mentioned by Cunningham et al., using the culture medium developed by Leeming et al. (12,13). They described three serotypes called serovars A, B, and C. They used a transferable solid phase (TSP) ELISA technique and found that three morphological types could be classified into three serological types. Howell and coworkers have shown, using pulsed-field gel electrophoresis, that the organism produced patterns containing seven chromosome bands (28). These bands could be separated into distinct groups, correlating to the three morphological groups described earlier (28).

V. GENOME ANALYSIS

Guero and Mayer showed in 1989 that *P. ovale* with different macromorphology had the same genetic characteristics with mol% G + C in the range of 65.9–66.7% (29). They also found DNA/DNA reassociation values of 84.5–100% between round and oval forms of the organism. However, later studies by Simons and Guero described a new member of the genus *Pityrosporum*, which they called *M. sympodialis* (30). Recently a molecular taxonomic revision of the genera *Pityrosporum* (*Malassezia*) was performed by means of nucleic acid comparisons (nDNA and rRNA) correlated to morphological, physiological, and biochemical characteristics (31,32). In this very elegant work, Guillot and Gueho, using the genus name *Malassezia*, were able to divide the genus into eight genetically distinct species. Each taxon was confirmed by a homogenous mol% G + C and percentages of DNA/DNA reassociations higher than 85%. The non-lipid-dependent *P. pachydermatis* (*M. pachydermatis*) was mentained as one species. However, lipid-dependent strains were shown to be distributed among seven species, which they named *M. furfur*, *M. sympodialis*, and *Malasezzia* species 1–5 (32). Obviously the final classification of the lipophilic member(s) of the organism is more complex than earlier thought and is still not completely clear.

VI. ISOLATION AND DISTRIBUTION

Pityrosporum ovale is a member of the normal human cutaneous flora, at least in adults (7). It can also been cultured from the skin of children; however, the number of yeasts is significantly higher in adults than in children, and it is also higher in middle-aged individuals than in 80-year-olds (24,33). There are great variations in the form of the organism (round or oval), the incidence, and the number of organisms isolated, depending on skin location, age, whether the skin is clinically normal or diseased, and the geographic source. Using both direct microscopy and culture, Roberts found the oval form to dominate on the scalp and the round form to be the predominant form on the chest and back (34). Ashbee and coworkers found no differences in distribution of serovars A, B, and C on the foreheads and cheeks in healthy individuals or patients with pityriasis versicolor and seborrheic dermatitis (14). However, serovar A was the predominant isolate on the chest and back in both healthy subjects and patients (14). We have, in another study, found the highest number on the upper trunk and the lowest on the hand (35). This distribution parallels regional variations in sebum excretion.

VII. SAPROPHYTE AND PATHOGEN

Pityrosporum ovale is not only a member of the normal human cutaneous flora but also an opportunistic pathogen. Under the influence of predisposing factors, the yeast changes from saprophyte to pathogen. These factors include high temperature, high relative humidity, and endogenic factors such as greasy skin, hyperhidrosis, hereditary factors, systemic corticosteroids, immunosuppressive treatment, or defect in cell-mediated immunity. In pityriasis versicolor, the organism changes from the blastospore form to the mycelium form. This is very much the same situation as that seen in cutaneous candidiasis. *P. ovale* is not only the etiological agent of pityriasis versicolor but is also involved in *Pityrosporum* folliculitis, seborrheic dermatitis, and some forms of atopic dermatitis. It has even been suspected to have a role in some forms of psoriasis and confluent and reticulate papillomatosis (Gougerot-Carteaud) (36). Even systemic infection with these yeast has been reported (36). In *Pityrosporum* folliculitis, the yeast increases in number in the hair follicles but usually remains in the blastospore form (34). In seborrheic dermatitis, predisposing factors are predominantly a defect in cell-mediated immunity and increased sebum production (36). In atopic dermatitis localized to the head and neck, a type I allergy against *P. ovale* have been found in the majority of patients (36).

REFERENCES

1. Rivolta S. Parassiti vegetali. Torino: Di Giulo Speiranai, F Figlo, 1874: 469–479.
2. Malassez L. Note sur le champignon du pityriasis simplex. Arch Physiol Norm Pathol (Series 2) 1974;1:451–464.

3. Castellani A, Chalmers AJ. Manual of tropical medicine. London: Ballieré and Cox, 1913.
4. Gordon MA. Lipophilic yeastlike organisms associated with tinea versicolor. J Invest Dermatol 1951;17:267–272.
5. Sloof WC. Genus Pityrosporum. In Lodder J, ed. The Yeasts, 2d ed. Amsterdam: North-Holland, 1971:1167–1186.
6. Faergemann J, Fredriksson T. Experimental infections in rabbits and humans with Pityrosporum orbiculare and P ovale. J Invest Dermatol 1981;77: 314–318.
7. Faergemann J. Lipophilic yeasts in skin disease. Semin Dermatol 1985;4: 173–184.
8. Keddie FM. Tinea versicolor: The electron microscopic morphology of the genera Malassezia and Pityrosporum. In: Jadassohn W, Schirre CG. eds. XIII Congressus Internationalis Dermatologiae. Vol 2. Berlin: Springer-Verlag, 1968.
9. Randjandiche M. Polymorphism de Pityrosporum ovale (Bizzozero) Casellani & Castellani & Chalmers in vitro et in vivo. Bull Soc Med 1976;5:79–84.
10. Salkin IF, Gordon MA. Polymorphis of Malassezia furfur. Can J Microbiol 1977;23:471–475.
11. Midgley G. The diversity of Pityrosporum (Malassezia) yeasts in vivo and in vitro. Mycopathologica 1989;106:143–153.
12. Leeming JP, Notman FH. Improved methods for isolation and enumeration of Malassezia furfur from human skin. J Clin Microbiol 1987;25:2017–2019.
13. Cunningham AC, Ingham E, Gowland G. Humoral responses to Malassezia furfur serovars A, B and C in normal individuals of various ages. Br J Dermatol 1992;127:476–481.
14. Ashbee HR, Ingham E, Holland KT, Cunliffe WJ. The carriage of Malassezia furfur serovars A, B, C in patients with pityriasis versicolor, seborrhoeic dermatitis and controls. Br J Dermatol 1993;129:533–540.
15. Dorn M, Roehnert K. Dimorphism of Pityrosporum orbiculare in a defined culture medium. J Invest Dermatol 1977;69:244–248.
16. Nazzaro-Porro M, Passi S, Caprilli F, et al. Induction of hyphae in cultures in Pityrosporum by cholesterol and cholesterol esters. J Invest Dermatol 1977;69:531–534.
17. Faergemann J, Aly R, Maibach HI. Growth and filament production of Pityrosporum orbiculare and P. ovale on human stratum corneum in vitro. Acta Derm Venereol (Stockh) 1983;63:388–392.
18. Porro MN, Passi S, Caprilli F, et al. Growth requirements and lipid metabolism of Pityrosporum orbiculare. J Invest Dermatol 1976;66:178–182.
19. Wilde PF, Stewart PS. A study of the fatty acid metablism of the yeasts Pityrosporum ovale. Biochem J 1968;108:225–231.
20. Catterall MD, Ward ME, Jacobs P. A reappraisal of the role of Pityrosporum orbiculare in pityriasis versicolor and the significance of extracellular lipase. J Invest Dermatol 1978;71:398–401.
21. Marples RR, Downing DT, Kligman AM. Influence of Pityrosporum species

in the generation of free fatty acids in human surface lipids. J Invest Dermatol 1972;58:155–159.
22. Faergemann K, Bernander S. Micro-aerophilic and anaerobic growth of Pityrosporum orbiculare. Sabouraudia 1981;19:117–121.
23. Faergemann J: Antibodies to Pityrosporum orbiculare in patients with tinea versicolor and controls of various ages. J Invest Dermatol 1983;80:133–135.
24. Bergbrant I-M. Seborrhoeic dermatitis and Pityrosporum ovale: Cultural, immunological and clinical studies. Acta Derm Venereol (Stockh) 1991;Suppl 167.
25. 25. Faergemann J, Tjernlund U, Scheynius A, Bernander S. Antigenic similarities and differences in genus Pityrosporum. J Invest Dermatol 1982;78: 28–31.
26. Tanaka M, Imamura S. Immunological studies on Pityrosporum genus and Malassezia furfur. J Invest Dermatol 1979;73:321–324.
27. Bruneau SM, Guinet RMF. Quantitative immunoelectrophoretic study of genus Pityrosporum Sabouraud. Mykosen 1984;27:123–136.
28. Howell SA, Quin C, Midgley G. Karyotypes of oval cell forms of Malassezia furfur. Mycoses 1993;36:263–266.
29. Gueho E, Meyer SA. A reevaluation of the genus Malassezia by means of genome comparison. Anton van Leeuwenhoek 1989;55:245–251.
30. Simmons RB, Gueho E. A new species of Malassezia. Mycol Res 1990;94: 1416–1149.
31. Guého E, Faergemann J, Lyman C, Anaissie EJ. Malassezia and Trichosporum: Two emerging pathogenic basidiomycetous yeast-like fungi. J Med Vet Mycol 1994;32(suppl 1):367–378.
32. Guillot J, Guého E. The diversity of Malassezia yeasts confirmed by rRNA and nuclear DNA comparisons. Anton v Leeuwenhoek 1995;67:297–314.
33. Faergemann J, Fredriksson T. Age incidence of Pityrosporum orbiculare on human skin. Acta Derm Venereol (Stockh) 1980;60:531–533.
34. Roberts SOB. Pityrosporum orbiculare: Incidence and distribution on clinically normal skin. Br J Dermatol 1969;81:264–269.
35. Faergemann J, Aly R, Maibach HI: Quantitative variations in distribution of Pityrosporum orbiculare on clinically normal skin. Acta Derm Venereol (Stockh) 1983;63:346–348.
36. Faergemann J. Pityrosporum infections. In: Elewski BI, ed: Cutaneous Fungal Infections. New York, Tokyo: Igaku-Shoin, 1992:69–83.

26

Pneumocystis Genetic and Antigenic Variation

SAUNDRA LEMASTER STRINGER
University of Cincinnati
Cincinnati, Ohio

I. INTRODUCTION

Pneumocystis is a prevalent microorganism, and serological evidence indicates that although most people are infected by 5 years of age, few develop clinically detectable disease (1,2). The number of patients with diminished immunoresponsiveness has drastically increased over the past few years due to aggressive treatment of cancers, organ transplants, and a rise in the number of patients with acquired immunodeficiency disease syndrome (AIDS). As a result, life-threatening and severe infections caused by *Pneumocystis* have steadily increased (3,4). Although most primary *Pneumocystis* infections are effectively treated with drugs and some of these drugs offer effective prophylaxis for patients at risk, *Pneumocystis* remains a major cause of morbidity and mortality in immunocompromised patients (reviewed in Ref. 5). Currently, the drugs of preference in treating *Pneumocystis* infections are pentamidine and trimethoprim sulfamethoxazole (TMP/SMX, a folate antagonist). In many patients, TMP/SMX is associated with adverse side effects including allergic reaction (6). Pentamidine treatment, which is better tolerated and safer, has been associated with pneumothorax (7). However, the primary concern is that a greater percentage of pentamidine-treated patients as compared with TMP/SMX treated patients tend to develop *Pneumocystis* pneumonia again (8). All patients have *Pneumocystis* in their lungs after treatment, and it is not known if these are dead or dormant organisms (9). Among the alternative drugs used for patients with moderate disease or who do not tolerate or are unresponsive to pentamidine or TMP/SMX are Dapsone, atovaquone, trimethytrexate, and 8-aminoquinole, which is in clinical trials (10,11). The iron chelator deferoxamine may be a promising drug in the future (12,13). Since the number of efficacious drugs is very limited, the possibility of drug resistance is a concern. Resistance to pentamidine has been reported in vitro for *Saccharomyces cerevisiae* (14). Classic microbiological research on *Pneumocystis* has been hampered by the lack of a continuous in vitro culture system (15,16), although Barlett and coworkers have achieved some success by cocultivation of rat *Pneumocystis* with mammalian cells (17). Consequently, progress in the understanding of the basic biology of this organism has been slow and drug testing is difficult to interpret. However, great progress has been made in the last 6 years in our understanding of *Pneumocystis*. Molecular genetic research has identified that *P. carinii* encompasses an antigenically and genetically diverse group of fungi. This reclassification of *Pneumocystis* from the Protozoa to the Fungi has expanded drug research to review antifungal drugs. In recognition of this diversity, I shall refer to these organisms simply as *Pneumocystis* preceded by its host origin. This review considers the evidence supporting inclusion of *Pneumocystis* in the Fungi, current thinking regarding the relationship between *Pneumocystis* and other fungi, as well as analysis of *Pneumocystis* from different host species and between *Pneumocystis* found in the same host species. My examination of variation among *Pneumocystis* focuses on a complex family of genes that encodes a variety of surface antigens (gpA). The implications of genetic and antigenic variation in human *Pneumocystis* in terms of human exposure and disease are discussed.

II. PHYLOGENETIC ASSIGNMENT

Pneumocystis was initially thought to belong to the subkingdom of the Protozoa. This assessment was based on morphological and ultrastructure studies (18–21), responsiveness to antiprotozoan drugs in disease treatment (22), chemical composition (23–25, reviewed in Ref. 26), lack of ergosterol in the plasma membrane, insensitivity to amphotericin B, and inability to develop an in vitro culture system (15–17). However, it was recognized early that *Pneumocystis* lacks phagocytic structures. This indicated that its mode of feeding is by absorption, which is typical of fungi, and not by phagocytosis (27,28). In addition, the cyst form of *Pneumocystis* resembles a fungal reproductive structure (spore capsule containing spores) with a dense cell wall containing 1,3-β-glucan (reviewed in Ref. 29). In 1988, Stringer et al. (30), Watanabe et al. (31), and Edman et al. (32) found that the 18S ribosomal gene (srRNA) sequence of *Pneumocystis* is more similar to sequences from fungi than to those from protozoa; therefore *Pneumocystis* was tentatively grouped with the Ascomycota (30). Assignment of *Pneumocystis* to the Fungi has been supported by analysis of other genes, including thymidylate synthase (TS) (33), dihydrofolate reductase (34), a P-type ATPase (35,36), and translation elongation factor 3 (37).

Some uncertainty remains as to which branch of the fungal phylogenetic tree *Pneumocystis* belongs in. Most genetic analyses and some morphological features would place it somewhat closer to the Ascomycetes (30, reviewed in Refs. 38 and 39). However, the sequence of the 5S ribosomal RNA resembled those of the "Rhizopoda/Myxomycota/Zygomycota group" (31), and a mitochondrial ribosomal RNA (mtrRNA) gene sequence suggested a closer relationship to red yeasts, which are Basidiomycetes (40). The lack of ergosterol in *Pneumocystis* suggested a close relationship to rust and smut fungi, whose sterol and lipid composition is unique among the fungi. In support of this, recent analysis of *Pneumocystis* showed that it contained a double bond at the $\Delta 7$ position in C:28 and C:29 sterols (41), and C9- and C10-epoxy fatty acids were present in low levels (E. S. Kaneshiro, personal communication). However, the srRNA sequences of two rust fungi, *Cronartiium ribicola* and *Peridermium harkenessia*, did not support this conclusion. The extensive analysis of srRNA gene sequences reported by Bruns et al. placed the rusts and smut fungi in the Basidiomycota and *Pneumocystis* low branching among the Ascomycota in support of the earlier results of Bowman and Taylor (42–44). Li and Edlind have reported, based on β-tubulin sequence analysis, that *Pneumocystis* was most closely related to *Taphrina deformans*, congruent with Berbee and Taylor (45,46). A possible complication in the phylogenetic analysis of *Pneumocystis* was the additional finding, by quantitative hybridization experiments, that rat *Pneumocystis* contains no more than two (if the restriction sites of two loci are identical) srRNA genes per genome (47). We know of no other eukaryote that lacks multiple copies of the srRNA genes (i.e., *S. cerevisiae*, 150 copies, and *Pachysolen tannophilus*, 28 copies), which are arranged as tandemly arrayed repeats of approximately 10 kb (48). An exception is the Ciliates, which contain only one srRNA gene cluster in the micronucleus, but these organisms amplify the srRNA locus in the macronucleus. A single copy gene may evolve faster than an array, thereby causing *Pneumocystis* to appear to be more distantly related to the Ascomycota. The precise phylogenetic assignment of *Pneumocystis* in relation to other fungi will necessitate more protein gene sequencing or the discovery of a fungus much closer to *Pneumocystis*, from which the srRNA sequence can be analyzed. The data suggest that *Pneumocystis* is a member of the Ascomycota, but we are not significantly closer to understanding precisely to which phylogenetic niche it belongs than we were in 1988. It is possible that *Pneumocystis* represents a new class or order of fungi.

III. PHYLOGENETIC RELATIONSHIPS AMONG *PNEUMOCYSTIS* ISOLATES

Superimposed on the question of *Pneumocystis* phylogeny is the phylogenetic relationships among *Pneumocystis* isolates from the same and different host species. *Pneumocystis* isolates from different hosts are morphologically very similar (49,50), although recent elegant electron microscopic studies by Dei-Cas and colleagues have shown that mouse *Pneumocystis* can be distinguished from rabbit *Pneumocystis* because the filopodia in the latter were found to be thicker and less numerous (51). The abundant proliferating vegetative form is referred to as a troph, which appears to divide by binary fission, and the spore capsule is referred to as a cyst (reviewed in Ref. 29). Essentially nothing is known about the sexual reproduction of *Pneumocystis*. There is one report of synaptonemal complexes in the nucleus of a sporocyte (precyst) (52). Although similar in appearance, *Pneumocystis* isolated from different mammalian hosts are distinct in several other characteristics including host range, antigens, chromosomal band migration patterns (karyotypes), and gene sequences.

Inability to propagate *Pneumocystis* isolated from one host in another host led many investigators to suspect that *Pneumocystis* exhibited host range restriction. There have been a few reports of successful transfers from one host to another, but none of these results were unequivocal. Experiments on host range conducted using DNA markers specific for different types of *Pneumocystis* indicated that *Pneumocystis* are host-specific, at least in so far as ability to grow to high numbers in immunoincompetent hosts (53,54). Apparent host specificity, along with polypeptide migration differences noted on SDS-PAGE gels, led Frenkel to suggest that human *Pneumocystis* be referred to as *Pneumocystis jiroveci* (55). Further, characterization of polypeptides separated by electrophoresis and detected by binding of antibodies showed polypeptides prepared from organisms from different host species displayed different band patterns and most antibodies were not cross-reactive (56–65). Since it is difficult to infer the degree of genetic divergence or host range restriction on this basis alone, the proposed name was not accepted.

The first genetic data that indicated differences in *Pneumocystis* isolated from different host species as well as from within the rat (prototype and variant) came from comparisons of chromosome sizes by field inversion gel electrophoresis (66). In *Pneumocystis* isolated from rats, the genome is organized into 15 to 17 chromosomes ranging from 250 to 900 kb, indicating that the genome size is approximately 2×10^7 bp pairs (66) (see Fig. 1). *Pneumocystis* from other host species (human, mouse, and ferret) show electrophoretic karyotypes that were similar to those of *Pneumocystis* from rats in terms of the number and the size-range of bands, but chromosomal profiles of *Pneumocystis* from each mammalian host species were different (66–71; reviewed in Ref. 72). In addition to chromosomal band pattern differences, the overall DNA homology was found to vary in *Pneumocystis* isolated from various hosts. Total DNA from rat *Pneumocystis* did not hybridize at high-stringency hybridization conditions to chromosomes from human *Pneumocystis* (73), the α-repeat DNA from rat *Pneumocystis* did not hybridize to mouse or human *Pneumocystis* chromosomes (74), and three cloned genes from rat *Pneumocystis* failed to hybridize to ferret *Pneumocystis* chromosomes (70). Subsequently, we found that if conditions are relaxed by 25%, cross-hybridization can be observed between human, mouse, rat (prototype and variant), and ferret *Pneumocystis* (75; G. A. Weinberg and S. L. Stringer, unpublished). Genetic differences among *Pneumocystis* species have been studied further by comparison of gene sequences. *Pneumocystis* species have been found to differ in sequences of genes encoding mtrRNA (76), α-tubulin (77), β-tubulin (78), TS (79,80), introns found in the 26S rRNA gene (81), and the internal spacer regions (ITS) of the srRNA genes (82).

Genetic diversity also occurs among *Pneumocystis* from the same host species. Minor variation has been seen among isolates from rats, humans, and mice. The *Pneumocystis* mtrRNA (79,83), the ITS regions (82,84,85), and srRNA (S. L. Stringer, unpublished) have 1 to 3 bp polymorphisms within the same host species isolates. These results have prompted many investigators to begin studies on transmission and epidemiology. Rat *Pneumocystis* has been most extensively studied, particularly by electrophoretic karyotyping, which showed that different rat colonies harbor *Pneumocystis* with different electrophoretic karyotypes (66). Figure 1 shows the chromosomal band patterns of rat *Pneumocystis* isolated from four different rat colonies. Lanes 2 through 7 show chromosomal band patterns of prototype rat *Pneumocystis* isolated from rat colonies A, B, and C. Although variation is observed in the karyotype pattern, band position, and molarity, each has approximately 15 chromosomal bands. At least 3 additional chromosomal bands can often be observed. Also, length polymorphisms have been observed among prototype strains by restriction enzyme analysis after hybridization to the α-repeat and gpA

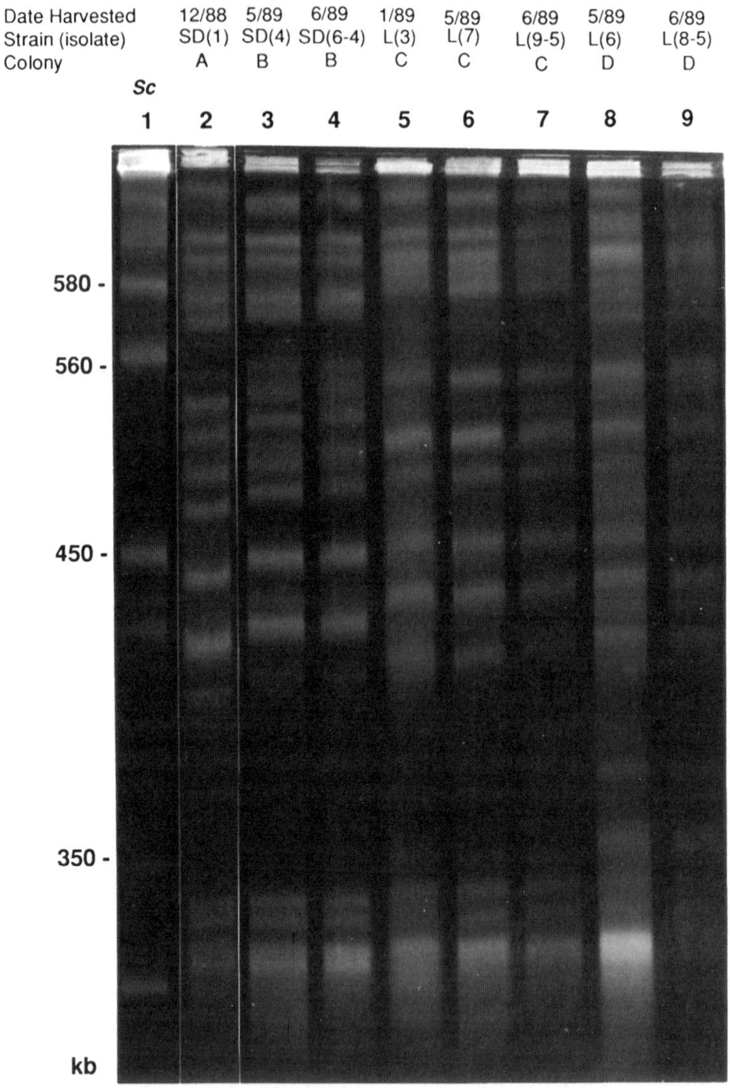

Figure 1 Variation of band patterns among rat *Pneumocystis* samples from different rat colonies. Rat *Pneumocystis* chromosomes were separated by field-inversion gel electrophoresis. Chromosomal patterns A, B, and C are from different rat colonies containing either Sprague Dawley (SD) or Lewis (L) rats. The colony D pattern contains chromosomes from rat prototype and variant *Pneumocystis*. Lane 2 was from an earlier gel, which comigrated with colony B bands in experiments in which both were run on the same gel. Sc = *S. cerevisiae*. Chromosomes were visualized after staining with ethidium bromide. (From Ref. 66.)

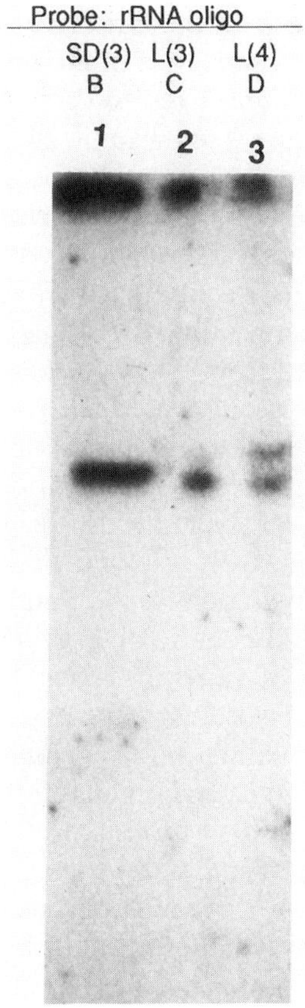

Figure 2 Mapping srRNA genes to chromosomal bands in two rat *Pneumocystis* strains. Rat *Pneumocystis* chromosomes, which were separated by field-inversion gel electrophoresis, were hybridized to a radioactive oligonucleotide complementary to a sequence in the gene encoding the rat *Pneumocystis* srRNA gene. Lanes 1 and 2 contain rat *Pneumocystis* that differ karyotypically, while lane 3 contains rat prototype and variant *Pneumocystis*. (From Ref. 66.)

(74; S. L. Stringer, unpublished). These results could be explained by rearrangements of a multigene family (gpA, discussed later).

Hong et al. first observed electrophoretic karyotypes suggesting that a single rat could be infected by two distinct strains of *Pneumocystis* (66). Figure 1 shows a complex chromosomal band pattern for rats from colony D, lanes 8 and 9, which is comprises at least 22 chromosomal bands. This observation suggested infection by two genetically distinct kinds of

Pneumocystis. To characterized this observation, a radioactive oligonucleotide complementary to a sequence in the gene encoding the rat *Pneumocystis* srRNA gene was hybridized to three karyotypically distinct rat *Pneumocystis* isolates. Figure 2 shows that two of these isolates showed hybridization to a single chromosome (lanes 1 and 2) while the third contained two chromosomes that hybridized to the gene probe (lane 3). The sequence of one of the genes was essentially the same as previously described (30), although bp 1687 can either be a G or an A (S. L. Stringer, unpublished). Further, I found that the sequence of the second srRNA gene was nearly as diverged from rat *Pneumocystis* as the rat and human *Pneumocystis* srRNA gene sequences were from each other (73,86). Subsequent experiments showed that this variant rat *Pneumocystis* also differs from the prototype at the ATPase (35,36), translation factor IID (35,87) mtrRNA (see Fig. 4; S. K. Keely and S. L. Stringer, unpublished), thymidylate synthase (see Fig. 3; S. Keely and S. L. Stringer, unpublished), inosine monophosphate deydrogenase (88), and gpA (89) gene loci. These data suggest that substantial genetic divergence among *Pneumocystis* is not solely a manifestation of isolation brought about by restriction to a particular mammalian host species. Prototype and variant occur separately (90) or can be found coinfecting the same rat (86), which raises the possibility of similar complexity in human infections. It has recently been reported that a similar "variant" form is present in ferret *Pneumocystis* (91). While these data clearly show differences, the relationship of these gene sequence differences to overall genotypic and phenotypic diversity is difficult to assess. To better understand this relationship, we have assessed the phylogenetic relationships of the srRNA, TS, and mtrRNA genes.

The srRNA gene sequence has been adopted as the standard for phylogenetic inferences. The percentage of pairwise comparison divergence between the rat and human *Pneumocystis* srRNA gene sequences was twice that between *Candida albicans* and *Candida tropicalis* and nearly as great as that between *S. cerevisiae* and *C. albicans*. The degree of divergence between the rat prototype and variant srRNA genes was at least as great as that between 14 pairs of Ascomycetes from different genera, such as *Podospora anserina* compared to *Neurospora crassa* and *Torulaspora delbrueckii* compared to *S. cerevisiae*. However, trees comparing 20 sequences from Fungi placed *Neurospora crassa* and a Basidiomycete in the middle of the *Pneumocystis* branch (from our analysis of the EMBL database). Pairwise comparisons of *Pneumocystis* to *C. albicans* and *S. cerevisiae* at the srRNA locus indicate that this gene is not evolving at an accelerated rate. However, similar molecular clock analysis of the protein sequence data from the entire TS, ATPase, and α-tubulin

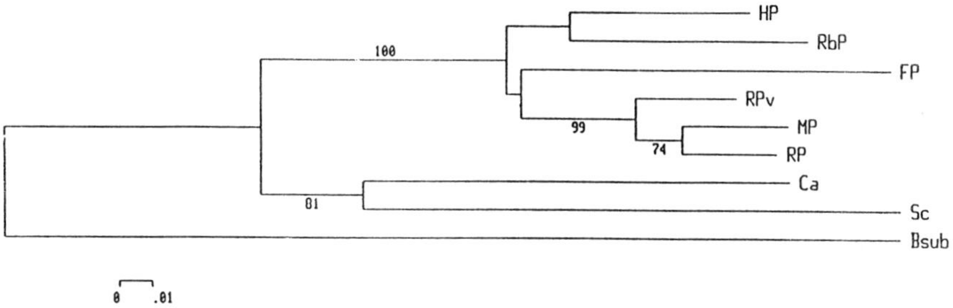

Figure 3 Neighbor joining tree of *Pneumocystis* TS genes. Phylogenetic relationships were generated with the MEGA program. The topology of the tree was supported by the bootstrap test (500 replications). Bar indicates horizontal branch length, corresponding to 1% divergence. Values less than 70 are of low confidence and are not shown. Alignments were done by eye for maximal identity, with gaps ignored. Bsub = *B. sublitis*; Sc = *S. cerevisiae*; Ca = *C. albicans*; P = *Pneumocystis*; H = human; R = rat; Rv = rat-variant; F = ferret; M = mouse; and Rb = rabbit. All sequences are from the EMBL data base except Rpv:AATTA TACAGGACAAGGAGTTGATCAATTAGCCAATATTATTAAAAAA-ATACAAACATCACCATATGATCTTCGACTTATTCTTTCAGCATGGA A TCCTGCAGATTTAGAAAAAATGGCATTACCTCCGTGCCACATGTTT T GTCAATTTTATGTTCATATATCATCGAATGATCACCGACCTGAACT T-TCATGTCAACTATA (S. Keely and S. L. Stringer).

genes indicated that even if only first and second base pairs were considered, that the distance was too great (in that saturation occurs) to predict accurate rates of evolution (S. L. Stringer, unpublished). Therefore this analysis was not helpful in indicating the actual distance of *Pneumocystis* to other fungi except to indicate that the distance is great. We concluded from this that this short region of the srRNA locus is either too small or too variable for accurate relationships to be generated. To better understand the implications of the srRNA data, we analyzed the TS and mtrRNA genes and compared these results to genes from other fungi.

Polymerase chain reaction (PCR) was used to obtain a 347-bp fragment of the human, mouse, ferret, and rat variant *Pneumocystis* (79), which starts in exon 1 and extends into exon 3 based on the rat *Pneumocystis* sequence (33). All of the *Pneumocystis* sequences differed from each other. The human and mouse *Pneumocystis* sequences were in agreement with those recently published by Mazars et al. (80). An identity of 80–96% was observed among *Pneumocystis* sequences, with the rodent *Pneumocystis* sharing the highest homology. Protein sequence identity values mirrored the nucleotide identity values. A neighbor joining tree was constructed using the MEGA program with *Bacillus subtilis* as the out group (92; Fig. 3). The topology of the tree was supported by the bootstrap test (500 replications). The *Pneumocystis* grouped together and the rodent *Pneumocystis* formed a subgroup or clade. The topology of the tree was not altered when only the first and second bp positions were considered. Since bootstrap values less than 70% are considered to be of low confidence, they are not noted on the tree and branches without values and may not be indicative of true phylogenetic relationships (93,94). The topology of the relationships of the nonrodent *Pneumocystis* could change with more sequence data. The branch lengths linking human and ferret *Pneumocystis* to rodent *Pneumocystis* were nearly as great as those linking *C.*

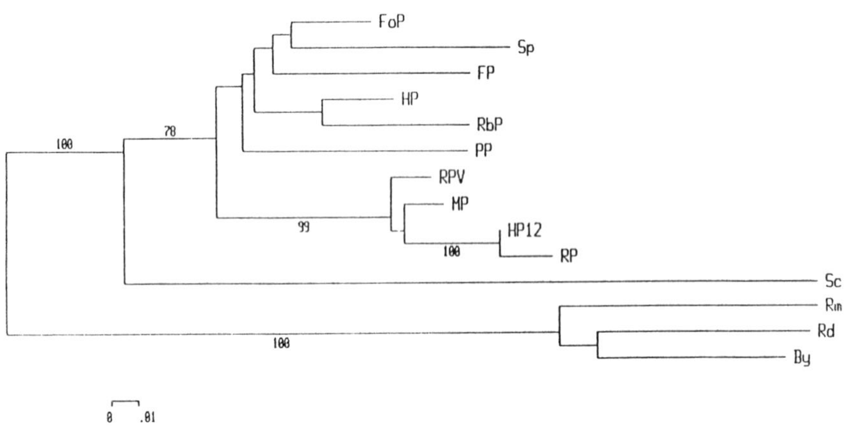

Figure 4 Neighbor joining tree of *Pneumocystis* mtrRNA genes. Phylogenetic relationships were generated with the MEGA program. The topology of the tree was supported by the bootstrap test (500 replications). Bar indicates horizontal branch length corresponding to 1% divergence. Values less than 70 are of low confidence and are not shown. Alignments were done by eye for maximal identity and all gaps were ignored. Ascomycetes: Sc = *S. cerevisiae*; Ca = *C. albicans*. Red yeasts: Rd = *Rhodosporidium diobovatum*; Rm = *Rhodotorula mucilaginosa*; By = *Bensingtonia yamatoana*; Pneumocystis: see Fig. 3 and HP12, human variant 12, Fo = horse, Sv = shrew, and P = pig. All sequences are from the EMBL data base except Rpv: G A T A T A G C T G G T T T T C T G C G A A A T C T A T T T A G G T A G A T A G C T T A A T A A G G A T G T T T A T T A G T G G G T A T A G C A C T G A A T A T C T A A T A T T A T T T G A A G G G A G T A T G A A A G T A C T T A C T T T G G A T A T T T A A T C T C A G A A T A A C T A A T A G A T G A AA G A T G A T T A A G T T G T C A G A C T TT T T G C G A T A A G G T G G G A A G T C A A A A G G G A A A C A G C C C A G A (S. Keely and S. L. Stringer).

albicans and *S. cerevisiae*, indicating that *Pneumocystis* comprises several species. Changes between *Pneumocystis* and other species were mainly transversions, which indicates that these distances are underestimates. Since a larger database exists for the mtrRNA, similar studies were done on these sequences to test the robustness of the tree. Very similar results were found as shown in Fig. 4. Parsimony analysis confirmed both neighbor-joining trees.

There are a number of possibilities to explain generation of a rodent clade and species level differences. Mutations occurred in a progenitor to allow organisms to invade a new host. One could theorize a progenitor in which host-cell receptor gene rearrangements isolated each daughter cell in a particular host. This frequency would be much lower than gpA rearrangements but possibly could be a summation of these rearrangements (see below). A variant and prototype *Pneumocystis* infected rats at a similar time but arose from different organisms. It is possible that one *Pneumocystis* organism sustained a mutation that prevented its mating to sister organisms. This variant organism grew clonally sustaining neutral mutations at a similar rate as its parent. It is not possible from the existing data to determine coevolution of the parasite with the host. Nor can it be discerned if *Pneumocystis* is an obligate or opportunistic parasite. Minimally, these results point to speciation of the various interhost species isolates of *Pneumocystis* based on comparisons to the phylogeny of other microorganisms. Subsequent phylogenetic analysis should point to a simplification of the provisional nomenclature adopted in 1994 (95).

IV. DIVERSITY IN GENES ENCODING gpA

Understanding host and parasite interactions is important for the development of means for prevention and treatment *Pneumocystis* infections. This requires detailed information specific to the organism infecting the host under study. This endeavor has focused attention on the glycosylated polypeptides of *Pneumocystis*.

Immunoreactive *Pneumocystis* proteins separated in one dimension by SDS polyacrylamide gel electrophoresis indicated at least 20 polypeptides. The highest-molecular-weight immunoreactive band, which also appears to be of high abundance based on Coomassie and silver staining, has garnered the most attention and is referred to as gp95-120, glycoprotein A (gpA), major surface glycoprotein (MSG), or gpA/MSG (75,96,97). I shall refer to this polypeptides as gpA preceded by a letter designation to indicate its host origin and followed by the specific name or number given by the authors who have reported on the gene sequence. To illustrate, MSG I from human *Pneumocystis* would be hgpA/I (98). This terminology is based on commonly used conventions used to name glycoproteins of unknown function based on relative electrophoretic mobility.

Iodination of *Pneumocystis* coupled with serum antibodies and monoclonal antibodies studies indicate that gpA is localized on the surface of the organism (59–61,99–102). The evidence that gpA is glycosylated has been derived from both direct and indirect analysis of associated oligosaccharide. The SDS-PAGE band of gpA is large and diffuse, suggestive of a glycoprotein. GpA binds a number of carbohydrate-specific lectins, including concanavalin A, wheat germ agglutinin, glycine max, *Ulex europaeus* agglutinin I, and tomato lectins (59–61,63,103,104). Chromatographic analysis of carbohydrates associated with partially purified gpA indicates that gpA polypeptides contain a variety of monosaccharides and notably lack or contain small amounts of neuraminic acid (60,63; reviewed in Ref. 26). Evidence for *N*-linked sugars is indicated by a reduction in apparent molecular weight following incubation of gpA with peptide-*N*-glycosidase F and endo-α-*N*-acetylgalactosaminidase specific for *N*-linked high mannose and complex oligosaccharides, respectively (60,63). Treatment with exoglycosidase mixtures result in a reduction of the molecular weight (59). The presence of O-linked oligosaccharides seems possible based on predicted polypeptide sequence data (see below). Direct demonstration of O-linked oligosaccharide has not been conclusive. It has been reported that reaction with gpA with trifluoromethanesulfonic acid (TFMS) reduced the molecular weight of rgpA to 68 kDa (59,105), but this is inconsistent with the recent gene sequence data, which predicts a size for unglycosylated gpA of approximately 116 kDa. TFMS is known to be difficult to control and peptide bonds were hydrolyzed in these experiments.

Immunoblotting studies have shown that polypeptides from different host species are distinct with respect to both epitopes and may vary in apparent molecular size. Some, but not all monoclonal antibodies raised against gpA from one *Pneumocystis* species cross react with similar polypeptides from other *Pneumocystis* species (56,62,64,97,106), and sera from infected hosts do not always show gpA to be the major reactive antigen (61,97). Results of gene sequence analysis are beginning to provide an understanding of the basis for the similarities and differences between gpA from different *Pneumocystis* and have revealed unexpected complexity in this glycoprotein.

GpA cDNAs from ferret and rat *Pneumocystis* have been isolated by screening expression libraries with monoclonal antibodies (96,97,107). GpA genes from human and rat *Pneumocystis* were isolated by screening genomic libraries for repetitive DNA (75,98,108). The gpAs of *Pneumocystis* from three host species—rat, human, and ferret—are encoded by families of polymorphic genes, some of which are organized as nonidentical repeated genes up to four times (75,109,110). The size of the gpA gene family is not known but is approximately 100 copies distributed on all of the chromosomes based on hybridization to a rat *Pneumocystis* genomic library (108). Genomic DNA from rat *Pneumocystis* fragmented by digestion with restriction enzymes and probed with the genomic clone Rp3-1 indicates that polymorphism of gpA loci is extensive (108). Figure 5 shows a schematic representation of a consensus predicted peptide sequence of rgpA. This composite was derived from two complete and 19 partial rgpA (96,97,107,110; S. L. Stringer and J. R. Stringer, M. L. Linke and P. D. Walzer, unpublished), one complete and three partial hgpA (75,98; S. L. Stringer and J. R. Stringer, unpublished), one fgpA (96), and one partial mgpA (111) gene sequence(s). We have found that gpA genes from rat prototype, rat variant, mouse, ferret, and human *Pneumocystis* hybridize to one only when low-stringency hybridization conditions are used (75; G. A. Weinberg and S. L. Stringer, unpublished). The nucleotide sequence of gpA from the same *Pneumocystis* hosts are approximately 80% identical and between host species approximately 40%. Despite this high degree of variation, fgpA DNA oligonucleotide primers have been designed that amplify gpA genes from a wide variety of *Pneumocystis* species (112).

There are three regions within the gpA sequence which are notable by their relatively simple sequence composition both at the amino acid and nucleotide level. A particularly striking region of sequence conservation is the threonine-rich motif, which varies from 17 to 34 residues (aa921–1024, Fig. 6A). This region is highly conserved between 19 rgpAs, hgpA/I, and fgpA. In rgpA class 1, only 5 of 103 amino acids vary, which is the longest area of conservation in the rgpA predicted peptide sequence. HgpA/I contains a run of 10 T residues followed by 56 amino acids, which are highly conserved between rgpA and hgpA, with an overall identity of 70%. Length variation in the T runs could have been caused by slipped mispairing of DNA strands during replication. The codons that encode T vary at the third position (average 50% identity), suggesting that maintenance of T runs is accomplished by selection. Four of 19 rgpA genes lack a T run but contain sequences comprising an 11-bp sequence repeated three times as a direct repeat followed by four degenerate repeats, which are 40% T. The second region in rgpA contains a domain composed primarily of E with K, G and D residues which differ in length, and a sequence which is rich in G-A (aa1029, Fig. 6B). This heterogeneity may have been generated by a combination of point mutations, primarily A $\Leftrightarrow$ G transitions, which change E $\Rightarrow$ K, and slipped mispairing events. The third region is composed of two sequence motifs with direct and redundant repeats (aa796–858, Fig. 6C). The second, GGAACACCA, is repeated

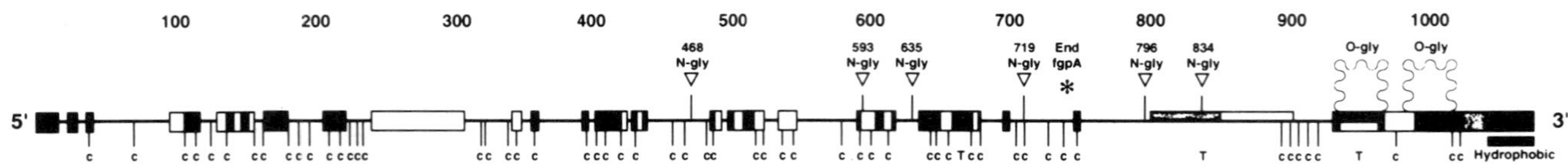

Figure 5 Consensus schematic representation of gpA. Predicted peptide sequences from 2 rgpA, 19 partial rgpA, 1 fgpA, 1 hgpA, and 3 partial hgpA polypeptides were aligned and a consensus sequence derived. Cysteine is represented by C. Since these are predicted peptide sequences, the carboxy and amino termini are indicated by 5′ and 3′ respectively. The sequences that are highly or 100% conserved are indicated by ■; approximately 85% conserved are indicated by □; and highly variable sequences are indicated by □. ∇N-gly and O-gly refer to a predicted N-glycosylation and O-glycosylation sites respectively. T indicates a predicted turn. The fgpA sequence comparison ends at *(see acknowledgments). Amino acid numbers refer to rgpA/B. (From Ref. 109.)

A

```
rgpA class1 PHHTETQKEISTTTTTTTTTTTTTTTTTTTTTT-5to+7--K(P,Q)GSGGKVTEECTMIQTTDTWVTSTSLHTSTTTSTSTVTSTVTLTSMRKCKPTKCTTDS 1024
rgpA class2 ......ITETKTETKTETKTETKTDGKADEKTVEKTVTETK  P  IG.......................................................
hgpA/I      ..E.V.ES---TTTTTTTTT-------------------  -  VTDP.A.-..KSL..Q.....Q..T....S.I......KI....T.R........GD  999
```

B

```
rgpA      CKPTKCTTDSKKETDKGGE5-8 ----------------------VKPNDGMKIRVPDMIKMILLGVIVMGMM  1065
                           -GGEEG1-2EED1-2
                           KE3-7
                           KEEDDEE
                           KEEG1-2KE2
rgpA/C    ----------VE..VEDKPAKEEEKKAEDKPAKEEEKQVEDKPSK....E.I..K.TE.....F.........
hgpA      ......R.GDDA..-------------------------------...SE.LRVSGWNVGRGV.VAMVISE.I  1031
```

C

```
rgpA/B    NGSAPVSPPAPESGSSPAVPPAVPPPPGS----PQNGTPGTPGGGSGGGSGTPGGSGTPSSGTT------NNAKLGLVKR  861
rgpA/A    ....SGPAPAPASRSSSASGPLPPPSP------PQDGTSDTPNGKPGTDASGKTPSTGDGTPGTSGSGTPYV.F......
rgpA/GP3  ...DSTLVPPPPQAPAGPPPPGSPPPPP-----SQNGTPGTPGGETGASGTPGTPGTPGTPTGPGMMK--..........
rgpA/GP14 ...DSVPAQVQDAPAGPPSAPGSPSSP------SQNGTPGTPGGETGTAGGTP-----------------..........
rgpA/GP22 ....SEQVLQPVQAPESGSSGSPSSPPGPPSAPPQNGTPATPGGAPKEAGTPNTTDETP-----------.P........
rgpA/GP46 ....SEQVLQPVQAPESGSSGSPSSPPGPPSAPPQNGPTATPGGADGTPSSGTT----------------P.........
rgpA/PC14 ....SAPPSAPAPESGSSGSPASGSPPASEP--STNGKVDTPAGGSQTQDKTSDASGQTT----------YT........
hgpA/I    ----SLPLSFVKK--------------------DGNNTPKNNSKSEDKNVVSNEKD--------------TIKHVKILR.  834
```

Figure 6 Sequence and length polymorphism of gpA attributable to slip-mispairing. Panel A. RgpA class 1 is a consensus sequence derived from 19 rgpA predicted peptide sequences. Amino acids in bold are those that showed 90% identity among all sequences compared. Amino acids in parentheses are all those that are seen at this position. RgpA class 2 is a consensus sequence derived from comparisons of four rgpA predicted peptide sequences. Amino acids shown in bold are those that varied. Panel B. RgpA is a consensus sequence derived from 19 rgpA predicted peptide sequences. Amino acids shown in bold are those that showed 38 to 89% identity. Variation in the $KGGE_{5-8}$ sequence is shown directly below this sequence. The hgpA sequence is a composite of three compared predicted peptide sequences. Amino acids shown in bold are those that showed 66 to 33% identity among all sequences compared. The direct repeats of rgpA/C are shown in italics. Panel C. Seven rgpA predicted peptide sequences are compared to a hgpA/I in a hypervariable and predicted turn region. Dots indicate identity and dashes indicate gaps that were introduced for maximal alignment. Amino acids not in bold showed 100% identity in the consensus sequences. Amino acid numbers refer to rgpA/B (109) and hgpA/I (98).

seven times and three more times as a redundant imperfect repeat in rgpA/GP3. There are additional smaller sequence areas that are similar to the above examples. The second and third regions are absent from the hgpA and fgpA sequences reported to date, and these genes may be nonfunctional. It is probable that the large number of repeated sequences arose by gene duplication. Much of this variation in sequence and length could be attributed to slip mispairing, neutral drift, or single events followed by homologous (equal and/or nonequal) recombination or gene conversion. The amino acid identity is twofold less than is seen in the nucleotide sequences, which suggests that gpA genes have undergone extensive genetic drift without strong selection against mutations that cause changes in peptide sequences. The selection for diversity in gpA polypeptides could be to evade the immune system or to provide the ability to invade new hosts.

GpA genes were analyzed for secondary structure using three computer programs, which are based on similar but different assumptions: (1) the Chou-Fasman analysis, which predicts α helix, β sheet, turn, and hydrophobic index (113,114); (2) the Kyte-Doolittle analysis, which predicts hydrophobic structure (115); and (3) the Eisenberg analysis, which produces a hydrophobic moment plot (116). The gpA polypeptides were predicted to be primarily globular structures. Turns were predicted at three rgpA conserved locations (Fig. 5). Another prominent conserved sequence was the hydrophobic termini, comprising of approximately 28 amino acids, which is unlikely to be a transmembrane domain. However, the short hydrophobic terminus is suggestive of a glycosyl-phosphatidylinositol-linked glycoprotein (117).

Our recent research and that of others has begun to resolve some of the above ambiguities and inconsistencies concerning gpA (118–120). Regulated gpA expression is suggested by the observation that the upstream sequence of every mRNA appears identical and maps to a unique chromosome (119). The upstream sequence is located near the telomere of the chromosomes, as demonstrated by BAL 31 digestion (120). It appears probable that each organism translates only one version of the gpA gene. This was indicated by indirect immunofluorescence using monoclonal antibodies (120). This explains the lack of reactivity from one preparation of antibodies to another. The gene sequences are translocated by recombination to the upstream sequences, which occurs by reciprocal exchange (Fig. 7). This could be mediated by a site-specific recombinase generating two or more possible gpA polypeptides, as shown in A1 and A2 of Fig. 7. Alternatively, the gpA polypeptide could be generated by homologous recombination in which only part(s) of the gpA peptide are changed to generate diversity as shown in B. Since we have found gpA genes that

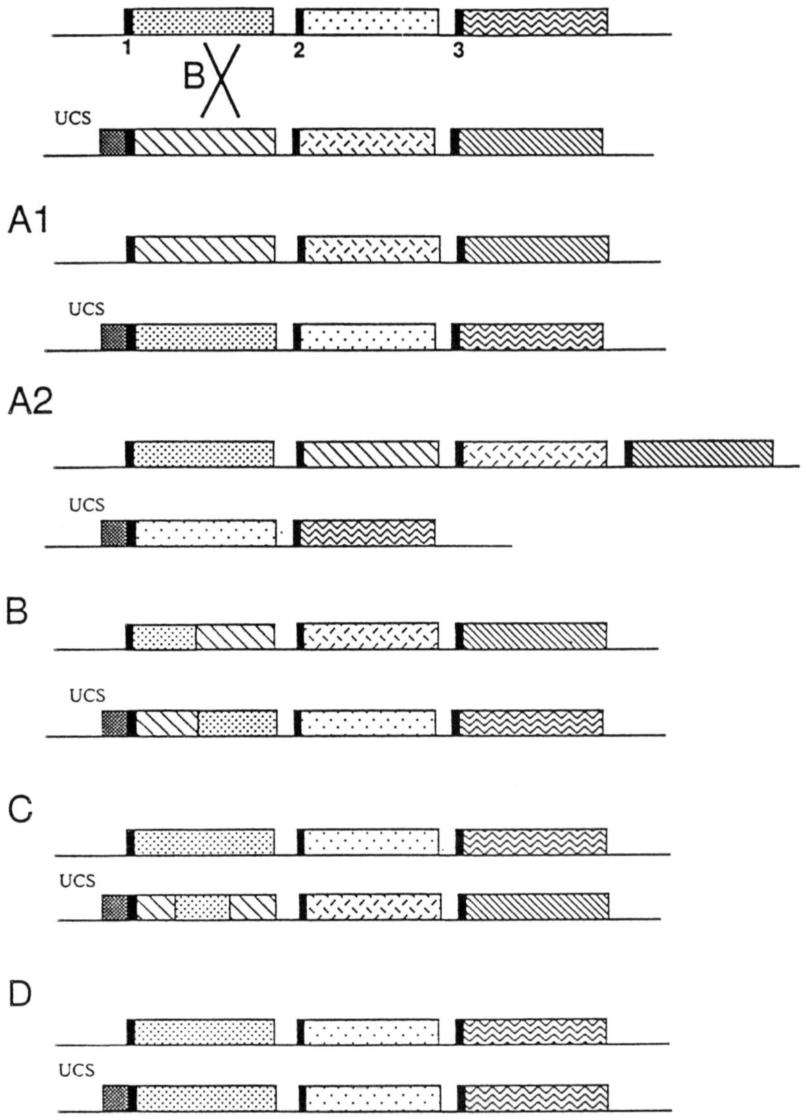

Figure 7 Reciprocal exchange model for generating different gpA arrays attached to the UCS. The UCS is as marked. Different gpA genes are represented by patterned rectangles and numbered. The narrow black bar at the beginning of each gpA gene represents the CRJE region. The top two schematics are the participants in recombination. A1 and A2 depict the products of reciprocal recombination between the CJRE linked to the UCS and CJREs, 1 and 2 respectively. B depicts the products of reciprocal exchange mediated by homology at the X marked B. C and D show products of gene conversion.

have large deletions, sometimes this could be nonequal homologous recombination. Shown in C and D are peptides generated by gene conversion limited to one part or extending downstream of the upstream sequences. Recombination is most likely the explanation for the heterogeneity in chromosomal band patterns that we have observed (66). Since some of the genes that were compared in Figs. 5 and 6 were derived from cDNA clones, it is likely that gpA function tolerates a high degree of sequence variability. It is those conserved sections that probably hold the key to function and to that prize of immunological protection which is being so avidly sought. Although desirable, this goal—by analogy to other biological systems—will probably take some time.

V. CONCLUSION

Genetic and antigenic variation in *Pneumocystis* has practical importance for understanding human exposure to the organism and for prevention and treatment of human disease. The genetic differences between *Pneumocystis* species are extensive, and this is advantageous for designing drugs. Current chemotherapy is usually effective, but the number of drugs is limited, and treatment regimens are relatively long-term, raising concerns about the possibility of the development of drug-resistance to *Pneumocystis*. In addition, there is a need for better drugs for prophylactic treatment of patients at high risk of developing *Pneumocystis* pneumonia (reviewed in Ref. 5). Development of better chemotherapeutic agents is proceeding through experiments with *Pneumocystis* enzymes produced from cloned genes. Based on the observed variation in *Pneumocystis*, it would seem advisable to focus efforts on the specific form of enzyme present in human *Pneumocystis* as well as to better understand the extent of genetic variation among *Pneumocystis* organisms found in humans. Molecular techniques have been important in the development of sensitive and specific methods of detection of *Pneumocystis* by DNA amplification using PCR. Oligonucleotide primers designed to a number of different loci of the *Pneumocystis* genome (srRNA, mtrRNA, TS) have been used in the diagnosis of *Pneumocystis* pneumonia (121–123). This is important to establish less invasive means of diagnosis. Immunological approaches to therapy have been explored with gpA to a limited extent in animal models (124,125). In light of recent results showing the high variability of this glycopeptide, it seems wise, by analogy to viral systems, to also focus such studies on other polypeptides whose sequence remains constant from preparation to preparation. Extrapolation of results obtained in laboratory animals to humans must incorporate recognition that each host species is infected by a distinct species of *Pneumocystis* and that a particular individual may be infected by more than one strain of *Pneumocystis*.

Investigation of genetic variation will also be important for development of methods for tracking *Pneumocystis* variants in a given host. There are still many open questions regarding the mode of transmission of *Pneumocystis*. In healthy humans, anti-*Pneumocystis* antibodies are detected in many individuals well into adulthood, suggesting either continual or episodic exposure to the organism. *Pneumocystis* infection can be transmitted through the air in rats, and the organism might persist in the lungs of immunocompetent rats (126–129). *Pneumocystis* has been detected in the air of patient rooms, but existence of the organism in healthy people has not been demonstrated (128). It is possible that people are constantly being infected with *Pneumocystis* and that the immune system is constantly eliminating the organism. Allele-specific PCR assays indicated that reinfection is the simplest explanation for the genetic variation seen in the human *Pneumocystis* organisms associated with recurrent pneumocystosis episodes and not quiescent organisms (130). The source of organisms infecting humans is not known. It is possible that infections are acquired by contact with individuals who carry the organism as a subclinical infection, and recent studies from Takashi et al. support this conclusion (131). Alternatively, airborne *Pneumocystis* may originate from an environmental reservoir, but we now know enough to conclude that animals probably do not carry *Pneumocystis* that can cause disease in humans. Many questions about the life-cycle of *Pneumocystis* remain unresolved, including the genetic stability of the different species, which may in part be dependent on whether the organism undergoes a sexual phase. Although this may be less important in the analysis of epidemiology, it has far greater impact on studies on long-term epidemiological tracking. Understanding these aspects of *Pneumocystis* will be crucial in evaluation of the appropriateness of current management of pneumocystosis patients and of individuals at high risk of contracting this disease.

ACKNOWLEDGMENTS

I thank James R. Stringer for his discussions, Bernard Roizman for his continued support and guidance, A. George Smulian for his advice on clinical studies, Barbara Bowman for her advice on phylogenetics, Frank Gigliotti and Geoff Weinberg for sharing their data prior to its publication.

The studies cited in this review attributed to the Stringer research group were supported by grants from the National Institutes of Health to JRS (RO1 A1 28471 and P01 AI 28932) and the National Science Foundation to SLS (MCB 94-07810).

Addendum: The completion of the fgpA sequence allowed insufficient time for modification of Fig. 7.

REFERENCES

1. Meuwissen JHET, Tauber I, Leeuwenberg ADEM, et al. Parasitologic and serologic observations of infection with Pneumocystis in humans. J Infect Dis 1976;136:43–49.
2. Pifer LL, Hughes WT, Stagno S, Woods D. Pneumocystis carinii infections: Evidence for high prevalence in normal and immunosuppressed children. Pediatrics 1978;61:35–41.
3. Mills J. Pneumocystis carinii and Toxoplasma gondii infections in patients with AIDS. Infect Dis 1986;8:1001–1011.
4. Kovacs JA, Hiemenz JW, Macher AM, et al. Pneumocystis pneumonia: A comparison between patients with AIDS and patients with other immunodeficiency. Ann Intern Med 1983;100:663–671.
5. Pneumocystis carinii pneumonia. In: Walzer PD, ed. Lung Biology in Health and Disease. Vol 69. New York: Marcel Dekker, 1994.
6. Ruskin J, LaRiviere M. Low-dose co-trimoxazole for prevention of Pneumocystis carinii pneumonia in human immunodeficiency virus disease. Lancet 1991;12:468–471.
7. Sepkowitz KA, Telzak EE, Gold JWM, et al. Pneumothorax in AIDS. Ann Intern Med 1991;114:455–459.
8. Hardy WD, Feinberg J, Finkelstein DM. A controlled study of trimethoprim/sulfamethoxazole or aerosolized pentamidine for secondary prophylaxis of Pneumocystis carinii pneumonia in patients with the acquired immunodeficiency syndrome. N Engl J Med 1992;5:1842–1848.
9. Colangelo G, Baughman RP, Dohn MN, Frame PT. Follow-up bronchoalveolar lavage in AIDS patients with Pneumocystis carinii pneumonia: Pneumocystis carinii burden predicts early relapse. Am Rev Respir Dis 1991; 143:1067–1071.
10. Walker RE, Mansur, H. In: Walzer PD, ed. Pneumocystis carinii Pneumonia. New York: Marcel Dekker, 1994;69:439–466.
11. Petty BG, Cornhauser DM, Shapiro TB. Multiple-dose pharmacokinetics, safety and tolerance of WR 6026 HCl in healthy subjects. Final report, task order 10, Contact No. DAmd17-C5133, 31 March 1990.
12. Weinberg GA. Iron chelators as therapeutic agents against Pneumocystis carinii. Antimicrol Agents and Chemothr 1994;38:997–1003.
13. Weinberg ED, Weinberg GA. The role of iron in infection. Curr Opin Infect Dis 1995;8:164–169.
14. Hatfield C, Kasarslis A, Staben C. Pentamidine sensitivity and resistance in Saccharomyces cerevisiae as a model for pentamidine effects on Pneumocystis carinii. J Protozool 1991;38:70S–71S.
15. Latorre CR, Sulzer AT, Norman LG. Serial propagation of Pneumocystis carinii in cell line cultures. Appl Eviron Microbiol 1977;33:1204–1206.
16. Armstrong MYK, Richards FF. Propagation and purification of rat Pneumocystis carinii in short term cell culture. J Protozool 1989;36:24S–27S.
17. Lee C-H, Bauer NL, Shaw MM, et al. Proliferation of rat Pneumocystis

carinii on cells sheeted on microcarrier beads in spinner flasks. J Clin Microbiol 1993;31:1659–1662.
18. Vossen MEMH, Beckers PJA, Meuwissen JHET, Stadhouders AM. Microtubules in Pneumocystis carinii. Z Parasitenkd 1976;49:289–292.
19. Vossen MEMH, Beckers PJA, Meuwissen JEHT, Stadhouders AM. Developmental biology of Pneumocystis carinii, an alternative view on the life cycle of the parasite. Z Parasitenkd 1978;55:101–118.
20. Bouton C, Kernbaum S, Christol D, et al. Diagnostic morphologique de Pneumocystis carinii. Pathol Biol 1977;25:153–160.
21. Balachandran IM, Jones DB, Humphrey DM. A case of Pneumocystis carinii in pleural fluid with cytologic, histologic, and ultrastructual documentation. Acta Cytol 1990;34:486–490.
22. Barton EG, Campbell WG. Pneumocystis carinii in lungs of rats treated with cortisone acetate. Am J Pathol 1969;54:209–236.
23. Kaneshiro ES, Jayasimhulu K, Ellis JE, Beach DH. Evidence for the presence of "metabolic sterols" in Pneumocystis: Identification and initial characterization of Pneumocystis carinii sterols. J Euk Microbiol 1994;41:78–85.
24. Zenghui G, Kaneshiro ES. Phospholipid composition of Pneumocystis carinii carinii and effects of methylrednisolone immunosuppression on rat lung lipids. Infect Immun 1995;63:1286–1290.
25. Florin-Christensen M, Florin-Christensen J, Kaneshiro ES. Uptake and metabolism of L-serine by Pneumocystis carinii carinii. J Eur Microbiol 1995; 42. In press.
26. Kaneshiro ES, Sleight RG. Biochemistry and metabolism. In: Walzer PD, ed. Pneumocystis carinii Pneumonia. New York: Marcel Dekker, 1994;69: 45–65.
27. Vavra J, Kucera K. Pneumocystis carinii Delanoe: its ultrastructure and ultrastructure affinities. J Protozool 1970;17:463–483.
28. ul Haque A, Plattner SB, Cook RT, Hart MN. Pneumocystis carinii: Taxonomy as viewed by electron microscopy. Am J Clin Pathol 1987;87:504–510.
29. Ruffolo JJ. Pneumocystis carinii cell structure. In: Walzer PD, ed. Pneumocystis carinii Pneumonia. New York: Marcel Dekker, 1994;69:25–39.
30. Stringer SL, Hudson K, Blase MA, et al. Sequence from ribosomal RNA of Pneumocystis carinii compared to those of four fungi suggests an ascomycetous affinity. J Protozool 1989;36:14S–16S.
31. Watanabe J, Hori H, Tanabe K, Nakamura Y. Phylogenetic association of Pneumocystis carinii with the "Rhizopoda/Myxomycota/Zygomycota group" indicated by comparison of 5S ribosomal RNA sequences. Molec Biochem Parasitol 1989;32:163–167.
32. Edman JC, Kovacs JA, Mansur H, et al. Ribosomal RNA genes of Pneumocystis carinii. J Protozool 1989;36:18S–20S.
33. Edman U, Edman JC, Santi D. Isolation and expression of the Pneumocystis carinii thymidate synthase gene. Proc Natl Acad Sci USA 1989;86: 6503–6507.
34. Edman JC, Edman U, Cao M, et al. Isolation and expression of the Pneumo-

cystis carinii dihydrofolate reductase gene. Proc Natl Acad Sci USA 1989; 86:8625–8629.
35. Meade JC, Smulian AG, Stringer SL, Stringer JR. Characterization of TFIID and ATPase from isolates of Pneumocystis. J Protozool 1991;38: 69S.
36. Meade JC, Stringer JR. Cloning and characterization of an ATPase gene from Pneumocystis carinii which closely resembles fungal hydrogen ATPases. J Euk Microbiol 1995;42:298–307.
37. Ypma-Wong MF, Fonz, A, Buck GA. Fungus specific translation elongation factor 3 gene present in Pneumocystis carinii. Infect Immun 1992;60: 4140–4145.
38. Stringer JR. Pneumocystis carinii: A fungus or a protozoan? Rev Iberoam Micol 1993;10:31–32.
39. Stringer JR. The identity of Pneumocystis carinii: Not a single protozoan, but a diverse group of exotic fungi. Infect Agents Dis 1993;2:109–117.
40. Wakefield AE, Peters SE, Banerji S, et al. Pneumocystis carinii shows homology with ustomycetous red yeast fungi. Molec Microbiol 1992;6: 1903–1911.
41. Kaneshiro ES, Jayasimhulu K, Ellis JE, Beach DH. Evidence for the presence of "metabolic sterols" in Pneumocystis: Identification and initial characterization of Pneumocystis carinii sterols. J Euk Microbiol 1994;41:78–85.
42. Bruns TD, Vigalys R, Barns SM, et al. Evolutionary relationships within the fungi: Analyses of nuclear small subunit rRNA sequences. Molec Phys Evol 1992;1:231–241.
43. Taylor JW, Bowman BH. Pneumocystis carinii and the ustomycetous red yeast fungi. Molec Microbiol 1993;8:425–427.
44. Bowman BH, Taylor JW, White TJ. Molecular evolution of the fungi: Human pathogens. Molec Biol Evol 1992;9:893–904.
45. Li J, Edlind T. Phylogeny of Pneumocystis carinii based on β-tubulin sequence. J Euk Microbiol 1994;1:97S.
46. Berbee ML, Taylor JW. Detecting morphological convergence in true fungi, using 18S RNA gene sequence data. Biosystems 1992;28:117–125.
47. Giuntoli D, Stringer SL, Stringer JR. Extraordinarily low copy number of ribosomal RNA genes in P. carinii. J Euk Microbiol 1994;41:88S.
48. Maleszka R, Clark-Walker GD. Yeast have a four-fold variation in ribosomal DNA copy number. Yeast 1993;9:53–58.
49. Palluault F, Slomianny C, Soulez B, et al. High osmotic pressure enables fine ultrastructural and cytochemical studies on Pneumocystis carinii: I. Epon embedding. Parasitol Res 1992;78:437–444.
50. Palluault F, Soulez B, Slomianny C, et al. High osmotic pressure for Pneumocystis carinii London resin white embedding enables fine immunocytochemistry studies: I. Golgi complex and cell-wall synthesis. Parasitol Res 1992;78:482–488.
51. Dei-Cas E, Mazars EC, Ferragut CÖ, et al. Ultrastructural, genomic, isoenzymatic, and biological features make it possible to distinguish rabbit

Pneumocystis from other mammal Pneumocystis strains. J Euk Microbiol 1994;41:84S.
52. Matsumoto Y, Yoshida Y. Sporogony in Pneumocystis carinii: Synaptonemal complexes and meiotic nuclear divisions observed in precysts. J Protozool 1984;31:420–428.
53. Gigliotti F. Host species restriction in rats, ferrets, and mice of Pneumocystis carinii. Infect Immun 1993;61:4140–4156.
54. Aliouat E-M, Mazars EC, Dei-Cas, et al. Pneumocystis cross infection experiments using SCID mice and nude rats as recipient host, showed strong host-species specificity. J Euk Microbiol 1994;41:71S.
55. Frenke JK, Good JT, Schultz JA. Latent Pneumocystis infection of rats, relapse, and chemotherapy. Lab Invest 1966;15:1559–1577.
56. Graves DC, McNabb SJN, Whorley MA, Downs TD, Ivey MH. Analysis of rat Pneumocystis carinii antigens recognized by human and rat antibodies by using Western immunoblotting. Infect Immun 1986;54:96–103.
57. Gigliotti F, Ballou LR, Hughes WT, Mosley BD. Purification and initial characterization of a ferret Pneumocystis carinii surface antigen. J Infect Dis 1988;158:848–854.
58. Walzer PD, Linke MJ. A comparison of the antigenic characteristics of rat and human Pneumocystis carinii by immunoblotting. J Immun 1987;138: 2257–2265.
59. Tanabe K, Takasaki S, Watanabe JI, et al. Glycoproteins composed of major surface immunodeterminants of Pneumocystis carcinii. Infect Immun 1989;57:1363–1368.
60. Fishman JA. Cross-reactive antigens of the rat and human Pneumocystis carinii. J Protozool 1989;36:66S–67S.
61. Kovacs JA, Halpern JL, Lundgren B, et al. Monoclonal antibodies to Pneumocystis carinii: Identification of specific antigens and characterization of antigenic differences between rat and human isolates. J Infect Dis 1989; 159:60–70.
62. Radding JA, Armstrong MYK, Ulu E, Richards FF. Identification and isolation of a major cell surface glycoprotein of Pneumocystis carinii. Infect Immun 1989;57:2149–2157.
63. Lundgren B, Lipschik GY, Kovacs JA. Purification and characterization of a major human Pneumocystis carinii surface antigen. J Clin Invest 1991; 87:163–170.
64. Roth A, Janitschke K. Detection of antibody formation in mice, rats, and rabbits immunized with different Pneumocystis carinii antigens. Zentralbl Bakteriol 1991;275:123–132.
65. Bauer NL, Paulsrud JR, Barlett MS, et al. Pneumocystis carinii organisms obtained from rats, ferrets, an mice are antigenically different. Infect Immun 1993;61:1315–1319.
66. Hong S-T, Steele PE, Cushion MT, et al. Pneumocystis carinii karyotypes. J Clin Microbiol 1990;28:1785–1795.
67. Fishman JA, Ullu E, Armstrong MYK, Richards FF. Organization of DNA and RNA from rat Pneumocystis carinii. J Protozool 1989;36:4S–5S.

68. Yoganathan T, Lin H, Buck GA. An electrophoretic karyotype and assignment of ribosomal genes to resolved chromosomes of Pneumocystis carinii. Molec Microbiol 1989;3:1473–1480.
69. Zhang J, Cushion M, Giuntoli D, et al. Localization of P. carinii genes to chromosomal bands. J Protozool 1991;38:69S–70S.
70. Weinberg GA, Bartlett MS. Comparison of pulse field gel electrophoresis karyotypes of Pneumocystis carinii derived from rat lung, cell culture, and ferret lung. J Protozool 1991;38:122S–123S.
71. Weinberg GA, Dylstra, CC, Durant PJ, Cushion MT. Chromosomal localization of 20 genes to five distinct pulsed field gel karyotypic forms of rat Pneumocystis carinii. J Euk Microbiol 1994;41:117S.
72. Stringer JR. Molecular genetics of Pneumocystis carinii. In: Walzer PD, ed. Pneumocystis carinii Pneumonia. New York, Marcel Dekker, 1993:73–90.
73. Stringer JR, Stringer SL, Zhang J, et al. Molecular genetic distinction of Pneumocystis carinii from rats and humans. J Euk Microbiol 1993;40: 733–741.
74. Zhang J, Cushion MT, Stringer JR. Molecular characterization of a novel repetitive element from Pneumocystis carinii from rats. J Clin Microbiol 1993;31:244–248.
75. Stringer SL, Garbe T, Sunkin SM, Stringer JR. Genes encoding antigenic surface glycoproteins in Pneumocystis from humans. J Euk Microbiol 1993; 40:821–826.
76. Sinclair K, Wakefield AE, Banerji S, Hopkin JM. Pneumocystis carinii organisms derived from rat and human hosts are genetically distinct. Molec Biochem Parasitol 1991;45:183–184.
77. Zhang J, Stringer JR. Cloning and characterization of an alpha-tubulin encoding gene from rat derived Pneumocystis carinii. Gene 1993;123:137–141.
78. Edlind TD, Barlett MS, Weinberg G, et al. The beta-tubulin gene from rat and human isolated of Pneumocystis carinii. Molec Microbiol 1992;6: 3365–3373.
79. Keely S, Pai K, Baughman R, et al. Pneumocystis species inferred from analysis of multiple genes. J Euk Microbiol 1994;41:94S.
80. Mazars E, Ödberg-Ferragut C, Dei-Cas E, et al. Polymorphisms of Pneumocystis carinii from different host species. J Euk Microbiol 1995;42:26–32.
81. Liu Y, Rocourt M, Pan S, et al. Sequence and variability of the 5.8S and 26S rRNA genes of Pneumocystis carinii. Nucleic Acids Res 1992;20: 3763–3772.
82. Lu J-J, Bartlett MS, Shaw MM, et al. Typing of Pneumocystis carinii strains that infect humans based on nucleotide sequence variations of internal transcribed spacers of rRNA genes. J Euk Microbiol 1994;41:102S.
83. Peters SE, English K, Laakkonen J, Gurnell J. DNA analysis of Pneumocystis carinii infecting Finnish and English shrews. J Euk Microbiol 1994; 41:108S.
84. Lu J-J, Bartlett MS, Shaw MM, et al. Typing of Pneumocystis carinii strains that infect humans based on nucleotide sequence variations of internal transcribed spacers of rRNA genes. J Clin Microbiol 1994;32:2904–2912.

85. Ortiz-Rivera M, Liu Y, Felder R, Leibowitz MJ. Sequence differences in the rRNA regions identify specific isolates of P. carinii. J Euk Microbiol 1994;41:107S.
86. Cushion MT, Zhang J, Kaselis M, et al. Evidence for two genetic variants of Pneumocystis carinii coinfecting laboratory rats. J Clin Microbiol 1993; 31:1217–1223.
87. Sunkin SM, Stringer JR. Sequence of transcription factor IID from prototype and variant Pneumocystis carinii. J Euk Microbiol 1994;42:12–19.
88. Weinberg GA, O'Gara MJ. Coinfection of rats with genetically diverse forms of Pneumocystis carinii demonstrated by P. carinii ionsine monophosphate dehydrogenase. J Euk Microbiol 1994;41:119.
89. Garbe TG, Stringer JR. Cloning and sequencing the gpA/MSG gene of Pneumocystis carinii rattus. J Euk Microbiol 1996. In press.
90. Liu Y, Leibowitz MJ. Variation and in vitro splicing of group I introns in rRNA. Genes of Pneumocystis carinii. Nuc Acids Res 1993;21:2415–2421.
91. Banerji S, Lugli EB, Wakefield AE. Identification of two genetically distinct strains of Pneumocystis carinii in infected ferret lungs. J Euk Microbiol 1994;41:73S.
92. Sudhir K, Tamura K, Masatoshi N. MEGA: Molecular Evolutionary Genetics Analysis, Version 1.0. University Park, PA: The Pennsylvania State University, 1993.
93. Hillis DM, Bull JJ. An empirical test of boostrapping as a method for assessing confidence in phylogenetic analysis. Syst Biol 1993;42:182–192.
94. Feldenstein J, Kishino H. Is there something wrong with the bootstrap on phylogenies: A reply to Hillis and Bull. Syst Biol 1993;42:192–200.
95. Stringer JR. Revised nomenclature for Pneumocystis carinii. J Euk Microbiol 1994;41:121S.
96. Haidaris PJ, Wright TW, Gigliotti F, Haidaris CG. Expression and characterization of a cDNA clone encoding an immunodominant surface glycoprotein of Pneumocystis carinii. J Infect Dis 1992;166:1113–1123.
97. Kovacs JA, Powell F, Edman JC, et al. Multiple genes encode the major surface glycoprotein of Pneumocystis carinii. J Biol Chem 1993;268: 6034–6040.
98. Garbe T, Stringer JR. Molecular characterization of clustered variants of genes encoding major surface antigens of human Pneumocystis carinii. Infect Immun 1994;62:3092–3101.
99. Yoshikawa H, Tegoshi T, Yoshida Y. Detection of surface carbohydrates on Pneumocystis carinii by fluorescein-conjugated lectins. Parsitol Res 1987;74:43–49.
100. Walzer PD, Rutledge ME. Comparison of rat, mouse, and human Pneumocystis carinii by immunofluorescence. J Infect Dis 1980;142:449–453.
101. Gigliotti F. Host species-specific antigenic variation of a mannosylated surface glycoprotein of Pneumocystis carinii. J Infect Dis 1992;165:329–336.
102. Gigliotti F, McCool T. Glycoprotein A is the immunodominant antigen of Pneumocystis carinii in mice following immunization. Parasitol Res 1995. In press.

103. De Stefano JA, Trinkle LS, Walzer PD, Cushion MT. Lectins as probes to Pneumocystis carinii glycocomplexes. J Protozool 1989;36:65S–66S.
104. Garner RE, Walker AN, Horst MN. Morphological and biochemical studies of chitin expression in Pneumocystis carinii. J Protozool 1991;6:12S–14S.
105. Linke MJ, Walzer PD. Identification and purification of soluble species of gp120 released by zymolyase treatment of Pneumocystis carinii. J Protozool 1991;38:176S–178S.
106. Smulian AG, Theus SA, Denko N, et al. A 55 kDa antigen of Pneumocystis carinii: Analysis of the cellular response and characterization of the gene. Molec Microbiol 1993;7:745–753.
107. Wada M, Kitada K, Saito M, et al. cDNA sequence diversity and genomic clusters of major surface glycoprotein genes of Pneumocystis carinii. J Infect Dis 1993;168:979–985.
108. Stringer SL, Hong S-T, Giuntoli D, Stringer JR. Repeated DNA in Pneumocystis carinii. J Clin Microbiol 1991;29:1194–1201.
109. Sunkin SM, Stringer SL, Stringer JR. A tandem repeat of rat-derived Pneumocystis carinii genes encoding the major surface glycoprotein. J Euk Microbiol 1994;41:292–300.
110. Wright TW, Bissondial TY, Haidaris CG, et al. Isoform diversity and tandem duplication of the glycoprotein A gene in ferret Pneumocystis carinii. DNA Res 1995;2:77–88.
111. Wright TW, Haidaris PJ, Gigliotti F, et al. Conserved sequence homology of cysteine rich regions in genes encoding glycoprotein A in Pneumocystis carinii derived from different host species. Infect Immun 1994;62: 1513–1519.
112. Wright TW, Gigliotti F, Haidaris CG, Simpson-Haidaris PJ. Cloning and characterization of a conserved region of human and rhesus macaque Pneumocystis carinii gpA genes. Gene 1996. In press.
113. Chou PY, Fasman G. Structural and functional role of leucine residues in proteins. J Molec Biol 1973;74:263–281.
114. Fasman GD. Protein conformation prediction. Trends Biochem Sci 1989; 14:295–259.
115. Kyte J, Doolittle RF. A simple method for displaying the hydropathic character of a protein. J Molec Biol 1982;157:105–132.
116. Eisenberg D. Three-dimensional structure of membrane and surface proteins. Ann Rev Biochem 1989;53:595–623.
117. Olson EN. Modification of proteins with covalent lipids. Prog Lipid Res 1988;27:177–197.
118. Wada M, Nakamura Y. Chromosomal organization of MSG antigen genes of rat Pneumocystis carinii: tandem repeat and unique 5′UTR sequence encoding intron. J Euk Microbiol 1993;41:115S.
119. Wada M, Sunkin SM, Stringer JR, Nakamura Y. Antigenic variation by positional control of major surface glycoprotein gene expression in Pneumocystis carinii. J Infect Dis 1995;171:1563–1568.
120. Sunkin SM, Stringer JR. Translocation of surface antigen genes to a unique

telomeric expression site in Pneumocystis carinii. Molec Microbiol 1996. In press.

121. Lipschik GY, Gill VJ, Lundgre JD, et al. Improved diagnosis of infection by polymerase chain reaction on induced sputum and blood. Lancet 1992; 340:203–206.
122. Wakefield AE, Guiver L, Miller RM, Hopkin JM. DNA amplification on induced sputum samples for diagnosis of Pneumocystis carinii pneumonia. Lancet 1991;337:1378–1379.
123. Gigliotti F, Haidaris PJ, Haidaris CG, et al. Further characterization of host species-specific variation in antigens of Pneumocystis carinii using polymerase chain reaction. J Infect Dis 1993;168:191–194.
124. Gigliotti F, Hughes WT. Passive immunoprophylaxis with specific monoclonal antibody confers partial protection against Pneumocystis carinii pneumonitis in animal models. J Clin Invest 1988;81:1666–1668.
125. Harmsen AG, Chen W, Gigliotti F. Active immunity to Pneumocystis carinii reinfection in T-cell depleted mice. Infect Immun 1995;63:2391–2395.
126. Hendley JO, Weller TH. Activation and transmission in rats of infection with Pneumocystis carinii. Proc Soc Exp Biol Med 1971;137:1401–1404.
127. Hong S-T, Ryu J-S, Chai J-Y, Lee S-H. Transmission modes of Pneumocystis carinii among rats observed by karyotype analysis. Kor J Parasitol 1992;30:283–288.
128. Bartlett MS, Lee C-H, Lu J-J, et al. Pneumocystis carinii detected in air. J Euk Microbiol 1994;41:75S.
129. Wakefield AE. Detection of DNA sequences identical to Pneumocystis carinii in samples of ambient air. J Euk Microbiol 1994;41:116S.
130. Keely S, Stringer JR. Change of Pneumocystis carinii genotype in recurrent episodes of pneumonia in AIDS patients. AIDS 1996. In press.
131. Takashi M, Kuramochi T, Hioki K, Nomura T. Effects of environmental factors and disinfectants on the survival of Pneumocystis carinii outside the host. J Euk Microbiol 1994;41:91S.

27

Animal Models for Fungal Infection and Therapy

JAN VAN CUTSEM
Janssen Research Foundation
Beerse, Belgium

I. INTRODUCTION

Fungi are widely spread in the environment. The majority of them live as saprophytes in nature; only a limited number may become opportunistic invaders for plants, animals, or humans if conditions for adaptation and infection are realized. Also, a few are considered as truly pathogenic.

Fungi that may be responsible for mycotic infections in animals or in humans have been studied in various animal species with and without predisposing or immunodepressing factors. The pathogenesis of the experimental mycosis may cover a broad range of aspects. One of those is the establishment of stable animal models for screening and detection of active new compounds and for evaluation of the activity of selected drugs in animal models, mimicking the clinical diseases and allowing extrapolation of the treatment of experimentally infected animals to treatment of patients.

The object of this study is restricted to a limited number of models that have been the basis for the evaluation, comparison, and selection of a number of antimycotics that are now used worldwide. These animal models were established on the basis of their reproducibility and have been repeated week after week for many years.

II. MATERIALS AND METHODS

Several animal species have been infected by various routes with a large number of fungi (Table 1). They were treated topically or orally for superficial infections, orally or parenterally (intraperitoneally) for disseminated and systemic diseases (1–10). Eventually, other treatment routes were used, such as, for example, inhalation of enilconazole from a smoke generator for aspergillosis or for disinfection of animal houses (11). For topical treatment, the compounds were mostly incorporated in polyethylene glycols or cyclodextrins. For oral treatment, they were administered in poly-

Table 1 Animal Models for Fungal Infection

Mycosis	Animal species	Route of infection	Route of treatment: Topical	Oral	Parenteral	Other
Cutaneous dermatophytosis	Guinea pig	Skin	X	X		
Disseminated dermatophytosis	Guinea pig	IV		X		
Cutaneous candidosis	Guinea pig	Skin	X	X		
Vaginal candidosis	Rat	Intravaginal	X	X		
Crop candidosis	Turkey	Gavage		X		
Oral and gastrointestinal candidosis	Guinea pig	Gavage		X		
Ocular candidosis	Guinea pig	Intracorneal	X	X	X	
Systemic and disseminated candidosis	Guinea pig, mouse, rabbit, chicken	IV		X	X	
Malasseziosis	Guinea pig	Skin	X	X		
Cutaneous cryptococcosis	Guinea pig	Skin	X	X		
Systemic and disseminated cryptoccocis	Guinea pig	IV		X	X	
Meningocerebral cryptoccosis	Mouse, guinea pig, rabbit	Intracerebral		X	X	
Pulmonary aspergillosis	Chicken	Lung, inhalation		X		X
Systemic and disseminated aspergillosis	Guinea pig, mouse, rabbit, chicken, pigeon	IV		X	X	
Ocular	Guinea pig	Intracorneal	X	X	X	
Others[a]	Various	Various		X	X	

[a] Others: By *Penicillium marneffei, Sporothrix, Histoplasma, Paracoccidioides, Fonsecaea, Rhizopus, Fusarium, Trichosporon, Pneumocystis carinii,* etc.

ethylene glycol 200, cyclodextrins, other solvents, or mixed as food additives. For parenteral (intraperitoneal) administration, the substances were prepared in cyclodextrins or other solvents. The compounds were always administered in solution or in microsuspension. Excipient-treated controls and reference-drug-treated animals were included (12).

A large number of predisposing factors and immunodepressing agents have been used (Table 2). In skin dermatophytosis, scarification or abrasion greatly improved the success of infection and the homogeneity of the lesions caused by the zoophilic fungi *Microsporum canis* and *Trichophyton mentagrophytes*. The guinea pig is the animal of choice for dermatophyte infections. In disseminated dermatophytosis, spores of a zoopathogenic *T. mentagrophytes* var. *granulare* were injected intravenously (IV) and produced granulomas in various internal organs, including the lungs, with dissemination to the skin, the hair, and the nails, corresponding to the "Maladie Dermatophytique" or disease of Hadida and Schousboe (dermatophyte disease) (4,13).

Candida albicans produced cutaneous candidosis lesions in adult guinea pigs, infected on the intact skin of the back, after induction of alloxan-diabetes (1 × 200 mg/kg). For *C. albicans* vaginal infection, female rats were ovariectomized and hysterectomized and maintained in permanent pseudestrus by weekly injections of estradiol undecyclate. But for vaginal infection with *C. glabrata*, the permanent pseudestrus had to be augmented with diabetes, induced with streptozotocin (120 mg/kg given singly or in three fractions at different times) (10). Oral and gastrointestinal candidosis could be induced by a combination pretreatment and continued administration, during the whole duration of the experiment, of corticosteroids and antibacterial antibiotics. Crop candidosis could easily be induced in young turkeys by gavage. The guinea pig is also particularly sensitive to *C. albicans* when injected IV (10). Invasion of most or all organs is common, including skin folliculitis with invasion of the hair shaft by *Candida*. Neutropenia induced by mechlorethamine hydrochloride (2 × 0.25 mg/kg on days 5 and 4 before infection) aggravates the disease. Systemic candidosis does not produce skin involvement in mice or rabbits.

Mild abrasion of the cornea is needed to obtain keratitis (keratoretinitis) with *C. albicans*, *Aspergillus fumigatus*, *A. flavus*, *Fusarium moniliforme*, or *F. solani (F. oxysporum)* (14).

Malasseziosis (pityrosporosis) can be induced on the occluded intact skin of the back of the guinea pig with a single inoculum application. However, a more acute infection is obtained with application of the inoculum on the intact skin for 7 consecutive days without occlusion. The chronic evolution of this infection leads to a seborrheic dermatitislike disease (7,10).

Table 2 Use of Predisposing and/or Immunodepressing Factors

Mycosis	Animal species	Factors	Need/effects on the severity of infection
Cutaneous dermatophytosis	Guinea pig	Scarification	Largely improved
Cutaneous candidosis	Guinea pig	Intact skin + IM alloxan	Needed
Vaginal candidosis by *C. albicans*	Rat	Castration + estrogens	Needed
Vaginal candidosis by other *Candida* spp.	Rat	Castration + estrogens + streptozotocin	Needed
Oral and gastrointestinal candidosis	Guinea pig	Corticosteroids + antibacterial antibiotics	Needed
Crop candidosis	Turkey	Young animals	Needed
Ocular candidosis	Guinea pig	Mild abrasion	Needed
Systemic and disseminated candidosis	Guinea pig	Immunodepression[a]	No need, slightly improved
Systemic and disseminated candidosis	Mouse, rabbit, chicken	Immunodepression	Improved
Malasseziosis	Guinea pig	Single infection + occlusion multiple inoculation	Needed (folliculitis) Needed (acute; seborrheic dermatitis)
Cutaneous cryptococcosis	Guinea pig	Intact skin	Slightly improved by immunodepression
Cutaneous cryptococcosis	Guinea pig	Scarification	Improved
Systemic and disseminated cryptococosis	Guinea pig	Immunodepression	No need, slightly improved
Pulmonary aspergillosis	Chicken	One day old	Largely improved
Systemic and disseminated aspergillosis	Guinea pig	Immunodepression	No need, slightly improved
Systemic and disseminated aspergillosis	Mouse, rabbit, chicken, pigeon	Immunodepression	Improved
Ocular aspergillosis	Guinea pig	Mild abrasion	Needed

Table 2 *(Continued)*

Mycosis	Animal species	Factors	Need/effects on the severity of infection
Penicilliosis	Guinea pig	Immunodepression	No need, slightly improved
Sporotrichosis	Guinea pig	Intratesticular or IV	No need
Chromoblasto-mycosis (*Fonsecaea*)	Guinea pig, rat	Various routes + immuno-depression	Poorly susceptible
Chromoblasto-mycosis (*Fonsecaea*)	Mouse	IV	No need, slightly improved
Mucormycosis (*Rhizopus*)	Guinea pig	Deferoxamine	Largely improved
Mucormycosis (*Rhizopus*)	Guinea pig	Streptozotocin	Improved
Pneumocystosis	Mouse	Corticosteroids + antibacterial antibiotics	Needed
Others[b]	Various	Immunodepression	Benefit

[a] Immunodepression: cyclophosphamide, hydrocortisone acetate, prednisolone acetate, mechlorethamine hydrochloride.
[b] Others: *Histoplasma, Paracoccidioides, Fusarium, Trichosporon,* etc.

Meningocerebral cryptococcosis is easily obtained in various animal species after intracerebral inoculation. Cutaneous cryptococcosis can be obtained with *Cryptococcus neoformans* serotype AD applied on the intact skin of the guinea pig, but skin lesions are more pronounced after scarification and dissemination in internal organs and meninges is increased. Immunodepression also promotes the spread of the yeast into the body. Systemic cryptococcosis with small inocula given IV in the guinea pig produced invasion of all organs, including meninges and lymph nodes, and the appearance of cryptococcal granulomas in the organs and the skin (6,12,14,15).

One-day-old chicks are highly susceptible to airborne *Aspergillus* spores. Infection is realized with an aerosol of *A. fumigatus* spores dispersed in an infection box (11). Direct inoculation of a spore suspension in the lungs or air sacs of chickens (100–300 g) is also very efficacious. Systemic aspergillosis with *Aspergillus fumigatus* or *A. flavus* can be produced successfully in various animal species, the guinea pig being very sensitive. Invasion can be increased with cyclophosphamide (leukopenia, neutrocytosis, and lymphopenia), hydrocortisone acetate (neutrocytosis and lymphopenia), and prednisolone acetate (leukocytosis, neutrocytosis, and lymphopenia); but the strongest immunodepression was obtained with mechlorethamine hydrochloride (leukopenia, neutropenia, lymphocytosis, and monocytosis) (9,10,14). In guinea pigs, the neutropenia is not reversible; in mice, however, it is reversible.

Penicillium marneffei infection in the guinea pig reproduced all aspects of penicilliosis in patients with acquired immunodeficiency syndrome (AIDS), including invasion of internal organs and skin eruptions (10,16).

The guinea pig is very susceptible to *Sporothrix schenckii* after intratesticular or IV infection (10).

Rats and guinea pigs are poorly susceptible to infection with *Fonsecaea pedrosoi*. In the mouse, infected intravenously, all aspects of chromoblastomycosis in humans can be reproduced: including lung invasion as well as black and granulomatous lesions of bones, legs, head, tail, etc., containing large amounts of sclerotic cells (2,10).

Mucoralomycosis by *Rhizopus arrhizus* and *R. microsporus* var. *rhizopodiformis* was enhanced in the guinea pig after a single IM dose of 100 mg/kg deferoxamine (DFO). The severity of the infection and rapid lethality are dependent on the total DFO dosage (17). Dermatophyte and *Candida* infections are not influenced by DFO, but *Cryptococcus* and *Aspergillus* infections are more severe (18,19). Diabetes induced by streptozotocin also enhanced mucoralomycosis in mice and rats.

A combined regimen of corticosteroids and broad-spectrum antibacterial antibiotics promotes *Pneumocystis carinii* infection in the mouse and the rat.

Histoplasmosis by *Histoplasma capsulatum* var. *capsulatum* can easily be induced in the mouse. The guinea pig is also highly susceptible to histoplasmosis, especially when the animal is infected with *H. capsulatum* var. *duboisii* (10).

The guinea pig infected IV or intratesticularly with *Paracoccidioides brasiliensis* presents suppurating ulceration affecting the mouth and nose and containing the specific multipolar budding yeasts. Bones and several internal organs are also invaded (10).

III. RESULTS

The results of topical and oral treatments of various superficial mycoses are summarized in Table 3. The results obtained in clinical trials and in

Table 3 Therapy of Experimental Superficial Mycoses

Mycoses caused by (infection site)	Animal species	Therapeutic activity												
		Nystatin	Miconazole	Terconazole	Griseofulvin	Ketoconazole		Terbinafine		Fluconazole		Itraconazole	
		T[a]	T	T	O	T	O	T	O	T	O	T	O
Microsporum	Guinea pig	1[b]	3	2	3	3	3	4	4	2	2	4	4+
Trichophyton	Guinea pig	1	3	2	3	3	3	4	4	3	3	4	4+
C. albicans (skin)	Guinea pig	2	3	3	0	4	4	1	1	4	4	4	4
C. albicans (vagina)	Rat	2	3	4	0	4	4	0	0	4	4+	4	4+
C. albicans (crop)	Turkey	2	2	1	0	—[c]	4	—	0	—	4	—	3
C. albicans (GI tract)	Guinea pig	2	2	—	0	3	3	0	0	—	—	4	4
Other *Candida* spp.	Rat	2	3	4	0	3	3	—	—	—	2[d]	3	3
Malassezia	Guinea pig	1	2	—	0	4	4	—	0	0	1	4	4

[a] T = topical; O = oral.
[b] Scores: from 0 (inactive) to 4; 4+ (the most efficacious).
[c] No data.
[d] Resistance to fluconazole of some species and strains.

the field largely confirmed the experimental data in vivo concerning spectrum as well as potency of the drugs (20).

The synthesis and selection in 1967 of miconazole, the first really broad-spectrum topical drug, opened new perspectives for the treatment of mycoses. The introduction of ketoconazole was a revolutionary step forward in the antimycotic armory, where griseofulvin, nystatin, and amphotericin B had been landmarks years before.

In a comparison of the activity and the spectrum of the three antifungals of the eighties, itraconazole emerges as the most potent drug with the broadest spectrum (21–24). For oral treatment, itraconazole was administered as a solution; for topical treatment, it was dissolved or in microsuspension.

The results of treatment of systemic and disseminated mycoses with itraconazole, fluconazole, or amphotericin B are given in Table 4, as well as combination therapy of itraconazole with flucytosine or with amphotericin B (9,14,25,26). The two azoles can be administered orally or parenterally (intraperitoneally, intravenously); amphotericin B (Fungizone Squibb), however, is always used parenterally (intraperitoneally, intravenously). The lipophilic triazole itraconazole was dissolved for parenteral use in hydroxypropyl-β-cyclodextrin. The hydrophilic triazole fluconazole is water-soluble.

Table 4 Therapy of Experimental Systemic and Disseminated Mycoses

	Therapeutic activity				
				Combination therapy	
Mycoses caused by	Itraconazole	Fluconazole	Amphotericin B	Itra + 5-FC	Itra + Ampho-B
T. mentagrophytes	4[a]	2	—[b]	—	—
C. albicans	4	4	3	4+	4+
C. neoformans	3	3	3	4+	4+
A. fumigatus—A. flavus	4	1	3	4+	4+
P. marneffei	4	—	—	—	—
Sp. schenckii	4	1	3	—	—
F. pedrosoi	3	—	—	4+	—
Histoplasma spp.	4, 4[c]	3[c]	4[c]	—	—
P. brasiliensis	4, 4[c]	3[c]	3[c]	—	—
B. dermatitidis	4[c]	4[c]	3[c]	—	—
C. immitis	3[c]	3[c]	3[c]	—	—
Rhizopus spp.	0	0	3	—	—
F. moniliforme	3	—	—	—	—
Other *Fusarium* spp.	1, 1[c]	1[c]	3[c]	—	—

[a] Scores: from 0 (inactive) to 4 (the most efficacious); + improved activity in combination therapy.
[b] No data
[c] Data from other investigators

In systemic dermatophytosis, itraconazole can eliminate the dermatophytes completely, not only from the skin and its appendages but also from the dermatophytomas in internal organs. Relapses are avoided as well.

In *Candida*, *Cryptococcus*, *Histoplasma*, *Paracoccidioides*, *Blastomyces*, and *Coccidioides* infections, all three drugs are active. Itraconazole clears skin as well as subcutaneous and deep organ lesions faster than fluconazole except for the kidneys when infected with *C. albicans*. In the meninges when infected with *C. neoformans* both azoles are equipotent. On the other hand, itraconazole is highly active in aspergillosis, sporotrichosis, penicilliosis, and chromoblastomycosis. Fluconazole may be considered as poorly active or not active in aspergillosis and sporotrichosis. The two triazoles have an excellent safety profile: amphotericin B, however, while active in several systemic mycoses, has its activity limited by side-effects and toxicity problems. In mucoralomycosis and in the majority of *Fusarium* infections, only amphotericin B can be considered as active, but the activity of amphotericin B is completely abolished in mucoralomycosis in kidney dialysis patients, treated with deferoxamine, due to antagonism and enhanced pathogenicity of the zygomycetes (17,19). Deferoxamine is also able to antagonize partially the potency of amphotericin B in cryptococcosis and aspergillosis but not in dermatophyte and *Candida* infections (18).

In combination therapy of low dosages of itraconazole with flucytosine (5-FC) or amphotericin B, additive if not synergistic effects were obtained in candidosis, cryptococcosis, and aspergillosis (9,14,25,26). Also, the combination of itraconazole with 5-FC in chromoblastomycosis has at least additive effects. The same interesting drug interactions of fluconazole with 5-FC and amphotericin B were observed (25). The activity data obtained in the experimental evaluation in various animal models were largely confirmed in the clinic and the incidence of negative drug-drug interactions and side effects was low (20,27–35).

REFERENCES

1. Gentles JC. Experimental ringworm in guinea-pigs: Oral treatment with griseofulvin. Nature 1958;182:476–477.
2. Van Cutsem J, Thienpont D. Experimental cutaneous Candida albicans infection in guinea-pigs. Sabouraudia 1971;9:17–20.
3. Polak A. Experimental infection of mice by Fonsecaea pedrosoi and Wangiella dermatitidis. Sabouraudia 1984;22:167–169.
4. Van Cutsem J, Fransen J, Janssen PAJ. Animal models for systemic dermatophyte and Candida infection with dissemination to the skin. In: Maibach HI, Lowe NJ, eds. Models in Dermatology. Vol 1. Basel: Karger 1985:196–201.

5. Brummer E, Clemons KV. Animal models of systemic mycoses. In: Miyaji M, ed. Animal Models in Medical Mycology. Boca Raton, FL: CRC Press, 1987:79–99.
6. Van Cutsem J, Van Gerven F, Fransen J, Janssen PAJ. New guinea-pig model of disseminated cryptococcosis associated with dermotropism. In: Maibach HI, Lowe NJ, eds. Models in Dermatology. Vol 3. Basel: Karger, 1987:180–189.
7. Yamaguchi H. Opportunistic fungal infections. In: Miyaji M, ed. Animal Models in Medical Mycology. Boca Raton, FL: CRC Press, 1987:101–158.
8. Van Cutsem J. Animal models for dermatomycotic infections. In: MacGinnis MR, Borgers M, eds. Current Topics in Medical Mycology. Vol 3. New York: Springer-Verlag, 1989:1–35.
9. Van Cutsem J. Fungal models in immunocompromised animals. In: Vanden Bossche H, Mackenzie DWR, Cauwenbergh G, et al, eds. Mycoses in AIDS Patients. New York: Plenum Press, 1990:207–222.
10. Van Cutsem J. Animal models of mycoses caused by fungi that produce yeast and hyphal forms. In: Vanden Bossche H, Odds FC, Kerridge D, eds. Dimorphic Fungi in Biology and Medicine. New York: Plenum Press, 1993; 341–360.
11. Van Cutsem J. Antifungal activity of enilconazole on experimental aspergillosis in chickens. Avian Dis 1983;27:36–42.
12. Van Cutsem J, Van Gerven F, Janssen PAJ. Activity of orally, topically and parenterally administered itraconazole in the treatment of superficial and deep mycoses: animal models. Rev Infect Dis 1987;9(S1):15–32.
13. Hadida E, Schousboe A. Aspects de la Maladie Dermatophytique. Algérie Méd 1959;63:303–316.
14. Van Cutsem J. Oral, topical and parenteral antifungal treatment with itraconazole in normal and in immunodepressed animals. Mycoses 1989;32(S1): 14–34.
15. Van Cutsem J. Therapy of experimental meningeal and disseminated cryptococcosis. Mycoses 1993;36:357–367.
16. Van Cutsem J, Van Gerven F. Activité antifongique in vitro de l'itraconazole sur les champignons filamenteux opportunistes: Traitement de la kératomycose et de la pénicilliose expérimentales. J Mycol Méd 1991;1:10–15.
17. Van Cutsem J, Boelaert JR. Effects of deferoxamine, feroxamine and iron on experimental mucormycosis (zygomycosis). Kidney Int 1989;36:1061–1068.
18. Boelaert JR, de Locht M, Van Cutsem J. Desferrioxamine and microorganisms: Studies on in vitro growth and on experimental infections. A review. Rev Med Microbiol 1993;4:171–175.
19. Boelaert JR, Van Cutsem J, de Locht M, et al. Deferoxamine augments growth and pathogenicity of Rhizopus, while hydroxypyridinone chelators have no effect. Kidney Int 1994;45:667–671.
20. Cauwenbergh G. Clinical efficacy of itraconazole: Focus on cutaneous infections. In: Rippon JW, Fromtling RA, eds. Cutaneous Antifungal Agents. New York: Marcel Dekker, 1993:295–308.
21. Odds FC, Van Cutsem J. Itraconazole: Preclinical data in vitro and in vivo

in cutaneous and other superficial mycoses. In: Rippon JW, Fromtling RA, eds. Cutaneous Antifungal Agents. New York: Marcel Dekker, 1993: 251–261.
22. Van Cutsem J. An investigation of the in vitro activity and antifungal spectrum of itraconazole and terbinafine in relation to in vivo efficacy in dermatophytosis and other mycoses. J Mycol Med 1994;4:737–744.
23. Balfour JA, Faulds D. Terbinafine. A review of its pharmacodynamic and pharmacokinetic properties, and therapeutic potential in superficial mycoses. Drugs 1992;43:259–284.
24. Grant SM, Clissold SP. Fluconazole: A review of its pharmacodynamic and pharmacokinetic properties, and therapeutic potential in superficial and systemic mycoses. Drugs 1990;39:877–916.
25. Walsh TJ, Van Cutsem J, Polak A, Graybill JR. Immunomodulation and antifungal therapy of experimental invasive candidosis, histoplasmosis and aspergillosis: Recent advances and concepts. J Med Vet Mycol 1992;30(S1): 225–240.
26. Van Cutsem J, Janssen PAJ. In vitro and in vivo models to study the activity of antifungals against Aspergillus. In: Vanden Bossche H, Mackenzie DWR, Cauwenbergh G, eds. Aspergillus and aspergillosis. New York: Plenum Press, 1988:215–227.
27. Lampo A, De Beule K, Cauwenbergh G, Van Cauteren H. Safety of itraconazole in animals and in man. In: Rippon JW, Fromtling RA, eds. Cutaneous Antifungal Agents. New York: Marcel Dekker, 1993:285–293.
28. Svejgaard E. Clinical experience with itraconazole. In: Rippon JW, Fromtling RA, eds. Cutaneous Antifungal Agents. New York: Marcel Dekker, 1993:309–322.
29. Dismukes W. Therapeutic considerations in aspergillosis therapy. Clinician 1993;11:37–40.
30. Galgiani JN. Current therapy for coccidioidomycosis. In: Vanden Bossche H, Odds FC, Kerridge D, eds. Dimorphic Fungi in Biology and Medicine. New York: Plenum Press, 1993:397–403.
31. Graybill JR, Sharkey PK. Treatment of sporotrichosis, blastomycosis and histoplasmosis. In: Vanden Bossche H, Odds FC, Kerridge D, eds. Dimorphic Fungi in Biology and Medicine. New York: Plenum Press, 1993: 381–389.
32. Negroni R. Azole compounds in the treatment of paracoccidioidomycosis. In: Vanden Bossche H, Odds FC, Kerridge D, eds. Dimorphic Fungi in Biology and Medicine. New York: Plenum Press, 1993:391–396.
33. Queiros-Telles F, Purim KS, Fillus GN, et al. Itraconazole in the treatment of chromoblastomycosis due to Fonsecaea pedrosoi. Int J Dermatol 1992; 11:805–812.
34. Stevens DA. Current status and future directions of antifungal therapy. Infect Dis Clin Pract 1994;3(S2):97–102.
35. Supparatpinyo K, Chiewchanvit S, Hirunsri P, et al. An efficacy study of itraconazole in the treatment of Penicillium marneffei infection. J Med Assoc Thai 1992;75:689–691.

28

Areas for Future Research in Antifungals and Molecular Basis for New Antifungal Therapy

GEERT CAUWENBERGH
Consumer Products Worldwide
Johnson & Johnson
Skillman, New Jersey

I. INTRODUCTION

Before 1980, the development of antifungal agents focused on topically active drugs in different delivery forms and, to a lesser extent, on systemically active agents, mainly for intravenous use. The oldest antimycotics, dating from the early 20th century, had a narrow spectrum (potassium iodide) or were topically active (Whitfield's ointment). Polyene antibiotics, e.g., nystatin and amphotericin B, were poorly soluble and not absorbed from the gastrointestinal tract. Depending on their spectrum, they were developed for topical use (nystatin against yeasts) or intravenous use (amphotericin against a large range of fungi causing systemic disease). Griseofulvin was the first orally active agent to come into routine use in dermatology. Discovered in the 1930s, but only introduced into human medicine in the second half of the 1950s, griseofulvin has remained the treatment of choice for recalcitrant dermatophytoses, onychomycoses, and tinea capitis for more than two decades.

Topical imidazoles entered the antifungal arena in the mid-1960s, initially in research and development, and later, from 1970 onwards, also in general clinical use. With their large spectrum, covering dermatophytes, yeasts, dimorphic fungi, and occasionally even some Gram-positive bacteria, they rapidly became the preferred treatment for a variety of superficial mycoses. Early attempts to turn them into systemically active drugs failed because of a lack of solubility and oral bioavailability (miconazole) or autoinduction of their metabolism (clotrimazole). The only imidazole that has made it into a systemically used drug has been miconazole, which was developed into an intravenous alternative for amphotericin B. Its dissolution in a cremophore basis, with the associated side effects, has, however, limited the widespread use of this form of miconazole.

The synthesis of ketoconazole in 1976, and its subsequent development from 1976 to 1980, has created a true revolution in the therapeutic thinking of many infectious disease specialists and dermatologists vis-à-vis fungal infections. As the first orally active broad-spectrum antifungal agent, ketoconazole has rapidly gained a prime place as a treatment of fungal infections of skin, nail, mucosa, and internal organs. Only in tinea capitis, griseofulvin remained preferred because of ketoconazole's limited effect in this disease when caused by *Microsporum canis*. Widespread use of the drug has, however, resulted in the reporting of rare but serious side effects. Ketoconazole has been associated with idiosyncratic hepatitis in rare instances. In addition, higher doses of the drug resulted in suppression of cortisol biosynthesis and androgen suppression. These "side effects" have resulted in new drug discoveries for treatment of Cushing's syndrome and prostate cancer.

Limited in systemic use by its relatively unselective inhibition of cytochrome P450 in mammalian cells, ketoconazole has become a treatment of choice as a topical agent for quasi-fungal conditions, such as seborrheic dermatitis and dandruff. In addition, the molecule has started a highly intensive search for more orally active antifungals, with an improved safety profile and an increased potency. This has resulted in the discovery and development of orally active triazole agents, such as itraconazole and fluconazole, but also in nonazole compounds, such as allylamines and morpholine derivatives.

II. AREAS FOR FUTURE RESEARCH IN ANTIFUNGALS

Looking at today's situation, it is clear that the mind-set of the researcher needs to adapt swiftly in the field of antimycotics. Since the beginning of the 1980s, several new challenges have appeared.

1. Fungal infections can be found on any part of the body. Whereas the conventional approach has been to develop an ointment or a cream as the unique therapeutic delivery form for topical antifungals, it cannot be denied that the patient's and the physician's expectations of topical drug delivery have evolved beyond this point. It has also become apparent that improved delivery forms may promote patient compliance and, as a

result, influence the therapeutic outcome. Formulations that have a longer retention time in the epidermis, and that as a consequence, can be applied once daily or even once weekly, will elicit more therapy loyalty from the patient. Also, improvement of the cosmesis of the delivery form has similar consequences.

2. Onychomycosis is an infection that has steadily increased in prevalence. The chronicity of the infection, the graying of our population with associated peripheral vascular problems, the inability to treat the infection topically with a reasonable chance for success, and the fear of toxicity associated with long-term oral treatment have made onychomycosis one of the more difficult bastions in superficial pathology that need to be conquered.

3. Immunosuppression of infectious or iatrogenic origin became more widespread during the 1980s. Selective immunosuppression, aggressive chemotherapy, long-term high-dose systemic steroids, and the AIDS pandemic have resulted in a dramatic rise in systemic life-threatening mycoses, requiring more potent and broader-spectrum agents.

4. Subtherapeutic use of narrow-spectrum antifungals in immunocompromised patients has resulted in the development of resistant strains in fungal organisms previously not recognized to have a resistance problem. Cross-resistance is as yet not frequent, but certainly exists.

5. Short (too short) courses of treatment in immunologically healthy women with vaginal candidosis have led to a shift in the vaginal flora of women. Yeasts, in particular *Candida* spp., are known to occur in the vagina as part of the natural flora. Frequent short-term use of a narrow-spectrum agent against *Candida albicans* has caused suppression of this organism in the normal vaginal flora, causing a disproportionate presence of non-*albicans* strains, with subsequent vaginitis unresponsive to conventional treatments.

6. A final challenge to the researcher in the antifungal domain is the change in the healthcare attitude. Economic pressure on health insurance and social security have been leading a trend toward autodiagnosis and self-medication. Today, patients with a superficial fungal infection (including vaginal and oral candidosis), coming to a physician, are more likely to have mistreated recalcitrant infections and have limited the available therapeutic armamentarium for the physician.

III. MOLECULAR BASIS FOR NEW ANTIFUNGAL THERAPY

The antifungals of the past have focused on two main families: the polyene antibiotics and the azole antifungals. The target of most available antifungals today is the cell membrane. The polyenes bind in a fairly unselective way to sterol components in the cell membrane, thereby causing destruction of that membrane, leading to permeability changes and ion leakage, resulting in cell death. The limited selectivity of the polyenes can be explained by their higher affinity for binding to ergosterol than to cholesterol.

The azole antifungals also target the fungal cell membrane, albeit through a more indirect mechanism. They bind to cytochrome P450, causing an inhibition of the ergosterol biosynthesis in the fungal cells. The accumulation of abnormal, lanosterollike structures in the cell causes leakage of cell constituents, ultimately leading to cell death. The indirect mechanism of azole antifungals means that the killing effect on fungi with this class of compounds takes longer to become apparent than with the polyenes.

Other molecular targets in antifungal therapy have included interference with nucleic acid synthesis and mitosis causing inhibition of hyphal cell wall material (griseofulvin), direct interference with protein synthesis (5-fluorocytosine), and interference with growing cells, having specific effects in hyphal growth of dermatophytes (tolnaftate). These mechanisms have been explored far less systematically than in the case of azoles and polyenes.

More recent antifungal research has brought to life two new chemical families of orally or topically active antifungals: the morpholin derivatives and the allylamines. Although both categories are chemically new, these molecules do not differ significantly in mechanism of action from the azoles, in the sense that both families interfere with the ergosterol biosynthesis, as do the azoles. The difference is that they do not inhibit cytochrome P450–mediated steps in this synthesis, but that they interfere at other different steps in the ergosterol biosynthesis pathway. The end result, however, is the same: inhibition of lanosterol incorporation in the membranes ultimately resulting in cell death.

In summary, the currently available antifungals have four more or less different targets:

1. Direct binding to ergosterol: polyenes
2. Interference with ergosterol biosynthesis: azoles, allylamines, and morpholines
3. Inhibition of protein synthesis: 5-fluorocytosine
4. Effects on mitosis resulting in impaired hyphal growth: griseofulvin (tolnaftate)

Recent years have seen a variety of attempts to arrive at new chemical classes of antifungals with the possibility of a new mechanism of action. Some of these are briefly commented on below.

A. Isoxazolidine Compounds

Quite some work has been done on these compounds in the second half of the 1980s. The aim has been to cover the same broad spectrum as the azole antifungals, but to have a faster killing effect on the fungi. The whole category, however, still builds on the azole ring as a key component of the structure, basically meaning that the primary molecular target for efficacy has not changed: cytochrome P450. These molecules have shown a variable degree of potency and a relatively broad spectrum, including even *Aspergillus fumigatus* for some of its derivatives. Clinical development of some selected molecules has focused on topical application. One of the compounds has been submitted for approval in the United States. It is not expected that these structures will fundamentally impact on the antifungal landscape.

B. Pyridotriazines

Also, primarily evaluated as topical agents, these compounds have a similar in vitro effect on dermatophytes and yeasts compared to micoazole. The mechanism of action of the molecules has not been documented extensively, and today no active development in this category is under way.

C. Lanosterol Derivatives

The idea with these structures has been to combine the membrane-disrupting effects of lanosterol accumulation with a heme-binding component (read imidazole) at the 14-methyl position. In vitro tests have shown that these compounds have indeed an antifungal effect, with a spectrum similar to that of the imidazoles themselves. Overall, the modern azoles ketoconazole and itraconazole were substantially more potent. The most interesting compound in this series of lanosterol derivatives did show some higher selectivity toward fungal cytochrome P450 than ketoconazole. Once again, however, the chemical class as such does not use a different molecular target in the fungus and consequently is not the appropriate category to face the therapeutic challenges ahead in the field of mycoses.

D. Polyacetylene Alcohols

Polyacetylenes have been reported in sponges and nudibranchs. Thus far, only a few substances in this category have been evaluated for biological activities. Substances in this category include petrosynol and siphonodiol. Only limited antifungal and antibacterial work has been done with these products. They only show moderate activity.

E. Phenolic Substances

Marine organisms also contain a variety of halogenated phenols, some of which have antifungal properties. The compounds are believed to act through an effect on the host defense mechanisms. Solid proof of this hypothesis does not exist, and considering the chemical origin of these structures, their toxicity should certainly be evaluated before human use could be considered.

F. Macrolides

Sponges of the genus *Theonella* have received more attention, because they contain unusual macrolides that have antifungal and antitumoral properties. As is the case with 5-fluorocytosine, the derivatives show considerable activity against *Candida* spp., but not against dermatophytes or molds. These macrolides (e.g., bistheonellide A and calculin A) also have a considerable degree of mammalian cell toxicity. Incorporation experiments in rat fibroblasts have shown an inhibition of the DNA synthesis, but no effect on RNA and protein synthesis.

G. Nitro-Containing Terpenes

These products too are derived from marine sponges, and they also have antimicrobial and cytotoxic effects. Lack of selectivity is the primary concern for this category.

H. Saponins

Antifungal saponins have been isolated from a variety of sea invertebrates as well as from certain plant sources. The saponins isolated from sea cucumbers are holotoxins and have good in vitro activity against dermatophytes and yeasts. A sea cucumber extract containing a mixture of saponins is available in Japan for treatment of tinea pedis. Saponins isolated from plants (e.g., *Sapindus* spp.) have also been described as pharmacologically active and have been used as spermicides, antibiotics, antifungals, and hair growth stimulants.

I. Other Marine Derivatives

Other natural antifungals include pyrole and indole compounds, tetradecapeptides, and kabiramides. Coming from a variety of marine invertebrate sources, they all have one thing in common: cytotoxicity. This common feature does make them less desirable, even for topical development, since the currently available azole and allylamine agents have an excellent side-effects profile after topical use. Some of these natural ingredients have interesting antiviral and antibacterial effects, however, which, in light of the recent surge in more resistant infections, could be a valuable source for new antimicrobial agents.

J. Antifungal Plant Proteins

Because of the lack of an immune system, plants tend to produce a variety of products that form their first line of defense against foreign invaders. Most of these products are enzymes that inhibit growth of parasitic invaders. Many of these enzymes act by synthesizing inhibitory compounds such as phytoalexins, phenols, lignins, tannins, and melanins. Other enzymes have direct growth-inhibiting effects. These enzymes belong to different groups, of which the most important are glucanases, chitinases, and ribosome-inactivating proteins. Studies with these plant enzymes have indeed confirmed antifungal effect, but in general this effect was relatively weak, had a fairly narrow spectrum, and did not match that of the currently existing synthetic antifungals.

K. Galbonolides

Galbonolides are antifungal macrolides derived from *Streptomyces galbus* and *Streptomyces eurythermus*. These structures have little or no antibacterial effect, and structural alterations of the original derivative from *S. galbus* has so far not resulted in a potentiation of the antifungal properties. The antifungal spectrum is relatively narrow, and does not include a significant number of pathogens of high pathogenic relevance to humans. Today, the mechanism of action has not been discovered as yet. There is no evidence of membrane destabilization, and there is no effect on the chitin biosynthesis or biosynthesis of DNA or RNA.

L. Echinocandins

Echinocandins are semisynthetic analogs of the antifungal lipopeptide echinocandin B. These molecules have a good activity on yeasts, both in vitro and in vivo, but are primarily active by the intravenous route, not by the oral route. Examples of members of this family are sporiofungin and mulundocandin. The mechanism of these agents is different from the conventional antifungals. They inhibit incorporation of glucose into the glucan fraction of the yeast cell wall. The echinocandins are consequently named glucan synthase inhibitors. The first molecules tested had some problems with hemolysis, but subsequent synthesis and screening has been able to overcome most of this problem. Today, the echinocandins are probably the only new and viable alternative (other than azoles and polyenes) for treatment of systemic yeast infections.

M. Enactins

Enactins are hydroxamic acid antimycotic antibiotics that were discovered in a screening effort to identify potentiators of polyene antifungal agents. Enactins are believed to act on the eukaryotic cell membrane and, in addition, to potentiate the activities of antitumor agents such as vincristine and bleomycin. The products in monotherapy do not have significant therapeutic potential, and seem to primarily focus on anticandidal activity.

N. Beta-Lactones

Beta-lactones are broad-spectrum antifungal antibiotics of fungal origin. They have been studied for spectrum and mechanism of action. The spectrum is similar to that of azoles, and the biochemical mechanism of action is the inhibition of mevalonate synthesis, resulting in an impaired ergosterol biosynthesis. Some of the beta-lactones also have a limited antibacterial spectrum against some Gram-positive bacteria. No significant clinical development activity has been shown so far with this category of drugs.

IV. DISCUSSION AND CONCLUSION

If one tries to match the areas for future research in antifungals with the molecular targets for new antifungal drug therapy, it becomes apparent that there is a disconnection between these two aspects today. The current challenges include more difficult-to-treat infections often caused by new pathogens, emergence of resistant strains, and economic realities. The survey of what exists today in terms of novel approaches in antifungal therapy reveals nothing new, or targets that do not allow for enough selectivity to differentiate between fungal and mammalian cells. This leads to drug categories that, once more, interfere with ergosterol biosynthesis, molecules that affect DNA or RNA synthesis and that often are quite unselective, or molecules that have vaguely documented mechanisms of action.

The only few interesting developments on the horizon in terms of antifungal agents seem to be the echinocandins, although they have limitations in administration (intravenous), spectrum, and potentially in toxicity. Considering the emergence of resistant strains of *Candida albicans*, it is certainly a development worth following in view of the AIDS pandemic and the increased prevalence of systemic candidosis in immunocompromised patients.

Other totally novel approaches, still in the experimental stage, deal with immunostimulating therapy in combination with antifungals as well as attempts to attack *Candida albicans* via the use of antisense. Whereas the first approach seems to yield some interesting therapeutic successes, the latter approach appears to have problems related to lack of penetration of the antisense into the yeast cells.

From the above, it is clear that the challenges posed to the medical community by an emerging world of pathogenic fungi will not be fully answered in the near future. Unless academic institutions and industrial laboratories start to focus on in-depth research into one of the possible new mechanisms, rather than constantly repeating their predecessors, fungal infections will become an increasingly problematic part of our daily life.

29

Mechanisms of Azole Resistance

KAZUO IWATA
University of Tokyo
Tokyo, Japan

I. INTRODUCTION

Until the advent of a novel antifungal, flucytosine, it had long been believed that human pathogenic fungi do not acquire resistance to antifungal agents (antifungals), in contrast to the critical importance of bacterial resistance frequently caused by a variety of antibacterial chemotherapeutic agents. As a matter of fact, the polyene group (for instance, amphotericin B) and some other classic antifungals have not as yet posed a broadly significant problem relative to drug resistance despite their long, widespread and frequent use (1–3). Fungal resistance had thus received little attention. Most initial reports on resistance to antifungals among human pathogenic fungi indicate that naturally occurring resistance is very rare and that the development of resistant mutants or variants in vitro and in vivo is much more difficult to achieve than that of resistant bacteria. A single exception to this generalization arose with the occurrence of high degree of resistance to flucytosine in yeasts, with a high frequency of isolation of resistant strains, which resulted in the unsuccessful treatment of mycoses with this drug (2,4,5). This new development has aroused great interest in the problem of antifungal drug resistance among medical mycologists. As illustrated by the case of flucytosine, inherently resistant mutants to antifungals occur within sensitive strains of pathogenic fungi with significant frequency. Given the relatively high degree of such primary resistance, these mutants should develop secondary resistance during therapy, leading to considerable limitations in the clinical usefulness of the antifungals.

It should also be noted that in recent years prolonged drug treatment of systemic mycoses, particularly in patients suffering from acquired immunodeficiency syndrome (AIDS) (6–10) and other serious diseases, has begun to increase the number of yeast and other fungal strains resistant to old and new antifungals, particularly azole antifungals (azoles) (6,11–15). Attention has also been directed to the fact that the recent extensive use of the newer azoles such as fluconazole appears to be selecting resistant strains of susceptible species and inherently resistant non-*albicans* species such as *C. glabrata* (16–18). Indeed, it is generally believed that fungi, like bacteria, are intrinsically capable of developing resistance to antifungals. The exploitation of new antifungals thus requires in vitro and in vivo investigations for the possible occurrence of resistance in their target fungi. Studies of drug resistance are also important in designing less toxic drugs and answering biological questions about pathogenic and nonpathogenic microorganisms.

As described above, resistance to the azoles appears to be increasing in clinical importance; nevertheless, the risk should not be overestimated, since the incidence of treatment failures and the frequency of isolation of resistant strains remain low at present.

This paper reviews the reports on fungal resistance to azoles, focusing on the mechanisms of resistance from biochemical and genetic points of view, with a brief description of the current status of the isolation of azole-resistant fungal strains and of azoles' mechanisms of action.

II. CURRENT STATUS OF THE ISOLATION OF AZOLE-RESISTANT FUNGI

Holt and Azmi (11) were the first to report the isolation of a strain of *C. albicans* resistant to miconazole, an imidazole antifungal, from a patient suffering from urinary candidiasis and other disorders who had been undergoing prolonged oral administration of miconazole. In 1980, Rosenblatt et al. (12) described the first instance of treatment failure of in a case of chronic mucocutaneous candidiasis due to the development of resistance to ketoconazole, the oral imidazole, in the course of long-term drug management. Subsequently, four ketoconazole-resistant strains of *C. albicans* (strains AD, KB, Darlington, and SH) were isolated by Horsburgh et al. (13), Warnock et al. (14), and Smith et al. (15), respectively, from two American and two British patients with chronic mucocutaneous candidiasis who relapsed during prolonged treatment with the drug. In 1986, Tavitian et al. (6) identified six patients, including two Tahitians with AIDS complicated by oral and esophageal candidiasis, who had been treated with ketoconazole for more than 2 months; they isolated two ketoconazole-resistant strains of *C. albicans* from two of these patients. More recently, several strains of *C. albicans* resistant to the oral *bis*-triazole fluconazole have been isolated from patients with or without AIDS, despite the relatively recent introduction of this drug (7–10). As described above, three non-*albicans* species resistant to fluconazole—namely, *C. glabrata* (16), *C. krusei* (17), and C. parapsilosis (18)—have been isolated. It is notable that a strain of *C. glabrata* resistant to fluconazole was isolated from a patient infected with the yeast as early as 9 days after treatment with the once-daily administration of 400 mg of this antifungal. Nevertheless, the isolation frequency of strains resistant to azoles is in general still small.

Cross-resistance, partial or complete, has been observed among most of these azole-resistant strains isolated from patients and those obtained in the laboratory by mutagenesis or ultraviolet irradiation. Phenotypic resistance of resistant fungal strains—pertinent to morphology, growth, biology, serology, virulence, and so on—has been proven to be more or less closely associated with the mechanisms of resistance.

III. AZOLES' MECHANISMS OF ACTION

Azoles are known to act as cytochrome P450 inhibitors through binding at the iron atom of the prosthetic heme group. Azoles, in other words, bind through *N*-3 of the imidazole ring or *N*-4 of the triazole ring to the heme moiety as a sixth ligand. The inhibition of 14α-sterol demethylase by these compounds results in the accumulation of methylated sterols, thus blocking the synthesis of ergosterol, the major membrane sterol (19). The accumulation of methylated sterols are thought to disrupt membrane structure, as pointed out by Yeagle et al. (20). There has been some evidence, however, that the inhibition of ergosterol biosynthesis relative to cytochrome P450 sterol demethylase may not be the primary mechanism of action in all cases, though the mechanism itself has been demonstrated in vitro for all azoles with antifungal activity. Hitchcock et al. (21) showed that in a *C. albicans* strain, the sterols are normally almost exclusively methylated. Yeagle et al. (20) and Uno et al. (22) stated that some imidazoles, including ketoconazole, may interact directly with cell membranes and affect other membrane-bound enzymes. Barug et al. (23) reported that effects associated with ergosterol depletion and the accumulation of undemethylated sterols were observed, indicating uncoordinated chitin distribution and cell growth. Shigematsu et al. (24) implicated cytochrome oxidase as the primary target for ketoconazole. Other effects of azoles, such as increased fatty acid synthesis and desaturation as well as direct membrane damage at higher levels, have been observed (19,25). Some other aspects of the azoles' mechanisms of action, however, remain to be elucidated.

IV. MECHANISMS OF AZOLE RESISTANCE

The fact that long periods of time are needed to isolate azole-resistant strains of *C. albicans* in clinics is paralleled by the difficulty in inducing resistance of this yeast—for instance, to clotrimazole (26–28) and miconazole (29) by successive passage in vitro through increasing gradients of the drugs, as in the case of *Cryptococcus neoformans* versus ketoconazole (30).

The major reason why resistant strains of *C. albicans* are not only rare in clinical practice but also difficult to induce in vitro and in vivo is believed to be the diploid nature of the yeast and the absence of a haploid stage in its life cycle (31,32). Contrary to this, resistance to azoles can more easily be induced in the haploid stage of *C. glabrata* (31–34). The various functions of the multiple targets of azoles—such as cell membranes, mitochondria, endoplasmic reticulum, cytochrome *b*, desaturase, and so on—all of which are essential for growth, are regarded as another factor (32).

It remains to be determined whether the therapeutic failures or relapses with ketoconazole or fluconazole are attributable to host factors associated with the immunodeficiency state or to fungal resistance to these drugs. In this respect, the report of Hughes et al. (35) is suggestive in that oral treatment with a large dose (80 mg/kg) of fluconazole resulted in significant fungistatic activity against the ketoconazole-resistant strains of *C. albicans* (13) in a subcutaneously infected neutropenic-site rabbit model, using semipermeable Visking chambers, but not with a small dose of fluconazole (20 mg/kg) or with ketoconazole (up to 67 mg/kg).

Vanden Bossche et al. (36) reported that the cellular fluconazole content of a fluconazole-resistant strain of *C. glabrata* (B57149), which had been isolated by Warnock et al. (14) from a patient with chronic mucocutaneous candidiasis after treatment with the drug, was from 1.5- to 3-fold lower than that of a sensitive strain of the same species (B57148) isolated from the same patient before treatment. They also showed that the growth inhibition of B57148 was about 50% at 43 μM of the drug, whereas that of B57149 was not measurably affected at a concentration as high as 100 μM. The authors stated that the fluconazole resistance of B57149 cannot be fully elucidated on the basis of such data, and that the difference in drug uptake between the two strains was smaller than the measured difference in susceptibility. Howell et al. (37) showed that the ketoconazole-resistant strains of *C. albicans* contain much larger amounts of fecosterol than the susceptible strains.

Vanden Bossche et al. (36) furthermore reported in the above paper that the microsomal cytochrome P450 content of a fluconazole-resistant strain of *C. glabrata* (B57149) was about twice that of a susceptible strain (B57148). This difference proved quantitatively similar to the increased subcellular ergosterol synthesis from mevalonate or lanosterol, suggesting that the level of P450-dependent 14α-demethylation of lanosterol is higher in the resistant strain. The increased ergosterol synthesis observed in the intact cells of the resistant strain was accompanied by a decreased susceptibility toward all three azoles tested—fluconazole, itraconazole, and ketoconazole—as well as toward amphotericin B. The strain, moreover, proved to have higher squalene epoxidase activity. Repeated subculture of this resistant strain on a drug-free medium resulted in a decrease of both P450 content and ergosterol synthesis and in a partial increase of its susceptibility to fluconazole as well as full restoration of its susceptibility to itraconazole.

Vanden Bossche et al. (38,39) implicated an altered cytochrome P450 with reduced affinity for miconazole, ketoconazole, itraconazole, and fluconazole in a resistant strain of *C. albicans*. This strain, which had been isolated by Smith et al. (15) from a patient with chronic mucocutaneous candidiasis, had less susceptibility to these azoles and had lessened pathogenicity in animal models.

The resistance mechanism of the ketoconazole-resistant strain of *C. albicans* (Darlington) was investigated in detail by Hitchcock et al. (40). The strain was characterized by susceptibility to both amphotericin B and azoles, the absence of ergosterol from its membrane fractions, and its consequent replacement by methylated sterol. Significant changes had also occurred in its total lipid content, which, in this strain, was about three times that of normal sensitive strains. In addition, it had a conspicuously lower ratio of polar to neutral lipid than other strains which were sensitive or resistant to azoles. Furthermore, Hichcock et al. (41) described differences in cellular permeability and the phospholipid/sterol ratio of *C. albicans* between two ketoconazole-resistant mutants (strains AD and KB) (13) and the Darlington strain. Both of the former strains proved impermeable to ICI 153,066 and had a much lower ratio. In contrast, the latter strain was permeable to the triazole and had a ratio similar to that of the sensitive strains. Perceiving an apparently different mechanism in the Darlington strain, these authors (21) determined in vitro the activity of 14α-sterol demethylase and its susceptibility to inhibition by ICI 153,066. The enzyme in this strain proved less sensitive to the drug than the azole-sensitive strains. There was no direct correlation, however, between the IC_{50} values for triazole inhibition of the enzyme and IC_{50} values for growth. They thus suggested that the azole resistance in the Darlington strain could not be explained solely on the basis of a lack of susceptibility of its 14α-sterol demethylase enzyme but that other target sites for azole may be altered or absent. Hitchcock et al. (41) earlier stated that, in four azole-resistant strains of *C. albicans* isolated from patients with chronic mucocutaneous candidiasis, resistance in each case was associated with failure of the drug to cross the cell envelope and reach its intracellular targets. They also demonstrated that in the Darlington strain, ICI 153,066 was taken up at a faster rate than in the three other sensitive strains. In this connection, Gale et al. (42) made an interesting report that in *C. albicans*, phenotypic resistance to miconazole develops after cessation of growth. They suggested that this change would derive from the alteration in the cell wall that prevented approach to the cell membrane.

Ryley et al. (43) reported that a ketoconazole-resistant strain of *C. albicans* manifested abnormal resistance to the inhibition of ergosterol biosynthesis in whole cells but not in cell-free systems and to inhibition of amino acid uptake. In contrast to normal isolates, these strains did not take up a radiolabeled ICI 153,066.

Kerridge et al. (31) investigated the influence of azoles on the inhibition of cytochrome P450 sterol demethylase by following acetate incorporation into the sterol fraction by intact cells of the miconazole-sensitive strain of *C. glabrata* (strain G4) and the resistant strains derived from it, particularly strain G4/M22, which had the highest degree of resistance to the drug. The incorporation of ^{14}C from radioactively labeled acetate into ergosterol was inhibited by miconazole at concentrations below those required to inhibit growth. On the other hand, in G4/M22, ergosterol biosynthesis was unaffected by the drug at concentrations of 3 μg/ml. An appreciable synthesis of ^{14}C-labeled ergosterol was observed even at a concentration of 30 μg/ml. These authors thus speculated that for strains G4/M22, at least, miconazole is prevented from reaching its targets in intact cells.

In an attempt to elucidate the primary cellular target for miconazole, Portillo and Gancedo (45) found that the mutation in a strain of *Saccharomyces cerevisiae*, which was resistant to the drug, was linked to a structural gene for a subunit of ATPase on mitochondrial DNA and that the drug inhibited the mitochondrial ATPase of the wild type, while the enzyme of the resistant mutant was not susceptible to this effect. In other words, the resistance was attributed to a mitochondrial gene mutation in subunit 9 of mitochondrial ATPase but not to an effect related to cytochrome P450. On the other hand, Kerridge et al. (32) reported that azole affected both mitochondrial functions and membrane biosynthesis. Mitochondrial ATPase and cytochrome oxidase in broken cell preparations from strain G4/M22 were remarkably inhibited by miconazole at concentrations lower than those required to inhibit oxygen uptake in vitro. Oxygen uptake was also inhibited in the miconazole-resistant strains, particularly strain G4/M22, by miconazole at concentrations similar to those required for inhibition of growth. On the basis of these results, Kerridge's group considered that azole resistance does not derive from a modification of cytochrome P450 sterol demethylase or mitochondrial ATPase and that in this respect, strain G4/M22 differs from a strain of *S. cerevisiae* where resistance was shown to be associated with a modification of the mitochondrial ATPase but not cytochrome P450 sterol demethylase, which had been reported by Portillo and Gancedo (44,45).

Watson et al. (46) showed that the mutation in the ketoconazole-resistant mutants of *S. cerevisiae* is nuclear in origin and allelic to *erg* 3, which gives rise to a block in the $\Delta^{5,6}$ desaturation step of ergosterol biosynthesis. They discussed the significance of this second site mutation at the point of inhibitory action of ketoconazole—that is, the P450-mediated ^{14}C demethylation of lanosterol. Kenna et al. (47) observed only slight increases in resistance to azoles under conditions that induced cytochrome P450 in several strains of *S. cerevisiae* from undetectable levels with strain variation. Two cytochrome P450-deficient mutants exhibited resistance to treatment with fluconazole and ketoconazole. They suggested that this effect could be attributed, at least in part, to an additional defect in sterol $\Delta^{5,6}$ desaturation and possibly to reduced cellular levels of azoles. Cytochrome P450-deficient mutants had already been reported (48,49). Kelly et al. (50) described two *S. cerevisiae* P450 mutant strains and showed them to be resistant to azole treatment. However, they found that this resistance was not associated with drastically reduced cellular levels of azole or with the alteration in the target enzyme but with a second sterol mutation in these strains in $\Delta^{5,6}$ desaturase, emphasizing that azole-resistant mutants were exclusively mutants in this latter sterol biosynthesis step. They suggested that it might be feasible to produce resistant enzymes through mutagenesis in vitro, which would have a lower affinity for azole and would indicate important domains and residues for azole/P450 interaction. Furthermore, they described, with two fluconazole-sensitive and less sensitive strains of *S. cerevisiae*, that the resistance level of transformants containing the episomal plasmid pEMBL Ye30 and the same plasmid with the *C. albicans* 14α-demethylase gene inserted. They thus stressed that *C. albicans* protein is overexpressed from this multicopy vector and that it can be placed in strains with undetectable or no levels of the corresponding *S. cerevisiae* protein.

Rine et al. (51) reported that the cloning of genes on a multicopy vector is capable of producing overexpression of the product of the cloned gene, leading to resistance to inhibitors of the gene product. Kirsch et al. (52) stated that a cloned sequence containing the structural gene of *C. albicans* for $P450_{14DM}$ produced increased levels of P450 and decreased susceptibility to econazole, ketoconazole, and fluconazole when present in multiple copies in *C. albicans* or *S. cerevisiae*. Overexpression of the *C. tropicalis* (53) or *S. cerevisiae* (54) P450 protein in *S. cerevisiae* was also proven to increase the cellular P450 content, resulting in a decrease in susceptibility to ketoconazole.

V. CONCLUSIONS AND DISCUSSION

Few or no reports have been published on antifungal-resistant isolates of fungi in the superficial mycoses of humans and animals upon topical application. Only in a few cases, griseofulvin-resistant isolates of dermatophytes and the therapeutic failures associated with the isolates having high MIC values have been described in cases where the antibiotic was administered orally but not applied topically (55), although griseofulvin has been used extensively for more than three decades. It is, however, significant that the spontaneous occurrence of resistant mutants of dermatophytes to this antibiotic have been observed (56). On the other hand, yeasts such as *C. albicans* and *C. glabrata*, which are responsible for systemic mycoses, appear to become resistant to antifungals in systemic application relatively more easily than do dermatophytes and other molds, as observed with flucytosine and even with ketoconazole or fluconazole, in particular, as therapeutic and prophylactic antifungals. Such differences in the occurrence of resistance to antifungals may depend on differences not only in routes of administration but also in the antifungal (static or cidal) activities themselves toward the target fungi, based on their chemical structure, distribution, and concentrations in tissues and body fluids, among other intrinsic factors.

In recent years, a variety of potential targets have been proposed for azole antifungals other than cytochrome P450 sterol methylase, which has been thought to be the primary target in their action mechanisms. This would make the analysis of the mechanisms of fungal resistance more complicated but would, in turn, provide important new findings in the mechanisms involved. In discussions on the mechanisms of fungal resistance, it is necessary to define precisely what is meant by fungal drug resistance. According to Kerridge et al. (32), a resistant fungus is one that will continue to grow and to produce clinical symptoms of disease in the presence of the drug at the maximum concentrations attainable at the site of infection. This view is considered pertinent from the clinical standpoint. The term *drug resistance* in itself may be defined more broadly, taking primary resistance in vitro and in vivo as well as other factors into consideration. In this sense, it would be important to consider the nature of resistance, as discussed on the nature of bacterial resistance, which occurs in two overall types, namely, "endogenous" resistance and "exogenous" or "positive-function" resistance (57).

This review has dealt with papers focusing on biochemical and genetic approaches to the analysis of azole resistance in yeasts, mainly *C. albicans* and *C. glabrata*, with reference to changes in susceptibility to drugs, cellular constituents, uptake of drugs, and essentials for growth, such as amino acids, permeability of the cell envelope, ergosterol biosynthesis, mitochondrial ATPase and other enzymes, gene mutation, and additional functions of resistant strains in comparison with susceptible strains. Some aspects, however, remain to be explored.

Resistance to some fungicides, for instance, benzimidazole compounds as well as pyrimidinemethanol compounds, has been demonstrated in *Aspergillus fumigatus, A. nidulans, Schizosaccharomyces pombe*, and other fungi. And the biochemical and genetic analysis of their resistance mechanism was well executed (58–60). For the purpose of reaching a comprehensive explanation of the resistance mechanisms of antifungals, including azoles, in human pathogenic fungi, comparative studies with agricultural fungicides and antibacterial agents are of paramount importance.

REFERENCES

1. Kerridge D. Antifungal drugs. Drugs Today 1988;24:705–715.
2. Iwata K. Drug resistance in human pathogenic fungi. Eur J Epidemiol 1992; 8:407–421.
3. Vanden Bossche H, Warnock DW, Dupont B, et al. Mechanisms and clinical impact of antifungal drug resistance. J Med Vet Mycol 1994;32(suppl 1): 189–202.
4. Atkinson GW, Israel HL. 5-Fluorocytosine treatment of meningeal and pulmonary aspergillosis. Am J Med 1973;55:496–504.
5. Block ER, Bennett JE. 5-Fluorocytosine resistance in Candida albicans infections in man. Am Rev Resp Dis 1974;109:723–724.
6. Tavitian A, Raufman J.-P, Rosenthal LE, et al. Ketoconazole-resistant Candida esophagitis in patients with acquired immunodeficiency syndrome. Gastroenterology 1986;90:443–445.

7. Willocks L, Leen CLS, Brettle RP, et al. Fluconazole resistance in AIDS patients. J Antimicrob Chemother 1991;28:937–939.
8. Kitchen VS, Savage M, Harris JRW. Candida albicans resistance in AIDS. J Infect 1991;22:204–205.
9. Dupouy-Camet J, Paugam A, Di Donato C, et al. Résistance au fluconazole en milieu hospitalier. Concordance entre la résistance de Candida albicans in vitro et l'échec thérapeutique. Presse Méd 1991;20:1341.
10. Dupont B. Antifungal therapy in AIDS patients. In: Bennett JE, Hay RJ, Peterson PK, eds. New Strategies in Fungal Disease. Edinburgh: Churchill Livingstone, 1992;290–300.
11. Holt RJ, Azmi A. A miconazole-resistant Candida. Lancet 1978;1:50–51.
12. Rosenblatt HM, Byrne W, Ament ME, et al. Successful treatment of chronic mucocutaneous candidiasis with ketoconazole. J Pediatr 1980;97:657–660.
13. Horsburgh CR, Kirkpatrick CH. Long-term therapy of chronic mucocutaneous candidiasis with ketoconazole: Experience with twenty-one patients. Am J Med 1983;74(suppl 1B):23–29.
14. Warnock DW, Johnson EM, Richardson MD, Vickers CFH. Modified response to ketoconazole of Candida albicans from a treatment failure. Lancet 1983;1:642–643.
15. Smith KJ, Warnock DW, Kennedy CTC, et al: J, Vanden Bossche H. Azole resistance in Candida albicans. J Med Vet Mycol 1986;24:133–144.
16. Hitchcock CA, Pye GW, Troke PF, et al. Fluconazole resistance in Candida glabrata. Antimicrob Agents Chemother 1993;37:1962–1965.
17. Marriott MS, Richardson K. The discovery and mode of action of fluconazole. In: Fromtling RA, ed. Resent Trends in the Discovery, Development and Evaluation of Antifungal Agents. Barcelona: Prous Science, 1987:81–92.
18. Nguyen MH, Yu VL, Morris AJ, et al. Fluconazole-resistant Candida parapsilosis isolated from candidemic patients receiving fluconazole prophylaxis. Abstr No F111. 95th ASM General Meeting, Washington, DC, May 21–25, 1995.
19. Vanden Bossche H. Biochemical targets for antifungal azole derivatives: Hypothesis on the mode of action. In: McGinnis MR, ed. Current Topics in Medical Mycology. Vol 1. New York: Springer-Verlag, 1985:313–315.
20. Yeagle PL, Martin RB, Lala AK, et al. Differential effects of cholesterol and lanosterol on artificial membranes. Proc Natl Acad Sci USA 1977;74: 4924–4926.
21. Hitchcock CA, Barrett-Bee KJ, Russel NJ. Inhibition of 14α-sterol demethylase activity in Candida albicans Darlington does not correlate with resistance to azole. J Med Vet Mycol 1987;25:329–333.
22. Uno J, Shigematsu ML, Arai T. Primary site of action of ketoconazole on Candida albicans. Antimicrob Agents Chemother 1982;21:912–918.
23. Barug D, Samson RA, Kerkenaar A. Microscopic studies of Candida albicans and Torulopsis glabrata after in vitro treatment with bifonazole: Light and scanning electron microscopy. Arzneim-Forsch 1983;33:528–537.
24. Shigematsu ML, Uno J, Arai T. Effect of ketoconazole on isolated mito-

chondoria from Candida albicans. Antimicrob Agents Chemother 1982;21: 919–924.
25. Sud IJ, Feingold DS. Heterogeneity of action mechanisms among antimycotic imidazoles. Antimicrob Agents Chemother 1981;20:71–74.
26. Plempel M, Bartmann K. Experimental studies on the antimycotic action of clotrimazole (Canesten) in vitro and after local application in vivo. Drugs Germ 1972;15:103–120.
27. Holt RJ, Newman RL. Laboratory assessment of the antimycotic drug clotrimazole. J Clin Pathol 1972;25:1089–1097.
28. Waitz JA, Moss EC, Weinstein MJ. Chemotherapeutic evaluation of clotrimazole. Appl Microbiol 1971;22:891–894.
29. Holt RJ. Recent developments in antimycotic chemotherapy. Infection 1974; 2:95–107.
30. Iwata K, Yamashita T, Ohsumi M, et al. Comparative morphological and biological studies on the itraconazole- and ketoconazole-resistant mutants of Cryptococcus neoformans. J Med Vet Mycol 1990;28:77–90.
31. Kerridge D, Nicholas RO. Drug resistance in the opportunistic pathogens Candida albicans and Candida glabrata. J Antimicrob Chemother 1986; 18(suppl B):39–49.
32. Kerridge D, Fasoli M, Wayman FJ. Drug resistance in Candida albicans and Candida glabrata. Ann NY Acad Sci 1988;544:245–259.
33. Nicholas RO, Burton JA, Kerridge D, Wayman FJ. Isolation of mutants of Candida glabrata resistant to miconazole. Crit Rev Microbiol 1987;15: 103–110.
34. Nobre G, Mendes E, Charrua MJ, Cruz O. Ketconazole resistance in Torulopsis glabrata. Mycopathologia 1989;107:51–55.
35. Hughes CE, Bennett RL, Tuna IC, Beggs WH. Activities of fluconazole (UK 49,858) and ketoconazole against ketoconazole-susceptible and -resistant Candida albicans. Antimicrob Agents Chemother 1988;32:209–212.
36. Vanden Bossche H, Marichal P, Odds FC, et al. Characterization of an azole-resistant Candida glabrata isolate. Antimicrob Agents Chemother 1992;36: 2602–2610.
37. Howell SA, Mallet AI, Noble WC. A comparison of the sterol content of multiple isolates of the Candida albicans Darlington strain with other clinically azole-sensitive and -resistant strains. J App Bacteriol 1990;69:692–696.
38. Vanden Bossche H, Marichal P, Gorrens J, et al. Mutation in cytochrome P-450-dependent 14α-demethylase results in decreased affinity for azole antifungals. Biochem Soc Trans 1990;18:56–59.
39. Vanden Bossche H, Marichal P, Gorrens J, et al. Interaction of azole derivatives with cytochrome P-450 isozymes in yeast, fungi, plants and mammalian cells. Pest Sci 1987;21:289–306.
40. Hitchcock CA, Barrett-Bee KJ, Russell NJ. The lipid composition and permeability to azole of an azole- and polyene-resistant mutant of Candida albicans. J Med Vet Mycol 1986;25:29–37.
41. Hitchcock CA, Barrett-Bee KJ, Russell NJ. The lipid composition of azole-

sensitive and azole-resistant strains of Candida albicans. J Gen Microbiol 1986;132:2421–2431.
42. Gale EF, Johnson AM, Kerridge D, Wayman FJ. Phenotypic resistance to miconazole and amphotericin B in Candida albicans. J Gen Microbiol 1980; 117:535–538.
43. Ryley JF, Wilson RG, Barrett-Bee KJ. Azole resistance in Candida albicans. Sabouraudia 1984;22:53–63.
44. Portillo F, Gancedo C. Mode of action of miconazole on yeasts: Inhibition of the mitochondrial ATPase. Eur J Biochem 1984;143:273–276.
45. Portillo F, Gancedo C. Mitochondrial resistance to miconazole in Saccharomyces cerevisiae. Mol Gen Genet 1985;199:495–499.
46. Watson PF, Rose ME, Kelly SL. Isolation and analysis of ketoconazole resistant mutants of Saccharomyces cerevisiae. J Med Vet Mycol 1988;26: 153–162.
47. Kenna S, Bligh HFJ, Watson PF, Kelly SL. Genetic and physiological analysis of azole sensitivity in Saccharomyces cerevisiae. J Med Vet Mycol 1989; 27:397–406.
48. Aoyama Y, Yoshida Y, Hata S, et al. Altered cytochrome P-450 in a yeast mutant blocked in demethylating C-32 of lanosterol. J Biol Chem 1983;258: 9040–9042.
49. King DJ, Wiseman A, Kelly DE, Kelly SL. Differences in the cytochrome P-450 enzymes of sterol C-14 demethylase mutants of Saccharomyces cerevisiae. Curr Genet 1985;10:261–267.
50. Kelly SL, Rowe J, Watson PF. Molecular genetic studies on the mode of action of azole antifungal agents. Biochem Soc Trans 1991;19:796–798.
51. Rine J, Hansen W, Hardeman E, Davis RW. Targeted selection of recombinant clones through gene dosage effects. Proc Natl Acad Sci USA 1983;80: 6750–6754.
52. Kirsch DR, Lai MH, O'Sullivan J. Isolation of the gene for cytochrome P450L1A1 (lanosterol 14α-demethylase) from Candida albicans. Gene 1988; 68:229–237.
53. Chen C, Turi TG, Sanglard D, Loper JC. Isolation of Candida tropicalis gene for P450 lanosterol demethylase and its expression in Saccharomyces cerevisiae. Biochem Biophys Res Commun 1987;146:1311–1317.
54. Kalb VF, Loper JC, Dey CR, et al. Isolation of a cytochrome P-450 structural gene from Saccharomyces cerevisiae. Gene 1986;45:237–245.
55. Michaelides P, Rosenthal SA, Sulzberger MB, Witten VR. Trichophyton tonsurans infection resistant to griseofulvin: A case demonstrating clinical and in vitro resistance. Arch Dermatol 1961;83:988–990.
56. Lenhart K. Griseofulvin-resistant mutants in dermatophytes: II. Physiological and genetic studies. Mykosen 1970;13:139–144.
57. Silver LL, Bostian KA. Discovery and development of new antibiotics: the problem of antibiotic resistance. Antimicrob Agents Chemother 1993;37: 377–383.
58. Van Tuyl JM. Genetic aspects of acquired resistance to benomyl and thiaben-

dazole in a number of fungi. Med Fac Landbouww Rijksuniv Gent 1975;40: 691–697.

59. Yamamoto M. Genetic analysis of resistant mutants to antimitotic benzimidazole compounds in Schizosaccharomyces pombe. Molec Gen Genet 1980; 180:231–234.
60. de Waard MA, Van Nistelrooy JGM. An energy-dependent efflux mechanism for fenarimol in a wild type and fenarimol resistant mutants of Aspergillus nidulans. Pest Biochem Physiol 1980;13:255–266.

30

Azole Drug Resistance as a Cause of Treatment Failure in Patients with Candidosis

DAVID W. WARNOCK and ELIZABETH M. JOHNSON
Public Health Laboratory
Bristol, England

I. INTRODUCTION

Candida albicans is found in the mouth and gastrointestinal tract of a significant proportion of the normal human population. This opportunistic pathogen can cause deep-seated infection, which may be localized or disseminated, but it is more often seen causing mucosal or cutaneous infection. Oral candidosis is a significant problem in patients undergoing treatment for cancer or organ transplantation and is one of the most common and persistent conditions encountered in individuals with human immunodeficiency virus (HIV) infection and acquired immunodeficiency syndrome (AIDS). Although *C. albicans* remains the predominant cause of all forms of human candidosis, *C. tropicalis* has emerged as an important pathogen in granulocytopenic patients, and *C. parapsilosis* infection is common in individuals receiving parenteral nutrition. Other *Candida* species, such as *C. krusei* and *C. lusitaniae,* have also been recognized as significant human pathogens.

Imidazole and triazole compounds are among the most useful drugs for the treatment of human candidosis. These compounds inhibit the cytochrome P450-dependent 14-α-sterol demethylation step in the formation of ergosterol, the principal sterol in the membrane of susceptible fungal cells. The consequent depletion of ergosterol and accumulation of methylated sterols leads to disruption of membrane structure and function (1). The earliest members of this large group of drugs, clotrimazole and miconazole, are useful for the topical treatment of superficial forms of candidosis, and this has remained the case for most of the similar imidazole compounds that have appeared since. However, some more recent compounds, such as the imidazole ketoconazole and the triazoles fluconazole and itraconazole, are effective after oral administration and can be used to treat both superficial and deep-seated infections.

Acquired drug resistance has long been identified as a major cause of treatment failure and relapse among patients with candidosis treated with flucytosine (2). In contrast, resistance to imidazole and triazole compounds has been regarded as an uncommon clinical problem, and other factors have been held to account for treatment failure or relapse. These include poor compliance with the treatment regimen, inadequate dosage or length of treatment, and drug interactions. However, recent reports of failures of azole treatment in patients with candidosis have given rise to increased concern about drug resistance. Acquisition of resistance to azole compounds has been recorded with several organisms, in particular *C. albicans,* in situations where the drugs have been given for long periods of time in the face of persistent infection. This is not a new problem but one that appears to be increasing in prevalence and importance. Another source of concern arising from the widespread use of triazole compounds as prophylactic and therapeutic agents in granulocytopenic patients has been an apparent increase in the number of infections due to less common organisms, such as *Torulopsis glabrata* (now reclassified as *C. glabrata*) and *C. krusei,* which appear to possess intrinsic resistance to particular azole compounds.

II. IN VITRO TESTING OF ANTIFUNGAL DRUGS

As with antibacterial compounds, tests designed to ascertain the minimum amount of drug needed to inhibit the growth of fungal strains in culture (the minimum inhibitory concentration, or MIC) are often used to determine the relative effectiveness of different azole compounds and to detect drug-resistant strains. One of the most popular methods is macrobroth dilution, but microbroth and agar dilution methods are also used. There are no defined standards to distinguish drug-resistant strains, but it is often assumed that strains possessing much higher MICs for a particular compound or group of compounds than other strains of the same organism, tested under similar conditions, can be regarded as resistant. The usefulness of this artificial distinction depends in major part on the extent of the correlation between MIC test results and clinical outcome.

There have been numerous attempts to assess the extent of the correlation between in vitro tests with azole antifungal drugs and the results of their administration in animal models of infection. Some have found a correlation (3–5) but others have not (6,7). Stiller et al. (8), using an animal model of candidosis, demonstrated that even with flucytosine, where there is a good general correlation, it is not possible to make individual predictions of in vivo outcome based upon in vitro findings. With ketoconazole, Polak et al. (6) found there was at best a poor correlation between tests in vitro and results in an animal model of candidosis. In contrast, in tests with fluconazole, Anaissie et al. (5) demonstrated a significant correlation between microbroth dilution MICs and outcome in mice infected with *C. albicans, C. lusitaniae,* or *C. krusei* strains.

In addition, there are several reports of strains of *C. albicans* from patients with chronic mucocutaneous candidosis (CMC) who relapsed following treatment with ketoconazole; these organisms were found to have high MICs in tests in vitro and were also found to be resistant to azole compounds in animal models of infection (9,10). More recent reports have demonstrated a definite correlation between clinical failure and the results of in vitro tests with ketoconazole and fluconazole for azole-resistant strains of *C. albicans* from AIDS patients with oral or esophageal candidosis (11).

The poor correlation that has sometimes been noted between in vitro tests and the clinical results of treatment with azole antifungal drugs has been due, at least in part, to the tremendous variation in MICs obtained under different test conditions (12). It is clear that the results are influenced by a number of technical factors, including the concentration of the fungal inoculum, the composition and pH of the medium, the incubation temperature, and the length of incubation (13–15). Another problem encountered with azole compounds results from the fact that these drugs often cause partial inhibition of growth over a wide range of concentrations, making visual determinations of endpoints in MIC tests difficult (16,17).

In the past, most laboratories with an interest in antifungal drug testing developed their own methods of MIC determination; there was considerable variation between them in the manner in which tests were performed and the results produced (12). In 1992 the U.S. National Committee for Clinical Laboratory Standards (NCCLS) published a proposed reference method for antifungal drug susceptibility testing with which other methods could be compared (18). As a result, MIC determinations with imidazole and triazole compounds can now be performed with greater confidence. However, because the conditions under which the tests are performed can have such a marked effect on the results obtained, a high MIC on its own is less than proof that treatment failure or relapse is due to drug resistance. Much more convincing is the demonstration that the MIC for the most recent strain is higher than that for strains obtained earlier during treatment (provided that identical test methods have been used). These latter reports provide much more credible evidence for emergent drug resistance.

III. EMERGENCE OF RESISTANCE

It is not surprising that initial reports of treatment failure attributable to the development of resistance to imidazole antifungal drugs were disputed, given the extent to which the results of MIC determinations with these compounds depend on the conditions under which the tests are done. In 1978 Holt and Azmi (19) described a strain of *C. albicans* resistant to miconazole (and cross-resistant to other imidazoles) recovered from an infant who had received oral treatment with this drug for 2 months. The MIC prior to treatment had been 100-fold lower. No further tests were performed on these strains and this initial report was never confirmed.

A. Ketoconazole

As the first oral imidazole compound to be introduced, ketoconazole altered the management of a number of different forms of fungal infection. It resulted in a dramatic improvement in the management of patients with chronic mucocutaneous candidosis, an uncommon condition that is often associated with congenital endocrinological and immunological defects. However, long-term treatment with ketoconazole was required if remission of infection was to be achieved and sustained; as might have been anticipated, this form of management soon led to reports of treatment failure or relapse due the apparent development of drug resistance. Rosenblatt et al. (20) were the first to mention such a case. Three more cases were reported in 1983 (21,22) and a fifth in 1986 (10).

Horsburgh et al. (21) reported the isolation of resistant strains of *C. albicans* from two patients with chronic mucocutaneous candidosis who had relapsed following prolonged treatment with ketoconazole. Although, much higher MICs were obtained with these strains than had been recorded for strains of *C. albicans* isolated at the beginning of treatment, the suggestion that resistance had developed was at first disputed on the grounds that different methods of MIC testing had been used to assess the strains obtained at the beginning and end of treatment (23). However, extensive testing of these strains of *C. albicans* and those from two other cases (10,22) has confirmed them as being much less susceptible to ketoconazole in vitro than other strains of this organism (9,10,14,24,25). These strains are also cross-resistant to a range of other azole drugs both in vitro (9,10,14,24,25) and in animal models of infection (9,10).

Until 1986, published accounts of acquired resistance to ketoconazole in *C. albicans* were confined to a small number of patients receiving long-term treatment for chronic mucocutaneous candidosis. Although it is probable that these reports represent a small number of instances of a more widespread phenomenon, it appears that the global clinical significance of the resistance phenomenon is not large. Moreover, no reports of emergent resistance to ketoconazole in *C. albicans* associated with courses of treatment lasting less than several months have been published.

Oral candidosis is one of the most common conditions encountered in patients with HIV infection, developing in over 80% of these individuals at some time during their illness. In noncompromised patients, this infection can often be eradicated with a short course of topical or oral treatment with an azole compound. However, because of the profound and sustained immunosuppression in patients with AIDS, persistent or recurrent oral infection with *C. albicans* is common and long courses of antifungal treatment are required if remission from infection is to be achieved and sustained. Oral ketoconazole has been used, but treatment failure and relapse have been reported. In most cases, this was associated with malabsorption of the drug, but in others drug resistance was suggested to be the cause (26).

B. Fluconazole

The triazole compound fluconazole has proved an effective, well-tolerated treatment for a wide range of mucosal and deep-seated forms of candidosis. It is more reliably absorbed than ketoconazole after oral administration and has been shown to be more effective in controlling oral candidosis in individuals with HIV infection (27). However, one consequence of the widespread use of fluconazole in these patients is that since 1991, numerous reports of apparent resistance to this compound have been published, almost all of which have concerned individuals with persistent oral or esophageal infection with *C. albicans*.

In most reported cases of fluconazole resistance in patients with AIDS, the individuals affected had low CD4 counts and were approaching the final stage of their illness (28–42). Many had received prior treatment with topical imidazoles or oral ketoconazole and had then been given repeated courses of low-dose treatment with fluconazole. For instance, Redding et al. (39) described a patient who responded to treatment with fluconazole (at a dosage of 100 mg) during nine episodes of oral candidosis. During these episodes, the MIC of the infecting strain of *C. albicans* rose from 0.25 to 8 mg/L. The MIC of the infecting strain continued to rise during five subsequent episodes of oral candidosis, but the patient responded to higher dosages of fluconazole (200, 400, and then 800 mg). However, after more than 2 years of successful treatment with fluconazole, the fifteenth episode of oral candidosis failed to respond to 800 mg of the compound and the patient required parenteral treatment with amphotericin B. The MIC of fluconazole for the infecting strain was >64 mg/L. Other authors have described a similar pattern of resistance development, with a gradual rise in MIC of the infecting *C. albicans* strain, and a period during which patients still respond to higher dosage treatment with fluconazole [30,31,35,40–42].

Molecular typing methods have demonstrated that there are two mechanisms by which these patients acquire their azole-drug-resistant strains of *C. albicans*. In some individuals, the original susceptible strain becomes resistant [31,39,41,43]. In others, a new resistant strain is acquired during treatment (31,38,41). Molecular typing has also demonstrated that transmission of strains between HIV-positive partners can occur (41,44), but it remains unclear whether azole-resistant strains of *C. albicans* persist if they are transmitted to noncompromised HIV-negative individuals.

Acquisition of drug-resistant strains of *C. albicans* does not appear to be a problem in clinical settings other than long-term treatment of AIDS patients with oral or esophageal candidosis. To date, there have been no verified reports of resistant *C. albicans* strains emerging during short-term treatment with fluconazole in patients with mucosal or deep-seated forms of candidosis. In vitro testing has demonstrated that most strains of *C. krusei* have much higher MICs for fluconazole than do *C. albicans* strains (45). It is therefore perhaps not surprising that there have been reports of patients developing infections with this organism while receiving prophylactic treatment with this drug (46,47) and of individuals with mucosal or deep-seated *C. krusei* infection who failed to respond to fluconazole (48–50).

Two case reports have appeared in which persistent *C. glabrata* funguria was associated with the rapid development of fluconazole resistance (51,52). In both cases, pre- and posttreatment strains were available for comparison. Unlike *C. albicans,* which has a diploid genome, *C. glabrata* is haploid, which favors the development of point mutations, some of which might confer resistance to azole antifungals (53). In one reported case (51), a 30-fold rise in MIC of fluconazole was recorded following 9 days of oral treatment. The pre- and posttreatment strains were found to be similar by restriction fragment length polymorphism (RFLP) analysis, suggesting the development of drug-resistant mutants during treatment

(54). In a second case (52), comparison of the pre- and posttreatment *C. glabrata* strains, using RFLP analysis, showed that the strains were unrelated. This suggests that the resistant organism was not a mutant derived from the susceptible strain but rather that it was selected from a mixed population of both strains as a result of the drug treatment. There have also been reports describing the failure of fluconazole treatment to suppress vaginal infection with *C. glabrata* (55,56), and it is recommended that the drug should not be used to treat this organism.

C. Itraconazole

There have been no verified reports of resistant strains of *C. albicans* developing during treatment with the triazole compound itraconazole. It is possible that this is simply a reflection of drug usage, because itraconazole has been used to treat fewer patients with mucosal forms of candidosis than has fluconazole. It is also possible, although it remains to be established, that itraconazole has a lower potential than fluconazole to induce the development of drug-resistant strains of *C. albicans*. It is interesting that tests on large numbers of fluconazole-resistant strains of *C. albicans* recovered from AIDS patients have demonstrated that fewer than 20% are cross-resistant to itraconazole in vitro (45) (see below). Tests in vitro have also indicated that, unlike fluconazole, itraconazole has similar MICs for strains of *C. albicans* and *C. krusei* (45). This suggests that the pathogen shift observed in granulocytopenic patients following prophylactic treatment with fluconazole (46) should not occur with itraconazole.

IV. MECHANISMS OF RESISTANCE

Imidazole and triazole compounds inhibit the 14-α-sterol demethylation step in the conversion of lanosterol to ergosterol (1). This leads to accumulation of methylated sterols with concomitant disruption of fungal cell membrane structure and function. Three distinct mechanisms of resistance to azole compounds have so far been described. One involves reduced intracellular drug accumulation. This has been demonstrated in two azole-resistant *C. albicans* strains from patients with chronic mucocutaneous candidosis (9,57,58) and in a strain of *C. glabrata* (54). The second mechanism, described for one azole-resistant *C. albicans* strain, is an alteration in the 14-α-demethylase enzyme that results in its decreased binding to azole drugs (59). This permits the organism to circumvent the azole-induced inhibition of ergosterol biosynthesis. The third mechanism is overproduction of the sterol 14-α demethylase; this has been found in one azole-resistant strain of *C. glabrata* (54).

The drug-resistant strains of *C. albicans* recovered from patients with chronic mucocutaneous candidosis who relapsed following long-term treatment with ketoconazole were also found to be resistant to other imidazole and triazole antifungal compounds in vitro (9,10,14,24,25). In contrast, recent reports have suggested that a significant number of fluconazole-resistant *C. albicans* strains from patients with AIDS are not cross-resistant in vitro to ketoconazole (42) or itraconazole (36,40,60,61). The present authors found that only 28 (17.5%) of 160 *C. albicans* strains classified as resistant to fluconazole were cross-resistant to itraconazole. In contrast, none of 28 *C. albicans* strains that were resistant to itraconazole in vitro were susceptible to fluconazole (45). These in vitro observations of apparent drug-specific resistance could help to explain those documented cases in patients with AIDS where treatment with other azoles has proved successful in oral *C. albicans* infections that had failed to respond to fluconazole (40,61).

Although their mechanism of action is identical, itraconazole and fluconazole differ in a number of important respects, and this may help to account for published reports of apparent drug-specific resistance. Itraconazole is a lipophilic compound, while fluconazole is hydrophilic, and this could affect their transport across fungal cell membranes. Differential intracellular accumulation of itraconazole and fluconazole has been demonstrated in fluconazole-resistant strains of *C. albicans, C. glabrata,* and *C. krusei* (54,62), although it is not clear whether the reduced accumulation of fluconazole is due to decreased uptake or increased outflow of the drug. Although reduced accumulation could account for drug-specific resistance, it remains to be established to what extent strains that exhibit this phenomenon occur in different patient groups.

V. CONCLUSIONS

Treatment failure among patients with candidosis, attributable to the development of azole-drug-resistant strains of *C. albicans,* appears to be becoming more common but still seems to be confined to individuals receiving long-term treatment. In view of the increasing number of patients requiring this form of management and the apparent potential of such treatment to select for resistance, it is becoming more important to investigate the effects of different therapeutic regimens. Although fluconazole has been implicated in instances of acquired resistance more often than ketoconazole and ketoconazole more often than itraconazole, it must not be assumed that the development of fluconazole resistance among *C. albicans* strains is a characteristic of this particular drug that is not shared with other azole compounds. Until proved otherwise, it must be regarded as an almost inevitable consequence of prolonged drug use. It is also apparent that even short courses of treatment can lead to the selection of organisms, such as *C. krusei,* that possess intrinsic resistance to particular azole compounds. This problem highlights the need for accurate speciation of organisms before deciding on treatment.

If treatment failure or relapse occurs during a course of treatment with an azole compound, a number of factors should be considered. First, cultures should be obtained to establish whether the diagnosis of fungal infection is correct. If this is confirmed, it is important to ascertain whether or not adequate drug concentrations are being achieved. Potential drug interactions should be investigated, because it is well recognized that serum concentrations of itraconazole and ketoconazole are reduced following concomitant administration of H2 antagonists or rifampin. If none of these factors are implicated, the infecting organism should be identified and MIC tests performed. If earlier strains are available for comparison, these should also be tested.

Management of oral candidosis in AIDS patients from whom fluconazole-resistant strains of *C. albicans* have been isolated is difficult. In the first instance, higher dosages of fluconazole (up to 800 mg) should be tried. If this is unsuccessful, itraconazole can be prescribed, as this has sometimes been found to be effective in patients who had earlier failed to respond to fluconazole (40). However, it is not unreasonable to expect these patients to need higher than usual dosages of itraconazole. Administration of an oral solution formulation of itraconazole has proved successful in AIDS patients with oral or esophageal candidosis that had failed to respond to fluconazole, ketoconazole, or the capsule formulation of itraconazole (63). This may reflect the improved absorption of the solution or an additional topical effect. As a last resort, patients with unresponsive azole-resistant oral or esophageal candidosis can often be managed with parenteral amphotericin B.

REFERENCES

1. Vanden Bossche H. Biochemical targets for antifungal azole derivatives: hypothesis on the mode of action. In: McGinnis MR, ed. Current Topics in Medical Mycology. Vol. 1. New York: Springer-Verlag, 1985;313–351.
2. Scholer H, Polak A. Resistance to systemic antifungal agents. In: Bryan LE, ed. Antimicrobial Drug Resistance. Orlando, FL: Academic Press, 1984; 393–460.
3. McIntyre KA, Galgiani JN. In vitro susceptibilities of yeasts to a new antifungal triazole, SCH 39304: Effect of test conditions and relation to in vivo efficacy. Antimicrob Agents Chemother 1989;33:1095–1100.

4. Velez JD, Allendoerfer R, Luther M, et al. Correlation of in vitro azole susceptibility with in vivo response in a murine model of cryptococcal meningitis. J Infect Dis 1993;168:508–510.
5. Anaissie EJ, Karyotakis NC, Hachem R, et al. Correlation between in vitro and in vivo activity of antifungal agents against *Candida* species. J Infect Dis 1994;170:384–389.
6. Polak A, Odds FC, Ludin E, Scholer HJ. Correlation of susceptibility test results in vitro with response in vivo: Ketoconazole therapy in a systemic candidiasis model. Chemotherapy 1985;31:395–404.
7. Fisher MA, Shen S-H, Haddad J, Tarry WF. Comparison of in vivo activity of fluconazole with that of amphotericin B against *Candida tropicalis*, *Candida glabrata*, and *Candida krusei*. Antimicrob Agents Chemother 1989;33: 1443–1446.
8. Stiller RL, Bennett JE, Scholer HJ, et al. Correlation of in vitro susceptibility test results with in vivo response: Flucytosine therapy in a systemic candidiasis model. J Infect Dis 1983;147:1070–1077.
9. Ryley JF, Wilson RG, Barrett-Bee KJ. Azole resistance in *Candida albicans*. Sabouraudia 1984;22:53–63.
10. Smith KJ, Warnock DW, Kennedy CTC, et al. Azole resistance in *Candida albicans*. J Med Vet Mycol 1986;24:133–144.
11. Rodriguez-Tudela JL, Martinez-Suarez JV, Dronda F, et al. Correlation of in vitro susceptibility test results with clinical response: A study of azole therapy in AIDS patients. J Antimicrob Chemother 1995;35:793–804.
12. Galgiani JN, Reiser J, Brass C, et al. Comparison of relative susceptibilities of *Candida* species to three antifungal agents as determined by unstandardized methods. Antimicrob Agents Chemother 1987;31:1343–1347.
13. Odds FC. Laboratory evaluation of antifungal agents: A comparative study of five imidazole derivatives of clinical importance. J Antimicrob Chemother 1980;6:749–761.
14. Johnson EM, Richardson MD, Warnock DW. In vitro resistance to imidazole antifungals in *Candida albicans*. J Antimicrob Chemother 1984;13:547–558.
15. Doern GV, Tubert TA, Chapin K, Rinaldi MG. Effect of medium composition on results of macrobroth dilution antifungal susceptibility testing of yeasts. J Clin Microbiol 1986;24:507–511.
16. Odds FC. Interactions among amphotericin B, 5-fluorocytosine, ketoconazole and miconazole against pathogenic fungi in vitro. Antimicrob Agents Chemother 1982;22:763–770.
17. Fromtling RA, Yu HP, Shadomy S. In-vitro inhibitory activities of 2 new orally absorbable imidazole derivatives: BAY n 7133 and BAY I 9193. Sabouraudia 1983;21:179–184.
18. National Committee for Clinical Laboratory Standards. Reference Method for Broth Dilution Antifungal Susceptibility Testing of Yeasts: Proposed Standard M27-P. Villanova, PA: NCCLS, 1992.
19. Holt RJ, Azmi A. Miconazole-resistant Candida. Lancet 1978;1:50.
20. Rosenblatt HM, Byrne W, Ament ME, et al. Successful treatment of chronic mucocutaneous candidiasis with ketoconazole. J Pediatr 1980;97:657–660.

21. Horsburgh CR, Kirkpatrick CH. Long-term therapy of chronic mucocutaneous candidiasis with ketoconazole: Experience with twenty-one patients. Am J Med 1983;74(suppl 1B):23–29.
22. Warnock DW, Johnson EM, Richardson MD, Vickers CFH. Modified response to ketoconazole of *Candida albicans* from a treatment failure. Lancet 1983;1:642–643.
23. Levine HB. Resistance to ketoconazole. Lancet 1982;2:211.
24. Rogers TE, Galgiani JN. Activity of fluconazole (UK 49,858) and ketoconazole against *Candida albicans* in vitro and in vivo. Antimicrob Agents Chemother 1986;30:418–422.
25. Hughes CE, Bennett RL, Tuna IC, Beggs WH. Activities of fluconazole (UK 49,858) and ketoconazole against ketoconazole-susceptible and -resistant *Candida albicans*. Antimicrob Agents Chemother 1988;32:209–212.
26. Tavitian A, Raufman JP, Rosenthal LE, et al. Ketoconazole-resistant Candida esophagitis in patients with acquired immunodeficiency syndrome. Gastroenterology 1986;90:443–445.
27. De Wit S, Weerts D, Goossens H, Clumeck N. Comparison of fluconazole and ketoconazole for oropharyngeal candidiasis in AIDS. Lancet 1989;1: 746–748.
28. Dupouy-Camet J, Paugam A, Di Donato C, et al. Resistance au fluconazole en milieu hospitalier: Concordance entre la resistance de *Candida albicans* in vitro et l'echec therapeutique. Presse Med 1991;20:1341.
29. Willcocks L, Leen CLS, Brettle RP, et al. Fluconazole resistance in AIDS patients. J Antimicrob Chemother 1991;28:937–939.
30. Barchiesi F, Giacometti A, Arzeni D, et al. Fluconazole and ketoconazole in the treatment of oral and oesophageal candidiasis in AIDS patients. J Chemother 1992;4:381–386.
31. Bart-Delabesse E, Boiron P, Carlotti A, Dupont B. *Candida albicans* genotyping in studies with patients with AIDS developing resistance to fluconazole. J Clin Microbiol 1993;31:2933–2937.
32. Boken DJ, Swindells S, Rinaldi MG. Fluconazole-resistant *Candida albicans*. Clin Infect Dis 1993;17:1018–1021.
33. Cameron ML, Schell WA, Bruch S, et al. Correlation of in vitro fluconazole resistance of Candida isolates in relation to therapy and symptoms of individuals seropositive for human immunodeficiency virus type 1. Antimicrob Agents Chemother 1993;37:2449–2453.
34. Heinec GS, Stevens DA, Greenspan D, et al. Fluconazole-resistant Candida in AIDS patients: Report of two cases. Oral Surg Oral Med Oral Pathol 1993; 76:711–715.
35. Troillet N, Durussel C, Bille J, et al. Correlation between in vitro susceptibility of *Candida albicans* and fluconazole-resistant oropharyngeal candidiasis in HIV-infected patients. Eur J Clin Microbiol Infect Dis 1993;12:911–915.
36. Baily GG, Perry FM, Denning DW, Mandal BK. Fluconazole-resistant candidosis in an HIV cohort. AIDS 1994;8:787–792.
37. Newman SL, Flanigan TP, Fisher A, et al. Clinically significant mucosal

candidosis resistant to fluconazole treatment in patients with AIDS. Clin Infect Dis 1994;19:684–686.
38. Pfaller MA, Rhine-Chalberg J, Redding SW, et al. Variations in fluconazole susceptibility and electrophoretic karyotype among oral isolates of *Candida albicans* from patients with AIDS and oral candidiasis. J Clin Microbiol 1994; 32:59–64.
39. Redding S, Smith J, Farinacci G, et al. Resistance of *Candida albicans* to fluconazole during treatment of oropharyngeal candidiasis in a patient with AIDS: Documentation by in vitro susceptibility testing and DNA subtype analysis. Clin Infect Dis 1994;18:240–242.
40. Ruhnke M, Eigler A, Tennagen I, et al. Emergence of fluconazole-resistant strains of *Candida albicans* in patients with recurrent oropharyngeal candidosis and human immunodeficiency virus infection. J Clin Microbiol 1994; 32:2092–2098.
41. Sangeorzan JA, Bradley SF, He X, et al. Epidemiology of oral candidiasis in HIV-infected patients: Colonization, infection, treatment, and emergence of fluconazole resistance. Am J Med 1994;97:339–346.
42. Johnson EM, Warnock DW, Luker J, et al. Emergence of azole drug resistance in *Candida* species from HIV-infected patients receiving prolonged therapy for oral candidosis. J Antimicrob Chemother 1995;35:103–114.
43. Millon L, Manteaux A, Reboux G, et al. Fluconazole-resistant recurrent oral candidiasis in human immunodeficiency virus-positive patients: Persistence of *Candida albicans* strains with the same genotype. J Clin Microbiol 1994; 32:1115–1118.
44. Boerlin P, Addo M, Boerlin-Petzold F, et al. Transmission of oral *Candida albicans* strains between HIV-positive patients. Lancet 1995;345:1052–1053.
45. Johnson EM, Davey KG, Szekely A, Warnock DW. Itraconazole susceptibilities of fluconazole-susceptible and -resistant isolates of five *Candida* species. J Antimicrob Chemother 1995;36. In press.
46. Wingard JR, Merz WG, Rinaldi MG, et al. Increase in *Candida krusei* infection among patients with bone marrow transplantation and neutropenia treated prophylactically with fluconazole. N Engl J Med 1991;325:1274–1277.
47. Casasnovas R-O, Caillot D, Solary E, et al. Prophylactic fluconazole and *Candida krusei* infection. N Engl J Med 1992;326:891–892.
48. Akova M, Akalin HE, Uzun O, Gur D. Emergence of *Candida krusei* infections after therapy of oropharyngeal candidiasis with fluconazole. Eur J Clin Microbiol Infect Dis 1991;10:598–599.
49. McIlroy MA. Failure of fluconazole to suppress fungemia in a patient with fever, neutropenia and typhlitis. J Infect Dis 1991;163:420–421.
50. Roder BL, Sonnenschein C, Hartzen SH. Failure of fluconazole therapy in *Candida krusei* fungemia. Eur J Clin Microbiol Infect Dis 1991;10:173.
51. Warnock DW, Burke J, Cope NJ, Johnson EM, von Fraunhofer NA, Williams EW. Fluconazole resistance in *Candida glabrata*. Lancet 1988;2:1310.
52. Hitchcock CA, Pye GW, Troke PF, et al. Fluconazole resistance in *Candida glabrata*. Antimicrob Agents Chemother 1993;37:1962–1965.

53. Kerridge D, Nicholas RO. Drug resistance in the opportunistic pathogens *Candida albicans* and *Candida glabrata*. J Antimicrob Chemother 1986; 18(suppl B):39–49.
54. Vanden Bossche H, Marichal P, Odds FC, et al. Characterization of an azole-resistant *Candida glabrata* isolate. Antimicrob Agents Chemother 1992;36: 2602–2610.
55. Arilla MC, Carbonero JL, Schneider J, et al. Vulvovaginal candidiasis refractory to treatment with fluconazole. Eur J Obstet Gynecol Reprod Biol 1992; 44:77–80.
56. White DJ, Johnson EM, Warnock DW. Management of persistent vulvovaginal candidosis due to azole-resistant *Candida glabrata*. Genitourin Med 1993; 69:112–114.
57. Hitchcock CA, Barrett-Bee KJ, Russell NJ. The lipid composition of azole-sensitive and azole-resistant strains of *Candida albicans*. J Gen Microbiol 1986;132:2421–2431.
58. Hitchcock CA, Barrett-Bee KJ, Russell NJ. The lipid composition and permeability to azole of an azole- and polyene-resistant mutant of *Candida albicans*. J Med Vet Mycol 1987;25:29–37.
59. Vanden Bossche H, Marichal P, Gorrens J, et al. Mutation in cytochrome P-450-dependent 14 alpha-demethylase results in decreased affinity for azole antifungals. Biochem Soc Trans 1990;18:56–59.
60. Barchiesi F, Colombo AL, McGough DA, et al. In vitro activity of itraconazole against fluconazole-susceptible and -resistant *Candida albicans* isolates from oral cavities of patients infected with human immunodeficiency virus. Antimicrob Agents Chemother 1994;38:1530–1533.
61. Newman SL, Flanigan TP, Fisher A, et al. Clinically significant mucosal candidiasis resistant to fluconazole treatment in a patient with AIDS. Clin Infect Dis 1994;19:684–686.
62. Vanden Bossche H, Marischal P, Odds FC. Molecular mechanisms of drug resistance in fungi. Trends Microbiol 1994;2:393–400.
63. Cartledge JD, Midgley J, Youle M, Gazzard BG. Itraconazole cyclodextrin solution—Effective treatment for HIV-related candidosis unresponsive to other azole therapy. J Antimicrob Chemother 1994;33:1071–1073.

31

Liposomes in Delivery of Antifungals

HANS CHRISTIAN KORTING and OTTO BRAUN-FALCO
Ludwig-Maximilians-Universität,
Munich, Germany

I. INTRODUCTION

Really effective treatment of severe fungal disease involving inner organs started with the development of amphotericin B in 1952 (1). Parenteral amphotericin B has become and remained the treatment of choice for systemic fungal infections of various types including candidosis, aspergillosis, and mucormycosis (2). Its spectrum of activity in fact still comprises more different fungi than demonstrated with any other type of antifungal so far (3). However, the high efficacy of systemic amphotericin B is also linked to a variety of unwanted effects, some of which are severe. The spectrum includes severe malaise, hyperpyrrhexia, hypotension, thrombophlebitis, anemia, hepatitis, hypokalemia, renal tubular damage, and azotemia (4). Clearly, nephrotoxicity is the core problem with side effects (5), often limiting the dose to be applied, which consequently can limit efficacy. Limited efficacy with usually effective doses is also of note; this has been explained by reduced bioavailability at the infection site (6). Thus, there is clearly a need for better treatment options.

Considering the high activity in vitro against so many fungal pathogens it has looked wise not only to develop new compounds with high antimycotic activity but also to try to improve galenics of amphotericin B, the more so as there have been galenical problems with the polyenes to which amphotericin B belongs. Thus, it does not come to us as a surprise that with the increased interest in drug delivery systems in general and in liposomes in particular, antimycotic treatment has become a major field of interest within drug delivery research (7). In practical terms this has led to the development of a commercial liposomal amphotericin B preparation called AmBisome (8). This drug represents the first systemic liposomal drug in general approved by drug regulatory authorities in various countries. Although the development of systemic antimycotics based on drug delivery systems has clearly attracted much interest in the recent past, it should not be overlooked that it was a topical liposomal drug incorporating econazole which came first: Pevaryl lipogel, launched in Switzerland as early as 1988, represents the first liposomal drug approved (9). Against this background, this report is a short overview of the current state of development of liposomes and related preparations in the delivery of antifungals.

II. LIPOSOMES

A. Characterization of Liposomes as Drug Carriers

Essentially, a liposome represents one or more spheric lipid bilayers separated by water or aqueous buffer. With respect to chemical composition and structure, the lipid bilayers correspond to biological membranes universally found with living cells. In fact, it was this aspect that originally attracted the interest of scientists when liposomes were first described by Bangham and his group (10). Corresponding to differing approaches to formation, there is a variety of structural possibilities, making nomenclature at first sight somewhat puzzling. Conventionally, the parameters considered most relevant for characterization comprise size and lamellarity. The span of possible sizes ranges from 80 nm to 100,000 nm, and there can be one, a few, or many lamellae. Basically, multilamellar vesicles (MLVs), small unilamellar vesicles (SUVs), and large unilamellar vesicles (LUVs) are of interest. The diameter of SUVs roughly ranges from 0.025 to 0.05 μm, of MLVs from 0.05 to 10 μm, while the approximate size of LUVs is 0.1 μm. Sometimes the method of preparation serves for characterization; e.g., REV stands for reward phase evaporation, and EIV for ether injection vesicles.

As is the case with biological membranes, phospholipids form the most important component of liposomes for pharmaceutical use. The typical core structure is glycerol and the prototypic chemical entity is phosphatidyl choline, which in the technological context is also called lecithin. It can be obtained by extracting egg yolk, but soybean oil is a much more relevant source. Figure 1 gives the chemical structure of phosphatidyl choline. With soy phosphatidyl choline linoleic acid is the most important fatty acid component while this is palmitic acid with egg phosphatidyl choline. Another important component of liposomes belongs to the steroids: cholesterol. As the phospholipids and steroids are widely distributed in nature, they also can easily be degraded both in man and in the environment. For metabolism of phosphatidyl choline, the ubiquitous enzyme phospholipase A2 plays an essential role. In some contexts synthetic phospholipids are considered such a dipalmitoyl phosphatidyl choline.

The crucial aspect of a lipid to be used for liposome formation is that there are two different head groups to it, a hydrophilic and a hydrophobic one. With phosphatidyl choline the "zwitterionic" head group seemingly can bind about 15 water molecules while the hydrocarbon fatty acid chains prefer to mix with one another.

For the use of liposomes as a drug carrier for a given compound, the chemical entity should either be polar to be incorporated into the aqueous compartment or nonpolar, to be attached to the lipid bilayers. For technological reasons, drugs with intermediate partition coefficients can prove particularly difficult when it comes to liposome encapsulation.

Practical use of liposomal drugs requires appropriate methods for quality assurance. In this context several methods are currently of interest. To detect the morphological structure freeze fracture electron microscopy clearly is helpful (Fig. 2). To address size in particular laser light scattering has also proven useful.

The easiest procedure to produce liposomes and multilamellar vesicles in particular is the one originally devised by Bangham and co-workers: a lipid mixture is deposited on the bottom of a round bottom flask. Then large amounts of water or aqueous buffer are added to the lipid film, which leads to the spontaneous formation of liposomes. Such liposomes do not, however, qualify for pharmaceutical use. Therefore other methods have been developed and introduced. In the given context the ethanol injection technique, which essentially is a solvent injection method, deserves partic-

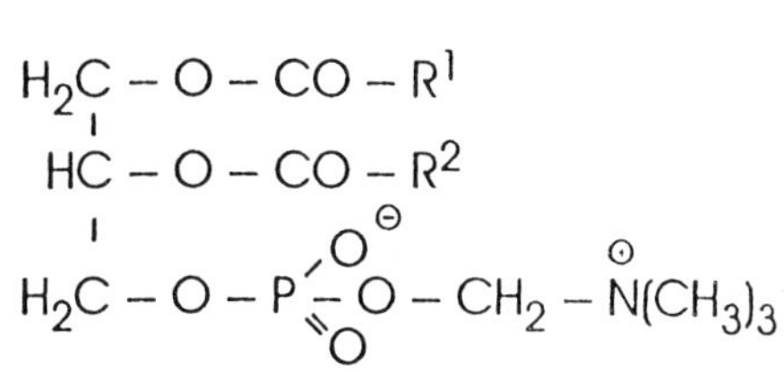

Figure 1 Chemical structure of phosphatidyl choline.

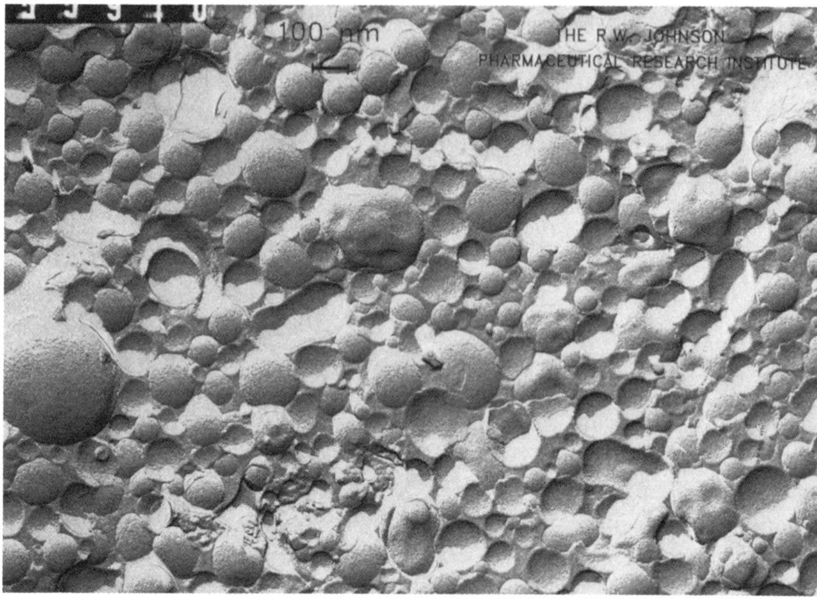

Figure 2 Freeze fracture electron micrograph of the liposomes used with a topical econazole gel preparation (from [9], with permission).

ular interest as it has been used to prepare the first liposomal drug produced on a large, i.e., industrial, scale. As originally described by Batzri and Korn (11), lipids dissolved in ethanol form small unilamellar vesicles when injected into large amounts of aqueous buffer. This method is both simple and comparatively harmless with respect to the integrity of the various chemical entities used. However, removal of ethanol for concentration can be very difficult. In particular with injectable drugs, long-term stability is clearly a problem. To make long-term stability of such drugs feasible, freeze-drying or lyophilization has proven extremely helpful (12). Liposomal vehicles are considered helpful both in the context of both systemic and, in particular, intravenous application of drugs and topical application, in particular to the lungs, eyes, and the skin.

Under the aspect of systemic application various ways of liposome cell interaction are considered relevant for the transfer of active compounds. There is evidence for at least three different mechanisms of interaction: (1) absorption, phagocytosis, and digestion within lysosomes; (2) lipid exchange between liposomal and cellular membranes; and (3) fusion between these elements (13). While the third possibility looks less well supported by experimental findings, the first two seem to be proven. This especially applies to hepatocytes. When liposomes are injected into the bloodstream, they are rapidly taken up by phagocytic cells belonging to the reticuloendothelial system. Macrophages play a major role with spleen and bone marrow, whereas in the liver the Kupffer cells are most relevant, although seemingly small liposomes can also be taken up by hepatic parenchymal cells via pinocytosis. The uptake by the liver in fact is so great that other organs than the liver and spleen might not be reached by a larger proportion of the injected liposomal preparation (14). Consequently, conventional liposomal preparations for parenteral application particularly apply for diseases of liver and spleen, and here primarily those involving phagocytic elements. Large liposomes are needed as their greater water content allows the incorporation of fairly large amounts of hydrophilic active compounds. Unfortunately, stable large liposomes rapidly disappear from the bloodstream. To overcome this problem the addition of polyethylene glycol seems to be rewarding (15).

The fate of liposomes upon topical application is still under debate. Yet more recent evidence makes the concept presented in the following most probable: if there is the possibility of direct interaction of liposomes with living skin cells, i.e., primarily keratinocytes, the liposomes can be attached, engulfed, and degraded within lysosomes. This makes release of active drug within cells highly probable which can be a prime target, e.g., with topical glucocorticoid treatment. In fact, as compared to a conventional form containing a higher concentration, liposomal betamethasone dipropionate has been proven more efficacious in atopic eczema where the stratum corneum representing the skin barrier is compromised. If liposomes are applied to skin commanding an intact stratum corneum, there is no uptake of intact vesicles into deeper strata, not even of the stratum corneum itself. Yet clearly there is a distribution of liposomal lipid at least in part forming elementary membranes resembling those that are genuine to the skin (16).

B. Current Role in Drug Treatment Beyond Mycology

While liposomes for a while were considered the magic bullet in targeted drug delivery, deception with initial results was so solid that later on, further practical development of liposomal drugs looked endangered. At the beginning of the 1990s, however, a variety of both systemic and topical liposomal drugs have been under clinical research. Apart from different amphotericin preparations, the focus in particular was on anticancer drugs with respect to systemic application. The active compounds investigated comprise daunorubicine (DaunoXome), doxorubicine (L-Dox, TLC D-

99), and muramyl tripeptide phosphatidyl ethanolamine. Not only in the context of systemic cytostatic agents, but also of antiinfectives, the challenge of treatment of HIV infection–associated diseases has contributed to the interest in liposomal drugs. For *Mycobacterium avium* intracellulare infection, a gentamycin preparation was developed: TLCG-65.

Interestingly, the systemic application of liposomal preparations is not confined to therapy. For diagnostic reasons ^{111} indium has been used in an liposomal formulation (Vescan) (14). So far, anthracycline preparations have been characterized best in relative terms. Judging from various mouse models this group of drugs, whose clinical application is limited by cardiotoxicity, profits from liposomal encapsulation both in terms of delivery and efficacy. While the improved pharmacokinetic behavior of the active substance has already also been demonstrated in man, final judgment on the relative efficacy and safety in tumor patients is still lacking (17). So-called long circulating heat-sensitive liposomes composed of dipalmitoyl phosphatidyl choline, distearoyl phosphatidyl choline, and amphipathic polyethylene glycol are considered particularly in conjunction with local hyperthermia in the area of the tumor (18). Clinically, at present probably anthracycline liposomal preparations are applied most often, in the context of AIDS-related Kaposi's sarcoma. Yet in spite of a fairly large amount of experience, the comparative benefit-to-risk ratio of liposomal and conventional forms has not been established (19).

With respect to topical drugs only lung and skin should be considered here in any detail. With the lung the focus is on beta-stimulators—i.e., isoprenaline and salbutamol (14). Addressing skin diseases a variety of compounds have been investigated. These range from glucocorticoid preparations for atopic eczema to the hair growth stimulant minoxidil for alopecia, local anesthetics such as tetracaine for minor surgery, retinoids and tretinoin in particular for acne, interferons for genital human papilloma virus infection, and methotrexate for psoriasis to antiinfectives, such as tobramycin and sulphadiazine silver for soft tissue infection including burn wounds (16).

III. SYSTEMIC LIPOSOMAL ANTIMYCOTICS AND RELATED PREPARATIONS

A. Structure

Facing the current benefit-to-risk ratio of available amphotericin B preparations for parenteral use, liposomal encapsulation was considered comparatively early. It was in 1982 that Graybill et al. (20) first reported on "treatment of murine cryptococcosis with liposome-associated amphotericin B.'' In the following, it was Lopez-Berestein and his group who forwarded evidence for the use of liposomes as drug carriers in the context of amphotericin B treatment. In 1983 Lopez-Berestein et al. (21) were able to demonstrate an improved therapeutic index with respect to liposomal as compared to conventional amphotericin B used for the treatment of disseminated *Candida albicans* infection in mice. They prepared multilamellar vesicles by the addition of a methanolic amphotericin B solution to lipids dissolved in chloroform. After evaporation of the organic solvents by the use of a rotary evaporator followed by vacuum desiccation physiologic saline solution was added to form the vesicles shaking by hand.

Later Lopez-Berestein et al. (22) were able to demonstrate in a group of 12 patients suffering from severe fungal infection associated with hematological malignancies that improvement or even cure was possible following the use of liposomal amphotericin B while conventional amphotericin B had failed before. The procedure for preparing liposomal amphotericin B was essentially the same as previously. As lipids, pure dimyristoyl phosphatidyl choline and dimyristoyl phosphatidyl glycerol (DMPC and DMPG) were chosen (molar ratio 7:3). The majority of liposomes could be shown to have a diameter between 0.5 and 3 μm the encapsulation efficiency amounting to more than 90%. While the so-called bedside preparations clearly paved the way for corresponding industrial ones, it was other groups who forwarded them. In fact, it became obvious that amphotericin B-loaded liposomes of the given type could not be produced on a large scale. Further development of the particular preparation, however, did not lead to a truly liposomal preparation of a different type but to the preparation of particulate carriers looking like ribbons. This preparation, called Amphotericin B Lipid Complex, still reflects the original lipid components and their molar ratio (DMPC and DMPG 7:3).

As shown in Table 1, the diameter of the ribbonlike structures still is large compared to newer liposomal and related preparations. The true liposome preparation now widely available on a commercial basis is represented by a SUV formulation now called AmBisome, initially characterized by Gondal et al. (25). With this preparation the main lipid components and their ratio are identical to the previous preparation. This, however, does not apply to another lipid drug carrier formulation, termed amphotericin B colloidal dispersion. The particulate drug carriers here are disk-shaped and essentially made of cholesterol sulfate. The two preparations share a fairly similar size of the carriers which is in the order of 100 nm.

B. Pharmacokinetics

Data on the pharmacokinetic behavior of liposomal amphotericin B in man were first provided by Lopez-Berestein in 1984 (26). Using Tc^{99m} as

Table 1 Lipid Formulations of Amphotericin B: Physicochemical Aspects

	Formulation (name)	Manufacturer	Structure	Size	Components
A	AmBisome	Vestar, Inc.	liposome	80 nm	dimyristoyl phosphatidyl choline:dimyristoyl phosphatidyl glycerol (7:3)
B	Amphocil (amphotericin B colloidal dispersion, A B C D)	Liposome Technology, Inc.	disk	122 ± 48 nm	cholesterol sulfate
C	Amphotericin B lipid complex (A B L C)	The Liposome Co.	ribbon	1.6–11 μm	dimyristoyl phosphatidyl choline:dimyristoyl phosphatidyl glycerol (7:3)

Adapted from (23) and (24).

a marker they found a very short distribution and elimination half-life amounting to about 5 min and 4–5 hr, respectively. Up to 15% of radioactivity was found in urine within the first 24 hr after application. With respect to the preparations available on a large scale, amphotericin B lipid complex has been looked at in particular (27). While serum C_{max} and AUC values were lower with the liposomal than with the conventional form, the opposite applied with respect to the volume of distribution. Elimination half-life also was longer with the liposomal preparation (second phase). Comparative data on the various preparations are given in Table 2, which is based on the overview by Janknegt et al. (23). The differences between the concentrations expressed as mg/kg tissue between various organs are remarkable. Data from three autopsy cases clearly show that these levels lie in the order of 10^2 mg/kg with liver and spleen, and 10^0 with other organs such as lung, kidney, and so on (28).

C. Activity In Vitro and In Vivo

Seemingly, liposomal encapsulation does not dramatically affect the in vitro activity of amphotericin B against common fungi such as *Candida albicans* and other *Candida* species, *Cryptococcus neoformans*, and *Aspergillus* or *Fusarium* species. According to Anaissie et al. (29), the minimum inhibitory concentration (MIC) for *Candida albicans*, e.g., ranges from 0.16 to 2.5 with conventional and 0.16 to 1.25 μg/ml for liposomal amphotericin B, the MIC 90 value amounting to 1.25 and 0.62 μg/ml, respectively. Accordingly, the minimum fungicidal concentration (MFC)

Table 2 Lipid Formulations of Amphotericin B: Pharmacokinetic Aspects

	Formulation (name)	Dose (mg/kg/d)	Peak serum level (C_{max}) (μg/ml)	Clearance (ml/min/kg)	Area under the serum level time curve (AUC) (mg/l h)
A	AmBisome	3.0	10–35	21	211
		4.0	11–35	21	419
		5.0	25–59	16	523
B	Amphocil	0.25		0.47	9.1
	(amphotericin	0.5		0.42	20
	B colloidal	1.0		0.36	45
	dispersion,	1.5		0.47	56
	A B C D)				
C	Amphotericin B	0.1	0.12	1.5	1.4
	lipid complex	0.25	0.21	1.2	4.3
	(A B L C)	0.5	0.26	1.3	7.0

Modified from (23).

90 is alike: 1.25 μg/ml. With respect to the uptake of *Candida albicans* blastospores by neutrophils in vitro, however, there is a clear-cut difference, free amphotericin B being much more active (30). In this context AmBisome was used.

In animal infection models AmBisome proved superior to conventional amphotericin B in systemic candidosis of leukopenic mice: only amphotericin B at a dose of 7 mg/kg/day could reduce the number of colony-forming units of *Candida albicans* in the kidney remarkably and thus prevent relapse a dose which is not tolerable with the conventional form (31). According to the findings by Van Etten et al. (31), it is clearly the better tolerability of amphotericin B liposomally encapsulated making high-dose treatment feasible which explains superiority of the liposomal drug. In parallel time-kill studies in vitro, these authors even found a clearly reduced activity of liposomal amphotericin B (31). A reduced activity of liposomal amphotericin B of the AmBisome type could also been demonstrated by Clemons and Stevens (32). Using 1.0 mg/kg comparatively, the conventional form influenced murine blastomycosis more than the liposomal one. However, only high-dose treatment with 7.5 mg/kg of AmBisome eradicated the fungus in the lungs of a majority of experimental animals, thus proving superior. Addressing amphotericin lipid complex it was also observed that at medium doses the liposomal formulation is less active than the conventional one (33). In this context experimental cryptococcal meningitis and disseminated candidosis of rabbits served as infection models.

D. Efficacy and Safety

For several reasons it is difficult to assess the clinical efficacy and safety of an amphotericin B preparation. Thus, the relative role of liposomal or other drug carrier formulations of amphotericin B has not yet finally been defined despite an increase of available data in recent years. Part of the problem of judging systemic antifungal drugs for life-threatening fungal disease is difficulty in the establishment of diagnosis, differences in the nature of fungal disease due to peculiarities of the given microorganism, and so on. Fortunately, a topical review by De Marie et al. is available (34). Table 3 cannot provide more than an initial orientation. However, it makes clear that comparative efficacy and safety data are still lacking, which makes final judgment impossible at this point of time (39). Nevertheless, the data on adverse events in the context of amphotericin B use, and in particular those reflecting renal damage, look advantageous.

With respect to efficacy the question of which type of amphotericin B treatment protocol to prefer has even become more difficult by the proposal to use conventional amphotericin B together with concomitant lipid

Table 3 Lipid Formulations of Amphotericin B: Efficacy and Safety Aspects

Formulation (name)	Indication	Efficacy	Safety in patients	Reference
A AmBisome	invasive candidosis;	response rate 84%;	decrease of serum potassium: 28%; rise of serum creatinine: 9%; nausea and vomiting: 3%, fever and chills: 1% each	28
	invasive aspergillosis	response rate 61%		35
B Amphocil (amphotericin B colloidal dispersion, A B C D)	coccidioidomycosis	response rate 84%		36
C Amphotericin B lipid complex (A B L C)	cryptococcal meningitis	mycological success rate 77%;		37
	coccidioidomycosis	complete response rate 55%		38

infusion. Originally proposed by Caillot et al. (40), more evidence on the subject has been forwarded later. In particular, Caillot et al. (41) were able to demonstrate that the use of a commercial lipid emulsion for infusion called Intralipid clearly reduces amphotericin B–linked unwanted effects related to renal damage, such as a 50% decrease of creatinine clearance.

IV. TOPICAL LIPOSOMAL ANTIMYCOTICS

At first sight the need for drug carriers such as liposomes might be less evident when it comes to topical treatment of cutaneous fungal disease. At first glimpse this might look particularly appropriate with respect to well-tolerated and highly efficacious antimycotics, as are the topical azoles. At second look, however, one might become aware of the fact that cure rates with conventional azoles, whatever the individual congener may be, only lie in the range of about 90% in both clinical and mycological terms. Moreover, suggested application periods of 2–3 weeks for common dermatoses such as tinea pedis or corporis might look long as compared to the expectations of today's patients; e.g., according to a recent controlled trial, using 1% econazole nitrate cream once a day for 28 days cured only 85% of the patients of the verum group compared to 41% with the so-called placebo or vehicle preparation. Furthermore, only 86% of mycologically cured patients remained so thereafter (compared to 55% in the control group) (42).

Against this background it is to be understood that topical antifungals have repeatedly been considered as candidates for liposomal encapsulation (43). As early as 1984 a European and a U.S. patent have been obtained by Mezei focusing on an econazole preparation made of multilamellar vesicles obtained by the film method using phospholipids, hydrogenated phospholipids, and cholesterol. Later Boller et al. described an econazole liposome gel preparation based on unilamellar vesicles made of phospholipids and cholesterol using the injection method. Based on the ethanol injection method described by Batzri and Korn 1973 (11), Cilag Corporation from Schaffhausen, Switzerland, was able to develop the first liposomal drug in general fit for production on a large scale (9). Introduced into the Swiss market at the end of the 1980s, econazole liposomal gel called Pevaryl Lipogel has proven once and for all that commercial liposomal drugs are feasible. In particular, it has been possible to demonstrate long-term stability with the use of an inexpensive regular aluminum tube for packaging. Unfortunately, comparative pharmacokinetic data have not been published so far although they seemingly have been obtained. About the same applies to clinical efficacy. While a formal publication is also missing, however, data are available from Cilag, Schaffhausen: according to a trial performed by Fritsch and Kokoschka, the onset of action was earlier with liposomal econazole compared to the potent antimycotic agent used for control, naftifin: after 1 week cultures were negative with the former agent in 48%, with the latter in 31%. After 3 weeks' time cure rates were similar, amounting to 92 in 90%. Tolerability was good with both drugs. Although this was not an equivalence trial in the modern sense, the results may serve as a sound basis for further investigations (Korting et al., in preparation).

V. OUTLOOK

Both systemic and topical liposomal antimycotics are feasible under technological aspects. Neither with the systemic nor with the topical route of application, has superiority of a liposomal formulation over a corresponding conventional one finally been proven. Yet there is reason to believe that there are possible advantages. With the systemic route and amphotericin B, it seems to be tolerability in particular that is increased using liposomes or other, similar lipoidal drug carriers. With topical forms, the progress may in particular lie in an early onset of activity and perhaps also in an increased overall cure rate. Thus, further investigations are clearly needed and promising. Fortunately, they are ongoing both with liposomal amphotericin B for systemic use (39) and with liposomal econazole for topical use (Korting et al., in preparation).

REFERENCES

1. Meunier F. Alternative modalities of administering amphotericin B: Current issues. J Infect 1994;28(suppl 1):51–56.
2. Medoff G, Brajtburg J, Kobayashi GS. Antifungal agents useful in therapy of systemic fungal infections. Annu Rev Pharmacol Toxicol 1983;2:303–330.
3. Medoff G, Kobayashi GA. The polyenes. In: Speller DCE, ed. Antifungal Chemotherapy. Chichester: John Wiley and Sons, 1980:3–34.
4. Miller R, Bates JH. Amphotericin B toxicity. A follow up report of 53 patients. Ann Intern Med 1969;71:1090–1095.
5. Butler WT, Bennett JE, Alling D, Wertlake PT. Nephrotoxicity of amphotericin B: Early and late effects in 81 patients. Ann Intern Med 1964;61:175–187.
6. Christiansen KJ, Bernard EM, Gold JWM, Armstrong D. Distribution and activity of amphotericin B in humans. J Infect Dis 1985;152:1037–1043.
7. Gregoriadis G, Florence AT. Liposomes in drug delivery. Clinical, diagnostic and ophthalmic potential. Drugs 1993;45:15–28.
8. Hay RJ. Liposomal amphotericin B, AmBisome. J Infect 1994;28(suppl 1): 35–43.

9. Kriftner RW. Liposome production: The ethanol injection technique and the development of the first approved liposome dermatic. In: Braun-Falco O, Korting HC, Maibach HI, eds. Liposome Dermatics. New York: Springer, 1992:91–100.
10. Bangham AD, Standish MM, Watkins JC. Diffusion of univalent ions across the lamellae of swollen phospholipids. J Mol Biol 1965;13:238–252.
11. Batzri S, Korn ED. Single bilayer liposomes prepared without sonication. Biochim Biophys Acta 1973;298:1015–1019.
12. Weiner N, Martin F, Riaz M. Liposomes as a drug delivery system. Drug Dev Indust Pharm 1989;15:1523–1554.
13. Ostro MJ. Liposomes. Sci Am 1987;256:102–111.
14. Fielding RM. Liposomal drug delivery. Advantages and limitations from a clinical pharmacokinetic and therapeutic perspective. Clin Pharmacokinet 1991;21:155–164.
15. Gregoriadis G. Overview of liposomes. J Antimicrob Chem 1991;28:39–48.
16. Schmid M-H, Korting HC. Liposomes: A drug carrier system for topical treatment in dermatology. Crit Rev Ther Drug Carr Sys 1994;11:97–118.
17. Gabizon AA. Liposomal anthracyclines. Hematol Oncol Clin North Am 1994;8:431–450.
18. Unezaki S, Maruyama K, Takahashi N, et al. Enhanced delivery and antitumor activity of doxorubicin using long-circulating thermosensitive liposomes containing amphipathic polyethylene glycol in combination with local hyperthermia. Pharm Res 1994;11:1180–1185.
19. Wagner D, Kern WV, Kern P. Liposomal doxorubicin in AIDS-related Kaposi's sarcoma: Long-term experiences. Clin Invest 1994;73:417–423.
20. Graybill JR, Craven PC, Taylor RL, Williams DM, Magee WE. Treatment of murine cryptococcosis with liposome-associated amphotericin B. J Infect Dis 1982;145:748–752.
21. Lopez-Berestein G, Mehta R, Hopfer RL, et al. Treatment and prophylaxis of disseminated infection due to *Candida albicans* in mice with liposome-encapsulated amphotericin B. J Infect Dis 1983;147:939–945.
22. Lopez-Berestein G, Fainstein V, Hopfer R, et al. Liposomal amphotericin B for the treatment of systemic fungal infections in patients with cancer: A preliminary study. J Infect Dis 1985;151:704–710.
23. Janknegt R, De Marie S, Bakker-Woudenberg IAJM, Crommelin DJA. Liposomal and lipid formulations of amphotericin B. Clinical pharmacokinetics. Clin Pharmacokinet 1992;23:279–291.
24. Khoo SH, Bond J, Denning DW. Administering amphotericin B—a practical approach. J Antimicrob Chemother 1994;33:203–213.
25. Gondal JA, Swartz RP, Rahman A. Therapeutic evaluation of free and liposome-encapsulated amphotericin B in the treatment of systemic candidiasis in mice. Antimicrob Agents Chemother 1989;33:1544–1548.
26. Lopez-Berestein G, Kasi L, Rosenblum MG. Clinical pharmacology of ^{99m}Tc labeled liposomes in patients with cancer. Cancer Res 1984;44:375–378.
27. Kan V, Bennett J, Amanthea M, Smolskis M, Grasela D. Comparative safety and pharmacokinetic study of amphotericin B lipid complex and amphoteri-

cin B deoxycholate in healthy young male volunteers. J Infect Dis 1991;164: 418–425.

28. Ringdén O, Meunier F, Tollemar J, et al. Efficacy of amphotericin B encapsulated in liposomes (AmBisome) in the treatment of invasive fungal infections in immunocompromised patients. J Antimicrob Chemoter 1991;28:73–82.
29. Anaissie E, Paetznick V, Proffitt R, Adler-Moore J, Bodey GP. Comparison of the in vitro antifungal activity of free and liposome-encapsulated amphotericin B. Eur J Clin Microbiol Infect Dis 1991;10:665–667.
30. Pallister CJ, Johnson EM, Warnock DW, Elliot PJ, Reeves DF. In-vitro effects of liposome-encapsulated amphotericin B (AmBisome) and amphotericin B-deoxycholate (Fungizone) on the phagocytic and candidacidal function of human polymorphonuclear leucocytes. J Antimicrob Chemother 1992;30: 313–320.
31. Van Etten EWM, Van den Heuvel–De Groot C, Bakker-Woudenberg IAJM. Efficacies of amphotericin B-desoxycholate (Fungizone), liposomal amphotericin B (AmBisome) and fluconazole in the treatment of systemic candidosis in immunocompetent and leucopenic mice. J Antimicrob Chemother 1993;32:723–739.
32. Clemons KV, Stevens DA. Therapeutic efficacy of a liposomal formulation of amphotericin B (AmBisome) against murine blastomycosis. J Antimicrob Chemother 1993;32:465–472.
33. Perfect JR, Wright KA. Amphotericin B lipid complex in the treatment of experimental crytococcal meningitis and disseminated candidosis. J Antimicrob Chemother 1994;33:73–81.
34. De Marie S, Janknegt R, Bakker-Woudenberg IAJM. Clinical use of liposomal and lipid-complexed amphotericin B. J Antimicrob Chemother 1994;33: 907–916.
35. Meunier F, Prentice HG, Ringdén O. Liposomal amphotericin B (AmBisome): Safety data from a phase II/III clinical trial. Antimicrob Chemother 1991;28:83–91.
36. Stevens A. Overview of amphotericin B colloidal dispersion (Amphocil). J Infect 1994;28(suppl 1):45–49.
37. Graybill JR, Sharkey PK, Vincent D, Johnson E, Havard PF. Amphotericin B lipid complex in treatment of cryptococcal meningitis in patients with AIDS. 31st Interscience Conference on Antimicrobial Agents and Chemotherapy, Chicago, September 29–October 2, 1991; Abstract No. 289, p. 147.
38. Sharkey PK, Lipke R, Renteria A, Galgiani J, Catanzarro A. Amphotericin B lipid complex in treatment of coccidioidomycosis. 31st Interscience Conference on Antimicrobial Agents and Chemotherapy, Chicago, September 29–October 2, 1991; Abstract No. 742, p. 222.
39. Meunier F. Alternative modalities of administering amphotericin B: Current issues. J Infect 1994;28(suppl 1):51–56.
40. Caillot D, Chavanet P, Casanovas O, Solary E, Zanetta G, Buisson M. Clinical evaluation of a lipid emulsion for administration of intravenous amphotericin B. Eur J Clin Microbiol Infect Dis 1992;11:722–725.

41. Caillot D, Reny G, Solary E, et al. A controlled trial of the tolerance of amphotericin B infused in dextrose or in intralipid in patients with haematological malignancies. J Antimicrob Chemother 1994;33:603–613.
42. Ison AE, Lufrano L, Thorne EG. Once-daily application of econazole nitrate in the treatment of tinea pedis. Adv Ther 1990;7:119–123.
43. Korting HC, Blecher P, Schäfer-Korting M, Wendel A. Topical liposome drugs to come: What the patent literature tells us. J Am Acad Dermatol 1991; 25:1068–1071.

32

Pharmacokinetics in Onychomycosis

PIET DE DONCKER
Janssen Research Foundation
Beerse, Belgium

I. INTRODUCTION

Nail kinetics of antifungal drugs have not until recently been a subject of intensive investigation. Moreover, a frequent reason given for the poor therapeutic response to antifungal drugs, such as ketoconazole or griseofulvin, is the failure to attain satisfactory plasma levels of the active agent. This may not be an accurate interpretation of the problem, because in skin and/or nail dermatophyte infections, where the infection is located in the stratum corneum and hard keratin structures, the plasma levels may not be directly linked to the expected clinical response. It is probably more important to consider the tissue levels achieved by the antifungal.

Traditionally, prolonged therapy was used for the treatment of onychomycosis. Today, new investigations with the latest antifungal agents have focused on the importance of nail pharmacokinetics in an attempt to develop the best possible treatment regimen in terms of efficacy, safety, ease of compliance, and cost. Specific studies have been performed to address the following important issues: (a) the mechanism by which the antifungal reaches the site of infection; (b) how quickly the antifungal achieves concentrations that are therapeutic for the broad range of fungi involved in nail infections; and (c) how long this effective concentration remains at the infection site post therapy. Answers to these questions should play a major role in the development of new oral drugs for onychomycosis or for any new treatment strategy with the existing drugs.

Furthermore, the thickness of the nail and its relatively compact construction make it a barrier to the entry of topically applied agents that is hard to overcome. As a result, effective topical treatment has been limited by the lack of penetration of the drug into the nail bed. Studies of the pharmacokinetic behavior of topically applied antifungal agents may lead to effective topical therapies for nail disease.

This chapter is a review of the data available on nail kinetics of topical and oral antifungals that are used for the treatment of onychomycosis and of the research carried out concerning itraconazole in the nail.

II. DISTRIBUTION OF TOPICAL ANTIFUNGALS IN THE NAIL

The topical delivery of chemicals to treat fungal nail disease effectively and noninvasively has been a challenge for years. It is obvious that any antifungal agent must reach the infected tissue in sufficient concentrations before it can exert its effect. One major problem associated with the treatment of fungal nail infections by the topical route is the lengthy duration of treatment, low incidence of cure, and high recurrence rates. This might be due to the fact that the nail plate is too thick for currently available topical agents to penetrate. Moreover, the drug should not only penetrate the nail plate but also reach the nail bed and matrix in sufficient concentration to stop the disease process effectively (Fig. 1).

The structures of the upper and lower parts of the nail plate are different from the stratum corneum. The nail plate is composed of layers flattened keratinized cells that have their origins in the nail matrix. The compactness of the plate is the result of tight binding of the cells, with numerous intercellular links (disulfide bridges). The nail plate is also much thicker than the stratum corneum. In chemical composition the nail plate is more like hair than stratum corneum (1–7).

As a consequence, the diffusion pathway for drug delivery into and/or through the nail plate is very long. In order to deliver a sufficient amount of drug into and/or through the nail plate, the permeability of the nail plate to the drug must be enhanced (6,7). In addition, several factors cause the permeation in the nail to differ from that in the stratum corneum: first, the nail contains less lipid. Lipids constitute up to only 5% of the weight of the nail plate, and the absence of sebaceous glands suggests that lipoidal pathways in the nail are less important than in the stratum corneum; second, the nail has a high sulfur content (cystine) in its hard keratin, whereas the stratum corneum does not; and third, the water content in the nail

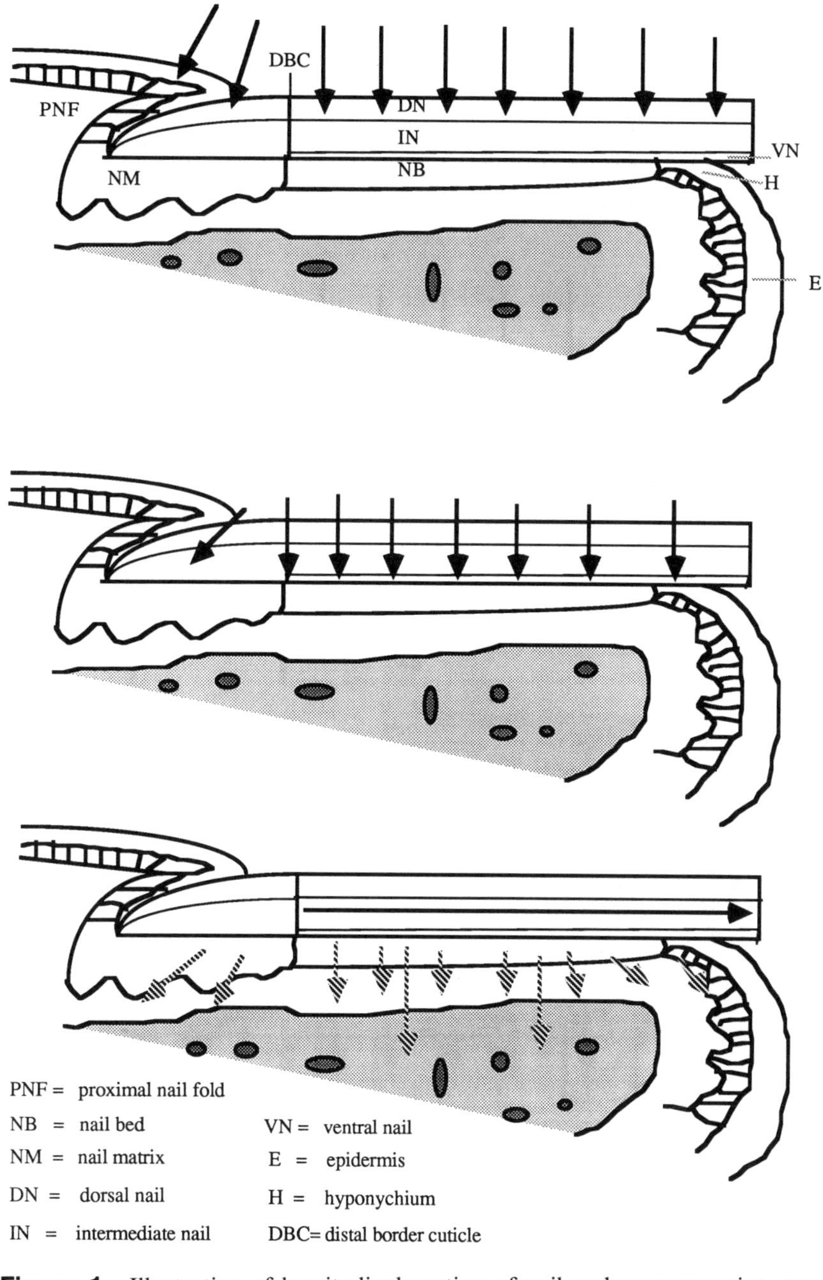

Figure 1 Illustration of longitudinal section of nail and accompanying structures. The arrows indicate the possible routes of topical antifungal nail penetration.

varies, but ideally it should be 18%, which is less than the >25% water content of the stratum corneum (4–7).

The strategy for antifungal drug delivery is to deliver an effective dose to the nail bed, nail matrix, and nail plate. The most effective way will most probably be by facilitating enhanced hydration and/or loosening the keratin structure. Today, a large number of topical antifungals are available or under development for the treatment of dermatomycosis. However, only a limited number of agents have been studied as topical nail formulations and even fewer have been evaluated for their intra- and transfungual penetration profile. So far no drug seems to produce complete cure by topical treatment alone. Therefore there is still room for major improvement, though interesting work has been carried out.

A. Miconazole

Miconazole is currently available in a 2% nail lacquer for the treatment of onychomycosis. However, no kinetic studies have been performed with this topical formulation. More recently, work by Walters et al. has demonstrated that the ionic form of miconazole dissolves as easily in the nail plate as the free base (8). It was concluded that the topical bioavailability of miconazole can be enhanced by decreasing the pH of the vehicle (Table 1).

B. Econazole

In vitro studies have shown that econazole penetrated the nail plate after topical application, and the penetration was clearly affected by the percentage of DMSO (9). The 1% econazole lotion with a higher percentage of DMSO (44–99%) resulted in higher uptake in the deeper layers and increased permeation time through the upper part than the 1% ointment (Table 1). Concentrations in the nail bed were 10–80 μg/ml; the highest concentration was reached with the formulation that contained 99% DMSO. A few clinical studies have been performed with the 1% econazole cream and with an alcohol solution. Success rates were variable (10).

C. Oxiconazole

A 1% oxiconazole tincture formulation proved to penetrate better into the deeper layers of the nails in comparison with the 1% ointment. In addition, concentrations of more than 10 μg/ml are achieved in the nail bed (Table 1) (9). Another study showed that oxiconazole in a formulation with *N*-acetyl-cysteine (NAC) has led to an improved penetration or uptake, even to the deeper nail layers (11).

Table 1 Penetration of Topical Antibiotics in the Human Nail

	Nail plate		Nail bed		
	Dorsal	Ventral	Upper layers	Deeper layers	Permeation
2% Miconazole (nail solution)	N/A[a]	N/A	N/A	N/A	Enhanced by ↘ PH
1% Oxiconazole (μg/ml)					
Exposure time: ±16.7 hr					
Ointment	1.000	15	5	7	
Tincture	1.500	50	80	80	Tincture > ointment
1% Econazole (μg/ml)					
Exposure time: ±16.7 hr					
Ointment	1.000	10	10	12	
Lotion (+49% DMSO)	800	70	20	10	
					↗ DMSO
Lotion (+99% DMSO)	1000	50	70	80	
8% Ciclopirox (relative % active drug in nail)	Layer 1	Layer 4			Max. conc. 3.4 μg/mg nail
7-Day sample	49.6	4.2	N/A	N/A	
14-Day sample	32	22.7	N/A	N/A	
30-Day sample	34.7	19.2	N/A	N/A	
5% Amorolfine (μg/ml)			End Rx	14 days post-Rx	Flux 10–40 ng/cm²/h
In a methylene chloride–based nail lacquer	N/A	N/A	31.4	17.4	
In a ethanol-based nail lacquer	N/A	N/A	28.1	15.4	

[a] N/A = not available
Source: From Refs. 9, 13, and 16.

D. Ciclopirox

The hydroxypyridone derivative ciclopirox has been studied in a nail lacquer formulation for onychomycosis (12). The penetration characteristics were recently investigated by Ceschin-Roques et al., who showed that cyclopirox in a 8% nail lacquer penetrates the nail (13). Concentrations reached a maximum of around 3.4 μg/mg nail after 30 days of treatment (Table 1). After 7 days of application, 49.6% of ciclopirox was found in the first layers, with a progressive decrease of active drug found in the deeper layers. During further therapy, penetration improved at the fourth layer to 19.2% of ciclopirox concentration (ventral side). No information on penetration through the whole nail plate into the nail bed has yet been reported.

E. Amorolfine

Amorolfine is the first representative of a new chemical group (phenyl-propyl-morpholin derivatives) and is an antifungal with a broad spectrum of activity (14). A 5% nail lacquer has been developed and several studies have evaluated the intra- and transungual penetration of this nail lacquer (15).

In vitro, one application of 500 μg/cm^2 amorolfine generates an amorolfine flux of 10–40 ng/cm^2/hr through the nail. It was also demonstrated that this formulation penetrates the keratin (±10% of the dose).

In a further study in onychomycosis patients (16), there was no significant difference in concentrations of amorolfine in the subungual grease between the methylenechloride- and the ethanol-based nail lacquers with a twice-weekly regimen for 1 month (Table 1). Maximum concentrations were around 31.4 and 28.1 μg/ml respectively just after therapy had been stopped. Amorolfine concentrations in the subungual region lasted for 14 days after cessation of 1 month therapy with concentrations of 17.4 and 15.4 μg/ml for the two formulations respectively. These amorolfine concentrations were still higher than the MIC to the different dermatophyte types. It was concluded from all these studies that the rapid and long-lasting penetration is responsible for the drug's efficacy in the treatment of onychomycosis.

F. Sodium Pyrithione

Sodium pyrithione is a metallic salt of the pyrithiones (2-1 pyridinethiol-1-oxide sodium salt), and has been investigated and registered as an antifungal, antibacterial and antiseborrhoeic agent (17). Although clinical results for the treatment of onychomycosis have not yet been reported, the local penetration into the nail has been studied in the rhesus monkey with a 3% radiolabeled sodium pyrithione solution applied once daily for 6 to 7 days (17). According to this study, absorption into and across the nail was slow, with the nails serving as a reservoir for the drug. Systemic absorption was also demonstrated after topical application of a film-forming solution on the nail, with peak plasma concentrations 1 day after the last dose has been removed. This indicates that it does accumulate to some extent in the nail bed before it is absorbed into the systemic route (less than 10% of a topically applied dose). Based on these results, a topically applied treatment in onychomycosis may be of use in the treatment of diseased nails. However, more studies are needed to determine the place of this new antimycotic agent in the treatment of onychomcyosis.

III. DISTRIBUTION OF ORAL ANTIFUNGALS IN THE NAIL

It is obvious that an antimycotic agent, before it can exert its effect, must reach the infected tissue in sufficient concentrations (Fig. 2). In contrast to skin, the nail plate is a slow-growing structure and is composed of layers of flattened keratinocytes. It takes several months to a year for a toenail outgrowth to be obtained (1,2).

This slow renewal of the nail will influence the ability of drugs to reach the site of action. If a systemic drug could be taken up in the newly formed nail, it would take a long time the nail to become fully impregnated with the drug. In addition, differences in growth speed between fingernails and toenails will have consequences in drug penetration into the nail, as will other factors that delay or increase the speed of the nail growth—such as age, psoriasis, yellow-nail syndrome, certain drugs etc.

Another difference between nails and the skin is that the nail is 10 times thicker than the stratum corneum and contains less lipid (1–6). This greatly affects drug penetration for the various oral drugs available.

To date, five oral agents have been explored in onychomycosis. However, extensive nail pharmacokinetic studies are not available for all five.

A. Griseofulvin

Although griseofulvin has long been used to treat tinea unguium, information on how and when it penetrates the nail and how much griseofulvin gets into the nail is not available.

Peak plasma levels of griseofulvin are achieved 2–4 hr after oral dosing. The mean peak plasma level following a single 330-mg dose of ultramicrosize griseofulvin (UMSG) was 1.25 μg/ml. Following a single dose of 500 mg microsize griseofulvin (MSG), the mean maximum concentration was 1.39 μg/ml (18). Moreover, it has been shown by Korting et al. that the plasma levels and skin-tissue drug levels after administration of the 330 mg of UMSG correspond to those following 500 mg of the microsize form (19).

Griseofulvin appears in the stratum corneum within 4–8 hr after oral administration. It is incorporated into the basal layer to some extent

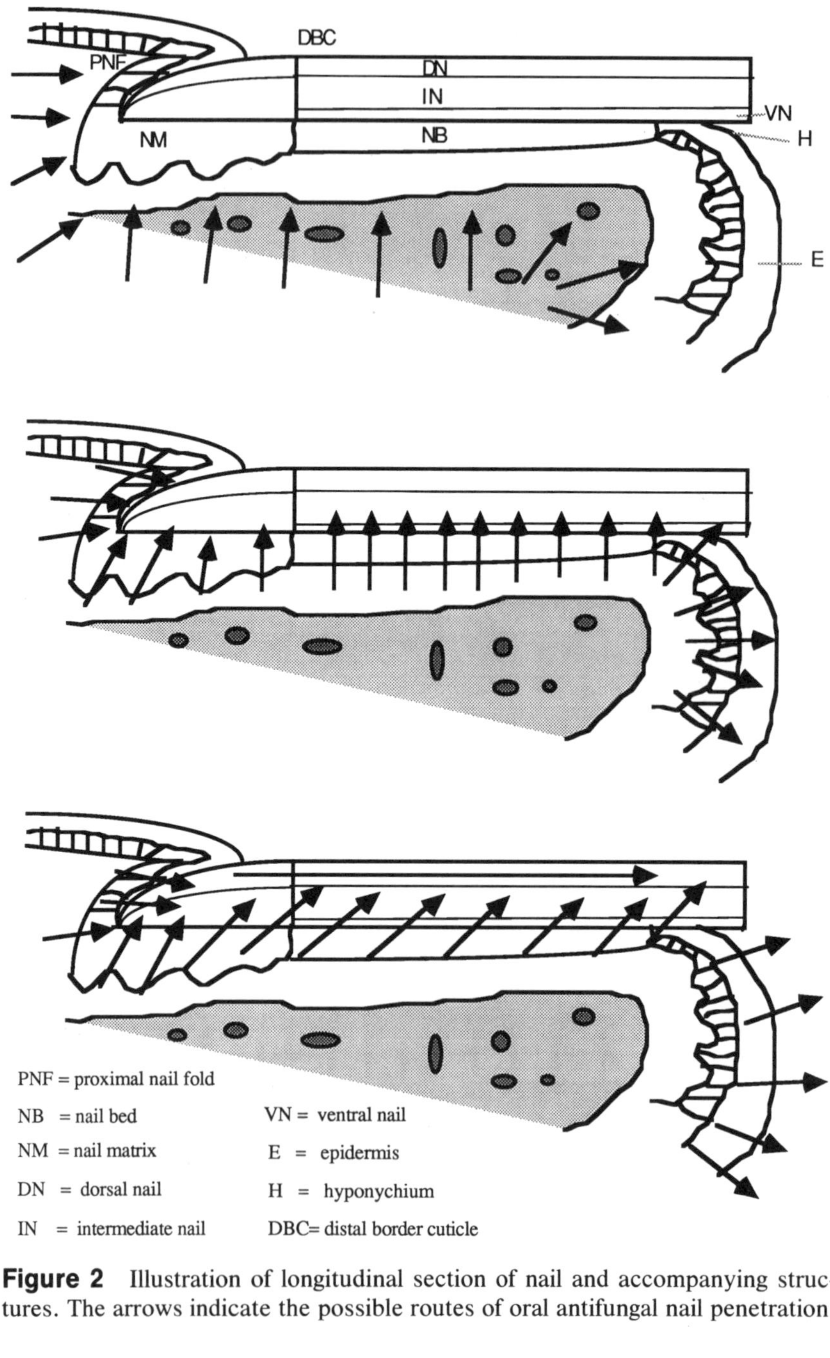

Figure 2 Illustration of longitudinal section of nail and accompanying structures. The arrows indicate the possible routes of oral antifungal nail penetration.

(20,21). However, sweat is the major route of griseofulvin delivery to the skin. Keratin adherence has been shown to be very weak. Studies by Epstein et al. have shown that drug levels in keratinized tissues decline in parallel with those in plasma and that the drug cannot be detected in the stratum corneum within 48 to 72 hr after discontinuation of therapy (22). Moreover, occlusion with absorbent material greatly reduced the concentration in the stratum corneum, with a further accumulation of griseofulvin in the absorbent material (23). These findings suggest that there is no special affinity for keratinized tissues.

Despite the fact that griseofulvin has been widely and safely used for the treatment of tinea unguium for years, there are no studies determining the penetration routes of griseofulvin in the nail. Therefore it has been assumed, on the basis of few or no data in humans from the early studies with griseofulvin, that the drug is taken up by the newly produced nail. Consequently, treatment of nail infections with griseofulvin was always continued until clinical and mycological cure (24). However, it is still possible that griseofulvin diffuses into the nail plate from the nail bed as suggested by Hägermark et al. (25). Therefore, the observation that in some cases the free distal end of the nails did not clear of infection in cases of onycholysis may be explained by the lower griseofulvin levels achieved in the distal part of the nail (25).

Lack of information makes it difficult to compare tissue levels to the minimal inhibitory concentration (MIC) for the infecting dermatophyte. The MIC for isolates from unresponsive nail infections has been reported to be less than 2 μg/ml. This finding suggests that much less active drug enters the hard keratin of the nail than is able reach the stratum corneum. It has been reported that high dosages (above 1 g/day) resulted in better cure rates (19,24), perhaps because higher tissue concentrations were achieved. Other dose regimens with griseofulvin, such as the use of a pulse regimen, might still be feasible for tinea unguium. However, to our knowledge, this regimen has not yet been explored.

B. Ketoconazole

Ketoconazole is an imidazole derivative and is the first orally active broad-spectrum antifungal agent (26). It is poorly soluble in water except at a pH below 3. Ketoconazole is well absorbed after oral administration of single doses of 100 to 800 mg (27). Peak plasma concentrations are generally attained within 1 to 2 hr of administration. After a single 400-mg oral dose, the drug was detectable within 1 hr and mean plasma concentrations reached peak values of between 5.5 and 6.5 μg/ml. It was found very rapidly in the stratum corneum (20). The plasma levels decreased to between 0.3 and 0.4 μg/ml after 12 hr (20,27).

Prolonged therapy with ketoconazole in onychomycosis owes more to tradition than to any data regarding its pharmacokinetics. This lack of information about the agent's pharmacology may have limited full exploration of its use in this disease. No information exists concerning the penetration route and the amount of the drug available in the nail.

As in the case of griseofulvin, sweat is the most important route of delivery of ketoconazole to the skin, while excretion in sebum and uptake or excretion in the basal layer is limited. In contrast to griseofulvin, ketoconazole has a strong adherence to keratin (28,29). That ketoconazole readily accumulates from sweat into keratinized structures (skin, hair, nails) was shown by partition experiments involving tritiated ketoconazole in which the accumulation into skin, hair, and nails was measured (28). From this study, it was shown that the affinity of hair and nails for ketoconazole partitioning from the fluid phase (ketoconazole's partition coefficients (KPC) are 77 and 79 for hair and nails, respectively) was good but that the KPC was much higher for stratum corneum (KPC = 680). As is the case with griseofulvin, there is surprisingly little information regarding the nail kinetics of ketoconazole. A possible new treatment strategy might involve a bolus dose of 400 mg ketoconazole once weekly (30). This pulse approach has been evaluated in dermatomycosis, with variable success rates for nail infections but with a potentially better safety profile than that found with the daily doses of long duration. These data suggest that prolonged once-daily therapy might not be the best way to treat fungal nail disease. Alternative approaches such as a pulse treatment with ketoconazole should be considered in the future.

C. Terbinafine

Terbinafine is an allylamine agent. In vitro data indicate that terbinafine is fungicidal for dermatophytes and for some *Candida* spp. However, in contact with serum or proteins, this activity is decreased and leads to reduced bioavailability (31,32). Therefore, the term *fungitoxic* may perhaps better describe the activity of terbinafine (as well as that of the other oral antifungal drugs) in the clinical situation (33). Extensive studies of the skin and nail pharmacokinetics of terbinafine have been performed. Terbinafine has a slow elimination, probably due to its strongly lipophilic nature, with good distribution in skin, adipose tissue, and nails (34–36). Terbinafine is well absorbed within 2 hr after ingestion, with plasma concentrations varying between 2.09 ± 0.78 μg/ml. After a single dose of 250 mg terbinafine, plasma concentrations are approximately 0.8 to 1.5 μg/ml. Urinary excretion is above 70% after 48 hr. The plasma elimination half-life is ±26 hr (35). However, other studies showed the elimination half-life to be increased to 100 hr (36). Low plasma levels can be measured for up to 8 weeks after discontinuation of therapy. This persistence in plasma may explain the residual effect sometimes observed in clinical trials.

Terbinafine is a lipophilic and keratophilic compound. The drug is delivered to the stratum corneum by a positive diffusion from the bloodstream through the dermis-epidermis. It is also excreted extensively via the sebum, but the drug is undetectable in eccrine sweat. It was shown in skin kinetic studies that tissue levels parallel plasma levels (37,38). In an ex vivo model using skin strippings, the lingering effect of terbinafine in human stratum corneum lasted for 2 weeks after cessation of therapy (33). Several studies, mainly done by the group of Finlay et al., have explored the nail kinetics of terbinafine (39,40). In an initial kinetic study (39), the mean time of appearance of terbinafine in the distal part of the nail was 7.8 weeks (range: between 3 and 18 weeks). It was also shown that the pharmacokinetics in the normal nail are analogous to those of the infected nail. The early detection of terbinafine in the distal portion of the nail leads to the conclusion that the diffusion of terbinafine is faster than the rate of nailgrowth and must also occur via the nail bed.

When terbinafine reaches the nail, a fast diffusion occurs, resulting in a steady state (39,41). During treatment, the levels of terbinafine in the nail do not increase with time (Fig. 3). This finding suggests that the mechanism of penetration is probably through both the nail matrix and nail bed and not by incorporation into the matrix cells. The mean terbinafine levels in the distal clippings of toenails were found to be between 250 and 550 ng/g. It was also shown that the nail concentration declines in parallel with the plasma level after completion of 3 months of therapy. This decline can take several weeks, as plasma elimination is very slow.

The relationships between an oral dose of terbinafine, nail plate levels during therapy, and posttreatment levels have also been investigated (42). Twenty-four patients with onychomycosis were treated in a double-blind study with either 125, 250, or 500 mg/day for 16 weeks and followed with a 32-week follow-up. Toenail levels of terbinafine reached a maximum at 8 weeks, whereas distal levels reached a maximum at 12 weeks. Nail levels in the 125 and 250 mg groups were lower, demonstrating a correlation between dosage and nail drug levels. After discontinuation of therapy, terbinafine persisted in distal nail clippings for at least 4 weeks but was not detectable after 8 weeks.

Recently, Effendi et al. presented the results of a new study (43) which were somewhat different from those of Finlay (39,41). Although diffusion into the nail was still evident, suggestive of a second penetration route, terbinafine continued to accumulate in the toenail instead of reaching a

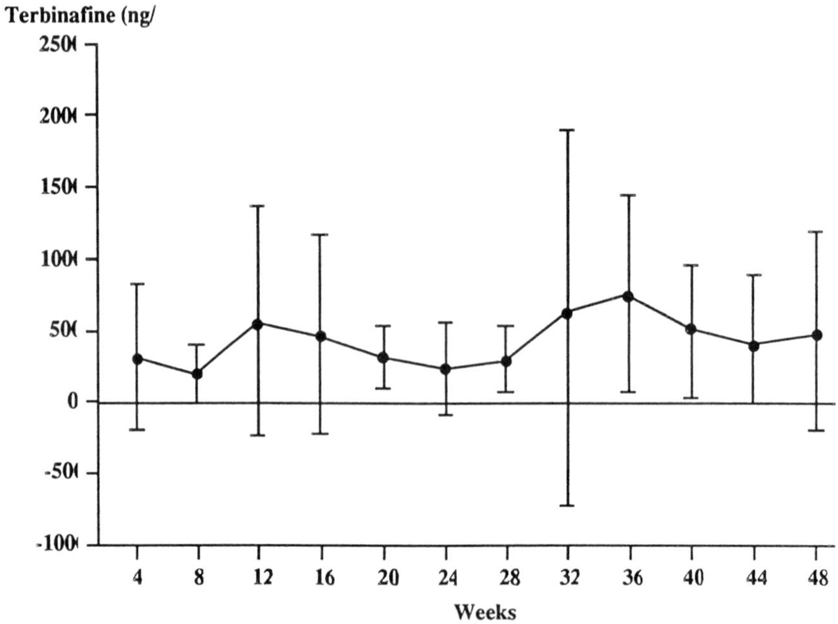

Figure 3 Terbinafine concentration in fingernail over 48 weeks (Mean values ± SD, ng/g). (Adapted from Finlay et al., Ref. 39.)

steady state. After the end of the 3-month treatment, drug levels persisted for several months, much longer than previously reported (42). These recent findings still need to be confirmed, but they suggest that terbinafine penetrates the nail not only by diffusion from the matrix and the nail bed but also by incorporation, to a certain extent, into matrix (43).

Another objective of pharmacokinetic studies is to provide information on the possible value of very short or single-pulse courses of therapy. Pulse therapy with terbinafine has been studied with some success in a few patients. No kinetic data are available from this limited study (44). More recent work by Faergeman et al. indicates that the length of therapy necessary to affect cure might be shorter than the currently recommended 12 weeks, since terbinafine is detected in distal nail clippings after 1 or 2 weeks of 250 mg daily and therapeutic concentrations persist for 2 to 3 months after medication is stopped (45). In the light of these new data, new dosing regimens may be explored in the future.

D. Fluconazole

Another drug in an advanced stage of clinical development for dermatomycosis or onychomycosis is fluconazole. This drug is a hydrosoluble bistriazole. The pharmacokinetic profile is different from that of the other azole derivatives. It is a hydrophilic compound with a low affinity for proteins (46). The unmetabolized drug is extensively absorbed. Its bioavailability exceeds 90%. Serum concentrations of 1.0 μg/ml are obtained after a single oral dose of 50 mg. The peak plasma concentrations achieved in healthy volunteers after single doses of fluconazole 100 mg and 400 mg are 1.9 μg/ml and 67 μg/ml respectively. Continued administration leads to an increase in peak plasma concentrations of 2.5-times that achieved after a single dose. Half-life is sufficiently long (±30 hr) to permit once-daily dosing. Fluconazole is metabolically stable and is excreted almost unchanged in the urine (91%) (47–49).

Fluconazole penetrates well into body fluids and tissues, including skin and nails (49). Tissue affinity is limited and keratin adherence is weak. Sweat is the most important route of delivery of fluconazole to the skin followed by excretion in sebum while uptake or excretion in the basal layer is limited (50–52). The ratio of the tissue/plasma concentration of fluconazole in skin blister fluid and nails was found to be 1/1. Two nail kinetic studies have so far been reported. In a first study by Hay, nine male volunteers were treated with 50 mg fluconazole daily (51). Mean plasma concentrations of fluconazole on days 1 and 14 of treatment were 760 and 2120 ng/ml. Mean nail concentrations were 1300 and 1800 ng/g, respectively (Fig. 4). The fast diffusion into the distal portion of nails within 48 hr of treatment onset suggests that diffusion from the nail bed is a key route of penetration in the nail.

In a second study, by Fraki et al., fluconazole was studied in onychomycosis patients, with 150 mg once-a-week-pulse dosing for a minimum of 6 months (53). In this study, fluconazole concentrations in the nail increased monthly, more quickly in healthy nails than in diseased nails. However at month 6 both healthy and diseased nails achieved similar concentrations—on average, 2000 ng/g. Long-term posttreatment data were not reported in this study. No data are available on how long fluconazole remains in the nail.

The use of a pulse regimen with a once-a-week treatment is realistic, but it appears as that this regimen must be given until the nail is completely mycologically and clinically healed (53,54). Pretreatment of the affected nails with urea clearly increased the cure rate (53).

Large-scale studies with these single-day pulses of fluconazole without

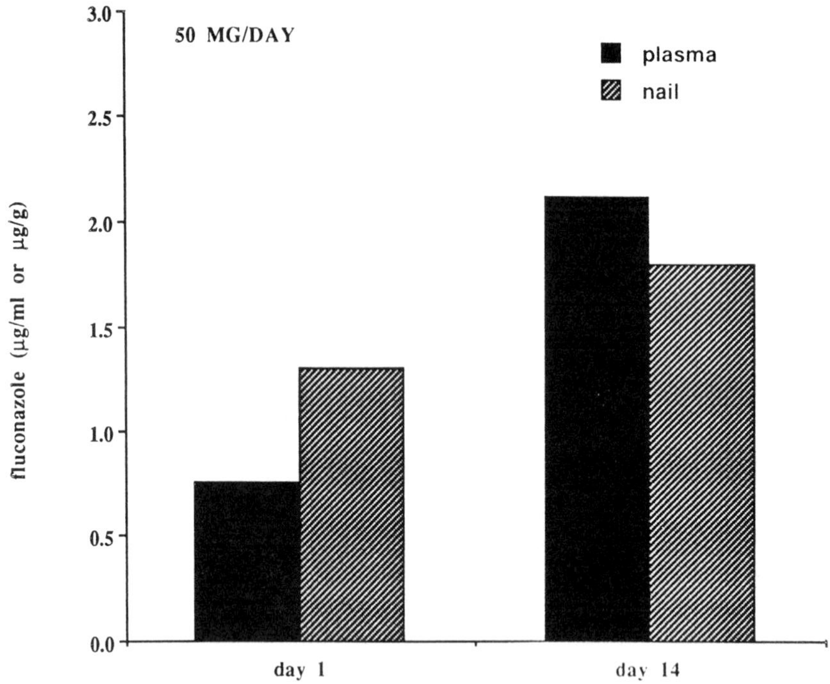

Figure 4 Fluconazole levels in nail and plasma on day 1 and day 14 during 50-mg once-daily administration (mean values, µg/ml or µg/g). (Adapted from Hay RJ, Ref. 51.)

beneficial adjunctive therapy in onychomycosis are warranted, as well as long-term safety studies at higher doses.

E. Itraconazole

Another option for treating fungal nail disease is itraconazole. Studies with this agent have created a breakthrough in relation to skin and nail pharmacokinetics, clearly demonstrating that awareness of the role of pharmacokinetic/pharmacodynamic studies in skin and nails has significantly increased.

Itraconazole is a broad-spectrum triazole derivative with high lipophilicity, good oral absorption, and extensive tissue distribution with a high affinity for keratinous tissues (55,56). Plasma half-life varies between 15 and 25 hr. After an oral 100-mg dose of itraconazole, the peak plasma level was 127 ng/ml (56). Steady-state is obtained within 2 weeks of treatment.

Plasma levels of the hydroxy metabolite of itraconazole, which is an antifungally active metabolite, exceed those of the parent drug (55,56). In comparison with itraconazole, peak plasma levels of hydroxy-itraconazole were on average 50% and area under the curve (AUC) 70% higher, but with a shorter half-life (14 hr) compared to the parent drug (15–25 hr). The in vitro antifungal activity of itraconazole and its hydroxy metabolite are similar (56). The in vitro antifungal activity of itraconazole is slightly increased when in contact with serum preparations in contrast to terbinafine (32).

Itraconazole binds strongly to protein. However, in spite of the fact that the drug binds strongly to plasma proteins, tissue concentrations of itraconazole are higher than those in plasma, indicating that the drug is extensively distributed to the tissues (29,56). Skin kinetic studies indicate that the major routes of itraconazole to the skin are probably passive diffusion from the blood in the keratinocytes, with strong adherence to keratin and incorporation into the basal layers and excretion by sebaceous glands. In contrast to ketoconazole, griseofulvin, and fluconazole, excretion in sweat is limited (29,56,57). Redistribution of itraconazole from the skin and appendages into the plasma appears neglible and renewal of the stratum corneum or growth of the hair and nails account for the disappearance of itraconazole from these tissues.

Several studies have been conducted to define and elucidate the kinetics of itraconazole in the nail. In these studies, itraconazole concentrations were determined by a specific high-performance liquid chromatographic method (58). The weight of the nail material was the critical factor in the assay. The detection limit was 2 ng per sample.

In one of the first nail pharmacokinetic studies conducted, which evaluated 100 mg daily for 4 weeks, itraconazole was detected in the distal nail clippings of volunteers within 7 days of beginning treatment (57) (Fig. 5A). This early detection suggests that itraconazole rapidly diffuses throughout the nail into the distal end, implying an alternate route via the nail bed. The latter penetration route may significantly contribute to the response to oral itraconazole therapy in onychomycosis. By 1 week after cessation of therapy, itraconazole had disappeared almost completely from plasma. A subsequent study in 19 patients with onychomycosis treated with itraconazole 100 mg/day for up to 7 months showed that the drug could be detected in the distal nail within 1 month after starting therapy and continued to be found throughout therapy (59) (Fig. 5A). At month 1, the mean itraconazole concentrations were about three times higher in fingernails than in toenails. The faster distribution of itraconazole into fingernails as compared to toenails may be due to differences in structure and thickness and faster outgrowth of the fingernails. Mean plasma levels of itraconazole

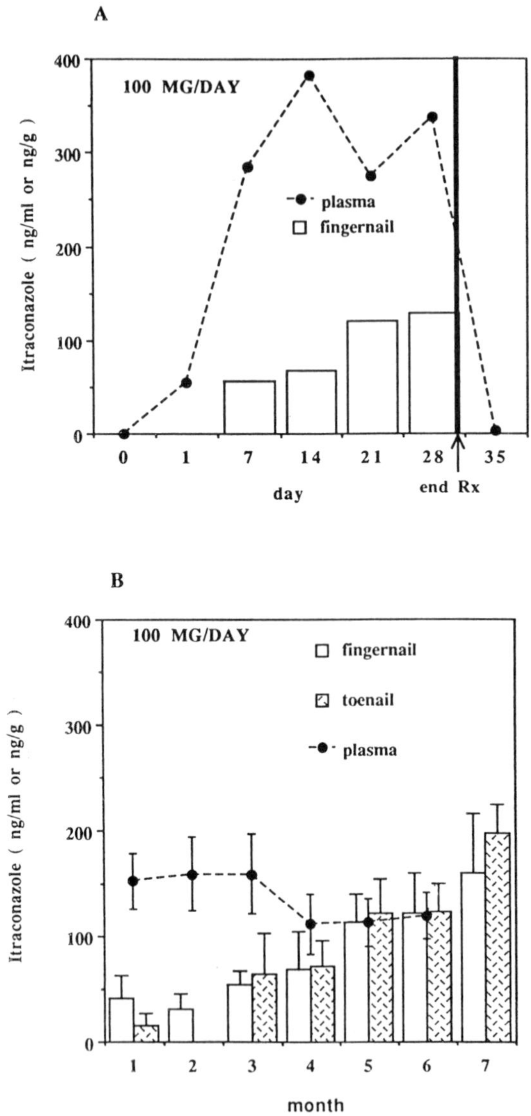

Figure 5 A. Plasma and fingernail levels of itraconazole (mean values, ng/ml or ng/g) during 4 weeks' administration of 100 mg daily. (Adapted from Cauwenbergh et al., Ref. 57.) B. Itraconazole concentrations (mean values ± SEM, ng/ml or ng/g) in fingernails, toenails, and plasma resulting during a 100 mg once daily administration. (Adapted from Matthieu et al., Ref. 59.)

oscillated between 152 ng/ml from the end of the first month and 119 ng/ml at month 6 of the treatment period, whereas in fingernails itraconazole (mean values) continued to accumulate from 42 ng/g at the first month to 160 ng/g at the end of the seventh month and in toenails from 16 ng/g at month 1 to 197 ng/g at month 7. The net increase between months 4 and 5 in itraconazole concentration in the distal nail can be explained by the contribution of the drug from the nail matrix. These pharmacokinetic findings suggest that if a dose of 100 mg is administered daily, a relatively long treatment time (i.e., more than 6 months) may be required to obtain therapeutic tissue levels and therefore a better cure rate.

In this study, the detection of the drug was related to nail growth and we could clearly show that itraconazole was recovered in the distal nail clippings before outgrowth of the fastest-growing toenail or fingernail in most of the patients. This is much earlier than would be expected if the drug were incorporated exclusively via the nail matrix, confirming an alternate route of penetration via the nail bed.

In the next stage of the development of itraconazole, the potential for shorter treatment schedules was investigated in onychomycosis, similar to the development of short and fixed dosage regimens in cutaneous mycoses, a study to determine the most efficacious itraconazole dose was begun. In this study, the results of treatment with daily doses of itraconazole 100 mg were compared with 200 mg administered for 3 months to 39 patients. Itraconazole concentrations in the toenails and fingernails were measured for up to 6 months after completion of therapy (60).

As shown in Fig. 6, the 200-mg group yielded severalfold higher concentrations in the distal nail plate throughout the 6-month follow-up period compared with the group treated with the 100 mg/day. In the toenail, mean itraconazole levels ranged from 84 to 149 ng/g of tissue for the 100-mg dosage group (mean maximum of 149 ng/g at month 5 after start of therapy) and from 490 to 990 ng/g for the 200-mg dosage group (mean maximum of 990 ng/g at month 5 after start of therapy). In 9 of 19 patients in the 200 mg group, concentrations of more than 1000 ng/g were found in the toenails. The toenail concentrations of itraconazole remained high throughout the 6-month follow-up period, while concentrations in fingernails declined faster. For at least 6 months after discontinuation of treatment, the mean itraconazole concentrations persisted more or less unchanged, with a mean of 149 ng/g for the 100-mg dose group and a mean of 670 ng/g for the 200-mg group 6 months after therapy. The mean levels for fingernails ranged from 35 to 111 ng/g in the 100-mg group and from 141 to 798 ng/g in the 200-mg group. In four patients in the 200-mg group, concentrations of more than 1000 ng/g were found in fingernails (one patient reached a maximum of 5 μg/g). These concentrations dropped from

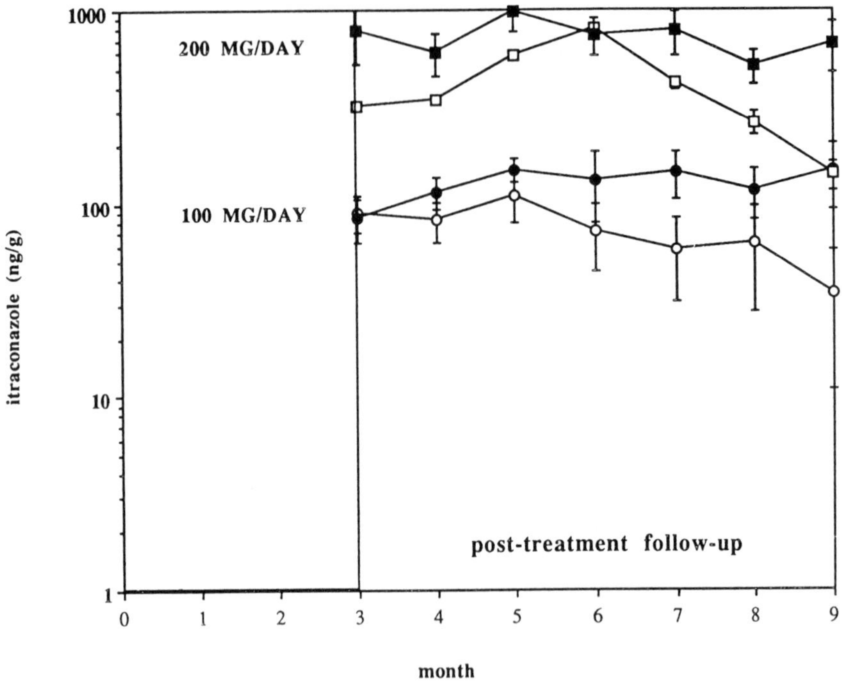

Figure 6 Posttreatment levels of itraconazole in the distal nail (mean values ± SEM, ng/g) after the end of a 3 months of treatment up to month 9. Key: open circles, fingernails, 100 mg; closed circles, toenails, 100 mg; open squares, fingernails, 200 mg; closed squares, toenails, 200 mg. (Adapted from Willemsen et al., Ref. 60.)

a peak concentration of nearly 800 ng/g at month 6 to 141 ng/g at the last follow-up visit at month 9 in comparison with the 100-mg group, in whom there was a reduction from maximum of 111 ng/g 3 months after therapy to 35 ng/g at the end of the follow-up period. This of, course, most probably correlates with the faster nail growth. This finding suggests that the mechanism of penetration is probably through both the matrix and the nail bed and by incorporation into the matrix cells. The route of penetration responsible for the slow delivery of the drug and for its long persistence of drug concentrations in the nail.

The difference in itraconazole content in the nail between the groups treated with 100 mg and the 200 mg affected the extent of cure in toenails, suggesting that the drug concentration in the nail is a good predictor of efficacy in fungal nail infections (Fig. 7A). The itraconazole concentra-

A

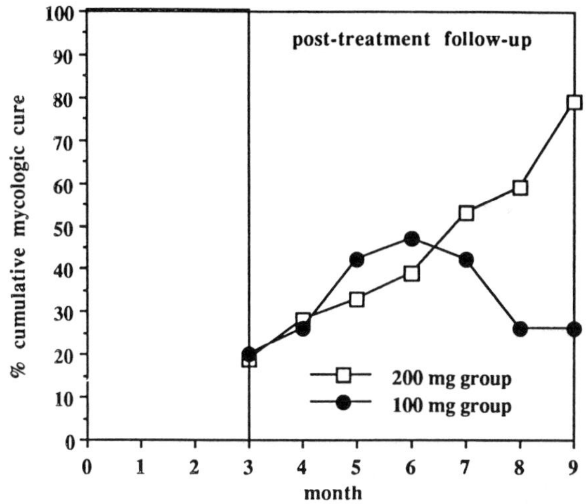

B.

itraconazole nail levels

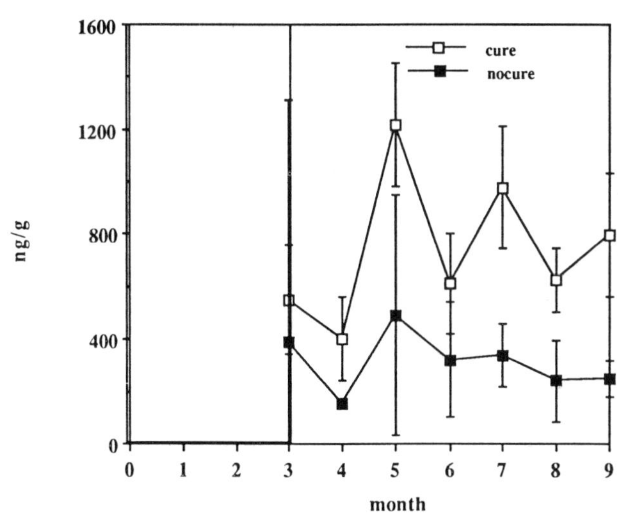

Figure 7 A. Percent cumulative mycological cure in patients treated with 200 mg or 100 mg itraconazole daily for 3 months. B. Itraconazole levels (median values ± SEM, ng/g) between cured or noncured patients treated with 200 mg daily.

tions in the nail reached with the 3-month 100 mg-treatment schedule appear to have been insufficient to result in mycological cure in most patients. Increasing the dosage to 200 mg daily resulted in a more-than-dose-proportional increase in drug levels (almost 10 times more). These increased tissue levels were associated with an increasing and superior cure rate with the 200 mg regimen, resulting in a mycological cure rate of 79%, versus the 26% achieved with the lower dosage. In addition, itraconazole levels achieved in the cured patients treated with 200 mg daily were higher compared with the noncured patients in the 200-mg group (Fig. 7b).

There are few data available relating to drug concentrations in the nail bed. It is very difficult to obtain such information without invasive procedures. However, the information is essential, because early fungal (primary or relapse) nail disease usually involves the nail bed and hyponychium itself.

So far, itraconazole levels have only been measured in distal nail material and subungual nail material from one sample, 10 days posttreatment of 1 month 200 mg daily.

Concentrations were more than double in the nail bed than in the distal nail clippings: 240 ng/g in nail plate and 567 ng/g in subungual hyperkeratotic nail material (61). A kinetic curve of itraconazole concentrations in nail bed is not available. However, since the nail bed takes part in nail formation or growth of the nail plate, as demonstrated by Johnson et al. (62), it can be expected that, as well as diffusing passively (as a fast process), itraconazole will be actively delivered at a slow rate from the nail bed into the nail plate.

Based upon these pharmacokinetics, the potential of itraconazole given as a pulse-dose regimen for 3 or 4 months was explored for the treatment of onychomycosis (64).

Intermittent pulse-doses of 1 week results in a rapid shunting of itraconazole into the distal nail, leading to a further progressive accumulation of itraconazole, which persists after discontinuation of the last pulse (64). In the group of patients receiving three pulses, mean toenail levels ranged from 67 ng/g (at month one after starting therapy) to a peak concentration of 471 ng/g (month 6) and persisted to month 11 with remaining concentrations of 186 ng/g. In fingernails, similar drug concentrations were found, but itraconazole decreased faster in the distal nail and the drug became undetectable from month 9 on. Mean toenail levels in patients receiving 4 pulses ranged from 32 ng/g (at month 1 after starting therapy) to a peak concentration of 623 ng/g (month 8) and persisted to month 13 with remaining concentrations of 165 ng/g. In fingernails, the drug became undetectable from month 9 on.

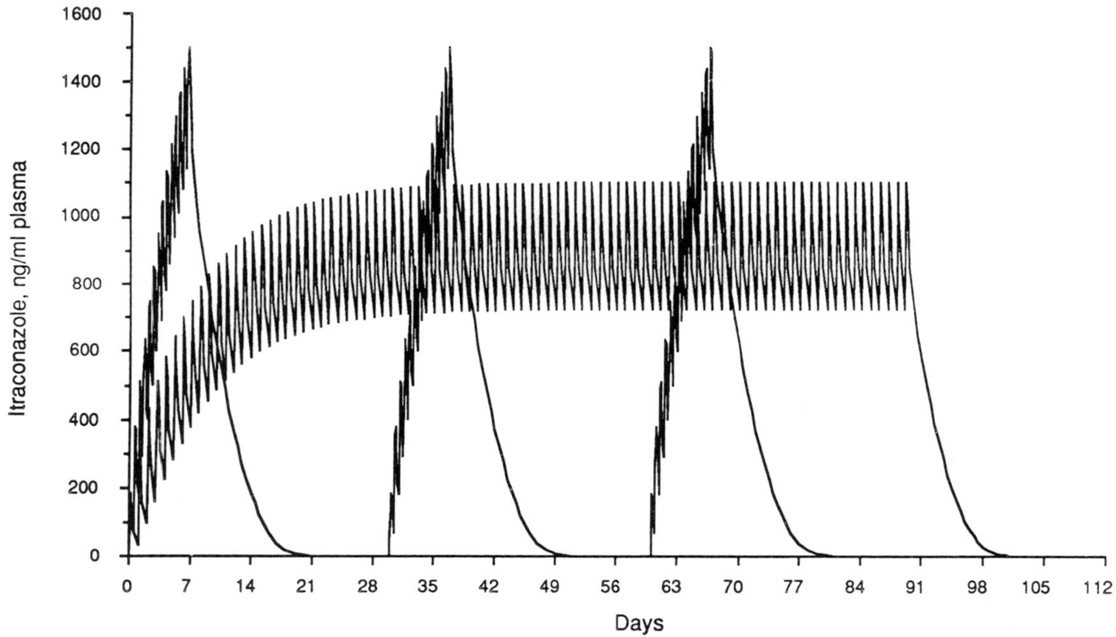

Figure 8 Plasma kinetics between a continuous treatment of 200 mg o.d. for 3 months and a pulse-dose regimen, monthly cycles of 1-week pulse 400 mg itraconazole.

In contrast to the nail levels, a decrease in the plasma levels after the 1-week treatment was noted with a complete elimination before the initiation of another pulse of 1 week. As a result, itraconazole disappears completely from the systemic circulation before the administration of another pulse (Fig. 8). In fact, total drug exposure for the patient, as expressed in area under the curve (AUC), is calculated to be three times less in the pulse therapy (743 μg·h/ml) compared with the continuous dosing for 3 months (1785 μg·h/ml). This reduction in total exposure may theoretically improve the safety profile and is currently investigated in clinical studies with itraconazole pulse therapy.

The clinical results of the different pulse studies are encouraging. Results from different clinical studies (n = 10) in 909 patients with toenail onychomycosis demonstrated a clinical and mycological cure of 79 and 85% for the three-pulse regimens (n = 673) and 76 and 77%, respectively for the 4-pulse group (n = 236) at the endpoint of the follow-up (month 12). Although further studies are required to confirm these results, the use of pulse therapy may offer a new option and represent the future for the treatment of onychomycosis. Further development in intermittent therapy is ongoing and is focusing on adaptation of dosing and/or frequency of pulses.

IV. DISCUSSION AND CONCLUSION

Topically applied antimycotic agents have the inherent advantage of local administration if the drug is able to penetrate the nail plate and if it can reach the nail bed, where the fungus is located. The addition of keratolytic compounds, like urea, salicylic acid, or penetration enhancers like dimethylsulfoxide (DMSO) has been shown to increase the effectiveness of topical antimycotics for the treatment of onychomycosis (65). One reason why complete cure is difficult to obtain with topical treatment might also be that insufficiently high concentrations are achieved by the topical route in the nail bed and nail matrix.

The nail plate is a difficult environment for oral drugs to penetrate, but after several years of intensive study with itraconazole, and, more recently, with terbinafine and fluconazole, results indicate that the behavior of these drugs in tissue will change the concept of treating onychomycosis by the oral route. For lipophilic antifungals such as itraconazole and terbinafine, the protein- or tissue bound concentration better reflects the availability and high affinity of these lipophilic compounds to the biophase. This biophase includes, beside keratin tissues, the fungal organisms as dermatophytes, yeasts, and moulds that may invade the nail. This means that drug availability at the infection site in the nail plate/nail bed is not necessarily related to the free concentration of drug in plasma and body fluids but rather to its tissue concentration. On the other hand, based on the in vitro activity, it is also clear that a drug like fluconazole must reach much higher concentrations in the nail than either itraconazole and terbinafine in order to exert its activity against dermatophytes. Therefore, the relative activity against fungi and the nail levels obtained with the various oral antifungal drugs should be considered together if one wishes to interprete the activity of these drugs in onychomycosis. Moreover the in vitro activity of an antifungal drug does not always reflect the reality. An example is terbinafine. This drug is fungicidal in vitro when inhibition is measured using medium containing aqueous solutions. However, it has been demonstrated that the presence of serum proteins reduces terbinafine's activity or its biological activity (30,31). In contrast, presence of serum has an increasing effect on itraconazole's activity. In view of the concentrations reached in the nail, it may be expected that both compounds are equipotent against dermatophytes in vivo.

In conclusion, we may state for the oral antifungal agents that penetration into the nail, combined with a good in vivo antifungal activity, an affinity for keratin, and a good safety profile, is certainly the key for success in onychomycosis. Oral antifungal agents are most likely more efficacious than topical therapy for the treatment of fungal nail infections, because systemic treatment should result in saturation of the nail bed and in diffusion and/or incorporation into the nail matrix. With the pharmacokinetic profiles of the currently available orally active antifungals, the advantages of taking a few high doses may increase patient compliance and safety, leading to better efficacy. This tendency toward shortening the treatment will also reduce the cost of treating this disease.

Finally, it becomes very clear that the role of nail pharmacokinetic studies has significantly increased during the last decade and has revolutionized the approach to successful treatment of a disease that, for years, was considered to be chronic and difficult to treat without an acceptable standard therapy and was associated with high recurrence rates. Today, as a contribution of these studies, a new concept has been developed specifically; now treatment can be tailored to the individual patient and the clinical presentation. Shorter treatments either orally or topically or perhaps in combination may also be possible.

REFERENCES

1. Runne U, Orfanos SE. The human nail: structure, growth and pathological changes. Curr Probl Dermatol 1981;9:102–149.
2. Baran R, Dawber RPR. Investigations and some physicochemical properties

of nails. In: 1984, 81–104. Baran R and Dawber RPR, eds. Diseases of the Nails and Their Management. Blackwell Scientific Publications, Oxford.
3. Parent D, Achten G, Stouffs-Vanhoof F. Ultrastructure of the normal human nail. Am J Dermatopathol 1985;6:529–535.
4. Baden HP, Kvedar JC. The nail. In: Goldsmith LA, ed. Physiology, Biochemistry and Molecular Biology of the Skin. Goldsmith 1992, 697–711.
5. Dawber RPR. The ultrastructure and growth of human nails. Arch Dermatol Res 1980;269:197–204.
6. Walters KA, Goldsmith LA, Fleming B. Permeability characteristics of the human nail plate. Int J Cosm Sci, 1983;5:231–246.
7. Walters KA. Penetration of chemicals into, and through, the nail plate. Pharm Int April 1985, 86–89.
8. Walters KA, Flynn GL, Marvel JR. Penetration of the human nail plate: The effects of vehicle pH on the permeation of miconazole. J Pharm Pharmacol 1985;37:498–499.
9. Stüttgen G, Bauer E. Bioavailability: Skin and nail penetration of topically applied antimycotics. Mycoses 1981;25(2):74–80.
10. Bazex A, Parent M, Ferrere J, et al. Infections à Scopulariopsis brevicaulis. Ann Derm Venereol 1977;104:254–255.
11. van den Hoven WE, de Wijn SR, Hall DWR. The use of n-acetyl-cysteine (NAC) in topical preparations for treating human nails. 18th World Congress of Dermatology, New York, June 12–18, 1992:242A.
12. Qadripur SA, Horn G, Hohler T. Zur Lokalwirksamkeit von Ciclopiroxolamin bei Nagelmykosen. Arzneim Forsch 1981;31:1369–1372.
13. Ceschin-Roques CG, Hänel H, Pruja-Bougaret SM, et al: Ciclopirox nail lacquer 8%: In vivo penetration into and through nails and in vitro effect on pig skin. Skin Pharmacol 1991;4:89–94.
14. Zaug M, Bergstraesser M. Amorolfine in the treatment of onychomycosis and dermatomycoses (an overview). Clin Exp Dermatol 1992;17(suppl 1): 61–70.
15. Pittrof F, Gerhards J, Erni W, Klecak G. Loceryl nail lacquer—Realization of a new galenic approach to onychomycosis therapy. Clin Exp Dermatol 1992;17(suppl 1):26–28.
16. Mensing H, Polak-Wyss A, Splanemann V. Determination of the subungual antifungal activity of amorolfine after 1 month's treatment in patients with onychomycosis: Comparison of two nail lacquer formulations. Clin Exp Dermatol 1992;17(suppl 1):29–32.
17. Mayer PR, Couch RC, Erickson MK, et al. Topical and systemic absorption of sodium pyrithione following topical application to the nails of the rhesus monkey. Skin Pharmacol 1992;5:154–159.
18. Schäfer-Korting M, Korting HC, Mutschler E. Human plasma and skin blister fluid levels of griesofulvin following a single oral dose. Eur J Clin Pharmacol 1985;29:109–113.
19. Korting HC, Schäfer-Korting M, Zienicke H, et al. Treatment of tinea unguium with medium and high doses of ultramicrosize griseofulvin compared with itraconazole. Antimicrob Agents Chemother 1993;37:2064–2068.

20. Artis WM. Final pathway for delivery of oral antifungals to keratinized cornified skin. In: Oral Therapy in Dermatomycoses: a Step Forward. Proceedings of a symposium held in Frankfurt, Germany, February 1985. The Medicine Publishing Foundation Symposium Series, 1985;16:61–70.
21. Shah VP, Riegelman S, Epstein WL. Determination of griseofulvin in skin, plasma and sweat. J Pharm Sci 1972;61:634–636.
22. Epstein WL, Shah VP, Riegelman S. Griseofulvin levels in stratum corneum: Study after oral administration in man. Arch Dermatol 1972;106:344–348.
23. Shah VP, Riegelman S, Epstein WL. Role of sweat in accumulation of orally administered griseofulvin in skin. J Clin Invest 1974;53:1673–1678.
24. Zaias N. Onychomycosis. Dermatol Clin 1985;3/3:445–460.
25. Hägermark O, Berlin A, Wallin I, Boréus LO. Plasma concentrations of griseofulvin in healthy volunteers and out-patients treated for onychomcyosis. Acta Derm Venereol 1976;56:289–296.
26. Van Cutsem J. The antifungal activity of ketoconazole. Am J Med 1983;74: 9–15.
27. Huang Y-C, Colaizzi JL, Bierman RH, et al. Pharmacokinetics and dose proportionality of ketoconazole in normal volunteers. Antimicrob Agents Chemother 1986;30:206–210.
28. Harris R, Jones HE, Artis WM. Orally administered ketoconazole: Route of delivery to the human stratum corneum. Antimicrob Agents Chemother 1983;24/6:876–882.
29. Cauwenbergh G. Skin kinetics of azole antifungal drugs. In: Borgers M, Hay R, Rinaldi MG, eds. Current Topics in Medical Mycology. Vol. 4. New York, Springer-Verlag, 1992;88–136.
30. Segal R, Trattner A, Alteras I, et al. Once-weekly treatment with oral ketoconazole for superficial fungal infections. J Am Acad Dermatol 1993;28: 126–127.
31. Ryder NS, Frank I. Interaction of terbinafine with human serum and serum proteins. J Med Vet Mycol 1992;30:451–460.
32. Van Cutsem J. An investigation of the in vitro activity and antifungal spectrum of itraconazole and terbinafine in relation to in vivo efficacy in dermatophytosis. J Mycol Med 1994;4:137–144.
33. Piérard GE, Arrese JE, de Doncker P. Antifungal activity of itraconazole and terbinafine in human stratum corneum: A comparative study. J Am Acad Dermatol 1995;32:429–435.
34. Jenssen JC. Pharmacokinetics in humans. J Dermatol Treat 1990;1(suppl 2): 15–18.
35. Kovarik JM, Kirkesselis, Humbert H, et al. Dose-proportional pharmacokinetics of terbinafine and its N-demethylated metabolite in healthy volunteers. Br J Dermatol 1992;126(suppl 39):8–13.
36. Samsoen M. Terbinafine (Lamisil): The first oral fungistatic and fungicidal allylamine. Nouv Dermatol 1992;11:743–762.
37. Lever LR, Dykes PJ, Thomas R, Finlay AY. How orally administered terbinafine reaches the stratum corneum. J Dermatol Treat 1990;1(suppl 2):23–26.

38. Faergemann J, Zehender H, Jones T, Maibach I. Terbinafine levels in serum, stratum corneum, dermis-epidermis (without stratum corneum), hair, sebum and eccrine sweat. Acta Derm Venereol 1990;71:322–326.
39. Finlay AY, Lever LR, Thomas R, Dykes PJ. Nail matrix kinetics of oral terbinafine in onychomysosis and normal nails. J Dermatol Treat 1990; 1(suppl 2):51–54.
40. Dykes PJ, Thomas R, Finlay AY. Determination of terbinafine in nail samples during systemic treatment for onychomycoses. Br J Dermatol 1990;123: 481–486.
41. Finlay AY. Pharmacokinetics of terbinafine in the nail. Br J Dermatol 1992; 126(suppl 39):28–32.
42. Finlay AY, Thomas R, Chawla M. Does the oral dosage of terbinafine influence its concentration in nail? Dermatology 2000, Vienna: Abstract Book, poster p 40.
43. Effendy I, Mensing H, Schatz MD, et al. Preliminary results of nail kinetics of terbinafine (abstr). In: International Summit on Cutaneous Antifungal therapy, San Francisco, October 21, 1993.
44. Shuster S, Munro CS. Single dose treatment of fungal nail disease. Lancet 1992;339:1066.
45. Faergemann J, Zehender H, Millerioux L. Terbinafine levels in plasma, stratum corneum, dermis-epidermis (without stratum corneum), hair and nails during and after 250 mg terbinafine orally once per day for 7 and 14 days. Dermatology 2000, Vienna, Abstract Book, poster p 37.
46. Hay RJ. New oral antifungals in dermatophytosis. Ann NY Acad Sci 1988; 544:580–585.
47. Humphrey MJ, Jevons S, Tarbit MH. Pharmacokinetic evaluation of UK-49858, a metabolically stable triazole antifungal drug, in animals and humans. Antimicrob Agents Chemother 1985;28:648–653.
48. Brammer KW, Tarbit MH. A review of the pharmacokinetics of fluconazole (UK-49-858) in laboratory animals and in man. In: Fromtling RA ed. Recent Trends in the Discovery, Development and Evaluation of Antifungal Agents. Barcelona, Spain, JR Prous, 1987;12(suppl 3):318–326.
49. Grant SM, Clissold SP. A review of its pharmacodynamic and pharmacokinetic properties and therapeutic potential in superficial and systemic mycoses. Drugs 1990;39(6):877–916.
50. Faergemann J, Laufen H. Levels of fluconazole in serum, stratum corneum, epidermis-dermis (without stratum corneum) and eccrine sweat. Clin Exp Dermatol 1993;18:102–106.
51. Hay RJ. Pharmacodynamic and pharmacokinetic evaluation of fluconazole in skin and nails. Int J Dermatol 1992;31(suppl 2):6–7.
52. Faergemann J, Godleski J Laufen H, Liss R. Intracutaneous transport of fluconazole to the stratum corneum (abstr). In: Interscience Conference on Antimicrobial Agents and Chemotherapy, New Orleans, October 17–20, 1993:382.
53. Fraki J, Heikkila H, Kero M, et al. Fluconazole in the treatment of onychomycosis: An open non-comparative study with oral 150 mg fluconazole once

weekly. In: Future Trends in the Treatment of Dermatomycoses. Dermatology 2000, Vienna, Abstract Book, poster p 14.
54. Monteiro-Gei F, Melendez M, Siles L. Fluconazole in the treatment of onychomycosis: Preliminary results. (abstr PS 3.84). In: Program and Abstracts: XI Cong Int Soc Human Animal Mycol, Montreal, 1991:142.
55. Van Cutsem J, Van Gerven F, Janssen PAJ. Activity of orally, topically and parenterally administered itraconazole in the treatment of superficial and deep mycoses: Animal models. Rev. Infect Dis 1987;9(suppl 1):15–32.
56. Heykants J, Van Peer A, Van de Velde V et al. The clinical pharmacokinetics of itraconazole: An overview. Mycoses 1989;32(suppl):67–87.
57. Cauwenbergh G, Degreef H, Heykants J, et al. Pharmacokinetic profile of orally administered itraconazole in human skin. J Am Acad Dermatol 1988; 18:263–268.
58. Woestenborghs R, Lorreyne W, Heykants J. Determination of itraconazole in plasma and animal tissues by high performance liquid chromatography. J Chromatogr Biomed Appl 1987;413:332–337.
59. Matthieu L, De Doncker P, Cauwenbergh G, et al. Itraconazole penetrates the nail via the nail matrix and the nail bed: An investigation in onychomycosis. Clin Exp Dermatol 1992;16:374–376.
60. Willemsen M, De Doncker P, Willems J, et al. Post-treatment itraconazole levels in the nail. J Am Acad Dermatol 1992;26:731–735.
61. De Doncker P. Pharmacokinetics: Basis for research in fungal nail disease. In: Issues in the modern management of onychomycosis: New approaches to diagnosis and management. Symposium Monaco, April 1993.
62. Johnson M and Shuster S. Continuous formation of nail along the bed. Br J Dermatol 1993;128:277–280.
63. De Doncker P, Cauwenbergh G. Intermittent itraconazole for onychomycosis (abstr). In: Annual meeting of the American Acad. Dermatol, San Francisco, 1992.
64. De Doncker P, Decroix J, Piérard GE, et al. Antifungal pulse therapy in onychomycosis: A pharmacokinetic/pharmacodynamic investigation of monthly cycles of 1 week pulse with itraconazole. Arch Dermatol 1996;132: 34–41.
65. Hay RJ. Treatment of dermatomycoses and onychomycoses–State of the art. Clin Exp Dermatol 1992;17(suppl 1):2–5.

33

Allylamine Antifungals

BONI E. ELEWSKI
Case Western Reserve University
Cleveland, Ohio

I. INTRODUCTION

In 1974, the allylamine naftifine was unexpectedly synthesized during a search for new psychotropic compounds.[1–3] Naftifine was later determined to be a novel, potent antimycotic with topical activity against dermatophytic fungi. The allylamine family thus began with this accidental, fortuitous, and unexpected discovery of naftifine. Subsequent investigations and modifications of the structure of naftifine led to the synthesis of additional allylamines that offer increased potency, increased bioavailability, and a broader spectrum of activity (Table 1).

This chapter reviews the chemistry, biochemical mode of action, and spectrum of activity of the allylamine antifungals. Clinical effectiveness, in vivo usage, and comparison with other antifungal agents will be emphasized.

II. PHARMACOLOGY OF ALLYLAMINES

A. Overview of Allylamines

The naftifine molecule is composed of a substituted naphthalene aromatic ring and an allylamine side chain (Fig. 1). The presence of the allylamine

Table 1 Overview the Availability of Allylamines

Topical	Oral
Naftifine	Terbinafine
Terbinafine	
Benzylamine—butenafine	
Investigational—SDZ-SBA-586	

side chain is pivotal to the antifungal function. Because of such importance, the designated chemical name of this antifungal family is allylamine. Alterations of the basic structure of naftifine led to the synthesis of its analogue terbinafine, which some classify as a second generation allylamine. As compared to naftifine, terbinafine has increased potency, broader spectrum of activity, and oral availability (Fig. 2). It should be noted that naftifine is converted to inactive compounds upon oral administration and therefore is limited to topical usage. Also related to the allylamine family is the topical benzylamine butenafine, available in Japan, and the benzylbenzylamine SDZ-SBA-586, which is currently under investigation by Sandoz researchers in Europe. The latter differs from the allylamine terbinafine by the benzylbenzylamine side chain (Fig. 2).

B. Mode of Action

The antifungal activity of the allylamines is a result of the inhibition of ergosterol biosynthesis. Ergosterol is a vital component of the cell membrane of fungi and is not present in human cells (Table 2). Although the azole antifungal family also inhibits ergosterol, the allylamines inhibit this

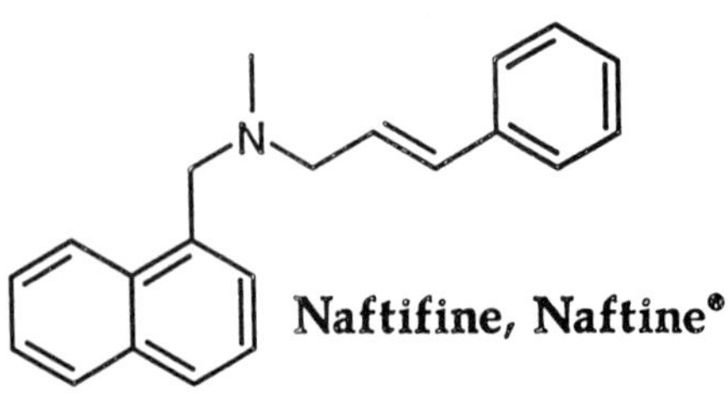

Figure 1 Naftifine molecule. The allylamine side chain is pivotal for antifungal activity.

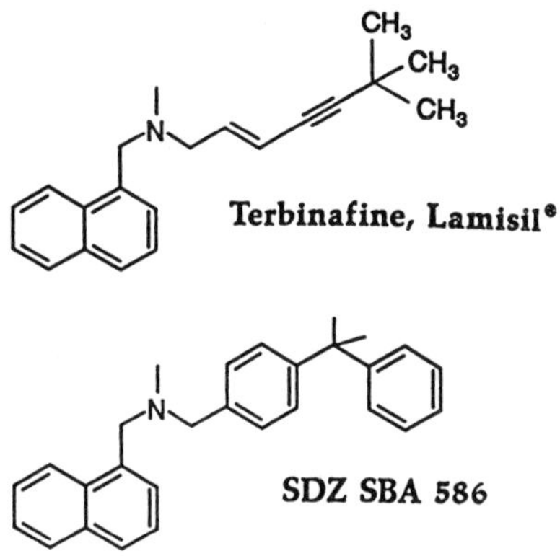

Figure 2 Terbinafine (upper), SDZ-SBA-586 (lower). Note benzylbenzyl side chain.

sterol at an earlier step than do the azoles.[4–6] The enzyme squalene epoxidase is inhibited (Fig. 3) by the allylamines, which results in a twofold cascade of events—the accumulation of squalene and the depletion of ergosterol. The accumulation of squalene is thought to result in fungicidal activity.[7–11] Squalene concentrates in lipid vesicles in the fungal cytoplasm, and cell death correlates with high intracellular levels of squalene. Presumably, these cytoplasmic, lipid-staining squalene vesicles cause weakening of the vacuolar membrane, with subsequent release of lytic enzymes into the fungal cytoplasm, followed by autolysis.[10] Based upon these observations, it is clear that ergosterol deficiency alone does not

Table 2 Site of Action of Systemic Antifungals

Cell membrane level	Nucleus level
Azoles	Griseofulvin
Ketoconazole	
Fluconazole	
Itraconazole	
Allylamines	
Terbinafine	
SDZ-SBA-586	

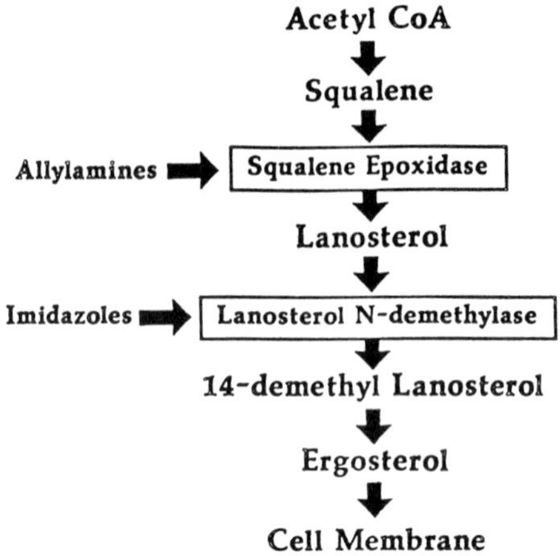

Figure 3 Biochemical pathway leading to synthesis of ergosterol. The allylamine family inhibits an earlier enzyme than do the azoles.

account for a fungicidal mode of action. Alternatively, the fungistatic mode of action of the azole antifungal family is thought to be due to depletion of ergosterol.

The mammalian enzyme squalene epoxidase plays a vital function in cholesterol synthesis. However, orally delivered terbinafine has no known effect on human or animal cholesterol levels.[6–7] From animal studies, it has been determined that human squalene epoxidase is less sensitive to terbinafine than is the fungal squalene epoxidase, and therefore no alteration in cholesterol levels occurs during therapy.[8–9]

Unlike lanosterol demethylase, the enzyme targeted by the azole antifungals, squalene epoxidase does inhibit cytochrome P450 enzymes.[4,5,11] As mammalian cytochrome P450 enzymes are involved in the synthesis of vital steroids including cortisol and testosterone, plus other essential physiological functions, drugs that inhibit or have affinity with this enzyme system may be associated with toxicity. This is illustrated by certain adverse events occasionally developing during ketoconazole therapy, including impotence, hypoadrenalism, and gynecomastia. Orally administered terbinafine elicits no inhibition of cytochrome P450 function, and—in contrast to the azoles—there have been no reports of adverse events related to cytochrome P450 inhibition such as depletion of cortisol synthesis. (Refer to the discussion of adverse events in Sec. VII.)

C. Pharmacokinetics

Oral terbinafine accumulates in sebum, stratum corneum, hair, and nail plate. It is highly bound to serum plasma proteins, including albumin and lipoprotein. Terbinafine also undergoes extensive hepatic metabolism; 80% is excreted in urine, the remainder via the gut.[16] Dosage may need to be altered if hepatic or renal function is impaired. Plasma half life ranges from 11–16 hr.

D. Resistance

As different enzymes are targeted, fungal pathogens resistant to the azole family of antifungals may not display cross resistance to the allylamines. This may have important ramifications in the future.

III. FUNGISTATIC VERSUS FUNGICIDAL ACTIVITY

The allylamines are considered to have a primary fungicidal effect in eradicating fungi, which contrasts with the fungistatic action associated with the imidazoles and griseofulvin.[12–15] Is this difference relevant? The terms *fungicidal* and *fungistatic* both refer to in vitro tests, based on laboratory MICs (minimum inhibitory concentrations) and MFCs (minimum fungicidal concentrations).[4] The MIC is defined as the lowest concentration of a drug that prevents visible fungal growth. Results can be influenced by methodology, size of inoculum, and other factors, so caution must be exercised in interpreting data.[4,13,16] The MFC is the concentration of a drug that reduces the viability of the original fungal inoculum by 99.9%, and, like the MIC, is greatly influenced by laboratory technique. The allylamines have an MIC against target dermatophytic organisms equal to the MFC, implying primary fungal cell death rather than inhibition.[4] However, as these are in vitro tests; the clinical significance or advantage of a fungicidal agent versus a fungistatic agent is unknown. Clearly, fungicidal activity in vitro is of practical relevance only if it also occurs in vivo.

The theoretical advantages of a fungicidal antimycotic over a fungistatic agent may include more rapid onset of action, shorter duration of therapy, more rapid time to mycological cure, and improved eradication of pathogenic fungi in the immunocompromised patient. Additionally, less relapse should occur with fungicidal agent if the ''spores'' are killed. There is no hard evidence that the currently available allylamines are fungicidal in vivo. However, as compared with clotrimazole, the prototypical azole, terbinafine has a more rapid onset of activity and exhibits mycological cure after 7 days in certain dermatophytic infections. Indeed, no other topical antifungal has been demonstrated to be clinically effective against dermatophytic fungi with 1 week of topical usage. This permits speculation that the allylamine terbinafine is fungicidal in vivo. Additionally, there are clinical supporting data that relapse of dermatophytic infection is less with terbinafine cream than with the azoles, which may be due to a sporicidal effect in vivo. Higher cure rates at follow-up than at discontinuation of therapy suggest residual fungicidal effect in tissue.

IV. SPECTRUM OF ACTIVITY OF THE ALLYLAMINES

In vitro, the allylamines are potent inhibitors of most fungi, including dermatophytes, a variety of yeasts, the dimorphic fungi, and many filamentous fungi.[13–17] They are more effective in vitro against filamentous fungi than yeast fungi. However the clinical usage of both topical terbinafine and naftifine is limited to those fungi causing superficial and cutaneous mycoses including the dermatophytes *Candida* and *Malassezia furfur*.[18–20] This underscores the point that in vitro susceptibility tests do not necessarily correlate with in vivo antifungal activity. Also, it is important to stress that when the drug is administered orally, the spectrum of activity differs. Terbinafine, the only currently available oral allylamine, is active topically against dermatophytic fungal infections as well as cutaneous infections with the yeasts *Candida* and *Malassezia furfur*. When it is orally administered, it appears limited to dermatophytic fungi (Table 3), with additional activity against *Candida parapsilosis* and cutaneous sporotrichosis. Presumably, orally administered terbinafine does not reach the stratum corneum in high enough concentrations to exceed the MIC of certain yeast fungi. It should also be stressed that terbinafine is significantly more effective in vitro than naftifine against most yeast fungi, which probably correlates with in vivo activity. However, there has been no clinical study comparing these two allylamines. The benzylamines ex-

Table 3 Spectrum of Activity of the Allylamines

	Naftifine, topical	Terbinafine, topical	Terbinafine, oral	Topical, azole	Oral, azole	Griseofulvin
Dermatophytes	+	+	+	+	+	+
Candida	+	+	–	+	+	–
Malassezia	+	+	–	+	+	–

Key: + = Effective, – = Not effective.

hibit comparable biological activity to the allylamines. The benzylbenzylamine SDZ-SBA-586 has in vitro fungicidal activity against dermatophytes, *Candida parapsilosis*, and the aspergilli.

The allylamines are potent antimycotics in vitro, with a broad spectrum of activity; however, it is puzzling that when delivered orally, they appear to be limited to integumentary fungi. Terbinafine is highly lipophilic and has great affinity for the lipophilic cells in the epidermis. The inability to eradicate systemic mycoses may be explained by impaired bioavailability due to metabolic degradation. Alternatively, the molecule may not reach the target site of infection in sufficient concentrations. Other factors influencing clinical efficacy may include absorption, drug interactions, rapid uptake into fatty tissue, interference by serum factors, and hepatic metabolism.[18] In vivo activity may be best predicted by animal models.

V. ROUTE OF DELIVERY TO THE INTEGUMENT

Topically delivered antimycotic drugs reach the stratum corneum in adequate concentration, and providing they persist in the integument, are generally effective in eliminating fungal pathogens. The topical allylamines naftifine and terbinafine persist on the stratum corneum and kill dermatophyte fungi and the yeasts *Candida* and *Malassezia*.

In order for a systemically delivered antimycotic to be effective in eradicating superficial cutaneous fungi, the drug must be delivered to the outer layers of the stratum corneum and its keratinized appendages. Possible routes of systemic antimycotic delivery include (1) passive diffusion through the dermis and epidermis; (2) delivery through eccrine sweat; (3) delivery via sebum; and (4) deposition in new epidermal cells.[4,20] The allylamines are delivered primarily to the stratum corneum by sebum, which differs from the mode of delivery of both griseofulvin and ketoconazole, which reach the outer integument by eccrine sweat. It should also be noted that the potent antidermatophyte azole itraconazole is similar to terbinafine in being delivered to the outer stratum corneum via sebum.[21]

VI. CLINICAL EFFECTIVE OF ALLYLAMINES VERSUS THE AZOLES

A. Topical Preparations

The topical allylamines, including naftifine and terbinafine, are broad-spectrum antifungals. They are effective against a variety of superficial fungi including dermatophytes, *Candida*, and *Malassezia*.[22–30] In this regard, they are similar to the topical azoles. However, terbinafine is effective in eliminating tinea pedis, tinea cruris, and tinea corporis after 1 week of topical usage. In a multicenter study comparing 1 week of terbinafine cream to 4 weeks terbinafine and 4 weeks clotrimazole cream in interdigital tinea pedis, the 1-week course of terbinafine was clinically and mycologically equivalent to a 4-week course and far superior to both 1- and 4-week courses of topical clotrimazole.[31] Additionally, the relapse rate with 1 week of terbinafine cream is low. Other topical antimycotic preparations generally require a 4-week minimal course for mycologic cure. The explanation of the quick cure rate of allylamine antifungals probably lies with the fungicidal mode of action, and may be clinical evidence of in vivo fungicidal activity. A particular advantage of the allylamines is their ability to eradicate *Microsporum canis*. Azole antifungals are less effective against this prevalent dermatophyte. When *M. canis* is suspected or cultured, topical naftifine or terbinafine would be a better choice than an azole antimycotic. However, based on recent data from Europe, terbinafine (oral) is *less* effective than oral itraconazole against *M. canis* tinea capitis infections.

B. Oral Usage

The oral allylamine terbinafine has demonstrated in vitro and in vivo activity against dermatophytic fungi (Table 3). At a dosage of 250 mg daily, terbinafine exhibits a spectrum of activity similar to that of griseofulvin. However, the impressive fungicidal in vitro potency sets it apart from griseofulvin. Terbinafine is rapidly delivered through the dermis and epidermis via the sebum and by rapid diffusion through the basal layers. Griseofulvin is delivered to the outer integument via eccrine sweat, and little data are available on its nail kenetics. Terbinafine reaches the nail plate from the nail bed, which probably attributes to its effectiveness in onychomycosis. Griseofulvin has limited potential in treating onychomycosis, with cure rates of only about 25% for toenail disease and slightly higher for fingernail disease. Additionally, griseofulvin must be given until the nails are clinically and mycologically normal, which is generally 6 months for fingernails, and 12–18 months for toenails.[4] These dismal facts have led to the search for other agents that would offer higher cure rates with a shorter duration of therapy. A dosage of 250 mg per day of terbinafine for 6 weeks is effective for fungal fingernail infections, and for 12 weeks is effective for mycotic toenails, with cure rates over 80%.[32–33] (Table 4). At the end of this period, the nail is not clinically normal, but the fungus is presumed "killed" and new healthy nail grows. It is important to stress to the patient that the nail will not appear normal until several weeks or months have elapsed after discontinuation of therapy. Terbinafine thus

Table 4 Dosage of Systemic Terbinafine

Onychomycosis	
Fingernails	250 mg/day—6 weeks
Toenails	250 mg/day—12 weeks
Tinea capitis	62.5—250 mg/day—4–6 weeks[a]

[a] Controlled studies are needed to confirm dosage and duration of therapy.

appears to be an ideal antimycotic for onychomycosis. This regimen resembles the short course of itraconazole in treating onychomycosis using 200 mg per day for 6 weeks for fingernails and for 12 weeks for toenail infection. A pulse dosage of 400 mg per day 1 week per month for 4 months (toenails) or 2 months (fingernails) is also effective. Approximately an 80% cure rate occurs with both protocols. As itraconazole is not considered fungicidal, the high cure rate obtained with terbinafine cannot be attributed solely to a fungicidal mode of action. Itraconazole, like terbinafine, penetrates in the nail plate via the nail bed. Both systemic itraconazole and terbinafine are clearly effective in dermatophytic fungal nail disease and elicit comparable cure rates.

Oral terbinafine may also be an effective therapy in tinea capitis, a common childhood infection where oral agents are essential. Griseofulvin-resistant *Trichophyton tonsurans* is emerging as a particular problem in the United States, and oral terbinafine may be an excellent alternative. There have been several reports of successful therapy of childhood endothrix and ectothrix tinea capitis. A study in Pakistan reported 10 children with noninflammatory tinea capitis caused by *T. tonsurans* (1/10) and *Trichophyton violaceum* (9/10).[34] Oral terbinafine, dosed according to body weight (range, 62.5 mg/d–250 mg/d) brought about mycologic cure in all patients and clinical cure in 9/10. No adverse events were reported. In this instance, the fungicidal activity may account for the short course and rapid onset of activity. Additionally, systemically delivered terbinafine demonstrates activity against *M. canis,* an organism particularly hard to eradicate with systemic or topical azoles. As *M. canis* is a frequently implicated in tinea capitis worldwide, terbinafine may usurp griseofulvin in therapy of this common childhood malady.

VII. ADVERSE EVENTS

The topical allylamines are generally well tolerated, and discontinuation due to irritation seldom occurs. However, if a patient is sensitive to a chemical in the vehicle, an alternative therapy is necessary. The pharmacokinetics of topically administered terbinafine shows less than 5% penetration into systemic circulation. Cautious use is indicated in pregnancy.[16]

Orally delivered terbinafine is generally well tolerated. The most common side effect is gastrointestinal. Nonspecific effects such as malaise may also occur.[16] Unlike the case with the azole ketoconazole, hepatic dysfunction is a rare occurrence.[34] Symptomatic hepatic cholestasis occurs 1 in 40,000 patients. A peculiar reaction attributed to terbinafine is reversible loss of taste. One patient in our clinic who experienced this reaction early in therapy did not wish to discontinue terbinafine and went on to successfully complete a 12-week course and eradicate his chronic onychomycosis. Morbilliform rashes have also been reported, as have rare occurrences of erythema multiforme and leukopenia.

Potential drug interactions need to be addressed. Terbinafine has less interaction with other agents than do the azoles. Ketoconazole can inhibit the metabolism of cyclosporin A, elevating cyclosporin blood levels and increasing potential nephroxicity.[35] In vivo studies in healthy volunteers showed minimal variation of cyclosporin A levels when coadministered with terbinafine. Thus, terbinafine does not appear to interfere with cyclosporin A metabolism in vivo, which is a distinct advantage over azole antifungals. This observation suggests that terbinafine may be a safe alternative antifungal in patients taking cyclosporin A. However, cautious monitoring of renal function and cyclosporin A levels is probably warranted until more data are available.[36]

The nonsedating antihistamines terfenadine and astemizole can also be administered safely with terbinafine. There appears to be no interaction with the metabolism of these compounds as occurs with systemic azoles, particularly ketoconazole. Ketoconazole inhibits cytochrome P450 metabolism, resulting in increased levels of the antihistamines metabolite. In the case of terfenadine, this can augment the drug's potential cardiotoxicity, causing prolongation of the QT interval and increased risk of fatal ventricular arrythmias.

Terbinafine dosage may need adjustment with cimetidine, which decreases its elimination, and rifampin, which increases its elimination.[16]

VIII. CONCLUSION

The allylamine family of antifungals represents an important contribution to our antimycotic armamentarium. They offer select advantages over the azole family and other antimycotics designed to treat cutaneous mycoses. The fungicidal activity displayed in vitro correlates on the clinical level with rapid onset of action, short time to mycologic cure, high cure rates, and low relapse rates. The Achilles heel of the allylamine family is their lack of potency against many yeast fungi, including *Candida albicans,* occurring particularily during oral therapy. Oral terbinafine has great potential in therapy of onychomycosis and tinea capitis. Further studies are required to determine benefit in systemic mycoses.

REFERENCES

1. Berney D, Schuh K. Heterocyclic spironaphthalenones: Part I. Synthesis and reactions of some spiro (1H-naphthalenone)-1,3-piperidines. Helv Chim Acta 1978;61:1262–1273.
2. Georgopoulos A, Petranyi G, Mieth H, Drews J. In vitro activity of naftifine, a new antifungal agent. Antimicrob Agents Chemother 1981;19:386–389.
3. Petranyi G, Georgopoulos A, Mieth H. In vivo antimycotic activity of naftifine. Antimicrob Agents Chemother 1981;19:390–392.
4. Elewski BE. Mechanisms of action of systemic antifungal agents. J Am Acad Dermatol 1993;28:528–534.
5. Ryder NS. Terbinafine: mode of action and properties of the squalene epoxidase inhibition. Br J Dermatol 1992;126(suppl 39):2–7.
6. Ryder NS. Specific inhibition of fungal sterol biosynthesis by SF 86-327, a new allylamine antimycotic agent. Antimicrob Agents Chemother 1985;27: 252–256.
7. Stütz A. Allylamine derivatives—a new class of active substances in antifungal chemotherapy. Angew Chem 1987;2:320–328.
8. Ryder NS, Dupont M-C. Inhibition of squalene epoxidase by allylamine antimycotic compounds: A comparative study of the fungal and mammalian enzymes. Biochem J 1985;230:765–770.
9. Ryder NS. Squalene epoxidase as the target of antifungal allylamines. Pest Sci 1987;21:281–288.
10. Long MT, Steel CC, Mercer EI. Location of squalene accumulation and physiological effects of ergosterol depletion in naftifine-grown yeast. Biochem Soc Trans 1988;16:1044–1045.
11. Ryder NS. Squalene epoxidase: Enzymology and inhibition. In: Kuhn PJ, Trinci APJ, Jung MJ, Goosey MW, Copping LG, eds. Biochemistry of cell walls and membranes in fungi. Berlin: Springer-Verlag, 1990:189–203.
12. Dismukes WE. Azole antifungal drugs: Old and new. Ann Intern Med 1988; 109:177–179.
13. Clayton YM. In vitro activity of terbinafine. Clin Exp Dermatol 1989;14: 101–103.
14. Petranyi G, Meingassner JG, Mieth H. Antifungal activity of the allylamine derivative terbinafine in vitro. Antimicrob Agents Chemother 1987;31: 1365–1368.
15. Shadomy S, Espinel-Ingroff A, Gebhart RJ. In vitro studies with SF 86-327, a new orally active allylamine derivative. Sabouraudia 1985;23:125–132.
16. Balfour JA, Faulds D. Terbinafine: a review of its pharmacodynamic and pharmacokinetic properties, and therapeutic potential in superficial mycoses. Drugs 1992;43:259–284.

17. Ryder NS. Mechanism of action and biochemical selectivity of allylamine antimycotic agents. Ann NY Acad Sci 1988;544:208–220.
18. Mieth H, Petranyi G. Preclinical evaluation of terbinafine in vivo. Clin Exp Dermatol 1989;14:104–107.
19. Petranyi G, Ryder NS, Stütz A. Allylamine derivatives: New class of synthetic antifungal agents inhibiting fungal squalene epoxidase. Science 1984; 224:1239–1241.
20. Harris R, Jones HE, Artis WM. Orally administered ketoconazole: Route of delivery in the human stratum corneum. Antimicrob Agents Chemother 1983;24:876–882.
21. Saul A, Bonifax A. Itraconazole in common dermatophyte infections of the skin: Fixed treatment schedules. J Am Acad Dermatol 1990;23:554–558.
22. Savin RC, Zaias N. Treatment of chronic moccasin-type tinea pedis with terbinafine: A double-blind, placebo-controlled trial. J Am Acad Dermatol 1990;23:804–807.
23. White JE, Perkins PJ, Evans EGV. Successful two week treatment with terbinafine (Lamisil) for moccasin tinea pedis and tinea manuum. Br J Dermatol 1991;125:260–262.
24. Smith EB, et al. Comparison of once- and twice-daily naftifine cream regimens with twice-daily clotrimazole in the treatment of tinea pedis. J Am Acad Dermatol 1990;22:1116–1117.
25. Zaias N, Astorga E, Cordero CN, et al. Naftifine cream in the treatment of cutaneous candidiasis. Cutis 1988;42:238–240.
26. Astorga E, et al: Naftifine cream 1% in cutaneous candidiasis. Curr Ther Res 1989;46:1106–1109.
27. El Darouti MA, Kalinka P. Naftifine cream 1% compared with miconazole cream 2% in dermatophytosis. Int J Dermatol 1990;29:521–522.
28. Jordon RE, Gordon RE, Rapin RP, et al. Once-daily naftifine cream 1% in the treatment of tinea cruris and tinea corporis. Int J Dermatol 1990;29: 441–442.
29. Dobson RL, et al. Naftifine 1% cream in the treatment of tinea cruris and tinea corporis. Drug Invest 1991;3:57–59.
30. Berman B, Ellis C, Leyden J, et al. Efficacy of a 1-week, twice-daily regimen of terbinafine 1% cream in the treatment of interdigital tinea pedis. J Am Acad Dermatol 1992;26:956–960.
31. Bergstresser PR, Elewski BE, Hanifin J, Lesher J, et al. Topical terbinafine and clotrimazole in interdigital tinea pedis: A multicenter comparison of cure and relapse rates with 1 and 4 week treatment regimens. J Am Acad Dermatol 1993;28:648–651.
32. Goodfield MJD, Andrew L, Evans EGV. Short term treatment of dermatophyte onychomycosis with terbinafine. Br Med J 1992;304:1151–1154.
33. Van der Schroeff JG, et al. A randomized treatment duration-finding study of terbinafine in onychomycosis. Br J Dermatol 1992;126(suppl 39):36–39.
34. Haroon TS, Hussain I, Mahmoud A, et al. An open clinical pilot of the

efficacy and safety of oral terbinafine in dry non-inflammatory tinea capitis. Br J Derm 1992;126(suppl 39):47–50.
35. Heiberg JK, Svejgaard E. Toxic hepatitis during ketoconazole treatment. Br Med J 1981;283:325–326.
36. Back DJ, Tija JF. Azoles and allylamines; the clinical implications of interaction with cytochrome P-450 enzymes. J Dermatol Treat 1990;1(suppl 2): 11–13.

Index

About the Editors

PAUL H. JACOBS is Professor Emeritus (Active) of Dermatology, Stanford University School of Medicine, Stanford, California, and an international lecturer on mycology. The coauthor or coeditor of over 70 journal articles and book chapters, as well as the coeditor of several books, including *Antigungal Drug Therapy* (Marcel Dekker, Inc.), Dr. Jacobs is a Fellow of the American Academy of Dermatology and the American College of Physicians, and a member of several other societies. He received the premedical degree (1949) from St. Procopius College, Lisle, Illinois, and the M.D. degree (1953) from Loyola University, Chicago, Illinois.

LEXIE NALL is Epidemiologist and Coordinator, National Epidermolysis Bullosa Registry, Stanford Clinical Site, Department of Dermatology, Stanford University School of Medicine, Stanford, California. Dr. Nall is the coauthor or coeditor of nearly 100 publications on epidemiologic methods for psoriasis, skin cancer, arthritis, closed ecological systems, aging, and mycology, including *Antifungal Drug Therapy* (Marcel Dekker, Inc.). A member of the Society of Applied Anthropology and the Society of Medical Anthropology, she received the B.S. degree (1958) in zoology from George Washington University, Washington, D.C., the M.A. degree (1966) in medical anthropology from Stanford University, Stanford, California, and the Ph.D. degree (1981) in epidemiology from Pacific Western University, Encina, California.